THE GUIDE TO CARDIOLOGY

THE GUIDE TO CARDIOLOGY

Edited by

Robert A. Kloner, M.D., Ph.D.
Assistant Professor of Medicine
Harvard Medical School
Associate Physician
Brigham and Women's Hospital
Boston, Massachusetts

A WILEY MEDICAL PUBLICATION
JOHN WILEY & SONS
New York · Chichester · Brisbane · Toronto · Singapore

Library of Congress Cataloging in Publication Data:
Main entry under title:

The Guide to Cardiology

  (A Wiley medical publication)
  Includes index.
    1. Heart—Diseases—Handbooks, manuals, etc.
2. Cardiology—Handbooks, manuals, etc. I. Kloner,
Robert A. II. Series.
RC681.M366 1984   616.1'2   83-16982
ISBN 0-471-09576-1

Printed in the United States of America

10 9 8 7 6 5 4 3 2 1

CONTRIBUTORS

Elliot M. Antman, M.D.
Assistant Professor of Medicine
Harvard Medical School
Director, Samuel A. Levine Cardiac Unit
Cardiovascular Division
Associate Physician
Brigham and Women's Hospital
Boston, Massachusetts

Edward J. Brown, Jr., M.D.
Assistant Professor of Medicine
State University of New York
Director, Cardiovascular Research Laboratory
Director, Nuclear Cardiology
Stony Brook Medical Center
Stony Brook, New York

Wilson S. Colucci, M.D.
Assistant Professor of Medicine
Harvard Medical School
Associate Physician
Brigham and Women's Hospital
Boston, Massachusetts

Victor J. Dzau, M.D.
Assistant Professor of Medicine
Harvard Medical School
Director of Hypertension
Associate Physician
Brigham and Women's Hospital
Clinical Associate in Medicine
Massachusetts General Hospital
Boston, Massachusetts

Brian G. Firth, M.D., Ph.D.
Assistant Professor of Internal Medicine
University of Texas Health Science Center
Associate Director, Cardiac Catheterization Laboratory
Parkland Memorial Hospital
Dallas, Texas

Peter L. Friedman, M.D., Ph.D.
Assistant Professor of Medicine
Harvard Medical School
Director, Clinical Electrophysiology
Associate Physician
Brigham and Women's Hospital
Boston, Massachusetts

Samuel Z. Goldhaber, M.D.
Instructor in Medicine
Harvard Medical School
Associate Physician
Brigham and Women's Hospital
Boston, Massachusetts

Lee Goldman, M.D.
Associate Professor of Medicine
Harvard Medical School
Physician and Assistant Physician-in-Chief
Brigham and Women's Hospital
Boston, Massachusetts

Thomas B. Graboys, M.D.
Assistant Professor of Medicine
Harvard Medical School
Associate Physician
Brigham and Women's Hospital
Boston, Massachusetts

Haim Hammerman, M.D.
Research Fellow
Harvard Medical School
Brigham and Women's Hospital
Boston, Massachusetts

Donald P. Harrington, M.D.
Associate Professor of Radiology
Harvard Medical School
Co-Director, Cardiovascular Radiology
Brigham and Women's Hospital
Boston, Massachusetts

L. David Hillis, M.D.
Associate Professor of Internal Medicine
University of Texas Health Science Center
Director, Cardiac Catheterization Laboratory
Parkland Memorial Hospital
Dallas, Texas

B. Leonard Holman, M.D.
Professor of Radiology
Harvard Medical School
Director of Clinical Nuclear Medicine Services
Brigham and Women's Hospital
Boston, Massachusetts

Robert A. Kloner, M.D., Ph.D.
Assistant Professor of Medicine
Harvard Medical School
Associate Physician
Brigham and Women's Hospital
Boston, Massachusetts

Richard R. Liberthson, M.D.
Assistant Professor of Medicine and Pediatrics
Harvard Medical School
Assistant Physician in Medicine and Associate Pediatrician
Massachusetts General Hospital
Boston, Massachusetts

Leonard S. Lilly, M.D.
Instructor in Medicine
Harvard Medical School
Associate Physician
Brigham and Women's Hospital
Boston, Massachusetts

James D. Marsh, M.D.
Assistant Professor of Medicine
Harvard Medical School
Associate Physician
Brigham and Women's Hospital
Boston, Massachusetts

Gilbert Mudge, M.D.
Assistant Professor of Medicine
Harvard Medical School
Director of Clinical Cardiovascular Service
Associate Physician
Brigham and Women's Hospital
Boston, Massachusetts

James E. Muller, M.D.
Assistant Professor of Medicine
Harvard Medical School
Associate Physician
Brigham and Women's Hospital
Boston, Massachusetts

Carl E. Orringer, M.D.
Staff Physician, Department of Internal Medicine
Section of Cardiology
Oschner Clinic
New Orleans, Louisiana

Marc A. Pfeffer, M.D., Ph.D.
Assistant Professor of Medicine
Harvard Medical School
Associate Physician
Brigham and Women's Hospital
Boston, Massachusetts

Joseph F. Polak, M.D.
Clinical Fellow in Radiology
Harvard Medical School
Brigham and Women's Hospital
Boston, Massachusetts

John D. Rutherford, M.D.
Cardiology Divison
Green Lane Hospital
Auckland, New Zealand

Neil J. Stone, M.D.
Associate Professor of Medicine
Section of Cardiology
Northwestern University School of Medicine
Chicago, Illinois

Peter H. Stone, M.D.
Assistant Professor of Medicine
Harvard Medical School
Associate Director, Samuel A. Levine Cardiac Unit, Cardiovascular Division
Associate Physician
Brigham and Women's Hospital
Boston, Massachusetts

Richard F. Wright, M.D.
Research Fellow in Medicine
Harvard Medical School
Associate Physician
Brigham and Women's Hospital
Boston, Massachusetts

Joshua Wynne, M.D.
Assistant Professor of Medicine
Harvard Medical School
Director, Noninvasive Cardiac Laboratory
Associate Physician
Brigham and Women's Hospital
Boston, Massachusetts

Eliot Young, M.D.
Assistant Clinical Professor of Medicine
Harvard Medical School
Chief, ECG Laboratory
New England Deaconess Hospital
Boston, Massachusetts

PREFACE

There are several excellent encyclopedic textbooks of cardiology. The busy schedule of the intern, resident, cardiology fellow, general practitioner, internist, and cardiovascular nurse does not always allow time for reading these books in their entirety. *The Guide to Cardiology* provides a broad overview of diagnostic testing and a synopsis of major topics in adult cardiology that can be read over a relatively brief period of time. This text is aimed primarily at interns, residents, cardiology fellows, internists, general practitioners, medical students on internal medicine or cardiology rotations, and cardiovascular nurses. The first eight chapters deal with diagnosis and contain separate sections on the cardiac history, physical examination, electrocardiography, chest x-ray, echocardiography and pulse-wave recordings, exercise testing, ambulatory electrocardiographic monitoring, nuclear cardiology, and cardiac catheterization. The remaining chapters deal with specific topics in adult cardiology, with emphasis on those diseases the health care professional is most likely to encounter, such as coronary artery disease. Thus, there are separate chapters on angina, coronary spasm, myocardial infarction, newer therapies for myocardial infarction, lipid abnormalities, and cardiac rehabilitation.

Recent advances covered include two-dimensional echocardiography, electrophysiologic testing for atrioventricular conduction abnormalities, calcium antagonists, streptokinase therapy for myocardial infarction, chronic beta-blockade postmyocardial infarction for reducing mortality, vasodilator therapy for congestive heart failure, newly released beta-blockers, coronary and renal angioplasty, and therapy for hyperlipidemia. There are separate chapters on the role of the cardiology consultant in caring for patients with cardiac and noncardiac surgery.

The diagnostics section of the book is heavily illustrated and contains many examples of typical echocardiographic, radiographic, and cardiac catheterization findings.

Cardiology is a rapidly moving field and therapeutic regimens, drugs, drug doses, and indications for drugs frequently change. The drugs, indications for drugs, and dosages throughout this book are those commonly used by practicing cardiologists, and have been recommended in the literature. Not all drugs, doses, and indications have at the time of this writing been FDA approved. Therefore, it is suggested that the package inserts or *Physicians' Desk Reference* be consulted as well for drug indications, contraindications, side effects, and dosages as recommended by the FDA. While the procedures and treatments in this text are based upon current standard practices, they should serve as a guide and not as the sole reference or sole determinant to practice and therapy of individual patients.

I wish to acknowledge Candy Gulko for help with the initial plans for the book, Dr. Leonard Lilly for review of the manuscript, Judith A. Kloner for help with proofreading and suggestions, Alexander Neumann and Drs. Kenneth M. Borrow and Laurence J. Sloss for help with the illustrations. To Mary Gillan for typing, to Laura Ducey, Nancy Watterson, and Ellen Holzman for secretarial assistance and to Cheryl Howell and Robert Hurley at John Wiley & Sons for their assistance with the organization and preparation of the book.

R.A.K.

CONTENTS

CHAPTER

1

THE CARDIAC HISTORY

Robert A. Kloner

Despite the recent surge in new cardiac diagnostic technology, the history and physical remain the cornerstones of the patient work-up. For example, the single most important aspect of diagnosing angina pectoris is the patient's history, as discussed in Chapter 9. The following chapter reviews the major symptoms directly related to the heart, including chest pain, shortness of breath (dyspnea), syncope, edema, palpitations, cough, hemoptysis, cyanosis, and fatigue.

Chest Pain

In most cases the etiology of chest pain can be derived from an adequate history. The patient should be questioned as to the quality, duration, radiation, exacerbating and ameliorating factors, and frequency of the pain. Chest pain due to angina pectoris is typically a dull substernal pain or pressure that radiates down the arms and up into the jaw; typically lasts a few to 15 minutes; is exacerbated by exertion, anxiety, and cold; and is relieved by rest and nitroglycerin. The chest pain of myocardial infarction usually is more severe than that of angina, is not relieved by rest or nitroglycerin, and lasts longer than an angina attack. Pericardial chest pain tends to be sharper than angina, positional (worse when the patient is lying down and often relieved by sitting up), and exacerbated by inspiration.

There are a number of cardiac conditions in which the chest pain of angina is mimicked, including that associated with hypertrophic cardiomyopathy, mitral valve prolapse, pulmonary hypertension, and myocarditis. Clues such as associated viral illness may help differentiate myocarditis from angina. The pain of mitral valve prolapse is often of shorter duration and may not be related to exertion.

There are many *noncardiac* causes of chest pain that may be confused with that of cardiac chest pain. Noncardiac causes of chest pain and their differentiating features are listed in Table 1.

Dyspnea

Dyspnea is defined as an uncomfortable awareness of breathing, with a need for increased ventilation. When dyspnea is due to chronic organic heart disease, it is typically exacerbated by exertion and develops gradually over weeks to months.

1

Table 1. Noncardiac Causes of Chest Pain that May Mimic Cardiac Pain

Disease Entity	Differentiating Features
Musculoskeletal	Pain tends to be exacerbated by motion of certain extremities and certain postures; often follows a nerve route distribution; point tenderness may be present in costochondritis
Herpes zoster	Chest wall pain occurs several days before development of typical rash; pain follows dermatome distribution

Pulmonary
  Pleuritis
  Pneumonitis
	Pain is sharp, worse with inspiration, associated with fever, cough

Pulmonary embolism	Pain is pleuritic when there is an associated infarction; shortness of breath is typically present; massive pulmonary embolus associated with cardiovascular collapse may be confused with myocardial infarction
Gastrointestinal Esophageal	Esophagitis and esophageal spasm often mimic angina; the latter may be relieved by nitroglycerin; patient may complain of regurgitation of food and have relief with antacids
Gastric and duodenal (gastritis, ulcers)	Epigastric discomfort typically is exacerbated by aspirin, alcohol and relieved by food, antacids
Gall bladder (cholecystitis)	Right upper quadrant cramping, pain exacerbated by fatty foods, occurs postprandial; there may be associated ECG abnormalities
Pancreatitis	Mid- and epigastric abdominal pain; possible history of associated alcohol ingestion; exacerbated by ingestion of food
Functional	Nonexertional chest tightness often associated with anxiety
Aortic dissection	Pain typically is sharp, tearing in nature, may radiate to the back; onset of pain is often as severe as pain ever becomes, in contrast to myocardial infarction, in which the pain has a crescendo-like onset

Dyspnea at rest is more common in lung disease but is also exacerbated by exertion, making the distinction between cardiac and pulmonary dyspnea difficult. Further differentiating features between these two types of dyspnea are discussed in Chapter 19. Both cardiac and pulmonary dyspnea should be differentiated from functional dyspnea, which occurs at rest and is often accompanied by anxiety. Normal subjects experience dyspnea upon extreme exercise.

Sudden onset of dyspnea at rest may be due to a variety of causes, including pneumothorax, pulmonary embolism, and pulmonary edema. End-stage heart disease is associated with chronic dyspnea at rest.

Syncope

The term *syncope* refers to a temporary loss of consciousness associated with muscle weakness and the inability to stand upright. Cardiac causes are usually due to a reduction of blood flow to the brain. Common cardiac causes include arrhythmias (both tachyarrhythmias and bradyarrhythmias including atrioventricular block and sick sinus syndrome). Stokes-Adams attacks are episodes of loss of consciousness due to asystole or ventricular fibrillation in the setting of high degrees of atrioventricular block. One form of cardiac syncope is due to episodic ventricular fibrillation associated with prolonged QT interval and may be familial. This is one condition in which ventricular fibrillation may spontaneously revert to sinus rhythm. Other causes of cardiac syncope include valvular heart disease (especially aortic stenosis), hypertrophic obstructive cardiomyopathy (also referred to as idiopathic hypertrophic subaortic stenosis), congenital heart disease (especially tetralogy of Fallot), atrial myxoma, cardiac tamponade, acute myocardial infarction, mitral valve prolapse, vasovagal attacks, and orthostatic hypotension, which is often associated with the administration of certain antihypertensive medicines. Cerebrovascular disease and subclavian steal syndrome may also result in syncope. A rare cause of syncope is excessive sensitivity of the carotid baroreceptor to pressure. In this condition, carotid sinus syncope, slight pressure to the neck (tight collar, rapid turning of the head) causes extreme bradycardia coupled with peripheral vasodilatation and hypotension. Another rare cause is associated with excessive coughing, resulting in increases in intrathoracic pressure large enough to reduce systemic venous return. Other causes of syncope include hypoglycemia, hyperventilation often associated with anxiety, syncope associated with migraine headaches, and micturition. Loss of consciousness may also occur with seizures and should be differentiated from cardiac causes of syncope.

The history may be extremely useful in differentiating the various causes of syncope, especially if a witness observed the patient during the event. For example, if the patient was observed to develop loss of consciousness associated with typical epileptiform movements and incontinence, then seizure is more likely to be the diagnosis. However, Stokes-Adams attacks may be associated with a few clonic jerks due to reduced perfusion to the brain. Patients should be questioned about the presence of an aura prior to the loss of consciousness, which would also favor seizures as a diagnosis. Loss of consciousness that occurs abruptly favors Stokes-Adams attacks, other cardiac arrhythmias, or seizures. A gradual onset is more suggestive of a vasodepressor reaction (the common faint) or syncope due to a metabolic cause, such as hypoglycemia or hyperventilation. The patient should be questioned about the presence of palpitations prior to syncope, which would favor arrhythmias as a cause.

A history of syncope associated with a change in body position from lying to standing would favor a diagnosis of orthostatic hypotension. Syncope associated with a change in body position, such as bending over or leaning forward, is suggestive of left atrial myxoma or ball-valve thrombus of the left atrium. Syncope independent of changes in body position occurs with arrhythmias, asystole, and hyperventilation; seizures also occur independent of body position. The patient should be questioned in detail about antihypertensive drugs, which may contribute to orthostatic hypotension as a cause of syncope.

Vasodepressor syncope, or the common faint, typically occurs in patients subjected to emotional or physical stress (such as pain). These patients often have a chronic history of such episodes. There is a peripheral vasodilatation plus a bradycardia, and episodes can be terminated by having the patient promptly assume a recumbent position.

The syncope of hypertrophic obstructive cardiomyopathy typically occurs after cessation of exercise while the patient is in an upright position or maintaining an erect posture for a long period of time, when standing suddenly, or after coughing. A family history of syncope is not uncommonly present.

A detailed past history is especially important. The patient should be questioned as to history of known valvular or congenital heart disease; history of transient ischemic attacks, which might suggest a cerebrovascular cause for syncope; epilepsy; migraine headaches; anxiety; and use of insulin.

Many of the same conditions that can cause syncope may cause dizziness, lightheadedness, or faintness (sense of impending loss of consciousness and sometimes referred to as presyncope). Vertigo due to disturbances of the inner ear is associated with a sense of "the room spinning" but rarely is associated with loss of consciousness.

Palpitations

The term *palpitation* refers to an uncomfortable awareness of the heart beat, which is usually associated with an arrhythmia. The patient may complain of a forcible pulsation of the heart, often with an increase in frequency, with or without irregularity of the rhythm. If patients describe a skipped beat or the heart stopping for an instant, they may be sensing the compensatory pause following a premature beat; it is not uncommon for patients to sense the postextrasystolic beat as a forceful contraction. Following strenuous exercise, palpitations due to rapid sinus tachycardia are common and normal.

Palpitations with sinus tachycardia at rest or with mild exertion may represent pathology, including high output states due to thyrotoxicosis, AV fistulas, anemia, beri-beri, and heart failure. Palpitations that come on suddenly and end abruptly may represent the diagnosis of paroxysmal atrial tachycardia, atrial fibrillation, atrial flutter, or paroxysmal junctional tachycardia whereas a gradual onset and end is more likely to reflect sinus tachycardia. The patient should be questioned as to whether the palpitations feel like a regular fast rhythm or irregular rhythm, as the latter would be more suggestive of atrial fibrillation. Palpitations may also be felt with very slow rates, as in atrioventricular block.

Patients should be questioned about concomitant symptoms. With very rapid heart rates of supraventricular or ventricular tachycardias, patients may describe lightheadedness or presyncope. Syncopal episodes following palpitations suggest asystole or severe bradycardia following a tachycardia (as in sick-sinus syndrome) or may be due to a Stokes-Adams attack. If the patient develops angina in association with rapid palpitations, the chest pain is likely to be ischemic and due to an increase in O_2 demand greater than O_2 supply to the heart.

Edema

Edema is described as a perceptible accumulation of fluid in the tissues. Questioning the patient on the location of the edema may be important in determining whether the edema is due to a cardiac or noncardiac cause. Common cardiac causes of edema include right heart failure, left heart failure, biventricular failure, constrictive pericarditis, restrictive cardiomyopathy, and tricuspid valvular disease. Peripheral edema due to a cardiac cause is usually distributed from the ankles upward; but in patients who are bedridden, the edema is more prominent in the presacral area. In patients who are upright during the day, edema of the lower extremities typically becomes more severe in the evening, a feature also common to peripheral edema due to venous insufficiency. Edema of the lower extremities associated with a history of prominent neck veins is suggestive of a cardiac cause rather than venous insufficiency alone. In adults, edema of the face and upper extremities without edema of the lower extremities is more suggestive of a noncardiac cause, such as superior vena caval syndrome (obstruction of this vessel due to carcinoma of the lung, lymphoma, or aortic aneurysm) or angioneurotic edema. Periorbital edema with edema of the face is often present in acute glomerulonephritis, the nephrotic syndrome, and myxedema but is not uncommon in children with cardiac edema. When edema of one extremity occurs, it is likely that local problems, such as thrombophlebitis, lymphatic obstruction, or varicose veins, are the cause.

Patients should be questioned about accompanying symptoms, such as dyspnea, ascites, and jaundice. Cardiac edema commonly associated with dyspnea includes mitral stenosis, left ventricular failure, and cor pulmonale due to chronic obstructive lung disease. Cardiac edema without a history of dyspnea is more suggestive of constrictive pericarditis, tricuspid stenosis or regurgitation, or right heart failure. Ascites is recognized by the patient as an increase in abdominal girth or a swelling of the abdomen. When ascites is of cardiac origin it is more common for the patient to give a history of peripheral edema prior to the development of ascites. Conversely, if the history of ascites occurs prior to peripheral edema, and especially if jaundice is present, the diagnosis is more likely to be hepatic dysfunction.

Cough and Hemoptysis

Cough is defined as a sudden explosive expiration, initiated by an effort to expel mucus or foreign material from the tracheobronchial tree, while hemoptysis is defined as coughing up blood. Causes of cough due to cardiac disorders include pulmonary edema, pulmonary hypertension, pulmonary emboli leading to infarction, and aortic aneurysms compressing the tracheobronchial tree.

Cough associated with dyspnea may be due to cardiac or pulmonary disease. Determining which of these is the cause may be difficult. A long history of productive cough in a patient who is a heavy smoker and a history of cough associated with wheezing in a patient with known allergic (extrinsic) asthma suggest a pulmonary cause. A cough that produces pink, frothy sputum is likely to be associated with acute pulmonary edema; a cough that produces thick yellow sputum is more likely to be of an infectious nature.

Hemoptysis may be due to a number of noncardiac causes, including pulmonary tuberculosis, pneumonia, bronchiectasis, carcinoma of the lung, and chronic obstructive lung disease. Cardiovascular causes include mitral stenosis, pulmonary emboli leading to infarction, Eisenmenger's physiology, pulmonary arteriovenous fistulas, and rupture of an aortic aneurysm into the tracheobronchial tree. Large amounts of blood (greater than one-half cup) due to brisk bleeding are more likely to be due to focal ulceration, as in bronchogenic carcinoma, bronchiectasis, presence of a foreign body, and rupture of an arteriovenous aneurysm; but it may occur, less frequently, in mitral stenosis and pulmonary infarction. Exsanguinating hemoptysis suggests rupture of an aortic aneurysm into the bronchi.

Associated symptoms may clarify the etiology of hemoptysis. Hemoptysis associated with pleuritic chest pain suggests pulmonary infarction; hemoptysis associated with chronic cough and grey sputum in a patient who smokes suggests chronic lung disease; hemoptysis associated with purulent sputum suggests pulmonary infection including abscess; hemoptysis associated with dyspnea on exertion or during pregnancy may be associated with mitral stenosis; episodes of hemoptysis in an otherwise healthy young woman may be due to pulmonary adenoma.

Other Symptoms Of Cardiac Disease

Although fatigue and weakness are not specific symptoms of cardiac disease, they do occur with decreased forward cardiac output, as in heart failure. These symptoms may occur following massive diuresis with orthostatic hypotension and hypokalemia. In addition, fatigue and weakness are side effects of some antihypertensive medications, such as alpha methyldopa and, occasionally, beta blocking agents.

Either the patient or the patient's family may note cyanosis, but cyanosis often goes unnoticed. For cyanosis to occur, 5 g or more of reduced hemoglobin must be present. Cyanosis occurs in certain forms of congenital heart disease with right to left shunts, pulmonary embolism, peripheral vascular disease, and low output states.

Gastrointestinal symptoms such as anorexia, nausea, and vomiting may occur in right-sided heart failure and be secondary to digitalis toxicity. Epigastric distress is a symptom not uncommonly associated with left ventricular inferior wall infarction or ischemia. Indigestion may occur as the sole symptom of angina pectoris or myocardial infarction. Hiccups may occur in patients with myocardial infarction or after cardiac surgery.

Although many of the common symptoms of heart disease have been discussed above, further details and other symptoms are discussed under specific disease states.

Bibliography

Braunwald E: The history, in Braunwald E (ed): Heart Disease:*A Textbook of Cardiovascular Medicine*. Philadelphia, Saunders, 1980, p. 3.

Fowler NO: The history in cardiac diagnosis, in Fowler NO (ed): *Cardiac Diagnosis and Treatment*. Hagerstown, Harper & Row, 1980, p. 23.

Hurst JW, Morric DC, Crawley JS: The history: Symptoms due to cardiovascular disease, in Hurst JW (ed): *The Heart Arteries and Veins*. New York, McGraw-Hill, 1982, p 151.

Wood P: *Diseases of the Heart and Circulation*, ed 3. Philadelphia, Lippincott, 1968.

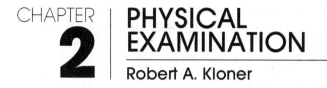

CHAPTER 2 | PHYSICAL EXAMINATION
Robert A. Kloner

A useful approach to the cardiac physical examination is to begin by recording the general appearance and vital signs, followed by examination of the patient from head downward.

General appearance of the patient may provide helpful clues as to the nature and severity of the cardiac illness. For example, cachexia is not uncommonly seen in end-stage heart disease. If the patient appears short of breath at rest or when walking from one end of the examining room to another, significant pathology is suggested. Body habitus should be noted. For example, long extremities and an arm span exceeding height, kyphoscoliosis, pectus excavatum, and pectus carinatum suggest Marfan's syndrome. Extreme obesity, somnolence, and cyanosis suggest Pickwickian syndrome.

Vital signs (pulse rate, respiratory rate, blood pressure, and temperature) are crucial to the cardiovascular physical examination. The pulse rate should be obtained by palpation of the radial pulse for a full minute, noting the strength of the pulse and any irregularities in rhythm. The apical rate, determined by cardiac auscultation should be measured as well.

Blood pressure is recorded with a sphygmomanometer and a stethoscope over the brachial artery. The standard size blood pressure cuff is designed for the average adult arm. In patients with large or obese arms, a standard cuff will overestimate arterial pressure and therefore a leg cuff should be used to measure pressure in their upper extremities. As the cuff is deflated the first appearance of clear tapping sounds (phase I of Korotkoff sounds) is the systolic pressure. Most physicians record the disappearance of sounds (phase V of Korotkoff sounds) as the diastolic pressure, but if phase IV (a sudden muffling of sounds prior to their disappearance) is heard and is greater than 10 mm Hg from phase V, then it should be recorded as well. An auscultatory gap is a period of silence occurring after phase I and before phase II of Korotkoff sounds. (Phase II is that period in which the clear tapping sounds of phase I are replaced by soft murmurs). If the reappearance of sound is read mistakenly as systolic pressure, then this pressure is underestimated. The auscultatory gap occurs when there is reduced velocity of blood flow through the arms (i.e., aortic stenosis) or when there is venous distension of the arms.

In order to determine blood pressure in the basal state, it is important to obtain multiple readings. Blood pressure should be obtained in both arms, as differences between extremities greater than 15 mm Hg may signify obstructive lesions in the arterial tree. It is useful to obtain both supine and standing blood pressures, especially in patients who have symptoms suggesting orthostatic hypotension and who are on antihypertensive medicines. Normally, there is only a small, transient decrease in systolic arterial pressure of 5 to 15 mm Hg and a rise in diastolic pressure when a person assumes the upright posture. Systolic blood pressure in the legs may be up

9

to 20 mm Hg higher than in the arms, but diastolic pressures should be the same. In patients with hypertension, pressures in the legs should be recorded to rule out coarctation of the aorta, in which case pressures are lower than in the arms.

Pulsus paradoxus is a fall in arterial pressure greater than 10 mm Hg during inspiration and is associated with pericardial tamponade but may also occur in chronic lung disease, asthma, pleural effusions, and pneumothorax. It may be appreciated by feeling the radial pulse diminish or disappear during inspiration. Pulsus alternans occurs during a regular rhythm when every other heart beat has a higher systolic pressure. This phenomenon is associated with end-stage left ventricular failure and can occur for several beats following a premature contraction.

Examination of the Head and Face

Facial edema may occur in myxedema, constrictive pericarditis, tricuspid valve disease, and superior vena caval syndrome. There are a number of structural facial abnormalities associated with various congenital cardiac diseases, as in Down's, Turner's, Hurler's, and Noonan's syndromes. In Down's syndrome, which is commonly associated with endocardial cushion defect and ventricular septal defect, there is a prominent medial epicanthus and large protruding tongue. Turner's syndrome is associated with coarctation of the aorta, bicuspid aortic valve, and other congenital cardiac abnormalities; these patients characteristically have webbing of the neck and widely set eyes (hypertelorism). In Hurler's syndrome, in which aortic and mitral regurgitation, cardiomyopathy, and coronary artery disease may be present, the facies exhibit coarse features and there is corneal clouding. Patients with Noonan's syndrome, in which a characteristic cardiovascular abnormality is pulmonic stenosis, have hypertelorism, webbing of the neck, small chin, low set ears, epicanthal folds, and ptosis. Patients with a nonfamilial form of supravalvular aortic stenosis may have a so-called "elfin facies," with a prominent, high forehead; low-set ears; hypertelorism; a small, pointed chin; epicanthal folds; overhanging upper lip; upturned nose; and dental abnormalities.

Examination of the eyes should include assessment for exophthalmos and stare, which occur in both hyperthyroidism and advanced right-sided heart failure. Arcus is a light colored ring around the iris associated with hypercholesterolemia in young adults but may be normal in the elderly. Xanthelasma are lipid-filled plaques which surround the eyes and also are associated with hypercholesterolemia.

Blue sclera can be seen in Marfan's syndrome, osteogenesis imperfecta, and Ehlers-Danlos syndrome; they are associated with aortic dilatation and dissection. Cataracts occur in a number of diseases associated with cardiovascular disorders, including Marfan's syndrome, myotonic dystrophy, homocystinuria, and rubella. Argyll Robertson pupils (small unequal pupils that do not react to light but do react to accommodation) are classic for central nervous system syphilis and may be associated with luetic aortitis.

Fundi should be examined for the presence of hypertensive and atherosclerotic arterial changes. Roth's spots are hemorrhages with a white center, which are observed on fundoscopic examination; they are usually due to infective endocarditis. Conjunctival hemorrhages also may be seen in cases of endocarditis.

A deep vertical crease in the earlobe in young patients has been associated with premature atherosclerosis but is non-specific.

Examination of the Neck

This exam includes assessing the jugular venous pressure and pulse, the carotid pulse, and examination of the thyroid gland.

THE JUGULAR VENOUS PULSE

The internal jugular vein should be examined for assessment of jugular venous pressure and is more reliable than the external jugular vein. The pulsations caused by this vein are best visualized with a flashlight shining tangentially across the neck. Jugular venous pulses are effectively examined with the patient lying at a 45° angle, but if venous pressure is high, a greater inclination is desirable (60–90°). If it is low, the patient should be positioned at a 30° angle. In order to estimate central venous pressure, the patient is placed at 45° and the height of the oscillating meniscus of the jugular pulse is determined. Normally the height of the pulse wave is less than 4 cm above the sternal angle. Since the sternal angle is approximately 5 cm above the right atrium, central venous pressure is normally less than 9 cm H_2O (4 cm above the sternal angle plus 5 cm above the right atrium). Thus, to determine central venous pressure in cm H_2O, one adds the number of centimeters the height of the jugular pulse is above the sternal angle to 5.

The wave form of the jugular venous pulse provides important information and should be examined. Details of the components of the pulses are described in Chapter 5. With the unaided eye, two waves per heart beat are visible: the a and v waves. The a wave reflects atrial contraction and occurs prior to the carotid pulse. Following the a wave, there is a drop in pressure called the x descent, due to atrial relaxation and occurring just prior to the second heart sound. The v wave follows and results from a rise in right atrial pressure as blood flows into the right atrium while the tricuspid valve is closed. The v wave occurs just after the carotid pulse. Following the v wave, there is a smaller fall in pressure, the y descent, which is due to the fall in right atrial pressure as the tricuspid valve opens, and which ends just after the second heart sound.

When the jugular venous pressure is elevated, the v wave becomes higher and the y descent more prominent. Conditions in which there is an increase in the jugular venous pressure reflect an increase in right atrial pressure, such as occurs in right heart failure, pericardial disease (cardiac tamponade and constrictive pericarditis), and restrictive cardiomyopathies. The jugular venous pressure is also elevated in superior vena caval obstructions.

With cardiac tamponade the x descent is prominent and the y descent is small; with constrictive pericarditis the y descent is prominent and deep. Large a waves are observed in pulmonary stenosis, tricuspid stenosis, right ventricular hypertrophy, pulmonary hypertension, and ventricular septal hypertrophy. In conditions of atrioventricular dissociation, when the atrium contracts against a closed tricuspid valve, giant or cannon a waves are observed. A prominent regurgitant v wave and absence of an x descent suggest tricuspid regurgitation. In tricuspid stenosis, the y descent is typically gradual.

THE CAROTID PULSE

Normally, the carotid pulse has a rapid rise to a rounded peak followed by a less rapid decline, which is interrupted in its early phase by an incisura or dicrotic notch (a sharp downward deflection representing closure of the aortic valve). As the pulse wave is transmitted from the ascending aorta to the peripheral vessels, the systolic upstroke becomes steeper and its amplitude higher; the incisura or dicrotic notch becomes smoother in configuration.

The carotid pulse contour is abnormal in a number of disease states. A delayed systolic peak (pulsus tardus) is typical of aortic stenosis, in which there may also be an accentuated anacrotic notch (a pause on the ascending limb of the pulse). A bisferiens pulse occurs when there are two systolic peaks; it is associated with aortic regurgitation, a combination of aortic regurgitation and aortic stenosis, and idiopathic hypertrophic subaortic stenosis. Pulsus paradoxus and pulsus alternans may be appreciated by palpation of the pulse and are described above. Pulsus alternans, which occurs with a regular rhythm, should be distinguished from pulsus bigeminus, which occurs with ectopic bigeminal rhythms, usually ventricular. In this latter condition, the weaker beat follows a shorter interval. Pulsus parvus refers to a weak pulse and can be encountered in any condition in which left ventricular stroke volume is reduced. The arterial pulse may be accentuated or bounding in cases of high cardiac output states (e.g., hyperthyroidism and arteriovenous fistulas), aortic regurgitation, and in patients with rigid, sclerotic arteries. Excessive carotid pressure during the physical examination should be avoided in elderly patients who might have atherosclerosis. Besides palpation of the carotid pulses, all peripheral pulses should be examined. Reduced, unequal pulses or bruits may signify significant obstructive disease due to atherosclerosis or other causes (dissection, aneurysm, aortitis, embolism).

Examination of the Lungs

Bilateral rales that are fine and crackling (like crackling cellophane) and that are often more prominent at the bases of the lungs occur in congestive heart failure. Rales, however, may be due to noncardiac causes (e.g., pneumonia), in which case they may be coarser in sound and unilateral. Auscultation of the lungs following deep breathing and coughing decreases false positive findings. Pleural effusions secondary to heart failure are commonly bilateral; but when they are unilateral, they tend to occur on the right side.

Examination of the Heart

Inspection and palpation of the precordium provide information concerning the location and quality of the left ventricular impulse. The examiner should palpate the precordial movements of the heart with the patient both in the supine and the left lateral decubitus position. This latter maneuver increases the ability to palpate the left ventricle. The apex beat is the lowest and most lateral point on the chest at which the cardiac impulse can be felt. Normally it is superior to the fifth left inter-costal space and within the left midclavicular line. It is often, but not always, the point of maximal impulse (PMI), since pulsations arising from other structures may be more forceful.

The normal precordial pulse is an outward systolic motion felt during isovolumetric contraction as the left ventricle rotates and strikes the anterior chest wall, followed by retraction of the left ventricle as blood is ejected from the cavity. With left ventricular hypertrophy, the outward systolic motion is exaggerated and sustained. Displacement of the left ventricular impulse downward and to the left suggests left ventricular dilatation, such as occurs in chronic aortic regurgitation or chronic congestive heart failure. Aneurysms of the left ventricle result in a large systolic bulge, which is felt above and often medial to the apex beat. Left ventricular dyskinesis may also be appreciated as two impulses separated by several centimeters. A presystolic impulse is felt when the atrial contribution to left ventricular filling is increased (in myocardial ischemia, left ventricular hypertrophy due to hypertension, aortic stenosis, myocardial fibrosis) and is associated with a fourth heart sound.

Double systolic impulses plus a presystolic impulse typically are felt in hyper-trophic obstructive cardiomyopathy (idiopathic hypertrophic subaortic stenosis). Parasternal lifts usually are due to right ventricular enlargement and/or left atrial enlargement in the setting of mitral regurgitation. Systolic retraction of the chest is associated with constrictive pericarditis. Prominent systolic pulsations in the left second intercostal space represent pulmonary hypertension or increased pulmonary blood flow. Finally, thrills may be palpated in association with loud murmurs (such as those resulting from aortic stenosis, ventricular septal defect, and pulmonary stenosis).

AUSCULTATION

The First Heart Sound

There has been ongoing controversy as to the exact origin of the first heart sound (S_1), but the classic theory holds that it is due to closure of the mitral and tricuspid valves. An alternative explanation holds that it is due to movement and acceleration of blood in early systole. S_1 is often split, with the first component representing mitral and the second component representing tricuspid valve closure. The two components are separated by a narrow interval of 0.02–0.03 second. The first heart sound is heard best at the mitral area.

Conditions that increase the intensity of S_1 include mitral stenosis (in cases where the valve is not extensively calcified and is still pliable), exercise, thyrotoxicosis, systemic hypertension, and a short PR interval, which results in the atrioventricular valves being widely separated at the beginning of ventricular contraction. Conditions that decrease the intensity of S_1 include a prolonged (>0.20 second) PR interval (atrioventricular valves have partially closed prior to a later onset of ventricular contraction), aortic insufficiency (also due to premature mitral valve closure), mitral insufficiency, and in cases of mitral stenosis in which the valve is severely calcified and rigid. The intensity of S_1 varies in complete heart block and in atrial fibrillation. Abnormally wide splitting of S_1 is unusual but may occur in Ebstein's anomaly when associated with right bundle branch block; occasionally in right bundle branch block alone, and in tricuspid stenosis.

The Second Heart Sound

The second heart sound (S_2) consists of two components: A_2 representing closure of the aortic valve and P_2 representing closure of the pulmonic valve (Fig. 1A). The two components normally fuse with expiration and are separated (by 0.02–0.06 second) with inspiration. Wide splitting of S_2 with preservation of respiratory variation occurs when P_2 is delayed relative to A_2. This situation occurs with complete right bundle branch block, occasionally in Wolff-Parkinson-White syndrome, with ventricular premature beats arising from the left ventricle, with pacing from the left ventricle, in pulmonic stenosis, and in severe mitral regurgitation in which the left ventricular ejection time is shortened. Broad fixed splitting of S_2 occurs in atrial septal defect with an average splitting interval of 0.05 second and a range of 0.03–0.08 second. Fixed splitting may also occur in right ventricular failure due to any cause, although the splitting interval is not usually wide in this situation.

Reversed or Paradoxial Splitting of S_2

When aortic valve closure is delayed, A_2 and P_2 are separated during expiration and come together during inspiration. Thus, the splitting is said to be reversed (Fig. 1A). The two most common causes of reversed splitting of S_2 are left bundle branch block and aortic stenosis. Other causes include right ventricular paced and ectopic beats, idiopathic hypertrophic subaortic stenosis, patent ductus arteriosus, and, less commonly, systemic hypertension and ischemic heart disease.

S_2 is single in tetralogy of Fallot, pulmonary atresia, hypoplastic left heart syndrome, and truncus arteriosus. S_2 may appear single when P_2 is very faint due to obesity or emphysema.

Intensity of S_2

A_2 is best heard in the second right intercostal space; P_2 is best heard in the second left intercostal space. In adults A_2 is normally louder than P_2. Hypertension within the aorta or pulmonary artery results in a loud A_2 or P_2 respectively. Dilatation of these vessels may also cause the second sound to be accentuated. Thin-chested individuals may have a louder second sound, which is a normal finding. A_2 is also accentuated in coarctation of the aorta and corrected transposition of the great arteries.

A_2 is reduced in intensity in aortic stenosis when the valve is rigid secondary to calcification; it may also be reduced in intensity in aortic regurgitation. P_2 is reduced in both valvular and infundibular stenosis. In patients with a greater distance between the origin of S_2 and chest wall, due to either a thoracic deformity or lung disease, especially emphysema, the intensity of S_2 is reduced.

The Third Heart Sound

The third heart sound (S_3) is a low-pitched sound occurring approximately 0.15 second (range of 0.1–0.2 second) after the second heart sound and is probably due to

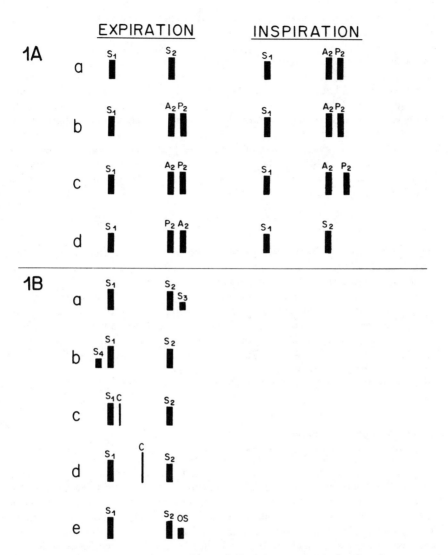

Figure 1A Respiratory variation of the second heart sound. S_1, first heart sound; S_2, second heart sound; A_2, aortic component of the second heart sound; P_2, pulmonic component of the second heart sound. (*a*) Normal splitting of S_2 in inspiration. (*b*) Fixed splitting of S_2, as in ASD. (*c*) Splitting in expiration enhanced with inspiration, as in RBBB. (*d*) Paradoxical splitting. Splitting in expiration but not in inspiration, as in LBBB and aortic stenosis.

Figure 1B Timing of extra heart sounds in relationship to S_1 and S_2. S_3, third heart sound; S_4, fourth heart sound; C, click; OS, opening snap. (*a*) Third heart sound. (*b*) Fourth heart sound. (*c*) Early systolic ejection click. (*d*) Midsystolic ejection click. (*e*) Opening snap.

rapid expansion and filling of the left or right ventricle in early diastole (Fig. 1B). An S_3 may be a normal finding in young people; but when it is associated with a pathologic condition, it is also termed a protodiastolic gallop or an S_3 gallop. Left-sided S_3's are heard best at the apical area with the bell of the stethoscope.

Frequent causes of an S_3 gallop include high cardiac output states, as in anemia or thyrotoxicosis; mitral insufficiency in which there is increased ventricular filling in early diastole; and congestive heart failure with a dilated ventricle. Other causes include atrial septal defect, ventricular septal defect, patent ductus arteriosus, and aortic insufficiency. S_3 should be differentiated from an opening snap of mitral stenosis, which tends to be a higher frequency sound and occurs 0.03–0.12 second— that is, earlier—after the second heart sound. S_3's may also be confused with the pericardial knock of constrictive pericarditis, which tends to be somewhat higher in frequency, occurs earlier than S_3's (0.09–0.12 second after A_2) and radiates more widely over the precordium.

The Fourth Heart Sound

The fourth heart sound (S_4), or presystolic gallop, is a low-frequency vibration that occurs when the atrium contracts into a ventricle (left or right) with reduced compliance. S_4 occurs when the ventricular walls are stiff due to hypertrophy, fibrosis, or ischemia. Thus, S_4's are a common feature of systemic hypertension and aortic stenosis with left ventricular hypertrophy, idiopathic hypertrophic subaortic stenosis, and coronary artery disease. Left-sided S_4's are best heard with the bell of the stethoscope at the apex; placing the patient in a left lateral decubitus position accentuates the S_4. S_4's originating from the right ventricle occur with pulmonary hypertension and pulmonary stenosis.

When heart rates are very rapid, S_3's and S_4's may merge to produce a "summation gallop."

Ejection Sounds and Clicks

Ejection sounds and clicks are high-frequency sounds that arise from the aortic or pulmonic valve areas and occur in early systole (Fig. 1B). Aortic ejection sounds occur in association with congenital aortic stenosis, bicuspid aortic valve, or acquired aortic stenosis; they imply that the valve is mobile and not heavily calcified. When due to an abnormal aortic valve, the sounds may radiate over the entire precordium. Ejection sounds also occur when the aortic root is dilated, as in systemic hypertension. Pulmonic ejection clicks are heard in cases of valvular pulmonic stenosis, pulmonary hypertension, and occasionally idiopathic dilatation of the pulmonary artery. In cases of pulmonary stenosis, the earlier in systole the ejection sound is heard, the more severe the stenosis. Pulmonary ejection sounds are absent in subvalvular pulmonic stenosis or when valvular stenosis is caused by severely immobilized valves. The pulmonic ejection sound is typically louder during expiration, unlike most other right-sided cardiac sounds. It tends to be localized to the left upper sternal border, in contrast to aortic ejection sounds, which are heard more widely over the precordium. Pulmonic ejection sounds also tend to occur slightly earlier than aortic ejection sounds, and, as noted vary with respiration, while aortic ejection sounds do not.

Midsystolic Clicks

A midsystolic click or multiple clicks that may be accompanied by a late systolic murmur occur in patients with mitral valve prolapse (Fig. 1B). Simultaneous echocardiographic and phonocardiographic studies have shown that the click or clicks correspond to the point of maximal prolapse of the valve.

Opening Snap

The opening snap (OS) is a high frequency sound heard in early diastole in patients with mitral or tricuspid stenosis and results from the stiff valve snapping into its respective ventricle during the early filling phase (Fig. 1B). The S_2–OS interval is important (see Chapter 13), in that severe stenosis is associated with a shorter S_2–OS interval. The OS due to mitral stenosis is heard best between the mid left sternal border and apex. Those due to tricuspid stenosis are heard at the lower left sternal border.

Murmurs

Murmurs are a series of vibrations due to turbulence of blood flow (Fig. 2). The intensity of a murmur depends upon blood velocity and volume of blood flowing across the sound-producing area and the distance from the sound-producing area to the stethoscope. The intensity of murmurs are graded on a scale of 1 to 6. Grade 1 is the faintest murmur that can be heard; grade 2 is faint but slightly louder; grade 3 is moderately loud; grade 4 is a loud murmur associated with a palpable thrill; grade 5 is a very loud murmur but still requires a stethoscope to be heard; a grade 6 murmur is so loud that it can be heard without the use of a stethoscope. Radiation of murmurs depends upon the direction of blood flow responsible for the murmur, site or origin, and intensity of the murmur. The duration of a murmur depends upon the duration of the pressure gradient that causes the murmur. Timing of murmurs during systole or diastole is aided by the simultaneous palpation of the carotid pulse.

Systolic Murmurs

Systolic murmurs are classified as midsystolic ejection murmurs or as pansystolic regurgitant murmurs (Fig. 2). Midsystolic diamond-shaped crescendo-decrescendo ejection murmurs occur as a result of the forward ejection of blood into the root of the aortic or pulmonary arteries. They begin after the first heart sound and end before the second. Pansystolic (or holosystolic) regurgitant murmurs occur due to backward flow of blood through the mitral or tricuspid valve or through a ventricular septal defect and have a more even intensity. They begin with the first heart sound and proceed to the second sound on their side of origin.

SYSTOLIC EJECTION MURMURS. Causes of systolic ejection murmurs include physiologic or functional ejection murmurs (not associated with any cardiac abnormality), aortic stenosis, pulmonic stenosis, idiopathic hypertrophic subaortic stenosis, ejection of blood through a normal valve into a dilated aorta or pulmonary artery, and increased rate of ejection of blood in otherwise normal individuals due to anemia, fever, thyrotoxicosis, and exercise. An ejection murmur originating from one side

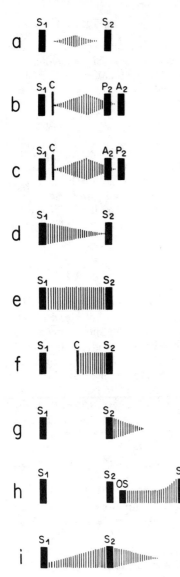

Figure 2 Principal cardiac murmurs. (*a*) Short midsystolic murmur as in innocent murmur. (*b*) Aortic stenosis. Aortic ejection click, mid to late peaking systolic murmur, delayed A$_2$. (*c*) Pulmonic stenosis. Pulmonic ejection click, systolic ejection murmur stops before P$_2$ but extends through A$_2$. (*d*) Holosystolic murmur decreases in late systole as in acute mitral regurgitation. (*e*) Pansystolic regurgitant murmur as in mitral regurgitation. (*f*) Midsystolic murmur due to mitral valve prolapse. (*g*) Diastolic decrescendo murmur due to semilinar valve insufficiency. (*h*) Diastolic murmur of mitral stenosis. (*i*) Continuous murmur as in patent ductus arteriosus.

of the heart always stops before the closure of the semilunar valve on that side but may continue through the closure of the semilunar valve on the other side of the heart. Thus the murmur of pulmonic stenosis continues through A$_2$ but stops before P$_2$. It is now felt that functional murmurs are probably aortic in origin. They tend to peak in early systole (less than 0.20 second after the QRS complex). Murmurs caused by high grades of aortic or pulmonic stenosis tend to be prolonged and peak in mid-to late systole (>0.24 second after the QRS complex). On the other hand, in tetralogy of Fallot the systolic ejection murmur becomes shorter with increased severity of the pulmonic stenosis as less blood crosses the pulmonary valve and more is ejected through the ventricular septal defect.

PANSYSTOLIC MURMURS. Causes of pansystolic regurgitant murmurs include blood flowing retrograde through the mitral and tricuspid valves and ventricular septal defect. The even intensity and long duration of the murmur corresponds to the duration of the pressure difference across the orifice producing the murmurs. These murmurs tend to have a higher frequency and a "blowing" quality when compared to systolic ejection murmurs, which in general tend to be harsher in quality. The murmur of tricuspid regurgitation increases with inspiration while that of mitral regurgitation does not.

EARLY SYSTOLIC MURMURS. Early systolic murmurs may be heard in acute mitral regurgitation due to rupture of a chordae tendineae or papillary muscle or in infective endocarditis. The murmurs may be confined to early and midsystole and taper off in late systole. Since a large volume of blood enters a small, previously normal left atrium during systole, the ventricular and atrial pressures equalize during the second half of systole, thus suppressing the murmur. Tricuspid regurgitation due to disease of the valve itself rather than related to pulmonary hypertension can cause an early systolic murmur. Early systolic murmurs are heard in very small ventricular septal defects or ventricular septal defects once the Eisenmenger's complex (pulmonary hypertension) develops. The murmur of patent ductus arteriosus becomes confined to early systole once pulmonary hypertension develops.

LATE SYSTOLIC MURMUR. Late systolic murmurs are most frequently due to mitral valve prolapse and often begin with a midsystolic click or clicks. These murmurs begin in mid- to late systole, continue to the second heart sound, and tend to be of relatively high frequency. Sometimes late systolic murmurs are musical in nature and sound like a honk or a whoop. Late systolic murmurs are rarely due to ventricular septal defect or coarctation of the aorta.

Diastolic Murmurs
Diastolic murmurs are classified as occurring due to regurgitation of blood across the aortic or pulmonic valves or to forward flow across the mitral or tricuspid valves (Fig. 2). When the etiology is regurgitation across the semilunar valves, the murmurs begin in very early diastole, just after S_2, while those due to flow across the atrioventricular valves tend to occur in middiastole.

DIASTOLIC MURMURS DUE TO INSUFFICIENCY OF THE SEMILUNAR VALVES. These murmurs begin with S_2, are high frequency, blowing, and decrescendo. When the aortic cusps are torn or perforated, the murmur of aortic regurgitation may have a musical or cooing quality. These murmurs are heard best with the diaphragm of the stethoscope in the third or fourth intercostal space at the sternal edge, while the patient is sitting upright and leaning forward. Aortic insufficiency due to disease of the valve leaflets typically radiates to the left sternal border, while that due to aortic root dilatation radiates to the right sternal border. It may be difficult to differentiate the murmurs of aortic from pulmonary regurgitation; however, inspiratory augmentation favors the latter. The pulmonary regurgitant murmur due to pulmonary hypertension (Graham Steell murmur) is higher in pitch and may be heard earlier in diastole than the murmur of pulmonary regurgitation due to primary valvular disease.

DIASTOLIC MURMURS DUE TO FORWARD FLOW THROUGH THE MITRAL AND TRICUSPID VALVES. Diastolic murmurs originating from the atrioventricular valves occur when forward flow through these valves is increased or when these valves become stenotic. The onset of these murmurs begins in early to mid-diastole, when ventricular pressure has fallen below atrial pressure and the valve opens, which may be associated with an opening snap. The murmur is low pitched, rumbling in quality and may intensify during atrial contraction just prior to the first heart sound of the next beat. This presystolic accentuation typically is absent in atrial fibrillation. However, occasionally mild accentuation of a mitral diastolic rumble may occur in the absence of atrial systole due to closer coaptation of the diseased mitral leaflets toward end diastole. The murmur of mild mitral stenosis is relatively short and may disappear in mid-diastole, reappearing with atrial contraction in late diastole, while the murmur of severe mitral stenosis tends to be longer in duration and more even in intensity. Mitral stenosis murmurs are best heard at the apex with the bell of the stethoscope. The murmur of tricuspid stenosis has similarities to that of mitral stenosis but is augmented with inspiration, has a higher frequency, is best heard at the left lower sternal border, and occurs slightly earlier in diastole. Murmurs due to left atrial myxoma often mimic those due to mitral stenosis but tend to change quality and intensity with alterations in body position.

There are a number of causes for diastolic murmurs that occur with increased blood flow across the mitral valve, including mitral regurgitation, ventricular septal defects, and patent ductus arteriosus. Increased flow across the tricuspid valve may result in a diastolic murmur as in tricuspid regurgitation and atrial septal defect.

An Austin Flint murmur is an apical diastolic rumbling murmur heard in aortic insufficiency due to "functional mitral stenosis," when the anterior leaflet of the mitral valve partially closes due to the regurgitant stream.

Continuous Murmurs

Continuous murmurs begin in systole and extend through the second heart sound into all or part of diastole. They occur when there is a continuous pressure difference between areas. Abnormal connections between the systemic arterial and systemic venous systems or between the systemic and pulmonary systems may cause such murmurs. Examples of conditions causing continuous murmurs include patent ductus arteriosus, rupture of a sinus of Valsalva into the right side of the heart, systemic or pulmonary AV fistulas, and man-made fistulas (Blalock, Potts procedure, shunts for hemodialysis). Abnormalities in arteries may cause such murmurs, as occur in constriction of a peripheral systemic artery, constriction of a pulmonary artery, and coarctation of the aorta.

The venous hum is a continuous murmur originating over the great veins of the lower part of the neck and is a normal finding. It can be obliterated by recumbency, pressure over the veins of the neck, and by Valsalva maneuver.

The Use of Maneuvers to Differentiate Different Types of Heart Sounds and Murmurs

Various physiologic and pharmacologic maneuvers can be useful in differentiating murmurs and sounds with similar characteristics.

Respiration

Inspiration results in increased right ventricular filling and stroke volume and decreased left ventricular filling and stroke volume. In general, the intensity of murmurs arising from the right side of the heart increases during inspiration, while the intensity of murmurs originating from the left side either does not change or decreases. In mitral valve prolapse, however, inspiratory decrease of left ventricular cavity size increases the redundancy of the valve, and the click occurs earlier and the murmur may become accentuated. S_3 and S_4 originating from the left side of the heart are increased during expiration, while those originating from the right side are increased during inspiration.

Valsalva Maneuver

This maneuver involves forced expiration against a closed glottis. During phase I of Valsalva maneuver, intrathoracic pressure rises and there is an increase in left ventricular output and blood pressure. During the strain phase (II), venous return is impaired, with a reduction in right ventricular filling followed by a reduction in left ventricular filling, and there is a fall in stroke volume and blood pressure. During this strain phase, almost all murmurs and heart sounds diminish in intensity except the murmurs of idiopathic hypertrophic subaortic stenosis, which increase in intensity due to the reduction in left ventricular volume, and occasionally the murmur of mitral prolapse, which increases or occurs earlier due to more severe prolapse. During phase III (release of respiratory pressure), flow to the right side of the heart increases first, followed by increased flow to the left side of the heart. Thus, murmurs originating from the right side of the heart return to normal (or may actually temporarily increase) one to two cardiac cycles after release of the maneuver, while murmurs from the left side require 4–11 cardiac cycles to recover their intensity. Thus Valsalva maneuver may aid in differentiating right-sided from left-sided murmurs.

When the cardiac cycle length varies, as in atrial fibrillation or with compensatory pauses following a premature contraction, systolic ejection murmurs following the pause are increased in intensity, whereas there is no change in left-sided pansystolic regurgitant murmurs or systolic murmurs due to ventricular septal defect. Therefore, this sign may be helpful in differentiating aortic stenosis from mitral regurgitation. There is, however, an increase in intensity following longer cycles in the murmur of tricuspid regurgitation.

Isometric Exercise

Isometric exercise consisting of hand grip for 30–40 seconds causes an increase in systemic blood pressure and heart rate, cardiac output, and left ventricular filling pressure. This maneuver should be avoided in patients with myocardial ischemia and ventricular arrhythmias. Isometric exercise helps differentiate systolic murmurs due to valvular aortic stenosis and idiopathic hypertrophic subaortic stenosis, which decrease during hand grip, from mitral insufficiency and ventricular septal defect, which increase with this maneuver. The diastolic murmur of aortic insufficiency increases with hand grip. The murmur of mitral stenosis increases with hand grip due to increased cardiac output. The systolic murmur and click of mitral prolapse is delayed by hand grip.

Squatting
Squatting increases systemic venous return; at the same time, it increases arterial blood pressure. The systolic murmur of idiopathic hypertrophic subaortic stenosis is characteristically reduced by squatting; the murmur of aortic insufficiency is accentuated. S_3's and S_4's are augmented during squatting.

Changes in Posture
Rapid changes in posture alter venous return. Lying down from a standing position and elevation of the legs increase right ventricular filling and hence right ventricular stroke volume, followed by an increase in left ventricular stroke volume. Murmurs of aortic and pulmonic stenosis, functional systolic murmurs, mitral and tricuspid regurgitation, and ventricular septal defect are increased by maneuvers that increase venous return, while the murmur of idiopathic hypertrophic subaortic stenosis is diminished and that of mitral prolapse is delayed or reduced. Gallop sounds are increased and the splitting of S_2 is widened with increased venous return.

Venous return is decreased by sudden standing, which has the opposite effect on murmurs. Specifically, the murmur of idiopathic hypertrophic subaortic stenosis is increased by sudden standing.

Pharmacologic Maneuvers
AMYL NITRITE. When amyl nitrite is inhaled, there is marked systemic vasodilatation with a fall in blood pressure and reflex tachycardia. This is followed by an increase in venous return and cardiac output. Because of the increase in forward flow, systolic murmurs of idiopathic hypertrophic subaortic stenosis, aortic stenosis, pulmonic stenosis, functional flow murmurs, and the diastolic murmurs of tricuspid and mitral stenosis are increased. An exception is the systolic murmur of tetralogy of Fallot, which is reduced in intensity. Blood flowing through the pulmonary outflow tract decreases in favor of increased flow through the right to left shunt, due to reduced systemic arterial pressure. The fall in systemic arterial pressure results in a diminution of the systolic murmur of mitral insufficiency, ventricular septal defect (less left to right shunting), patent ductus arteriosus, and the diastolic murmur of aortic insufficiency. Increased pressures on the right side of the heart and a slight increase in pulmonary artery pressure cause the murmur of tricuspid and pulmonic insufficiency to increase. The murmur of mitral valve prolapse occurs earlier, which lengthens the duration of the murmur; however, the intensity of the murmur may have a variable response to amyl nitrite. Amyl nitrite is especially useful in differentiating the murmur of mitral insufficiency (decrease) from aortic stenosis (increase), differentiating the murmur of rheumatic mitral stenosis (increase) from an Austin Flint murmur due to aortic insufficiency (decrease); differentiating right-sided regurgitant murmurs (increase) from left-sided regurgitant murmurs (decrease), and differentiating small ventricular septal defects (decrease) from pulmonary stenosis (increase).

VASOPRESSORS.   The vasopressors commonly used to assess murmurs include phenylephrine (0.5 mg IV) and methoxamine (3–5 mg IV). These drugs increase systemic and vascular resistance, increase systolic and diastolic arterial pressure, and increase systolic pressures within the ventricles. Phenylephrine is preferred, since it elevates pressure for only 3–5 minutes compared to methoxamine, which has a duration of action for up to 15–20 minutes. The increased systemic pressure causes an increase in regurgitant flows, thus increasing the diastolic murmur of aortic insufficiency and the systolic murmur of mitral regurgitation. The systolic murmurs due to left to right shunts through ventricular septal defects and patent ductus arteriosus also are increased. Because these agents cause an increase in left ventricular size, they reduce the systolic murmur of idiopathic hypertrophic subaortic stenosis and delay the onset of the click and murmur of mitral prolapse.

Other Heart Sounds and Rubs

Artificial cardiac valves are associated with various heart sounds not normally heard. The caged ball or disc valve has an opening sound and closing sound. Early evidence of valve dysfunction may result in a change in intensity or timing of these sounds. Pacemakers may produce a presystolic extra sound due to skeletal muscle contraction; and occasionally the pacemaker wire causes a late systolic musical murmur due to its position across the tricuspid valve. Pericardial friction rubs are variously described as scratching, grating, or squeaking sounds heard between the left sternal border and apex of the heart. The quality of the sound has been likened to the noise produced when two pieces of leather are rubbed together. These sounds may be inconstant, appearing or disappearing depending upon the patient's position. They are easiest to hear with the diaphragm of the stethoscope pressed tightly against the chest while the patient is sitting up and leaning forward. Since the sound occurs as the heart moves within an inflamed pericardium, the rubs often have three components, reflecting movement of the heart during atrial systole, ventricular systole, and ventricular diastole. Three component rubs are diagnostic of pericarditis; however, pericardial rubs may only have one or two components, in which case they may be confused with systolic or to and fro murmurs, respectively.

The Abdominal Examination

Valuable clues to the cardiac status may be derived from the abdominal exam. The liver may be enlarged and tender to palpation, due to venous congestion in cases of right heart failure or constrictive pericarditis. Pulsation of the liver occurs in severe tricuspid regurgitation, but can also be due to transmitted pulsations, such as occur in aortic aneurysms. Palpation of the spleen may reveal enlargement when there is concommitant hepatomegaly. The abdomen should be palpated for the presence of aortic aneurysms; and if these are found, an attempt should be made to estimate their width. Auscultation should be performed to assess for bruits which can be heard in cases of renovascular hypertension.

Skin and Extremities

Reduction of blood flow may result in cool, cyanotic extremities. Cyanosis is particularly marked in the nailbeds. The term *peripheral cyanosis* refers to cyanosis in this setting of reduced flow secondary to peripheral vascular disease or heart failure. Central cyanosis refers to that which occurs with intracardiac or intrapulmonary right to left shunting and is more prominent in the conjunctiva and mucous membranes. Differential cyanosis is cyanosis in the lower but not the upper extremities and is associated with patent ductus arteriosus with right to left shunting.

Raynaud's phenomenon is recognized as the presence of cold-induced pallor of the fingers or toes followed by intense cyanosis and pain. During the recovery period, there may be a hyperemic phase, in which case the digits appear bright red. Raynaud's phenomenon is associated with certain collagen vascular diseases, atherosclerosis, and primary pulmonary hypertension.

With long-standing arterial vascular insufficiency, atrophic skin changes include a thin, shiny appearance to the skin, loss of hair on the backs of hands and feet, and dry brittle nails containing transverse ridges. Small round scars, ulcers, and in severe cases gangrene of the skin develop. Venous insufficiency is associated with vericose veins, edema, brownish pigmentation and induration of the skin, and stasis ulcers. Stasis ulcers due to chronic venous insufficiency of the lower extremity typically occur in the area of the internal malleolus.

The skin should be examined for the presence of petechiae and the nailbeds for splinter hemorrhages, both of which are signs associated with bacterial endocarditis. Xanthomas are cholesterol-filled nodules located subcutaneously or along extensor surfaces of tendons and occur in certain types of hyperlipidemias (see Chapter 26).

Clubbing of the fingers and toes is seen with right to left shunts, pulmonary disease, and endocarditis as well as a number of noncardiac conditions.

There are a number of congenital diseases in which bony abnormalities are associated with heart disease. Patients with Holt-Oram syndrome have a thumb with an extra phalynx and atrial septal defect. Ellis-van Creveld syndrome includes polydactyly, hypoplastic fingernails, and atrial or ventricular septal defects. Long, thin, spiderlike fingers—arachnodactyly—are seen in Marfan's syndrome (see Chapters 28, 29).

Bibliography

Braunwald E: The physical examination, in Braunwald E (ed): *Heart Disease: A Textbook of Cardiovascular Medicine*. Philadelphia, Saunders, 1980, p 13.

Criscitiello M: Physiologic and pharmacologic aids in cardiac auscultation, in Fowler NO (ed): *Cardiac Diagnosis and Treatment*. Hagerstown, Harper & Row, 1975.

Dohan MC, Criscitiello MG: Physiological and pharmacological manipulation of heart sounds and murmurs. *Mod Con Cardiovasc Dis* 39:121, 1970.

Harvey WP: Gallop sounds, clicks, snaps, whoops and other sounds, in Hurst JW (ed): *The Heart*. New York, McGraw-Hill, 1978, p 255.

Leatham A: The first and second heart sounds, in Hurst JW (ed): *The Heart*. New York, McGraw-Hill, 1978, p 237.

Leatham A, Leech GJ, Harvey WP, et al: Auscultation of the heart, in Hurst JW (ed): *The Heart, Arteries and Veins*. New York, McGraw-Hill, 1982, p 203.

Levine SA, Harvey WP: *Clinical Auscultation of the Heart*. Philadelphia, Saunders, 1959.

Perloff JK: Systolic, diastolic and continuous murmurous, in Hurst JW (ed): *The Heart*. New York, McGraw-Hill, 1978, p 268.

Perloff WP: *Physical examination of the heart and circulation*. Philadelphia, Saunders, 1982.

Tavel ME: *Clinical phonocardiography and external pulse monitoring*. Chicago, Yearbook Medical Publishers, Inc., 1978.

CHAPTER 3

ELECTRO-CARDIOGRAPHY

Eliot Young

Many aspects of electrocardiography are easy to understand and are quickly learned. Nevertheless, some criteria for clinical diagnosis are controversial or nondiagnostic. Poorly recorded tracings and the use of only one or a limited number of leads may also contribute to difficulties in interpretation.

P Wave

The P wave represents the spread of depolarization throughout both atria. The sinus node does not directly contribute to the electrocardiogram (ECG), but its activity is deduced from the presence of a normal P wave. Recently, Cramer et al. used a transvenous catheter to record sinus node potentials in the intact canine heart. This technique may prove to be clinically useful in the future.

The normal P wave is positive in leads 1, 2, aV_F and left precordial leads. It is negative in aV_R and variable in leads 3, aV_L and V_1. The P wave amplitude should not exceed 2.5 mm in any lead.

Electrocardiographic criteria for atrial enlargement are not always associated with such a morphological change. Many laboratories now prefer using the nonspecific term *atrial abnormality*. Nevertheless, certain P wave changes are useful in suggesting left atrial enlargement (LAE) or right atrial enlargement (RAE).

The criteria for LAE include (1) P wave duration equals 0.12 second or longer, (2) P wave is notched with the duration between peaks more than 0.04 second (Fig. 1), or (3) P wave is diphasic in V_1, with the late deflection negative and at least 1 mm deep and 0.04 second wide.

Criteria for LAE are at least associated with conduction delay between right and left atria. However, left atrial dilatation, hypertrophy, or increased pressure in the left atrium may or may not be present (Josephson et al.). The criteria for LAE may even be due to a very enlarged right atrium (Marriot et al.). In these latter cases, this "pseudo-LAE" pattern may be due to the right atrium enlarging to the left and posteriorly.

Criteria for RAE include (1) P wave is positive, peaked, and at least 2.5 mm in 2, 3, or aV_F (Fig. 2), (2) the initial positive deflection of the P wave in V_1 or V_2 is at least 1.5 mm, or (3) P wave axis is greater than $+75°$. Criteria for RAE may not necessarily be associated with right atrial hypertrophy, dilatation, or increased pressure in the right atrium. As shown by Chou et al., it may be due only to delay in conduction within the right atrium, vertical heart position, sinus tachycardia, low K, or even hypertensive heart disease.

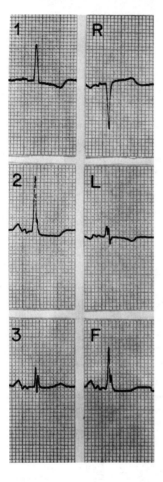

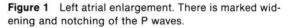

Figure 1 Left atrial enlargement. There is marked widening and notching of the P waves.

Criteria for biatrial enlargement (BAE) include one or more of the criteria for both RAE and LAE.

Atrial Arrhythmias

Junctional rhythm with retrograde atrial conduction usually results in negative P waves in 2, 3, aV$_F$ (Fig. 3) and biphasic (negative-positive) or positive P waves in V$_1$. Occasionally retrograde P waves may even be biphasic (negative-positive) in 2, 3, and aV$_F$. The initial negative part of the P wave may be buried within the preceding QRS, thus simulating a normal upright P wave. It is now established that the diagnosis of upper, middle, or lower AV nodal rhythm is not based solely on the P wave's appearing before (with short PR interval), within, or after the QRS. The PR or RP interval also depends on the difference in conduction antegrade into the ventricles and retrograde into the atria. Recent evidence indicates that cells in the more proximal parts of the AV node (AN and N regions) show no inherent automaticity. As described by Cranefield et al., so-called junctional rhythms arise from the low atria, low AV nodal region (NH), His bundle, or coronary sinus. Thus, it has now become customary to use the less specific term *AV junctional* rather than *AV nodal rhythm*.

The mechanism of atrial flutter remains somewhat controversial, but it is generally thought to be due to reentry. Atrial flutter rates usually range from 220–350, but generally are about 300 beats a minute. A supraventricular tachycardia with an apparent rate of about 150 beats a minute should be carefully evaluated in order to rule out atrial flutter with 2 : 1 AV block. The F wave is diphasic (negative-positive) or entirely negative in 2, 3, aV$_F$ in 85% of cases and entirely upright in 15% of cases. Electrophysiologic differences in these two types of flutter have not been completely delineated. Atrial flutter may be precipitated by rapid atrial pacing or stimulated atrial premature beats. It may also be terminated by rapid atrial pacing or multiple stimulated atrial premature beats, but not by a single stimulated atrial beat. Rapid atrial pacing may partially change the contour of flutter waves (fusion). This suggests

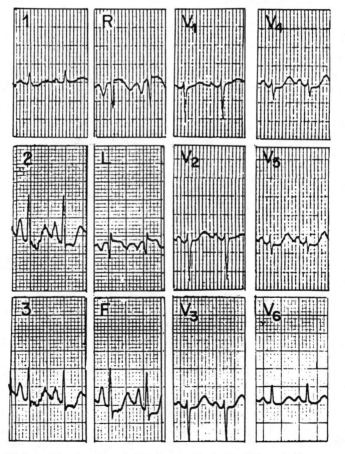

Figure 2 Right atrial enlargement. The P waves in leads 2, 3, and aV$_F$ are very tall and peaked.

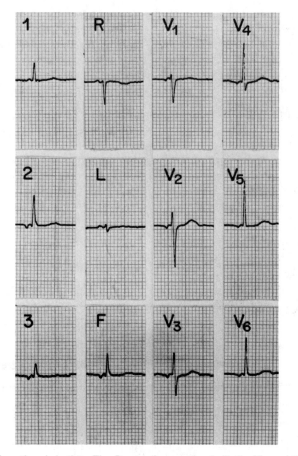

Figure 3 AV junctional rhythm. The P wave is negative in 2, 3, aV$_F$ and the PR interval is 0.10 second.

that atrial flutter, though it may be due to reentry, must involve a small circuit and not circulate around the orifices of the venae cavae (macro reentry) as Sir Thomas Lewis concluded (Waldo et al.). The most common AV conduction ratio in the untreated patient is 2:1; 3:1 block is rare. Higher degrees of block may also be seen. Frequently, flutter waves may not be apparent especially when 2:1 or even 1:1 AV conduction is present. Often flutter will reveal itself spontaneously and by carotid pressure or drugs causing a higher degree of AV block and thus separating F waves from the QRS and T waves.

The mechanism of atrial fibrillation is not entirely settled, but the theory of multiple reentry circuits is most popular. Distinct and similar type f waves and regular f-f intervals are not present. Atrial activity is represented by f waves of varying rate, amplitude, and morphology that cause an oscillatory baseline (Fig. 4). At times some of these f waves may be quite prominent and somewhat regular, so-called flutter-fibrillation. If f waves in V$_1$ measure 1.5 mm or more from top to trough, left atrial

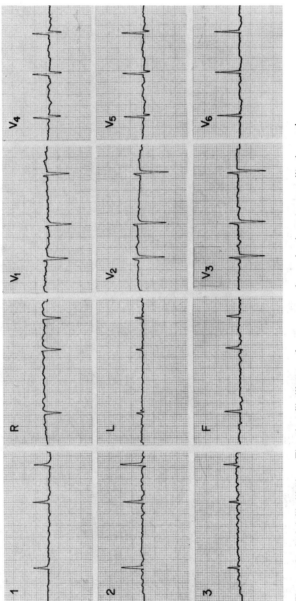

Figure 4 Atrial fibrillation. The tiny fibrillatory, f, waves are irregular in rate, amplitude, and direction. Ventricular rate is also irregular.

enlargement is suggested. Generally, flutter-fibrillation may also be distinguished from pure flutter by causing a totally irregular ventricular response. However, it has been shown that pure atrial flutter may be associated with a totally irregular ventricular rate in 12% of cases and thus may simulate flutter-fibrillation (Besoain-Santander et al.)

PR Interval

The PR interval is measured from the beginning of the P wave to the beginning of the QRS. It is usually measured in the standard leads. It is derived by subtracting

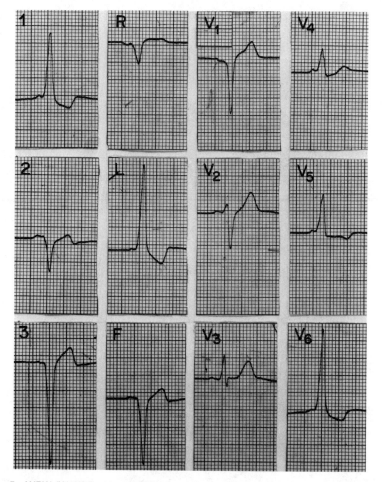

Figure 5 WPW (Wolff-Parkinson-White) syndrome. PR interval is very short and there is a marked delta wave on V_4–V_6, 1, and aV_L. Note similarities to left ventricular hypertrophy and inferior infarction.

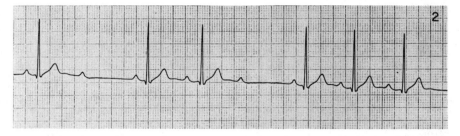

Figure 6 Type 1 second-degree AV block (Wenckebach). The first two cycles show 2:1, 3:2 AV block.

the widest QRS duration in any one of these leads from the longest P to J point in any one of these leads. Lead 2 is most apt to show the earliest onset of the P wave and particularly if a Q wave is also present in this lead, it will accurately display the PR interval. The PR interval represents the sum of conduction time from upper right atrium through AV node, bundle of His, bundle branches, and distal Purkinje fibers.

The normal PR interval in the adult varies from 0.12–0.20 second. The PR interval usually shortens slightly with exercise, because of catecholamine stimulation, which causes faster conduction in the AV node. Short PR interval with normal P and QRS may be due to posterior internodal tract bypass, atrio-His bypass, and congenital small or absent AV node. Short PR interval with anomalous QRS is most apt to be due to bundle of Kent bypass, or Wolff-Parkinson-White (WPW) syndrome (Fig. 5), but infrequently may be due to one of the above causes of short PR associated with Mahaim fibers. Both short PR interval with normal or anomalous QRS may be associated with supraventricular tachycardia. The former has been popularly called the Lown-Ganong-Levine (LGL) syndrome.

Prolonged PR interval may be due to excessive vagal tone and occurs in athletes or during sleep. It may also be due to drugs (digitalis), as well as disease of the AV node, His bundle, or simultaneous involvement of both bundle branches.

AV block may be 1° (prolonged PR interval), 2° (some P waves are not conducted), and 3° (no P waves are conducted into the ventricles). In type I AV block (Wenckebach), consecutive P waves are associated with a progressive increase in the PR interval until a P wave is not conducted (Fig. 6). Usually only one P wave is dropped. This type of block generally occurs in the AV node. However, in about 10% of cases, type I AV block occurs in the His bundle or bundle branches. Type II AV block (dropping of P wave without progressive increase in PR interval) occurs in the His bundle or bundle branches. In type II AV block, it is common for two or more consecutive P waves to be dropped, and therefore it may cause syncope. Two to one AV block may be due to type I or II AV block. Three to one AV block may be due to 3:1 AV nodal block or type II block in the His-Purkinje system. The former is due to concealed conduction of two consecutive P waves in the AV node, but only the third P wave is conducted into the ventricle (Langendorf et al.). However, it is not the type of block but where the block occurs that determines whether a pacemaker is necessary to prevent syncope. For example, patients with type I block of the His-Purkinje system usually require a pacemaker; in contrast, patients with type I block in the AV node usually do not require pacemaker therapy.

QRS, ST SEGMENT, T WAVE

The QRS represents depolarization of the ventricular myocardium. It does not include depolarization of the His-Purkinje system. If the first deflection of the QRS is negative, it is called a Q wave. If the QRS is entirely negative, it is a QS. The first positive deflection is an R wave. A negative deflection following the R wave is an S wave. Subsequent positive and negative deflections following R and S are R′ and S′, R″ and S″, etc. A capital letter indicates a deflection of large amplitude; a small letter, a deflection of relatively low amplitude.

The normal QRS duration varies in the adult from 0.05–0.10 second. The QRS is usually measured in the limb lead that shows the widest QRS and may be 0.02 second or so longer in the precordial leads. A wide QRS, 0.12 second or longer, may be normal in duration in a given lead because a portion of its vectors are perpendicular

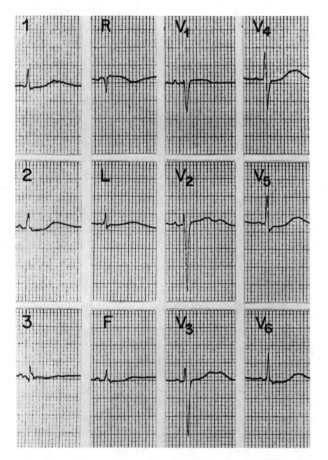

Figure 7   Prolonged QT-U interval. The U waves fuse with the T waves in some leads, making it difficult to determine where the T wave ends. This patient had a potassium level of 2.7.

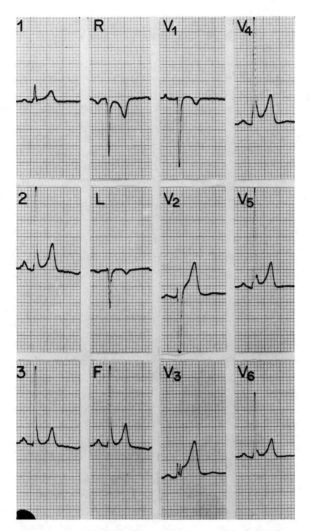

Figure 8 Normal early repolarization. The patient was a thin and tall normal 19-year-old man. ST elevation is present in all leads except aV_L, where it is isoelectric and depressed in aV_R.

to that lead. The QRS may be increased in duration in hypertrophy, bundle branch block, hyperkalemia, myocardial infarction (peri-infarction block), and by drugs.

QRS voltage is greater in childhood. Adult criteria for left ventricular hypertrophy in either limb or precordial leads may be found in normal individuals up to 35 years or even older. In the normal adult, the S wave in V_2–V_3 may be 25–30 mm, due to the dipole having twice as much strength in these leads as compared to lead V_6. Therefore, the use of V_2 and V_3 in diagnosing left ventricular hypertrophy is less specific than using V_1.

Low voltage, 5 mm or less, in the standard leads is most commonly found in the normal person but may be seen in obesity and in pulmonary, myocardial, or pericardial disease.

The ST segment and T wave represent repolarization of the ventricles. It is thought that the U wave represents repolarization of the His-Purkinje system. Repolarization is effected by many causes both functional and organic.

The QT interval represents the duration of electrical systole. QT interval is determined in the lead that shows the longest measurement but with a T wave that has a distinct end point. The normal QT interval $= K\sqrt{RR}$, where K is a constant and is equal to 0.37 for men and children and 0.40 for women, and RR is the interval in seconds between two consecutive QRS cycles (Bazett formula). The QT interval corrected for heart rate (QTc) may be obtained by dividing the QT interval by the square root of the RR interval. The upper limit for men is 0.39 second and for women,

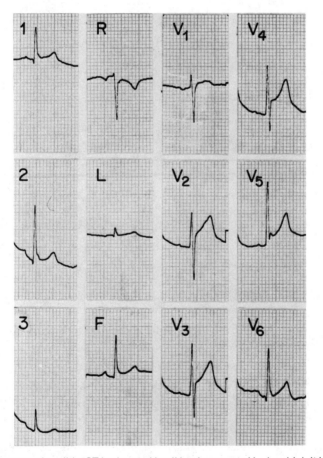

Figure 9 Acute pericarditis. ST is elevated in all leads except aV$_R$, in which it is depressed below the baseline.

0.41 second. Because of difficulties in obtaining an exact measurement of QT interval, it is customary to consider a QTc of more than 0.44 second as abnormal. Prolonged QTc may be caused by ischemia, hypertrophy, electrolyte disturbance, surdocardiac syndrome, and drug effect, especially quinidine and similar type I drugs (Fig. 7). Short QTc may be due to very early acute ischemia, electrolyte abnormalities (such as hypercalcemia), and drugs (especially digitalis).

ST elevation may be due to normal early repolarization that may be as much as 3–4 mm in some precordial leads (Fig. 8). Often a fast heart rate will normalize these changes. Acute pericarditis may also cause ST segment elevation and its contour is similar to normal early repolarization, forming an upward directed concavity (Fig. 9). Ischemic current of injury forms a convex upward ST segment; but during its very early onset, it may simulate pericarditis or normal early repolarization. AV junctional rhythm with retrograde P waves in 2, 3, aV_F may cause ST elevation due to abnormal atrial repolarization occurring at the time of the ST segment. Other causes of ST elevation include hyperkalemia, hypothermia, cardiac tumor, and acute cor pulmonale (ST elevation in inferior and anteroseptal leads).

ST segment elevation due to ischemic current of injury may be due to coronary artery spasm as well as obstructive organic coronary artery disease. If ST segment elevation persists for more than two weeks after acute myocardial infarction, it is probably due to an extensive infarction (aneurysm) as described by Mills et al.

The ST segment may be depressed by hypertrophy, ischemia, drugs (especially digitalis), electrolyte imbalance, and sinus and ectopic tachycardias. The reference point for determining ST depression and elevation is the end of the PR segment. This reference point is especially important in evaluating an exercise test in order to avoid making a false diagnosis of ischemia. [See Chapter 29 for discussion of effects of electrolytes on ECG].

Left Ventricular Hypertrophy (LVH)

The fact that there are so many QRS voltage criteria for LVH suggests that all of these criteria have limitations. Ralph Scott, who has devoted much time to the correlation of ECG with autopsy findings, favors the following criteria: R in 1 + S in 3 >25 mm, R in aV_L >7.5, R in aV_F >20, S in aV_R >14, R in V_5 or V_6 + S in V_1 or V_2 >35, R in V_5 or V_6 >26, R + S in any precordial lead >45 (Fig. 15). These criteria apply only to adults. In LVH the ST-T may be directed opposite to the QRS and in some cases may not be associated with increased QRS voltage. In the presence of left anterior hemiblock, an S in III of 15 mm suggests LVH. However, LVH is often masked by left anterior hemiblock. It is difficult to diagnose LVH in the presence of left bundle branch block (LBBB). There is some evidence that (R-S in I) + (S-R in III) = 19 mm or more indicates LVH in the presence of LBBB. A very deep S wave in V_1–V_3 may be found in uncomplicated LBBB and should not be used in diagnosing LVH. However, a tall R wave of >25 mm or even less in V_5–V_6 indicates LVH in the presence of LBBB.

Right Ventricular Hypertrophy (RVH)

The most common criteria used for diagnosing RVH are incomplete right bundle branch block (RBBB) pattern with QRS between 0.08 and 0.1 second, right axis deviation of $+110°$ or more, R/S ratio in $V_1 > 1$, qR in V_1, and R in $V_1 \lessgtr 7mm$ (Fig. 10). The first three criteria may be found as normal variants. In RVH, ST-T may be directed opposite to the QRS, especially in inferior leads and V_1.

Bundle Branch and Fascicular Blocks

Complete bundle branch block is usually diagnosed if QRS is 0.12 second or longer. However, in contrast to incomplete right bundle branch block, incomplete left bundle

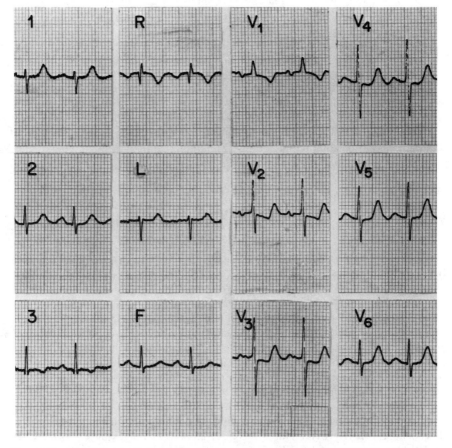

Figure 10   Right ventricular hypertrophy. There is marked right axis deviation. R wave is entirely upright and T wave negative in V_1. ST is depressed in leads V_1–V_5.

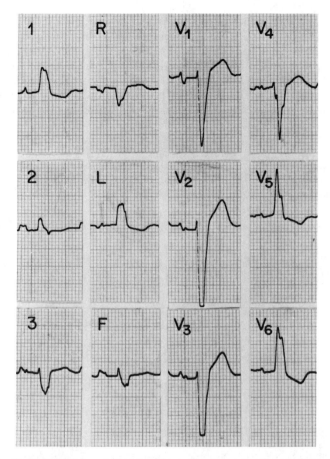

Figure 11 Complete left bundle branch block. There is a notch near the summit of the R wave and the QRS is 0.13 second in duration. Left atrial enlargement is present.

branch block may be present even when the QRS is as long as 0.15 second. It has been shown that it is not the duration of the QRS but its contour that characterizes complete LBBB.

Sodi-Pallares described three degrees of LBBB. In first degree LBBB the initial Q wave may or may not be present and there is a slur confined to the lower part of the R wave in left ventricular leads. The intrinsicoid deflection is delayed >0.04 second. In second degree LBBB, an initial Q is always absent; the slur involves most of the R wave, which is slightly rounded; and the intrinsicoid deflection is further delayed. In third degree (complete LBBB), there is a notch on the summit of the R wave (Fig. 11). The notch is supposed to occur during spread of excitation across the septal barrier from right to left ventricle.

In RBBB, the right precordial leads show a late R wave with the intrinsicoid deflection at least 0.03 second (Fig. 12). Incomplete RBBB may occur with the duration of QRS between 0.08–0.11 second.

In complete bundle branch block, the ST and T waves are opposite the R wave (secondary changes). If these ST-T changes do not occur (primary changes), ventricular disease in addition to conduction disease should be considered. Right bundle branch block tends to accentuate the axis that was present prior to development of block. There is evidence that LBBB with an axis more negative than $-30°$ indicates underlying ventricular muscle disease. In the presence of RBBB, voltage criteria for RVH (or posterior infarct) based on height or R wave in right precordial leads is unreliable.

Uncomplicated left anterior hemiblock (LAH) and posterior hemiblock should not have a QRS duration more than 0.10 second. If the QRS is more than 0.10 second underlying infarction, LVH or further peripheral conduction disease should be considered. Both the characteristic sequence of depolarization and axis must be considered in diagnosing hemiblock.

In left anterior hemiblock there is usually a qR in 1, aV_L, and an rS in 2, 3, aV_F. Mean axis is more negative than $-30°$. If RBBB is associated with LAH, there may

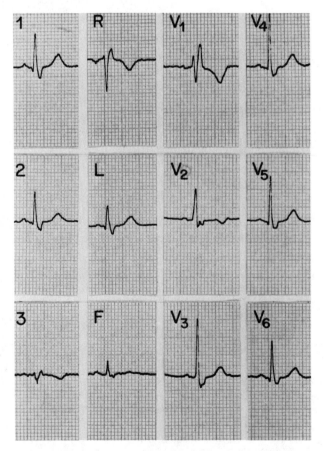

Figure 12   Complete right bundle branch block. QRS is 0.12 second in duration. There is an RSR′ complex in V_1 and the intrinsicoid deflection is delayed to 0.09 second.

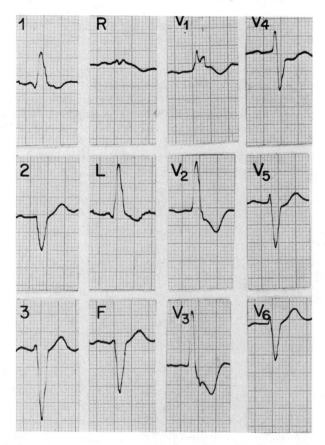

Figure 13 Left anterior hemiblock masking right bundle branch block in standard and unipolar limb lead. There is no S wave in 1, aV_L, but V_1 shows right bundle branch block.

not be a late S in 1, aV_L (masquerading pattern, Fig. 13); and in the case of incomplete RBBB, there may be no late R in V_1.

In posterior hemiblock, there is an rS in 1, aV_L, and qR in 3, and aV_F. Mean axis is +110° or more. The diagnosis of posterior hemiblock should not be made without clinical correlation. RVH, vertical heart position, and extensive anterior infarct may simulate posterior hemiblock.

Hemiblock may mask or simulate myocardial infarct or ventricular hypertrophy.

Myocardial Infarction

When a patient with acute myocardial infarction is first examined, his ECG may show any combination of changes in the QRS, ST, or T wave. Changes in any of these and particularly in the QRS may not appear for hours or days. In some cases the ECG may never show distinctive changes. The QRS changes generally last longer than ST and T changes and may remain for the rest of the patient's life. In the laboratory, the earliest change is T wave inversion (ischemic), followed by elevation of RS-T segment (current of injury) and tall upright T waves. Sometimes the very earliest change in the nonanesthetized closed-chest dog may be tall upright T waves; thus, resembling the tall upright T waves (hyperacute changes) seen in patients as described by Bayley et al. As the process in the laboratory progresses, there occur changes in the QRS with development of Q waves that are indicative of myocardial necrosis.

It is difficult to diagnose myocardial infarction in the absence of Q changes because ST and T changes may only be due to reversible ischemia. These reversible changes have been shown to occur in the laboratory. Nevertheless, when they are associated with a suggestive history or elevated enzymes, they may be accepted as evidence that some myocardial infarction has occurred.

Subendocardial infarction is usually associated with ST and/or T changes that persist for more than 24 hours. There are insufficient data to justify the use of the term *intramural* infarction in the presence of T changes. Large nontransmural infarctions (extending from one-half to three-quarters of the distance from endocardium to epicardium) may be associated with QRS changes (abnormal Q waves) that are commonly found in transmural infarction as described by Cook et al.

Diagnostic Q wave criteria for transmural myocardial infarction are often lacking even when such an infarction is present. It is common practice to diagnose infarction by the ST-T changes that are associated with any Q wave, even though the latter may be within normal limits. It has been shown that nondiagnostic Q waves may occur in up to 50% of infarctions. Indeed, in some cases of very extensive infarction with very poor ejection fraction, Q waves may not even be present (Young et al.).

In spite of the lack of sensitivity of the ECG in diagnosing infarction, Q wave criteria for infarction may be useful in the clinic. The following are suggested criteria for nomenclature of infarcts.

ANTEROSEPTAL INFARCTION. (1) QS is seen in V_1–V_2, occasionally also in V_3; (2) QS is seen in V_1 with QR or QRS in V_2–V_3. Occasionally a qrS may be seen in any of these three leads. QS in V_1–V_2 and even in V_3 may be occasionally seen as a normal variant, especially in women and in pulmonary disease.

ANTERIOR INFARCTION. (1) QS or QR is seen in V_2–V_4 with Q wave 0.04 second or longer and magnitude greater than 25% of the R wave. Patients with left ventricular hypertrophy may also show these changes; (2) poor R wave progression or even reversed R wave progression is seen in V_1 or V_2 to V_3 or V_4. Poor R wave progression may be seen in the normal, especially in women and in pulmonary disease.

ANTEROLATERAL INFARCTION. Q waves in V_4–V_6 are equal to or greater than 0.04 second in duration and 15% or more of the total amplitude of the QRS.

EXTENSIVE ANTERIOR INFARCTION. Abnormal Q waves are seen in leads V_1–V_5 and even in V_6 (Fig. 14).

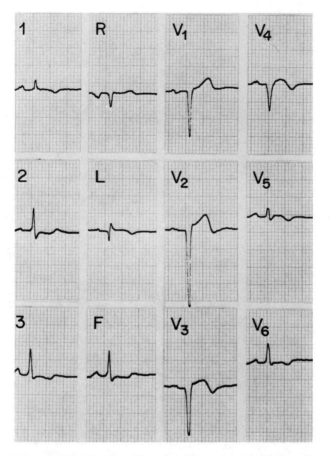

Figure 14 Acute anterior infarction. There are QS waves with ST elevation in V_1–V_4 and negative T waves V_4–V_6. The R wave is small in V_5–V_6.

HIGH LATERAL INFARCTION.   (1) Q in aV_L is equal to or greater than 0.04 second in duration and amplitude equal to or greater than 50% of the R wave. If the P wave is negative and even if the T wave is also negative, this rule cannot be used. (2) Q in lead 1 0.04 second or longer and greater than 10% of the total QRS voltage.

INFERIOR INFARCTION.   Q wave in aV_F is equal to or longer than 0.04 second and amplitude 25% or more of the R wave (Fig. 15). Any Q wave criterion applied to lead 3 is not sufficiently specific to be useful by itself. Ten to 15% of inferior infarctions may have an initial r wave in lead 3 or aV_F.

POSTERIOR INFARCTION.   Initial R in V_1–V_2 $\lessgtr$ 0.04 second and R/S ratio is > 1. These criteria may be fulfilled by normal subjects, especially in the younger age group, and by right ventricular hypertrophy.

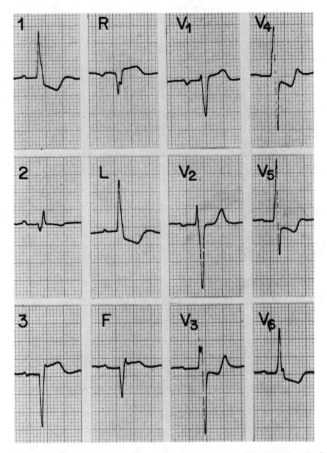

Figure 15 Acute inferior infarction. There are Q waves and ST elevation in 2, 3, and aV$_F$. Also present is left ventricular hypertrophy by voltage criteria and marked ST-T changes in V$_2$–V$_6$, suggesting active ischemia.

Myocardial infarction may be masked or simulated by both left anterior or posterior hemiblock, left bundle branch block, WPW, left or right ventricular hypertrophy. It may be simulated by idiopathic hypertropic subaortic stenosis.

Bibliography

Bayley RH, LaDue JS, York DJ, et al: Electrocardiographic changes (local ventricular ischemia and injury) produced in the dog by temporary occlusion of a coronary artery, showing a new stage in the evolution of a myocardial infarction. *Am Heart J* 27:164, 1944.

Besoain-Santander M, Pick A, Langendorf R, et al: AV conduction in auricular flutter. *Circulation* 2:604, 1950.

Chou T, Helm R: *Clinical Vectorcardiography*, New York, Grune and Stratton, 1967.

Chou TC, Helm R: The pseudo P pulmonale. *Circulation* 32:96, 1965.

Constant J: Learning electrocardiography, ed 1. Boston, Little Brown, 1973, p. 321.

Cook RW, Edwards JE, Pruitt RD: Electrocardiographic changes in acute subendocardial infarction: I. Large subendocardial and large nontransmural infarcts. *Circulation* 18:603, 1958.

Cramer M. Hariman PJ, Boxer RA, et al: Catheter recordings of sinoatrial node potentials in the in situ canine heart. *Am J Cardiol* 41:374, 1978.

Cranefield PF, Wit AL, Hoffman BF: Genesis of cardiac arrhythmias. *Circulation* 47:24, 1973.

Josephson ME, Kastor JA, Morganroth J: Electrocardiographic left atrial enlargement. Electrophysiologic, echocardiographic, and hemodynamic correlates. *Am J Cardiol* 36:967, 1977.

Langendorf R, Cohen H. Gozo EF: Observations on second degree atrioventricular block, including new criteria for differential diagnosis between type I and type II block. *Am J Cardiol* 29:111, 1972.

Lengyel L, Caramelli Z, Monfort J, et al: Initial electrocardiographic changes in experimental occlusion of the coronary artery in nonanesthetized dogs with closed thorax. *Am Heart J* 53:334, 1957.

Lown B, Ganong WF, Levine SA: The syndrome of short PR interval, normal QRS complex and proxysmal rapid heart action. *Circulation* 5:693, 1952.

Marriott HJ: Workshop in electrocardiography. Tampa Tracings, Oldsmar, Florida, 1972.

Mills RM, et al: Natural history of S-T segment elevation after acute myocardial infarction. *Am J Cardiol* 35:609, 1975.

Puech P: *Cardiovascular clinics*, Vol 6, No. 1. Philadelphia, F.A. Davis, 1974, p 58.

Scott R: *Cardiovascular clinics*, Vol 5, No. 3. Philadelphia, F.A. Davis, 1974.

Sodi-Pallares D: *New basis of electrocardiography*, St. Louis, C.V. Mosby, 1956, p 254.

Waldo A: Entrainment and interruption of atrial flutter with atrial pacing. Studies in man following open heart surgery. *Circulation* 56:737, 1977.

Young E, Cohn PF, Gorlin R, et al: Vectorcardiographic diagnosis and electrocardiographic correlation in left ventricular asynergy. *Circulation* 51:467, 1975.

4 THE CHEST RADIOGRAPH IN THE EVALUATION OF ACQUIRED CARDIAC DISEASE

Donald P. Harrington

After the discovery of x-rays by Konrad Roentgen, the chest radiograph was rapidly incorporated into the evaluation of cardiac disease and became an essential component of that evaluation. For many years, all diagnostic efforts in cardiac disease were based on the triad of clinical examination, electrocardiogram, and chest radiograph. Beginning with the era of cardiac catheterization and followed by the widespread use of echocardiography, the usefulness of the plain film has been questioned, but chest radiography survives despite newer technological advances. The purpose of this chapter is to review the basic principles of plain chest film examination in cardiac disease and to look at this safe, inexpensive, and reproducible screening procedure in the context of other tests that are more sophisticated but often more invasive.

Types of Plain Film Examinations

Plain films may be divided into three categories. The first is the posteroanterior (PA) and lateral chest radiograph, which represents the most basic and useful examination of the heart by plain radiographic means; in both positions the patient is upright with deep inspiration (Fig. 1). The second examination (four views of the heart with barium) is an extension of the first; the presence of barium within the esophagus provides a posterior cardiac marker, and the right and left oblique views of the heart (Figs. 2 and 3) provide a greater appreciation of cardiac structures. This examination is also made in the upright position with deep inspiration. The third examination is the supine chest radiograph, which is sometimes confused with the portable film. The term *portable* refers to the x-ray equipment that is used to perform the study. In fact, the portability of this equipment limits the power and flexibility of the system, and portable film examinations may not be as useful as the standard PA chest radiograph, particularly when the patient is very obese. The term *supine* refers only to the position of the patient when the radiograph is taken. The limitation of this study is the heightened position of the diaphragm because of the lessened ability of the patient to take a deep breath. By necessity, the view is anteroposterior (AP) in direction, which also tends to widen the mediastinal and cardiac outline as compared to the PA upright chest. In a portable x-ray examination the PA position cannot be

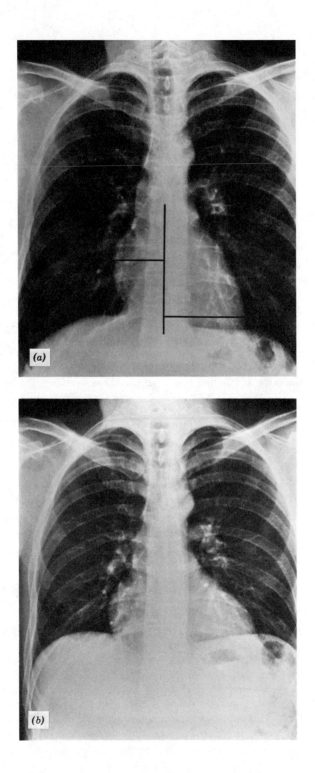

48

Figure 1 Normal posteroanterior, PA, chest radiographs. (a) PA inspiration film with markings for calculation of the cardiothoracic ratio. The verticle reference line is established using the spinous processes. The numerator of the cardiothoracic ratio is established by adding the longest distance to the right and left heart border from the reference line. The denominator is the longest length between the inner aspect of the rib cage. Note also the normal distribution of the pulmonary vascularity, with pulmonary venous vessels seen in the lower lung fields but none in the upper lung fields. (b) Normal expiration film for comparison with *a*. The normal value of 50% cardiothoracic ratio is not valid with an expiration film.

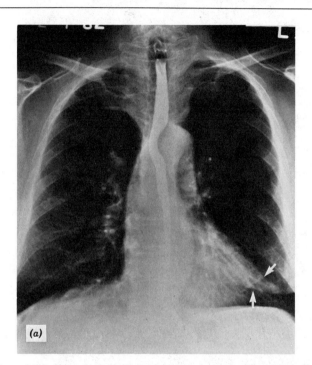

Figure 2 Four views of the heart with barium in a patient with mild aortic stenosis. (*a*) PA radiograph. The heart size is normal. A fat pad is present at the cardiac apex, accentuated by the density of the overlying left breast (arrows). Some rounding of the left ventricular contour is present, consistent with left ventricular hypertrophy. The ascending, arch, and descending portions are dilated and ectatic due to a combination of aortic stenosis and aging. If poststenotic dilatation were the only factor, the arch and descending portion of the aorta would be normal. (*b*) Lateral radiograph. Minimal aortic calcification is visualized (arrows). This calcification was better seen fluoroscopically at the time of cardiac catheterization but was identified first by plain film examination. The ascending aorta is prominent above the aortic valve. The retrosternal space is clear. The left ventricle does not extend beyond the IVC, and the esophagus is not significantly displaced posteriorly.(*c*) Left anterior oblique radiograph, LAO. Aortic calcification is obscured by overlying lung markings. The right atrial and right ventricular margin has a normal straight line configuration (arrows). The normal clear space is present between the right atrium and the left main stem bronchus. (*d*) Right anterior oblique radiograph, RAO. No deviation of the esophagus is present, and the right ventricular out-flow tract is normal (arrows).

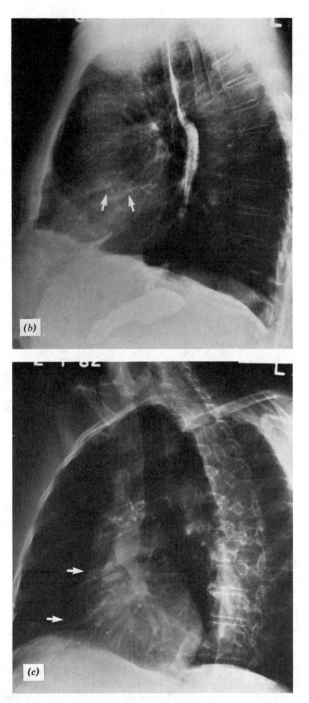

Figure 2 (Continued)

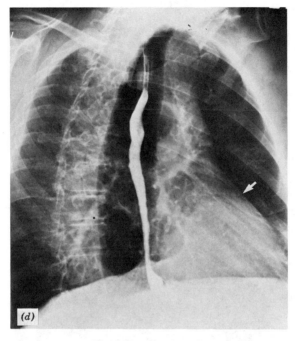

Figure 2   (Continued)

achieved, but the patient can be seated in an upright position for an AP radiograph. The position in which the examination is performed should always be clearly identified on the film itself.

Cardiac Contours and Overall Size

Any discussion of the chest radiograph might well begin with what is immediately apparent on the film. For the most part, the heart itself appears totally homogeneous; muscle and blood are indistinguishable. Calcification within the heart shadow can be distinguished from soft tissue, as can concentrations of normal fat around the heart; both may be significant clues to pathology. The contours of the heart are seen most readily in relationship to the air-filled lungs that surround it on two sides. We are easily able to distinguish the heart from aerated lung. This, in turn, allows a preliminary judgment about heart size, as a first step in the evaluation of the heart.

The simplest method for assessing overall heart size involves the use of what is termed the *cardiothoracic ratio*. This parameter, illustrated in Figure 1, is obtained by first establishing a vertical line through the heart, using the spinous process as a guide, and then assessing the longest displacement of the heart contour to the right and left of this line. The sum of these two lines represents the numerator of the cardiothoracic ratio. The denominator is obtained by determining the longest horizontal distance between the inner aspects of the rib cage. The cardiothoracic ratio is generally expressed as a percent, with any value below 50% considered to be within normal limits; some authors have suggested that 55% represents a more precise assessment. Although the number of true positives increases, so does the rate of false negatives. This value should be increased to 60% when dealing with children and infants.

Care must be taken in the use of the cardiothoracic ratio in several common situations. The heart appears larger in both the supine and the AP position in comparison with the standard upright PA positioning. There may also be a 1.0 to 1.5 cm

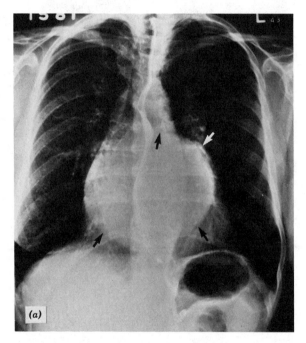

Figure 3   Four views of the heart with barium in a patient with severe mitral stenosis. (*a*) PA radiograph. Cardiothoracic ratio is just above 50%. The left atrium is massively enlarged, causing a double density within the cardiac contour (lower black arrows). The left atrial appendage is dilated (white arrows). The left main stem bronchus is markedly elevated by the left atrial enlargement (upper black arrows). Upper lobe vascularity on the right is easier to visualize than the left because it is not obscured by the heart. In this case, the heart contour is displaced to the right by the left atrial enlargement and not right ventricular or right atrial dilatation. (*b*) Lateral radiograph. There is marked posterior deviation of the esophagus by the enlarged left atrium. The retrosternal clear space is still present despite the distortion caused by the enlarged left atrium, suggesting that right side enlargement is not present. Calcification (black arrow) is noted in the wall of the left atrium. (*c*) LAO radiograph. The left main stem bronchus (arrows) is in contact with the enlarged left atrium and elevated. No vascular calcification is seen. (*d*) RAO radiograph. Further illustration of the size of the left atrium and deviation of the trachea. This series of films illustrates how the cardiothoracic ratio may underestimate the extent of cardiac enlargement, particularly when the dilatation is in the posterior direction with left atrial enlargement.

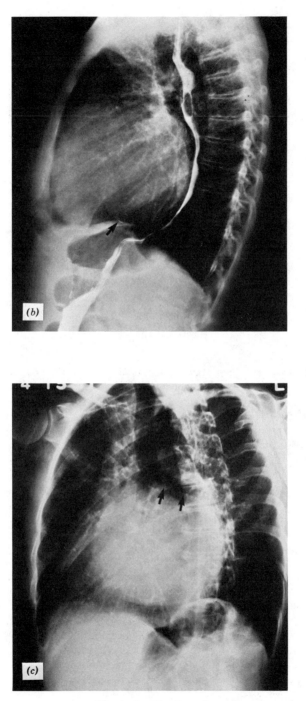

Figure 3 (Continued)

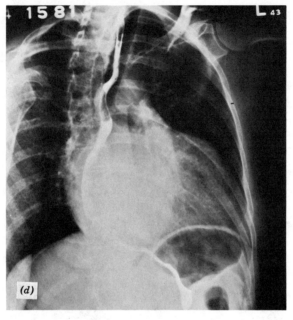

Figure 3 (Continued)

difference in heart size between systole and diastole in the same patient. Abnormalities of the spine, such as kyphosis and scoliosis, and of the sternum, as exemplified by pectus excavatum, preclude the use of the cardiothoracic ratio as an assessment of cardiac size. Finally, the established norms for the cardiothoracic ratio assume a deep inspiration on the part of the patient, so that an expiration film will tend to overestimate heart size (Fig. 1b). This fact affects the supine radiograph as well, because of the difficulty with a standardized deep inspiration in this position.

Several other methods of evaluating cardiac size have been developed, but those that provide the most precise measurements of heart volume also require complex analyses of both PA and lateral projections. They are seldom used in routine clinical work, and no method has received the same wide acceptance as the cardiothoracic ratio.

Lesions associated with moderate to severe cardiomegaly include the volume overload lesions of mitral, aortic, and tricuspid regurgitation, as well as congestive cardiomyopathy and pericardial effusion. Those acquired cardiac diseases, in which the patient is not in heart failure and which show normal or only slight enlargement of the heart, include all pressure overload lesions such as mitral and aortic stenosis and systemic hypertension. Other disease processes in this group include acute myocardial infarction, hypertrophic cardiomyopathy, and constrictive pericarditis. Left ventricular failure from any of these or any etiology results in cardiomegaly with left ventricular enlargement, left atrial enlargement, and pulmonary venous changes. An exception is if left ventricular failure is acute, as in acute myocardial infarction; then hours are needed for ventricular and atrial dilatation, whereas the pulmonary vasculature changes can be seen acutely.

Cardiac Configuration and Heart Borders

Our next step in assessment of the heart is related to cardiac configuration and individual chamber enlargement. As previously stated, it is important to look at changes at the interface between the heart and the lung. These can be seen most readily at the points where the right and left heart borders are outlined by the lungs. The PA radiographs in Figures 1 and 2 will serve as the visual reference for evaluation of the normal heart contours, since the first is normal and the second is an example of mild aortic stenosis, which only slightly alters cardiac configuration. Beginning at the left cardiophrenic angle, the apex of the heart is gently rounded and sharply delineated. Fat, a normal finding, can be seen in this area because fat is less dense than the heart and more dense than the lung (Fig. 2a). The presence of fat at the cardiophrenic angle may blunt the distinction between these organs and falsely increase the cardiothoracic ratio. An extension of the cardiac contour outward and downward suggests left ventricular enlargement; when severe, the air bubble within the stomach will be indented by the heart, since an enlarged left ventricle will press through the diaphragm. This can best be evaluated in the lateral projection. When

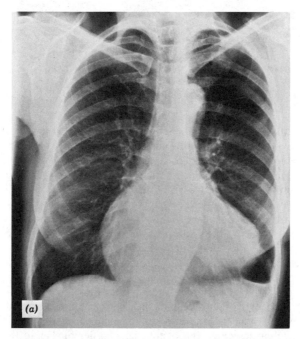

(a)

Figure 4   PA and lateral chest radiograph in a patient with combined mitral and tricuspid valvular disease, in whom tricuspid disease is the major component of the process. (a) PA radiograph. Cardiomegaly is present with prominence of the right heart border. No double density of left atrial enlargement is present. The pulmonary vascularity is normal. (b) Lateral radiograph. Filling in of the retrosternal clear space, with no abnormal posterior displacement of the left ventricle or left atrium. The findings are specific for right-sided enlargement due to the patient's predominant tricuspid valvular disease.

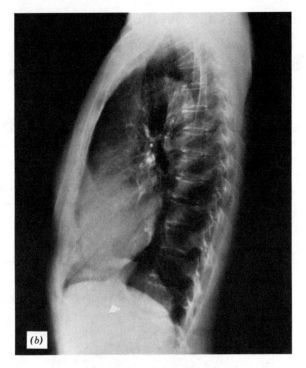

Figure 4   (Continued)

the right ventricular chamber is enlarged, there may also be leftward extension of the ventricular contour, but the apex tends to be deviated upward rather than downward, giving the appearance of a boot-shaped heart.

Localized bulging of the cardiac contour on the left lateral and posterior aspects of the cardiac border is frequently seen in aneurysms of the left ventricle. Ascending toward the pulmonary hilum, the left heart border rises diagonally as a line which either remains straight or becomes slightly concave in the region of the left atrial appendage, before reaching the main pulmonary artery segment. A bulging of the segment is noted when the left atrium and its appendage are dilated. This is seen particularly well in Figures 3 and 10. The main pulmonary artery followed by the aortic knob form the final two structures along the left mediastinal border.

In assessing the right heart border, we begin at the cardiophrenic angle on the right. A small portion of the right side of the heart is usually seen beyond the vertebral bodies; this represents the right atrium. Enlargement of either the right atrium or the right ventricle causes extension of the right border further to the right of the spine so that it appears more prominent than normal (Fig. 4). Advancing further up the right side of the heart, the junction between the right atrium and the superior vena cava may be noted as a change in direction of these structures as they form a small niche. The superior vena cava is the only border-forming element above this level. Just above the right main stem bronchus and right hilum lies the azygous vein, which is seen as a small mass density in supine radiographs (or in the upright radiograph whenever there is systemic venous distension). Overall, there are no absolute normal values for the extensions of these structures to the right or the left of the heart shadow, but experience differentiates between the normal and abnormal.

Pulmonary Vascularity

The evaluation of the pulmonary vascularity is an essential and rewarding part of the cardiac examination. An understanding of the radiographic changes and their functional significance has only come about since the widespread use of cardiac catheterization. Thus, in effect, a more invasive, more sophisticated procedure has actually enhanced the plain film examination, rather than replacing it.

The main pulmonary artery segments should be evaluated first, followed by the right and left pulmonary arteries and hilum, continuing into the smaller, more peripheral veins and arteries, and ending with the pulmonary parenchyma and pleural space. Enlargement of the main pulmonary artery segment is generally caused either by increased flow through the pulmonary artery, as in a left-to-right shunt, or by

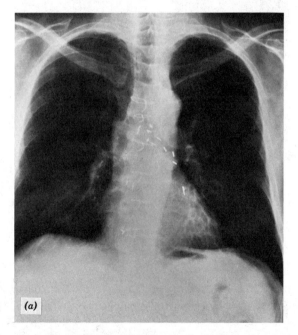

Figure 5 PA and lateral chest radiographs in a patient who had a previous myocardial infarction and coronary artery bypass graft. (a) PA radiograph. Postsurgical changes and normal heart size are present. No calcification or abnormalities of the left heart border are present. (b) Lateral radiograph. There is calcification in an area of left ventricular infarction (arrows). At the time of cardiac catheterization, a contrast left ventriculogram demonstrates an aneurysm in the region of calcification. This calcification is more centrally located than in patients with pericardial calcification.

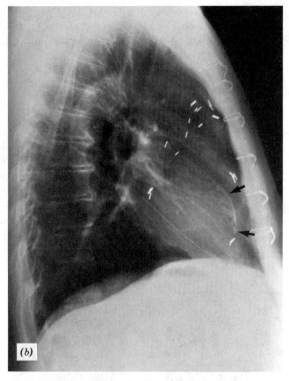

(b)

Figure 5 (Continued)

pulmonary hypertension. A third and uncommon cause of arterial prominence is poststenotic dilatation of this segment due to pulmonary stenosis. Idiopathic dilatation of the pulmonary artery without pulmonary stenosis may occasionally be seen in women under the age of 30. Increased blood flow or increased pressure can also cause enlargement of the right and left pulmonary artery segments. The vascularity in the more peripheral portions of the pulmonary arteries is helpful in differentiating between these two causes. This vascularity is best evaluated by covering over the hilum and proximal pulmonary arteries and viewing only the vessels in the outer two-thirds to one-half of the lung. Normal pulmonary vascularity is defined by experience; but except in the base of the lungs, only small, well-delineated vessels are to be seen. Increased vascularity or larger peripheral vessels are seen in high-flow shunt lesions (Fig. 9), whereas no vessels are seen in pulmonary hypertension because of pruning of the peripheral pulmonary vessels.

Differentiation between arterial and venous vascularity is difficult at first. In the normal patient in the upright projection, an increased number of vessels may be seen in the lower lung fields. These are both arterial and venous, and the difference will become apparent on close inspection. The arterial vessels tend to be vertical, while the venous tend to be horizontal in their passage into the left atrium. In the normal upper lobe, there is less arterial and venous vascularity than in the lower lobe (Fig.

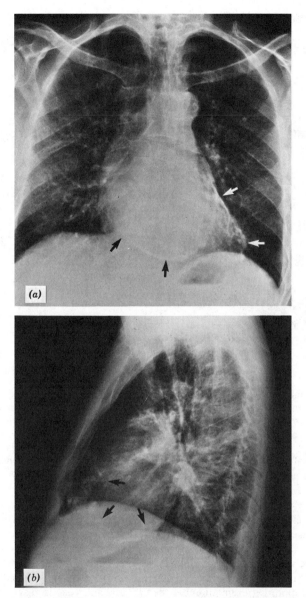

Figure 6 PA and lateral chest radiograph in a patient who is suspected of having constrictive pericarditis. (*a*) PA radiograph. Marked calcification of the entire pericardium (arrows). The overall heart size is normal, as is the pulmonary vascularity. Diffuse pulmonary parenchymal disease is noted. (*b*) Lateral radiograph. The lateral film confirms the previous findings of extensive pericardial calcification. Cardiac catheterization did not demonstrate evidence of pericardial constriction, and no other cardiac abnormalities were noted. The calcification is unequivocal evidence of previous pericarditis, but it is not specific for the present activity of the disease process or its etiology, although most cases of calcific pericarditis are tubercular in nature.

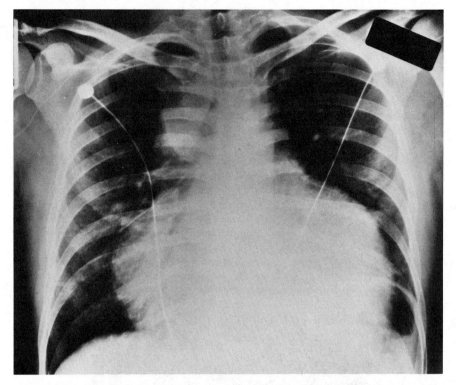

Figure 7 Portable AP chest radiograph in patient with pericardial effusion and mediastinal mass lesion. Obvious cardiomegaly is present, with uniform distribution that has been termed the *water bottle heart*. The pulmonary vascularity is normal in distribution, but the hila of the lung are obscured by the enlarging pericardial space. Cardiomegaly, other than from pericardial effusion, will not obscure the pulmonary vessels and hila. Also present is a mediastinal mass lesion just above the right main stem bronchus. This mass was a mediastinal tumor with pericardial metastasis, which led to the pericardial effusion.

1). As pulmonary venous pressure rises (15–20 mm Hg), no matter what the cause, the visible vascularity in the upper and lower lungs tends to equalize (Fig. 11). As pressure rises further in the venous system (20–25 mm Hg), there is a tendency for the lower lobe veins to disappear while those in the upper lobes become more prominent (Figs. 3 and 10a). This change occurs entirely on the venous side of the pulmonary circulation. Differentiation between arterial and venous vascularity is somewhat more difficult in the upper lung than in the lower; but here, too, the arteries tend to have a more vertical orientation than the veins, as in the lower lung fields. One note of warning: pulmonary vascular changes are only valid in the upright position.

As pressure rises within the pulmonary venous bed, the capillary oncotic pressure is exceeded and pulmonary edema occurs above 25 mm Hg. The first manifestation of this is generally a bilateral haziness and confluence of structures within the pulmonary hila. Normally, structures in the hila are clearly distinct. A second sign is the appearance of short, horizontal lines at the costaphrenic angles, representing interstitial edema; these are the classical Kerley B lines, illustrated in Figure 10. The next step in the process is haziness throughout the lung fields with frank pulmonary edema, also indicated by the so-called alveolar pattern and pleural effusion. Pulmonary edema of cardiac origin is usually associated with an increase in the cardiothoracic ratio, caused by left ventricular dilatation. This is not true when edema is rapid in onset, such as in an acute myocardial infarction, or when it is noncardiac in origin, as in the case of drowning or overhydration.

Cardiac Calcification

As illustrated in Figure 5, calcification within the left ventricular muscle is an accompaniment of the injury and repair after myocardial infarction. In general, this

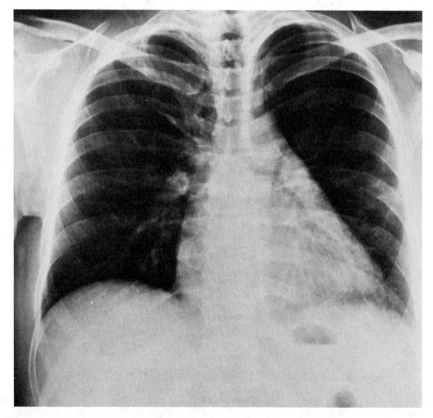

Figure 8   PA chest radiograph in a patient with idiopathic pericardial effusion. The overall heart size is only slightly larger than normal, but the left hila and pulmonary vessels are totally obscured, while the right hila is partially obscured. The pulmonary artery and pulmonary vascularity are normal.

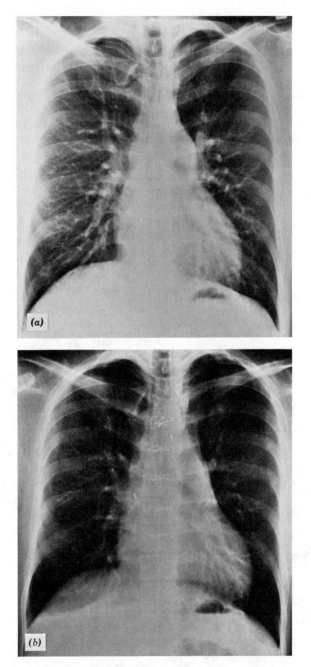

Figure 9 PA and lateral chest radiograph in a patient with an ASD. (*a*) Normal heart size in a patient with a large ASD. The increased pulmonary arterial vascularity is evident in both lungs, as is prominence of the main pulmonary artery segment. Note the vertical orientation of the vessels. (*b*) PA radiograph after surgical closure of the ASD. The sternal sutures and slightly larger heart size are consistent with the preceding surgical procedure. The pulmonary vascularity is now normal and in striking contrast to *a*.

calcification is more localized than pericardial calcification and may be associated with a bulging of the ventricular contour in aneurysm formation.

Cardiac calcification is useful in delineating specific pathological processes within the heart. As exemplified in Figure 6, calcification occurring within the pericardium is indicative of pericarditis. In this example, the calcification involves the entire pericardial space, whereas the calcification is usually seen in only parts of the pericardium. While calcification is a good indication of old pericarditis, only half the patients with constrictive pericarditis have evidence of calcification. Tuberculous pericarditis is the most frequent etiology for pericardial calcification.

Valvular calcification of the aortic and mitral valves is another common pathologic and radiologic phenomenon. Frequently, these valves are not seen clearly in the PA

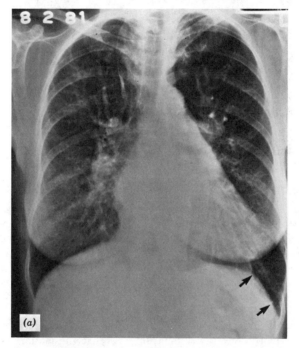

Figure 10 PA chest radiograph before and after replacement of the mitral valve in a patient with mitral stenosis. (a) PA radiograph preoperatively shows mild cardiomegaly, double density of enlarged left atrium, and prominent left atrial appendage. The left main stem bronchus is only minimally elevated. These factors are consistent with mitral stenosis. The pulmonary vascular changes also demonstrate the classical changes of this disease process. There is a shift of the pulmonary vascularity to the upper lung fields, with diminution of the venous pattern in the lower lungs. There is diffuse blurring of the pulmonary hila. Kerley B-lines (arrows) are noted at the left costaphrenic angle. Increased density throughout both lung fields indicates early pulmonary edema. (b) Postop PA chest radiograph after replacement of the mitral valve. All of the previously noted pulmonary changes have been reversed. The normal prominence of the lower lobe venous vascularity has returned. There is some mild residual atelectasis in the left lower lung. The Kerley B-lines are no longer present. Overall heart size and slight prominence of the left atrial appendage remains.

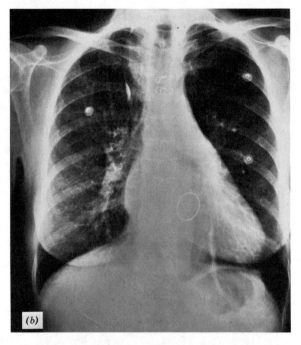

(b)

Figure 10 (Continued)

projection because they overlap the spine and tend to be superimposed on one another. The lateral and oblique projections are more useful in delineating valvular calcifications. In the lateral projection, the calcified aortic valve tends to be horizontally located in the middle third of the cardiac shadow, whereas the calcified mitral valve is in the posterior third and obliquely oriented. C-shaped calcification is frequently seen in the mitral anulus and while the mitral valve is not directly calcified, mitral insufficiency is associated with this phenomenon. Valvular calcification itself is usually irregular and spiculated and is more extensive in the aortic as opposed to the mitral valve. Calcification of any cardiac structure is better appreciated using fluoroscopy rather than films because the motion of the calcified structure enhances visualization. Pathological calcification of cardiac valves is far more frequent than radiologically evident calcification.

Calcification of the coronary arteries is a frequent accompaniment of atherosclerotic coronary artery disease but is usually too small to be seen on the plain chest radiograph. When it is seen, its linear arrangement and railroad-track configuration are good indications of its origin.

Other Cardiac Densities

Fat densities within the heart are normal findings—for example, in the lateral film, a radiolucent stripe of epicardial fat can frequently be seen in the retrosternal area, or the slight radiolucent density of a cardiac fat pad may be found at the left cardiophrenic angle. The retrosternal fat stripe is indicative of pericardial effusion if it lies well within the cardiac shadow in the lateral projection and away from the normal retrosternal location. As the pericardial fluid accumulates, it does so outside the epicardium, thus displacing the fat into a more central location in the overall cardiac shadow.

Specific Chamber Enlargement

The pathophysiologic response of the heart to a volume overload, such as aortic insufficiency, is chamber dilatation; whereas the response to a pressure overload, such as aortic stenosis, is myocardial hypertrophy. Dilatation of the ventricles will result in cardiomegaly and an abnormal cardiothoracic ratio, whereas ventricular hypertrophy generally only rounds out the left ventricular contour. Isolated dilatation of the left atrium does not result in cardiomegaly. Right atrial enlargement is difficult

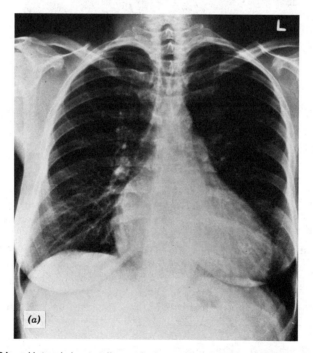

Figure 11   PA and lateral chest radiography in a patient with hypertrophic cardiomyopathy and clinical evidence of intermittent congestive heart failure. (a) PA chest radiograph. Cardiomegaly with left ventricular and left atrial dilatation. The pulmonary vascularity was normal to slightly increased upper lobe vascularity. (b) Lateral chest radiograph. The retrosternal clear space is still present. The enlarged left ventricle is displaced posteriorly to the inferior vena cava (arrow).

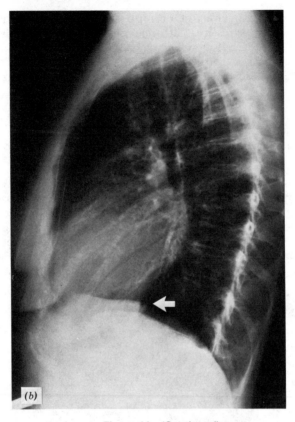

(b)

Figure 11 (Continued)

to distinguish from right ventricular enlargement; the two phenomena are usually considered together as right-sided dilatation. Ventricular hypertrophy subtly changes the cardiac contour but does not increase the size of the heart or of the cardiothoracic ratio.

Differentiation between right and left ventricular enlargement is somewhat difficult. One must first establish whether or not the right ventricle is enlarged. (Fig. 4). Such an enlargement is seen as the abnormal displacement of the cardiac shadow to the right of the ventral bodies and as a filling in of the retrosternal clear space in the lateral projection. There is also extension of the heart upward and to the left, into the shape of a boot. The left anterior oblique (LAO) projection can also be used to evaluate the right ventricle. In this projection, the right heart border is seen as a relatively vertical line as it rises to meet the superior vena cava (Fig. 2). If there is a step formed between the right side of the heart and the superior vena cava, right-sided enlargement is present. Right ventricular enlargement can mimic all the signs of left ventricular enlargement, so the latter cannot be adequately determined. If right ventricular enlargement is *not* clearly shown, evaluation of the left ventricle can proceed. Extension of the ventricle downward and outward to the left is one indication of enlargement. Another radiographic sign involves extracardiac organ relationships. In the lateral projection, one normally sees the posterior wall of the inferior vena cava as it rises from the abdomen. This is seen as a vertical structure arising from the diaphragm into the heart, and normally no cardiac shadow will be seen posteriorly. However, left ventricular enlargement will cause a portion of the left ventricle to extend beyond this vertical line (Fig. 11). The outward and downward expansion of left ventricular dilatation will also encroach on the left diaphragm and, in extreme cases, indent the gastric air bubble.

Of all radiographic signs of chamber enlargement, those involving the left atrium are the most reliable. Left atrial enlargement is indicated in the PA projection by the formation of a double density as the left atrium expands posteriorly and by prominence of the left atrial appendage on the left heart border (Figs. 3 and 10). As the left atrium enlarges, it tends to encroach upon and elevate the left main stem bronchus. This encroachment is especially clear in the LAO projection, where there is normally a clear space between the upper portion of the cardiac shadow and the left main stem bronchus (Fig. 2c). As the left atrium increases in size, this space is encroached upon by the cardiac silhouette until finally the left main stem bronchus is displaced upward by the cardiac mass (Fig. 3c). The LAO projection is also useful for separating the calcified mitral and aortic valves.

Specific Pathological Processes

A number of specific diseases may be identified on chest radiograph. Aortic valvular disease can present as aortic stenosis, as aortic insufficiency, or as a combination of these two. When aortic stenosis is the predominant lesion, the overall cardiac size is not increased. The result is a pressure overload of the left ventricle, which leads to myocardial hypertrophy. Myocardial hypertrophy may cause subtle changes in cardiac contour, but it does not lead to an increased cardiothoracic ratio. Calcification of the aortic valve frequently accompanies aortic stenosis, whether the underlying process is rheumatic heart disease or a congenital bicuspid aortic valve. Isolated dilatation of the ascending aorta, which results in an apparent increased density of the retrosternal space above the heart and a deviation of the superior vena cava to the right, is a further indication of aortic stenosis. This poststenotic dilatation is caused by turbulent blood flow through the stenotic valve (Fig. 2).

Dilatation of the ascending, arch, and descending portion of the aorta may result from the normal aging process or from sustained systemic hypertension.

When aortic regurgitation is the predominant lesion, there is a volume rather than a pressure overload of the left ventricle. This results in dilatation of the left ventricle and an increase in the cardiothoracic ratio (Fig. 12).

Mitral valve disease is another example of a process that is usually a combination of stenosis and insufficiency. When stenosis predominates, the left atrium dilates because of pressure overload, while the left ventricle tends to remain normal in size. Left atrial enlargement is indicated by prominence of the left atrial appendage along the left heart border, a double density in the PA projection with posterior extension of the left atrial chamber, and—in the most severe cases—elevation of the left main stem bronchus in the PA projection. In the LAO projection, the clear space between the cardiac shadow and the left main stem bronchus is obliterated, with ultimate elevation of the main stem bronchus. Also in the most severe enlargement, the left atrium can extend beyond the right heart border and thus give the impression of right-sided enlargement (Fig. 3). With left atrial hypertension, the pressure is transmitted into the pulmonary venous bed, and there is a shift of pulmonary venous vascularity from the lower lung fields to an equal balance between upper and lower vessels, finally giving marked prominence to those in the upper lobe (Figs. 3 and 10). In the presence of mitral regurgitation, left ventricular enlargement is added to

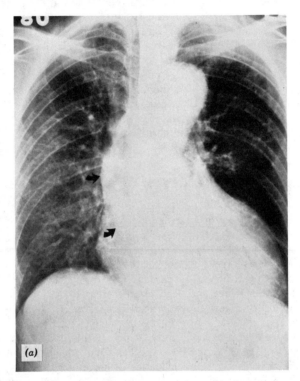

(a)

Figure 12 PA and lateral chest radiograph in a patient with signs and symptoms of aortic insufficiency. (a) PA radiograph. The heart is enlarged, with outward and downward displacement of the left heart border. The right heart border appears normal. The aortic knob is prominent, which may relate to patient age or to preexisting chronic hypertension, but the dilatation of the ascending aorta (arrows) suggests aortic valve disease, although an aneurysm involving the ascending aorta is a possibility. Equalization of the upper and lower pulmonary vascularity is present. (b) Lateral radiograph. The retrosternal clear space is maintained, with marked enlargement of the heart posteriorly beyond the inferior vena cava, where it passes through the diaphragm (arrows). No calcification of valves or of the ascending aorta is noted. Blunting of the posterior angle of the left diaphragm is incidentally noted. The overall cardial enlargement and configuration of the ventricles indicate left ventricular dilatation. Prominence of the ascending aorta suggests aortic valve disease. Together these observations suggest that aortic regurgitation is the predominant element. Increased pulmonary venous pressure is indicated by the shift of venous vascularity.

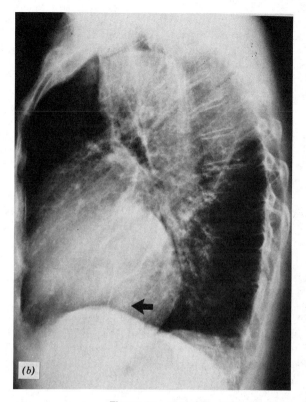

Figure 12   (Continued)

these findings, reflecting the volume overload of the left ventricle by the regurgitation.

Tricuspid valve disease, regardless of its etiology, is usually not associated with radiographically identifiable calcification, as is mitral or aortic valve disease; rather, it is indicated by enlargement of the right side of the heart without the evidence of pulmonary arterial or venous hypertension (Fig. 4).

When any valvular disease is combined with ventricular failure, or when multiple valves are involved, the previously noted distinctions are blurred and generally unreliable. The greatest value of the chest x-ray in these cases is its ability to delineate the progressive physiologic and pathologic changes that lead to ventricular failure.

In patients with coronary artery disease, the most frequently encountered acquired heart disease, the chest radiograph is usually normal. This is true for both acute and chronic myocardial ischemia. When ventricular failure results from myocardial ischemia, cardiomegaly, left ventricular and left atrial enlargement, and the accompanying signs of increased pulmonary venous hypertension are evident. Myocardial infarction may lead to aneurysm formation, which may be identifiable on chest radiographs as a localized bulging of the left ventricle, which ultimately may calcify. Other complications of myocardial infarctions, such as papillary muscle infarction and acute mitral regurgitation or septal infarction with ventricular septal defect (VSD) formation, are evident radiographically, though congestive heart failure is frequently the most obvious finding in these severe complications.

Other myocardial disease processes such as myocarditis can only be identified as the myocardium fails with resultant left ventricular dilatation. This is a late sign, and such a limitation in radiographic identification also holds true for the various forms of cardiomyopathy, whether they are restrictive or hypertrophic (Fig. 11).

Pericardial disease processes may be identified if calcification is present in pericarditis (Fig. 6) or, in the case of pericardial effusion, when the effusion is large enough to give identifiable cardiomegaly and to displace the retroperitoneal fat stripe (Figs. 7 and 8). Pericardial effusion is one disease process in which echocardiography has superseded all other diagnostic methods for its identification. This is particularly true when the effusion is small. Large amounts of pericardial effusion are necessary to increase the overall cardiac silhouette. Once pericardial effusion has been established, the chest radiograph can be used to follow resolution of this process by changes in cardiac size.

Supine and Portable Chest Films

The supine chest film is used to evaluate patients in the intensive care area and recovery room, when standard radiographic views cannot be obtained. As noted earlier, one limitation of this technique is that the standard cardiothoracic ratio cannot be used. But in spite of this, the serial nature of the film provides much diagnostic information. First, it shows increasing or decreasing cardiac size on a day-to-day basis; second, it shows change in the pulmonary venous vascularity, which can indicate cardiac function and/or pulmonary venous pressure. Portable chest films taken in the intensive care unit are limited by the variations in technique, patient positioning, and the respiratory cycle from one film to the next. However, when this drawback is taken into account, the chest film can provide a good anatomic and physiologic study.

Bibliography

Baron MG: Radiological and angiographic examination of the heart, in Braunwald E (ed): *Heart Disease: A Textbook of Cardiovascular Medicine* Vol I, Philadelphia, Saunders, 1980, p 147

Battler A, Karliner JS, Higgins CB, et al: The initial chest x-ray in acute myocardial infarction: Prediction of early and late mortality and survival. *Circulation* 61:1004, 1980.

Cooley RN, Schreiber MH: Radiology of the heart and great vessels, in ed 3: *Golden's Diagnostic Radiology*. Baltimore, Williams and Wilkins, 1978.

Higgins CB, Lipton MJ: Radiography of acute myocardial infarction. *Radiol Clin North Am* 18:359, Dec. 1980.

Newell JD, Higgins CD, Kelley MJ: Radiographic-echocardiographic approach to acquired heart disease: Diagnosis and assessment of severity. *Radiol Clin North Am* 18:387, Dec. 1980.

CHAPTER 5 | ECHOCARDIOGRAPHY; JUGULAR, AND ARTERIAL PULSE RECORDINGS

SECTION 1

ECHOCARDIOGRAPHY

Joshua Wynne

Technical Considerations

Echocardiography is the most widely utilized noninvasive cardiac diagnostic method available (aside from the chest x-ray and electrocardiogram), and it may provide definitive information in a wide variety of valvular, pericardial, myocardial, and congenital disease states. It utilizes short pulses (1–2 μsec duration) of high frequency (1.9–5 million cycles/sec or MHz) sound waves, repeated many times each second (typically 1000 Hz). Because of the short duration of the ultrasound pulses, no deleterious effects are found with echocardiography. The sound waves are generated by a piezoelectric crystal, which has the unique property of transforming electrical energy into mechanical (i.e., sound) energy, and vice-versa. A transducer containing the crystal is placed on the chest wall and it acts as both a transmitter and receiver of the short pulses of ultrasound that reflect off surfaces of the heart and return to the crystal for detection. Ultrasound waves are reflected when they strike an interface composed of two tissues of differing acoustic impedance (which is related to tissue density).

In the traditional M-mode (or "motion") study, the sound waves are transmitted and received along a single line; the resulting image has been called an "ice-pick" view of the heart (Fig. 1). Identification of cardiac structures requires careful, and sometimes tedious, positioning of the transducer on the patient's chest by the operator, who must change the orientation and position of the transducer in order to see different parts of the heart. Newer echocardiographic machines provide a cross-sectional or two-dimensional view by steering the echocardiographic beam through an arc of up to 90°, producing a tomographic image of excellent spatial resolution (Fig. 2). By obtaining many such images each second (typically 30–60 images/sec), the motion of the heart can be viewed in real time. In clinical practice, it is usually best to be able to perform both M-mode as well as two-dimensional echocardiographic studies, since these methods are complementary, rather than exclusive—

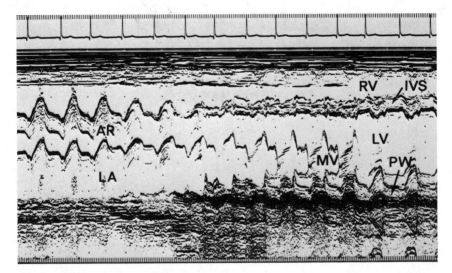

Figure 1 M-mode echocardiographic sweep in a normal subject, obtained by rotating the transducer so that various cardiac structures come into view. AR, aortic root; IVS, interventricular septum; LA, left atrium; LV, left ventricle; MV, mitral valve; PW, posterior wall; RV, right ventricle.

the two-dimensional technique provides high spatial resolution (because of its wide field of view), while the M-mode technique provides high temporal resolution (as a consequence of its high pulse repetition rate of 1000 Hz). The *primary* modality, however, is the two-dimensional one, which usually provides the more definitive data.

Clinical Applications

Echocardiography is probably the best method currently available (either invasive or noninvasive) for evaluating *structural* cardiac abnormalities larger than 1–2 mm (limited by the resolution of ultrasound). Because the air within the lungs disperses echocardiographic signals, it may be difficult or impossible to obtain adequate imaging in about 10% of patients in whom an optimal transducer position cannot be found, particularly those with obstructive lung diease. All four cardiac valves and chambers usually can be seen, as well as the interventricular and interatrial septum (particularly with the two-dimensional technique). The inferior vena cava and proximal aortic root usually are easy to image. Except for the proximal left coronary artery system, it usually is not possible to image the coronary arteries directly. Thus, unless a coronary stenosis has resulted in abnormal left ventricular wall motion as a consequence of myocardial ischemia or infarction, the echocardiogram typically is normal in coronary artery disease.

VALVULAR HEART DISEASE

Echocardiography permits evaluation of the *site, cause,* and *severity* of a variety of forms of valvular heart disease. Differentiation of subvalvular, valvular, and supravalvular involvement is usually easily determined, although this is usually a consideration only with the aortic valve. The *cause* of valvular disease can often be ascertained or at least suggested by echocardiography, since the echocardiogram can identify thickening and calcification of the valve (e.g., rheumatic disease) or its supporting structures (e.g., calcified mitral anulus); disruption of the valve (e.g., ruptured chordae tendineae); abnormal motion of the valve (e.g., mitral valve prolapse); or other disease processes (e.g., vegetations of infective endocarditis). The *severity* of valvular disease is determined by both direct imaging of the valve and by evaluation of the secondary functional and structural abnormalities produced by the valve lesion, such as left atrial and left ventricular enlargement and volume overload in mitral regurgitation. The clinical utility of the echocardiogram in the diagnosis of valvular heart disease varies from *definitive*, when cardiac catheterization is rarely

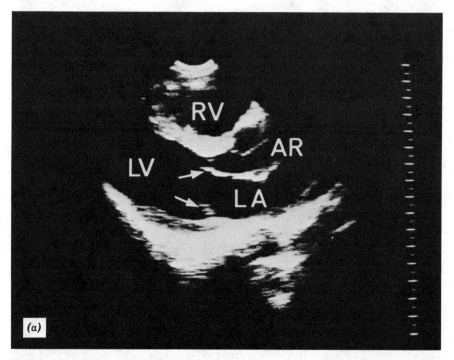

Figure 2   Two-dimensional echocardiographic views in a normal subject. (*a*) Long-axis parasternal view, demonstrating the coaptation in diastole of two of the aortic valve leaflets in the center of the aorta. (*b*) Short-axis parasternal view at the level of the papillary muscles, which are the indentations within the LV at 3 and 8 o'clock. (*c*) Apical four-chamber view, showing the normal dropout of echo signals from the region of the septum primum (asterisk). AR, aortic root; LA, left atrium; LV, left ventricle; RA, right atrium; RV, right ventricle. The arrows indicate the anterior and posterior mitral valve leaflets.

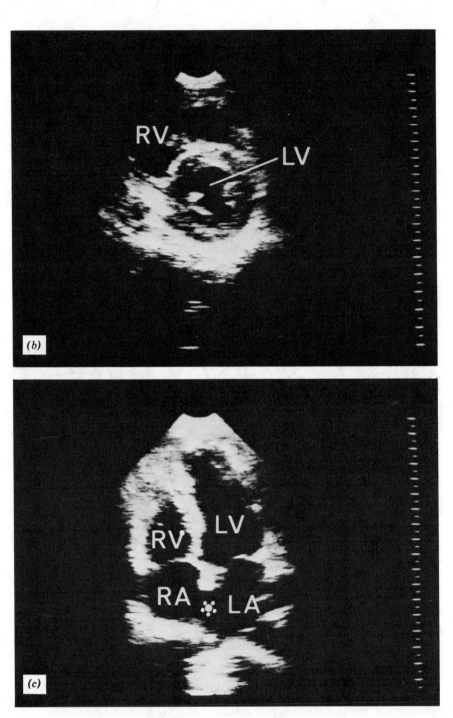

Figure 2 (Continued)

required, to *useful*, when, although the echocardiogram provides helpful information, cardiac catheterization frequently is required for complete evaluation (Table 1).

In addition to evaluating suspected diseases, echocardiography is also useful in *excluding* significant valvular involvement. Although there are exceptions, the presence of an apparently normal valve and supporting apparatus in a technically adequate two-dimensional echocardiogram essentially excludes hemodynamically significant involvement in most forms of valvular heart disease.

Mitral Valve

The appearance of the normal mitral valve is that of two thin mobile leaflets with the anterior leaflet demonstrating the larger excursion (Fig. 1). The motion of the posterior leaflet is a mirror-image of the anterior leaflet, although its excursion is substantially less. The pattern of motion of the leaflets is one of rapid opening in diastole (during the period of rapid ventricular filling), with anterior and posterior leaflets moving in opposite directions. With the termination of the rapid filling phase and the start of the slow filling phase, the leaflets float toward each other, assuming a more neutral position. With left atrial systole, transmitral flow again increases, and the leaflets are driven further apart, only to coapt completely with ventricular systole.

Table 1.   Utility of Echocardiography in Valvular Heart Disease

---

Definitive[a]
   Mitral stenosis
   Left atrial myxoma
   Ruptured chordae tendineae with disruption of mitral valve
   Aortic valve vegetation with early closure of mitral valve
   Presence of tricuspid regurgitation
   Exclusion of significant valvular stenosis
Highly useful[b]
   Vegetations
   Mitral valve prolapse
Useful[c]
   Aortic stenosis
   Pulmonic stenosis
   Tricuspid stenosis
   Pulmonary regurgitation

---

[a] Definitive implies that the echocardiogram provides sufficiently acurate and reliable information so that a clinical decision may be formed without cardiac catheterization in almost all patients.

[b] Highly useful indicates that the echocardiogram may provide unique information that is difficult or impossible to obtain by other techniques but that cardiac catheterization is often required to be certain of the severity of the lesion (typically regurgitant).

[c] Useful indicates that while the echocardiogram provides important anatomic information, assessing the severity of disease (typically stenosis) usually requires cardiac catheterization.

Mitral Stenosis

FEATURES. In mitral stenosis there is thickening of the leaflets; fusion of the commissures; and shortening, fusion, and thickening of the chordae tendineae (Fig. 3). The excursion of the valve typically is reduced, and there is concordant motion of the anterior and posterior leaflets due to the fibrotic process that joins them. Ventricular filling continues throughout diastole.

Two-dimensional echocardiography permits direct measurement of the mitral valve orifice. The valve is imaged in cross-section during diastole, the orifice planimetered, and the valve area calculated. Agreement with the actual orifice area determined at the time of cardiac surgery has been excellent. Other associated echocardiographic findings that may be of interest to the cardiac surgeon include a determination of the mobility and degree of calcification of the valve (to aid in the decision of commissurotomy or valve replacement), and whether there is an associated left atrial thrombus.

DIFFERENTIAL DIAGNOSIS. Diminished compliance (increased stiffness) of the left ventricle, usually as a consequence of left ventricular hypertrophy, may result in prolongation of the period of rapid filling, and the M-mode echocardiographic appearance may superficially simulate that of mitral stenosis. In such a case of diminished compliance, the mitral leaflets continue to move independently, rather than concordantly as in mitral stenosis. The two-dimensional echocardiogram demonstrates a normal mitral valve orifice size. Other less common causes of pulmonary venous hypertension can usually be distinguished by echocardiography, including a

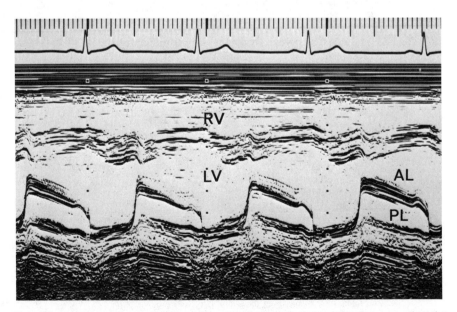

Figure 3 M-mode echocardiogram of a patient with mitral stenosis, demonstrating the thickening, shortening, and distortion of the leaflets. There is concordant anterior leaflet, AL, and posterior leaflet, PL, motion. LV, left ventricle; RV, right ventricle.

left atrial myxoma, supravalvular ring, cor triatriatum, and congenital mitral stenosis ("parachute" valve).

UTILITY OF ECHOCARDIOGRAPHY.   The noninvasive assessment of isolated mitral stenosis is so reliable that cardiac catheterization often is not required in the evaluation of these patients, and many patients may be sent directly to cardiac surgery for mitral valve commissurotomy or replacement on the basis of the two-dimensional echocardiographic and clinical findings alone. A normal echocardiographic study (M-mode or two-dimensional) *excludes* valvular mitral stenosis.

Mitral Regurgitation

FEATURES.   It is unusual to be able to directly identify mitral regurgitation on the echocardiogram. Only when gross disruption of the valve is found (as in rupture of chordae tendineae or papillary muscle) can one be certain of mitral regurgitation. In most other forms of mitral regurgitation, indirect signs must be employed to implicate mitral regurgitation, including an enlarged left ventricle (often with preserved systolic function); a dilated left atrium; and systolic left atrial expansion.

There has been increasing interest recently in using Doppler echocardiography to identify the presence and potentially the severity of regurgitant lesions such as mitral regurgitation. Doppler echocardiography analyzes the frequency shift which results when ultrasound strikes moving red blood cells; by determining the intracardiac location of this Doppler shift, it is possible to evaluate the presence of valvular regurgitation. Although not yet part of routine clinical practice, future developments are anticipated, particularly in further characterizing the significance of different patterns of Doppler signals.

Mitral valve prolapse may or may not be associated with mitral regurgitation. The absence of a reliable "gold standard" has hindered the identification of firm echocardiographic criteria for the diagnosis of prolapse, and even with two-dimensional echocardiography (which optimally should be obtained in conjunction with M-mode echocardiography), equivocal cases occur. Echocardiography may be useful in identifying prolapse of the tricuspid or aortic valves, since some patients have multiple valve involvement. (This syndrome has been called the "multiple floppy valve syndrome.")

DIFFERENTIAL DIAGNOSIS.   Mitral regurgitation may result from either structural deformity of the valve and/or its supporting apparatus, or from functional abnormalities of the valve apparatus and papillary muscles (grouped under the term *papillary muscle dysfunction*). The functional abnormalities typically are associated with normal appearing mitral valve leaflets, although LV wall motion abnormalities can often be identified. Pathologic deformity of the valve itself may be due to a variety of causes, the principal ones being rheumatic disease, rupture of chordae tendineae, infective endocarditis, obstructive hypertrophic cardiomyopathy, calcified mitral anulus, and mitral valve prolapse. Thickening of the valve is found in rheumatic disease, while calcification of the anulus presents a distinctive echocardiographic appearance, with a shelf of calcium behind the posterior mitral valve leaflet (Fig. 4). In ruptured chordae tendineae, hypermobile and flail components can be identified. In mitral valve prolapse, one or both leaflets bow posteriorly and cephalad into the left atrium, often commensing in midsystole, but sometimes occurring throughout systole (Fig. 5).

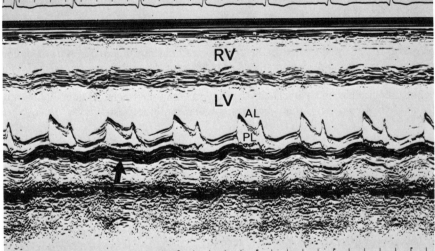

Figure 4 M-mode echocardiogram in a patient with severe calcification of the mitral anulus (arrow). The posterior leaflet, PL, of the mitral valve moves independently from the anulus. AL, anterior mitral valve leaflet; LV, left ventricle; RV, right ventricle.

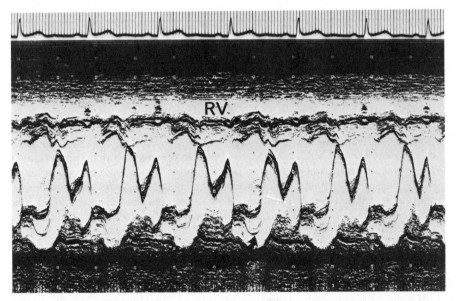

Figure 5 M-mode echocardiogram in a patient with marked mitral valve prolapse. Note the striking mid- and late systolic posterior motion of the mitral valve (arrow). RV, right ventricle.

UTILITY OF ECHOCARDIOGRAPHY.   The major use of echocardiography is in identifying the presence or absence of *structural* abnormalities of the mitral valve. It is less useful in assessing the *severity* of the resultant regurgitation; cardiac catheterization is often required for this purpose. The magnitude of enlargement of the left atrium and especially the left ventricle is, however, a general guide to the severity of regurgitation. Since the development of left ventricular dysfunction is a dreaded outcome in this condition, echocardiography is often used to monitor left ventricular function over time. Screening for mitral valve prolapse is one of the major reasons echocardiograms in general are ordered; however, careful cardiac auscultation by an experienced physician is probably as reliable as echocardiography for the diagnosis of *clinically significant* mitral valve prolapse. It has been suggested that mitral valve prolapse occurs more frequently than usual in young patients with focal cerebral ischemic events, and that the two may be etiologically related; it probably is reasonable to obtain echocardiograms in this group of patients, although the best management strategy for these patients remains unclear.

Aortic Valve

The aortic valve cusps, only two of which (the right and noncoronary) are imaged with the M-mode technique, are normally thin, symmetrical, and mobile. In diastole, they meet in the center of the aorta, and during systole they open until they are adjacent to the aortic wall (Figs. 2 and 6).

Aortic Stenosis

FEATURES.   In younger adults, a bicuspid aortic valve may not be thickened or calcified, while these changes are the rule in older patients with bicuspid or acquired

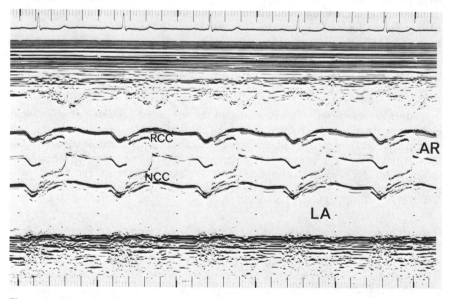

Figure 6   M-mode echocardiogram of a normal aortic valve. Note the movement of the right coronary cusp, RCC, and noncoronary cusp, NCC. AR, aortic root; LA, left atrium.

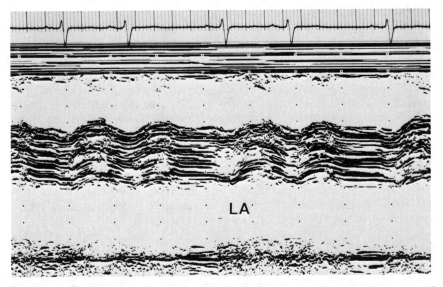

Figure 7 M-mode echocardiogram in calcific aortic stenosis. No cuspal movement is appreciated in this particular imaging plane. LA, left atrium.

aortic stenosis (Fig. 7). Identification by M-mode echocardiography of an uncalcified bicuspid stenotic valve may be difficult if the narrowed orifice at the free edge of the valve is not demonstrated; the pliable valve domes into the aorta, and the movement of the valve may be misinterpreted as separation of the cusps. The two-dimensional echocardiogram is usually able to demonstrate such doming of the valve when present (Fig. 8). Since bicuspid valves are usually asymmetric with one larger and one smaller cusp, the closure of the valve may be eccentrically located within the aortic root. However, this is not a foolproof echocardiographic sign for identifying a bicuspid aortic valve and provides no information as to the severity of stenosis.

DIFFERENTIAL DIAGNOSIS. Determination of the site of left ventricular outflow tract obstruction usually is determined easily by echocardiography, particularly the two-dimensional technique. Subvalvular stenosis may be either fixed or dynamic. The fixed variety may be caused by a fibrous or muscular membrane or channel, while the dynamic is caused by systolic anterior movement (SAM) of the mitral valve toward the septum. Two-dimensional echocardiography permits the determination of the extent, location, and type of supravalvular stenosis.

UTILITY OF ECHOCARDIOGRAPHY. The demonstration of normal cuspal appearance and motion on two-dimensional echocardiography essentially excludes valvular aortic stenosis. The technique is also highly reliable in identifying the *site* of outflow obstruction (subvalvular, valvular, supravalvular). While two-dimensional echocardiography can identify patients with severe aortic stenosis based on markedly reduced cuspal excursion, it has not been very useful in determining the severity of obstruction. In aortic stenosis, in contrast to mitral stenosis, the planimetered aortic valve area correlates poorly with catheterization findings, as does the degree of cuspal separation. The echocardiogram tends to overestimate the severity of stenosis, particularly in patients with left ventricular dysfunction. While adult patients without stenosis can be reliably distinguished from those with severe stenosis, the separation of patients with moderate from severe stenosis is more equivocal.

Aortic Regurgitation

FEATURES. Mitral regurgitation cannot be positively identified by any specific echocardiographic feature. In contrast, the presence of aortic regurgitation is confirmed in three-quarters or more of patients by high frequency diastolic vibration of the anterior leaflet of the mitral valve or interventricular septum (Fig. 9). This sign bears no relationship, however, to the severity of aortic regurgitation. As in mitral regurgitation, the extent of left ventricular enlargement is a rough guide to the severity of isolated aortic regurgitation. Once again, as in mitral regurgitation, Doppler echocardiography may provide additional information regarding the presence of regurgitation.

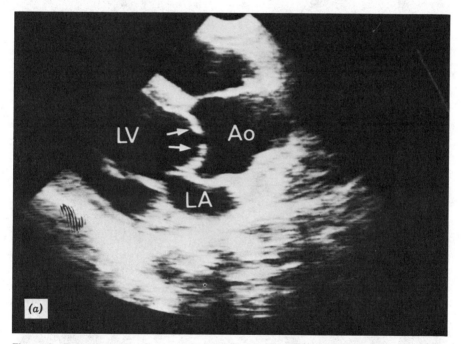

Figure 8 Two-dimensional echocardiographic studies of a bicuspid aortic valve. (a) Recorded during systole with the transducer in the long-axis parasternal position; demonstrates leaflet doming and thickening (arrows). The ascending aortic root is mildly dilated. Panels b and c were recorded using a short-axis parasternal transducer position. (b) During diastole, the leaflet, L, closure line is seen to be somewhat eccentric. (c) During systole, there is compromise of valve leaflet opening with a stenotic orifice, O. Ao, aorta; LA, left atrium; LV, left ventricle. (Used with permission from Borow KM. Congenital aortic stenosis in the adult. *J Cardiovasc Med*, in press, 1983.)

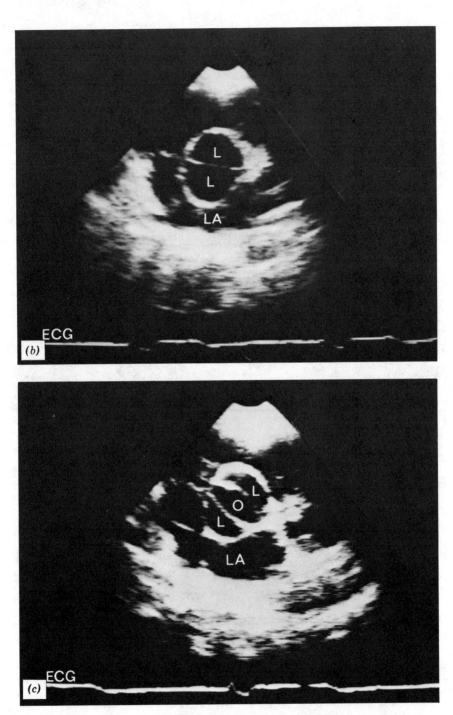

Figure 8 (Continued)

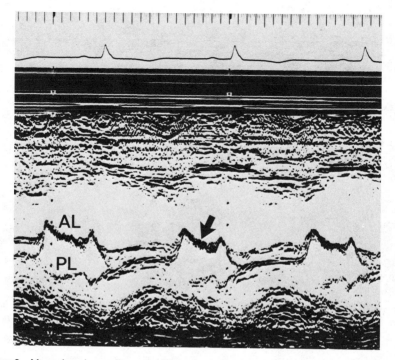

Figure 9 M-mode echocardiogram of the mitral valve in a patient with aortic regurgitation. High-frequency diastolic vibration (arrow) of the anterior leaflet, AL, of the mitral valve is found. PL, posterior leaflet.

DIFFERENTIAL DIAGNOSIS. The echocardiogram usually is able to distinguish between the two principal causes of aortic regurgitation: disease of the aortic cusps (typically due to rheumatic or calcific disease or to infective endocarditis); and enlargement of the aortic root (due to hypertension, aortic aneurysm, or anuloaortic ectasia) without direct involvement of the cusps themselves (Fig. 10). Acute severe aortic regurgitation as a consequence of endocarditis may result in early closure of the mitral valve as a result of the marked elevation of the left ventricular diastolic pressure; such patients are often in severe congestive heart failure and usually require immediate aortic valve replacement.

UTILITY OF ECHOCARDIOGRAPHY. The echocardiogram is quite reliable in distinguishing among the various causes of aortic regurgitation. It is less useful in estimating the *severity* of regurgitation, although, as in mitral regurgitation, the degree of left ventricular enlargement is a general guide. It has been suggested that asymptomatic patients with aortic regurgitation undergo serial echocardiographic evaluation, and those developing evidence of left ventricular dysfunction (manifested by an end-systolic dimension of >55 mm) be considered for valve replacement. The echocardiographic appearance of acute severe aortic regurgitation with an aortic vegetation due to endocarditis resulting in early closure of the mitral valve is sufficiently di-

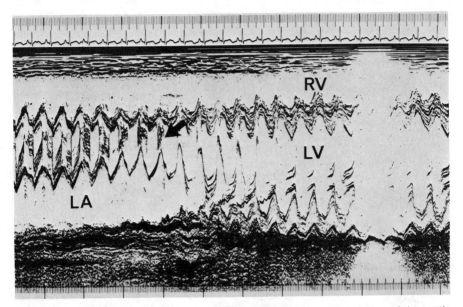

Figure 10   M-mode echocardiogram from a patient with a large vegetation of the aortic valve. A portion of this bulky, shaggy vegetation prolapses into the left ventricular outflow tract (arrow). LA, left atrium; LV, left ventricle; RV, right ventricle.

agnostic that aortic valve replacement can usually be undertaken without cardiac catheterization.

Tricuspid Valve

The normal tricuspid valve is similar in echocardiographic appearance to the mitral valve, although it is more anteriorly situated. The M-mode technique usually results in only partial imaging of the valve, and it is best seen in systole. Two-dimensional echocardiography affords a more complete evaluation of the valve, and is the preferred method of examining the valve.

Tricuspid Valve Disease

FEATURES.   Tricuspid stenosis, typically due to rheumatic valve disease, presents a similar echocardiographic appearance to rheumatic mitral stenosis, although the abnormalities are less severe. Tricuspid regurgitation is suggested by the presence of right ventricular and right atrial enlargement and by abnormal systolic movement of the interventricular septum as a consequence of the volume overload on the right ventricle. The presence of tricuspid regurgitation may be demonstrated by the abnormal movement of contrast material visible on echocardiography. Following the intravenous injection of saline (and other materials), a dense cloud of echoes normally appears in the right heart chambers. Reflux of these signals into the inferior vena cava and hepatic veins during systole is indicative of tricuspid regurgitation (Fig. 11).

DIFFERENTIAL DIAGNOSIS. There are three important causes of structural tricuspid valve disease: rheumatic tricuspid stenosis; involvement by vegetative endocarditis (typically in drug addicts or patients with central intravenous catheters); and Ebstein's anomaly of the tricuspid valve. Thickening of the valve with rheumatic involvement is similar to that seen with rheumatic mitral stenosis. A vegetation presents a distinctive appearance as a shaggy mass attached to the valve. Ebstein's anomaly is best appreciated on two-dimensional echocardiography, where the tricuspid valve is situated more apically in the right ventricle than usual.

The most common cause of tricuspid regurgitation, however, is right heart dilatation and failure, often due to mitral or pulmonary disease; the tricuspid valve is normal in appearance.

UTILITY OF ECHOCARDIOGRAPHY. The use of contrast or Doppler echocardiography is the most reliable method available for diagnosing tricuspid regurgitation. Echocardiography is also quite reliable in identifying the presence of tricuspid stenosis, and it provides an approximate qualitative estimation of its severity. However, the lack of a precise quantitative estimate of stenosis is usually not an important limitation, since rheumatic tricuspid stenosis virtually never occurs in the absence of rheumatic mitral stenosis. Thus, echocardiographic demonstration of tricuspid stenosis demands exploration of the tricuspid valve at the time of mitral valve surgery.

Pulmonary Valve

The pulmonary valve is the most difficult of all the cardiac valves to image and the least likely to be structurally abnormal in an adult patient. If the valve could be seen

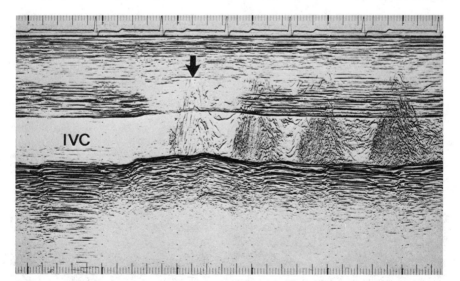

Figure 11 M-mode echogram of the inferior vena cava, IVC, in a patient with severe tricuspid regurgitation. Following the injection of saline into an arm vein, there is the appearance of the echo signal in the IVC (arrow) during each ventricular systole, indicative of tricuspid regurgitation. Notice also the systolic expansion of the IVC.

in its entirety, its appearance would resemble that of the aortic valve. However, imaging is usually limited to the cuspal closure line in diastole and the movement of the posterior cusp in early systole (Fig. 12).

Pulmonary Valve Disease

FEATURES AND DIFFERENTIAL DIAGNOSIS.   Structural abnormalities of the pulmonary valve are unusual, except for mild thickening with congenital pulmonic stenosis. They may rarely occur from a vegetation involving the cusps or with the carcinoid syndrome. Abnormalities of motion of the valve are more common. Doming of the valve on the two-dimensional study (or an abnormally prominent movement of the valve on M-mode echocardiography as a consequence of forceful right atrial contraction) indicates the presence of congenital pulmonic stenosis. Enhanced imaging of the valve, with systolic fluttering of the valve cusps, and ablation of the movement of the valve after right atrial systole often indicate pulmonary hypertension.

UTILITY OF ECHOCARDIOGRAPHY.   While the echocardiogram can determine the presence and location of right ventricular outflow tract obstruction, the echocardiographic estimation of the severity of valvular pulmonic stenosis is only a rough semiquantitative guide, and cardiac catheterization is often required in the adult patient for the physician to be confident of the degree of obstruction. Significant valvular pulmonic stenosis probably is excluded by a normal two-dimensional study of adequate technical quality. While the echocardiogram may suggest the presence

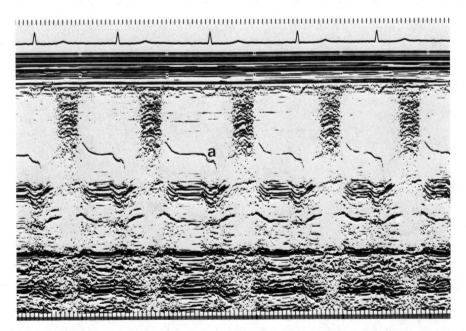

Figure 12   M-mode echocardiogram of a normal pulmonary valve. Atrial systole, a, partially opens the valve before the vigorous posterior movement of the cusp as a consequence of ventricular systole.

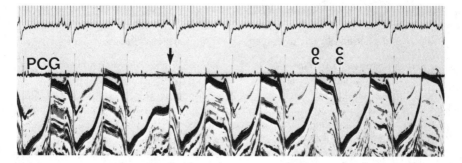

Figure 13 M-mode echocardiogram of a mechanical mitral prosthesis, which sticks in the closed position on one cycle (arrow), opening only after the subsequent atrial systole. OC, opening click; CC, closing click; PCG, phonocardiogram.

of pulmonary hypertension, the echocardiographic prediction of pulmonary artery pressure is only approximate.

Prosthetic Valves

Two principal forms of prosthetic valves are used: an entirely mechnical one, with a rigid ball or disc occluder; and a bioprosthetic type, with a rigid or semirigid prosthetic base and cusps composed of human or animal tissue (most commonly the cusps from the aortic valve of a pig). Because of the large difference in density between the mechanical occluder and human tissue, the occluder typically is easy to image. Consequently, the function of the mechanical valve is easy to evaluate echocardiographically, particularly in view of the precise timing of cardiac events possible with M-mode echocardiography. Movement of the occluder within its cage or supporting base is easily evaluated. Conversely, it may be difficult, on occasion, to image adequately the normally thin cusps of a bioprosthesis—although, when visualized, the cusps move in a pattern quite similar to that of native valves.

Prosthetic Dysfunction

FEATURES AND DIFFERENTIAL DIAGNOSIS. Stenosis and/or regurgitation may be seen with each type of valve. Partial dehiscence of the sewing ring of either type of valve from its anulus leads to *paraprosthetic* regurgitation. There are typically no specific echocardiographic findings to indicate this abnormality, aside from the secondary changes that may occur (such as ventricular enlargement). If the valve prosthesis is sufficiently detached, abnormal rocking of the valve may be demonstrable echocardiographically.

Dysfunction of a mechanical prosthesis may be caused by thrombosis, or ingrowth of fibrous tissue onto the valve. If motion of the occluder is disturbed as a result, echocardiography is often able to show such an abnormality of motion (Fig. 13). It is typically more difficult to identify the thrombus or fibrous tissue itself.

Acquired bioprosthetic dysfunction is usually heralded by thickening and, at times, calcification of the cusps. Diminished or abnormal motion of the leaflets may be identified when stenosis is present. Spontaneous tearing of a leaflet (or dysfunction as a consequence of endocarditis) usually results in a dramatic and virtually diagnostic echocardiographic appearance, with the flail portion of the valve vibrating violently and chaotically in the associated regurgitant jet of blood.

UTILITY OF ECHOCARDIOGRAPHY.   When the echocardiogram demonstrates major prosthetic dysfunction (such as sticking of the occluder or disruption of a bioprosthetic leaflet), further evaluation (including cardiac catheterization) is not required. Conversely, the failure to identify an abnormality may be misleading, and substantial prosthetic dysfunction may occur on occasion despite the lack of diagnostic echocardiographic abnormalities. An echocardiographic evaluation should be routine in cases of suspected prosthetic valve dysfunction, although simply fluoroscoping a mechanical valve may reveal definitive evidence of dysfunction in some cases. The echocardiogram is often critical in identifying other causes of symptoms in patients with suspected prosthetic valve dysfunction, including unappreciated left ventricular dysfunction, progression of disease in other native valves, and postoperative pericardial effusion or constriction.

AORTA

The proximal few centimeters of the ascending aorta above the aortic valve can usually be imaged echocardiographically; by placing the transducer in other locations, portions of the aortic arch and descending aorta often can be visualized.

Aortic Aneurysm
FEATURES.   Enlargement of a *visualized* portion of the aorta can be determined by echocardiography; assessment of the size of a dilated aorta has shown excellent agreement with catheterization findings. It is possible to image the false lumen of a dissecting aortic aneurysm as an extra channel located adjacent to the true lumen. Portions of the intimal flap itself may be identified in some patients with dissections.

DIFFERENTIAL DIAGNOSIS.   Because tangential imaging with the M-mode method may simulate a dissection when none is present, two-dimensional echocardiography with its wide field of view is required for optimal evaluation of the aorta.

UTILITY OF ECHOCARDIOGRAPHY.   Since failure to demonstrate an aneurysm of the aorta echocardiographically may be due to failure to image the involved segment, an aneurysm, particularly a localized one, cannot be excluded by echocardiography. Conversely, demonstration of aortic root enlargement by echocardiography is quite accurate. In patients with echocardiographically demonstrated aortic aneurysms, the distinction between a saccular aneurysm and a dissection may be difficult. The extent of the aneurysm may be difficult to determine if technical considerations limit imaging portals. Thus, most patients with suspected aortic aneurysms who require more definitive evaluation will need to undergo computed tomography and/or aortography.

INTRACARDIAC MASSES

The most noninvasive, safe, and reliable method of directly identifying intracavitary cardiac tumors, valvular vegetations, and atrial and ventricular thrombi is through the use of echocardiography, particularly two-dimensional.

Tumors

FEATURES.   The most common intracavitary cardiac tumor by far is the myxoma, which typically is found in the left atrium, but occasionally is seen in the right atrium and rarely in other locations. It may grow quite large and virtually fill the left atrium. The myxoma appears as a mass, often somewhat heterogeneous in appearance, that usually is pedunculated and attaches to the interatrial septum in the region of the septum primum (fossa ovalis) (Fig. 14). Frondlike protuberances from the mass are common.

DIFFERENTIAL DIAGNOSIS.   Other tumors beside myxomas may be found within a cardiac chamber; hypernephromas may extend up the inferior vena cava and fill the right atrium in a manner reminiscent of a myxoma. Left atrial thrombi may also simulate a myxoma; they are seen in patients with rheumatic mitral valve disease, and may be pedunculated. Very large myxomas rarely may be missed entirely by M-mode echocardiography, and a two-dimensional study always should be obtained, particularly in equivocal cases.

UTILITY OF ECHOCARDIOGRAPHY.   The echocardiographic identification of a suspected left atrial myxoma is almost always definitive; the next step is removal of the tumor at cardiac surgery. Cardiac catheterization is rarely necessary and, in fact, is probably contraindicated in most patients, for fear of dislodging a portion of the tumor with resultant embolization. While the symptoms of a myxoma may be quite protean (fever, malaise, etc.), an echocardiogram ordinarily should not be ordered unless there are specific factors suggesting a myxoma (diastolic murmur, embolization, etc.), or unless more common clinical entities have been excluded.

Vegetations

FEATURES.   Vegetations are identified echocardiographically on the basis of morphologic as well as functional features. They appear as masses associated with the

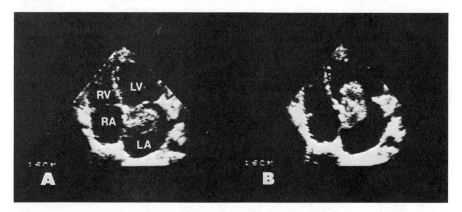

Figure 14 Apical four-chamber, two-dimensional echocardiogram in a patient with a large left atrial myxoma attached to the interatrial septum. (a) Systole. (b) Diastole, during which the myxoma prolapses through the mitral orifice into the left ventricle. LA, left atrium; LV, left ventricle; RA, right atrium; RV, right ventricle.

valve leaflets and are typically hypermobile (Fig. 10). M-mode echocardiography often shows them to vibrate violently as a consequence of the attendant valve destruction and regurgitation.

DIFFERENTIAL DIAGNOSIS. It may not be possible to differentiate a vegetation from an avulsed or disrupted portion of valve leaflet that is hypermobile. Except for rupture of mitral chordae tendineae, however, most disrupted valves result from endocarditis. The redundant and thickened valve seen in the mitral valve prolapse syndrome without endocarditis may simulate involvement by a vegetation; one should be cautious about diagnosing a vegetation in this setting unless there are unequivocal findings, or a *change* in the echocardiographic appearance is noted.

UTILITY OF ECHOCARDIOGRAPHY. Roughly half the patients with endocarditis have echocardiographically demonstrable vegetations. Patients with vegetations form a high risk group, and often require valve replacement; they are at risk of complications and death. Conversely, patients without visible vegetations infrequently develop complications, require surgery, or die. One should not, however, use the mere presence of a vegetation to decide about surgery; the usual clinical criteria (congestive heart failure, embolization, uncontrolled sepsis) remain operant. Vegetations may persist despite apparent bacteriologic cure, and the size or appearance of the vegetation does not appear to provide specific prognostic information.

Thrombi

FEATURES AND DIFFERENTIAL DIAGNOSIS. Thrombi may be encountered within all four cardiac chambers, as well as within the pulmonary artery; they are most commonly seen in the left ventricle. Left ventricular thrombi usually are located at the cardiac apex, and usually are seen following a myocardial infarction. Thrombi are found overlying dyskinetic or "paradoxically" moving left ventricular segments; a left ventricular thrombus is not found when normal wall motion is present in all left ventricular regions. Left atrial thrombi are seen on occasion but usually only when mitral stenosis is present; even then, a visualized thrombus is unusual.

UTILITY OF ECHOCARDIOGRAPHY. Although it is a frequently cited reason for ordering echocardiograms, the attempt to identify an intracardiac thrombus ultrasonically is often not worth the effort. Patients with manifestly normal left ventricular function and without mitral stenosis are at exceedingly low risk of harboring a thrombus in the heart. Similarly, even identifying a group of patients with visible ventricular thrombi after a myocardial infarction does not appear to identify patients at particularly high risk of embolization. While future developments may require modification of these principles, we employ anticoagulants when indicated by clinical imperatives, rather than based on echocardiographic findings.

LEFT VENTRICLE

Left ventricular (LV) cavity size, contour, orientation, and thickness are easily obtained with echocardiography. A variety of indices of function may be calculated with M-mode echocardiography, including the ejection fraction, mean velocity of circumferential fiber shortening (Vcf), and percent fractional shortening (%ΔD). Because the M-mode echocardiogram images a limited portion of the ventricle, assessment of left ventricular performance with this technique requires that function be uniform throughout the ventricle. When there are regional variations in left ventricular function (occurring most commonly in coronary artery disease), the two-dimensional technique is required to obtain an estimate of overall function; an M-mode study done through the best functioning portion of the ventricle may be completely misleading as to global function. Because the two-dimensional echocardiogram obtains a tomographic image of the ventricle, it is necessary to obtain at least two orthogonal views so that the proper three-dimensional contour of the ventricle can be estimated.

A major use of echocardiography is in evaluating a patient with an enlarged cardiac silhouette on chest roentgenography; the principal issue is whether the cardiac chambers are dilated, or if there is a pericardial effusion. Echocardiography is unparalleled in this role. When the heart itself is enlarged, the left ventricle is commonly the most dilated chamber (although patients with mitral stenosis or an atrial septal defect may present with a dramatically increased cardiac silhouette due to right ventricular enlargement, despite a small left ventricle).

Left Ventricular Enlargement

Left ventricular enlargement is usually due to one of three principal causes: volume overload (due to aortic or mitral regurgitation); coronary artery disease with myocardial infarction; or primary myocardial disease (dilated or congestive cardiomyopathy). Volume overload is characterized by an enlarged ventricle with preserved or increased systolic function; the stroke volume is thus increased. Evidence of valvular disease may be found. This distinctive pattern may become less clear once left ventricular dysfunction supervenes, and the pattern then approximates that of dilated cardiomyopathy, characterized by a dilated, hypokinetic ventricle.

The unique feature of LV dysfunction due to coronary artery disease and myocardial infarction is its focal and regional nature, although an end-stage patient with multiple myocardial infarctions may have diffuse abnormalities of wall motion that are indistinguishable from a cardiomyopathy or volume overload with dysfunction.

Coronary Artery Disease

It has been long known that a severe reduction in coronary perfusion results in cessation of systolic motion of the resultant ischemic myocardium. However, most patients with coronary artery disease have near-normal coronary blood flow at rest, and these patients demonstrate normal left ventricular wall motion. With stress, such as exercise, the limited coronary reserve cannot keep pace with the increased demand for nutrients and ischemia results. Variable success has been reported with imaging patients with two-dimensional echocardiography during and after exercise, largely because of the difficulty in maintaining an adequate imaging portal. When imaging is successful, however, the development of a regional wall motion abnormality is strong evidence of ischemia.

Most studies are performed at rest, however, commonly after a myocardial infarction. Some success has been reported in quantitating wall motion in different left ventricular regions, and formulas have been devised for estimating global left ventricular function. While the accuracy of such quantitative evaluations has not been completely accepted (and most studies are performed at academic centers) there is no question that left ventricular function can be categorized adequately by visual assessment into clinically useful groups (e.g., poor, fair, good). Patients in whom severe left ventricular dysfunction is demonstrated echocardiographically probably can be spared further invasive evaluation.

Two-dimensional echocardiography is also quite useful in evaluating the complications of myocardial infarction, both acute and chronic. Acute complications that can be imaged include ventricular septal rupture, papillary muscle rupture, and pericardial effusion. Chronic complications that can be evaluated include identification and differentiation of true and false left ventricular aneurysms, papillary muscle dysfunction, and left ventricular thrombi.

Cardiomyopathy

It is often useful to divide the cardiomyopathies into groups with similar echocardiographic, hemodynamic, and clinical findings, rather than grouping them etiologically. Echocardiography permits definitive evaluation of some of these cases, although the precise causal factor rarely is apparent from the echocardiogram.

The three principal functional groups are *dilated* (formerly called congestive), *restrictive*, and *hypertrophic* (Table 2). The primary feature of the dilated form is left ventricular dilatation and dysfunction; of the restrictive type, increased wall stiffness producing elevated filling pressures; and of the hypertrophic form, inappropriate myocardial hypertrophy. The distinctions are not absolute, and a given disease may have features of two of the functional groups.

DILATED CARDIOMYOPATHY. Although caused by a variety of toxic substances (alcohol, drugs such as Adriamycin, etc.), this cardiomyopathy is most frequently of unknown cause. Although four-chamber cardiac enlargement is the rule, the left ventricle typically is most involved, demonstrating enlargement and hypokinesis. The asynergy commonly is diffuse and involves all left ventricular segments, distinguishing dilated cardiomyopathy in many cases from coronary artery disease. However, end-stage left ventricular damage due to multiple infarctions also may appear

Table 2. Echocardiographic Features of the Cardiomyopathies

	Dilated	Restrictive	Hypertrophic
LV size	↑	N	N or ↓
LV systolic function	↓	N (or ↓)	N or ↑
LV wall thickness	N	↑	↑
Other features		PE	ASH
			SAM

ASH, asymmetric septal hypertrophy; LV, left ventricular; N, normal; PE, pericardial effusion; SAM, systolic anterior motion of the mitral valve; ↑, increased; ↓, decreased.

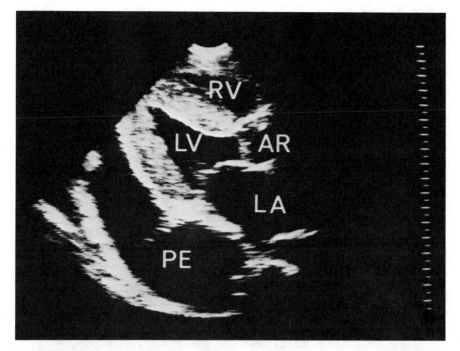

Figure 15   Long-axis parasternal two-dimensional echocardiogram in a patient with cardiac amyloidosis. Note the marked increase in thickness of the left ventricular (LV) walls, and the unusually echo-dense appearance. There is also a large pleural effusion, PE.

diffusely hypokinetic. Wall thickness is typically normal, and left ventricular thrombi may be found. No intrinsic valvular pathology is seen.

RESTRICTIVE CARDIOMYOPATHY.   Grouped in this category are primary restrictive processes and secondary diseases, most frequently infiltrative diseases of the myocardium (e.g., amyloid, sarcoid, iron overload, etc.). The typical echocardiographic feature is a normal-sized left ventricle with increased wall thickness. While the rigorous classification of the restrictive cardiomyopathies excludes secondary types (i.e., infiltrative diseases), these, in fact, are the most commonly encountered form of restrictive disease. Although systolic function is normal in idiopathic restrictive cardiomyopathy, it often is depressed in the infiltrative diseases. One striking feature of these diseases (particularly with amyloid involvement of the myocardium) is an unusual sparkling, echo-dense appearance (Fig. 15).

HYPERTROPHIC CARDIOMYOPATHY.   The characteristic feature in this category is inappropriate left ventricular hypertrophy. In 95% of cases, there is asymetric involvement of the septum (asymmetric septal hypertrophy, ASH), with the septum 1.3 to 1.5 or more times the thickness of the posterior wall (Fig. 16). The septum can reach dramatic widths; we have seen patients whose septa were 25 mm or more thick (normal 11 mm or less). In rare patients, other left ventricular locations are preferentially involved, including the anterolateral wall and apex. In about 5% of cases, symmetric hypertrophy is noted. Wall motion typically is normal or increased, and the left ventricular cavity size is small.

When dynamic obstruction is present, systolic anterior motion (SAM) of the anterior leaflet of the mitral valve is found (Fig. 16). The subaortic pressure gradient produces turbulent blood flow, which causes the aortic valve to vibrate violently. The severity of SAM and aortic valve fluttering bear a good relationship to the degree of outflow gradient. The M-mode technique on occasion may suggest ASH when the septum is imaged tangentially, but the two-dimensional technique usually removes any doubt. Since the magnitude of the pressure gradient is of little clinical importance except when surgery is being considered, we do not ordinarily perform catheterization, unless there are other unanswered questions (such as whether coronary artery disease is contributing to the patient's symptoms).

PERICARDIUM

The posterior pericardium generates a strong echocardiographic signal and usuallly is easily identified. A minimal separation may normally be found between the epi-

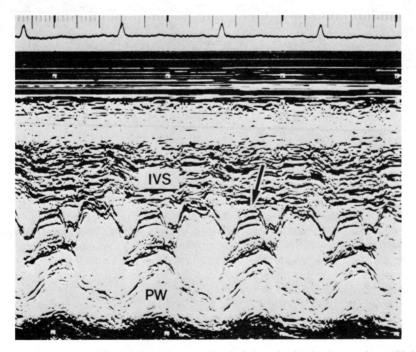

Figure 16 M-mode echocardiogram at the level of the mitral valve in a patient with hypertrophic cardiomyopathy. Asymmetric hypertrophy of the interventricular septum (IVS) is present. The arrow indicates systolic anterior motion of the mitral valve. PW, posterior wall. (Used with permission from Wynne J. Hypertrophic cardiomyopathy: A Broadened concept of the disease and its management, in Isselbacher KJ, Adams RD, Braunwald E, Martin JB, Petersdorf RG, Wilson JD, eds: *Update III: Harrison's Principles of Internal Medicine*, New York, McGraw Hill, 1982, p 129.)

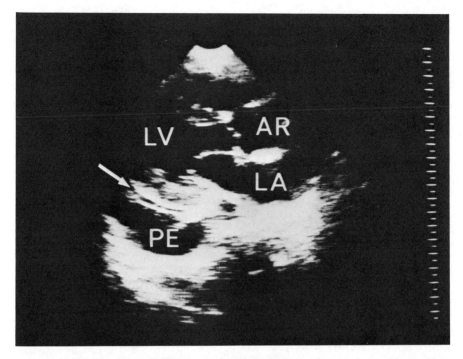

Figure 17   Long-axis parasternal two-dimensional echocardiogram in a patient with a large pleural effusion, PE. The arrow indicates minimal amount of pericardial fluid between the posterior left ventricular, LV, wall and the pericardium. AR, aortic root; LA, left atrium.

cardial and pericardial surfaces, and represents less than 15 ml of pericardial fluid (Fig. 17).

Pericardial Effusion

FEATURES.   More than a minimal separation of epicardium and pericardium identifies a pericardial effusion. Free-flowing fluid will move to dependent locations within the pericardial space, so the apparent size of an effusion is dependent upon the position of the patient during imaging. Precise estimation of the size of a pericardial effusion is probably both unnecessary and unreliable, but semiquantitative distinctions (trivial, small, medium, large) are clinically meaningful; these estimates are based on the degree of epicardial/pericardial separation. Both M-mode and two-dimensional techniques are quite useful for detecting and sizing effusions, although loculated effusions are best evaluated with the two-dimensional technique. Pericardial thickening is suggested by an unusually broad and prominent pericardial signal, and is often associated with concordant movement of the epicardium and pericardium, suggesting symphysis of these structures as a consequence of fibrosis.

In large pericardial effusions, fibrous strands and masses can be imaged within the pericardial fluid, as can tumor masses with neoplastic involvement of the pericardium.

DIFFERENTIAL DIAGNOSIS. There are numerous technical pitfalls in the evaluation of the pericardium, but strict adherance to proper techniques eliminates most spurious impressions. The differentiation of a left pleural effusion from a pericardial effusion may be difficult on occasion with the M-mode technique; two-dimensional echocardiography is almost always definitive in forming this distinction (Fig. 17).

While echocardiography is highly reliable in detecting pericardial effusions, it is less useful in establishing the hemodynamic burden caused by the fluid. Specific echocardiographic signs (such as gross cardiac oscillation, respirophasic variation in right and left ventricular chamber dimensions, and phasic changes in the mitral valve pattern of motion) may suggest pericardial tamponade, but this diagnosis usually rests more solidly on clinical and hemodynamic considerations than on ultrasonic findings.

UTILITY OF ECHOCARDIOGRAPHY. Echocardiography is the procedure of choice for detecting and obtaining a semiquantitative estimate of the size of pericardial effusions. Should pericardiocentesis be necessary, it is often advisable to perform this under two-dimensional echocardiographic guidance; the path of the needle can be imaged, and as a result the incidence of cardiac puncture is reduced. The diagnosis of tamponade remains a clinical one, although its presence may be suggested by certain echocardiographic abnormalities.

CONGENITAL HEART DISEASE

The development of two-dimensional echocardiography had its earliest and perhaps its most profound influence in the evaluation of congenital cardiac anomalies. Because of its wide field of view, two-dimensional echocardiography permits the analysis of often complex spatial relationships and orientations. Atrial, ventricular, and great vessel anatomy, orientation, and connections can be evaluated with a high degree of accuracy and reliability. Cardiac catheterizations have become more stylized since the introduction of two-dimensional echocardiography, since now the anatomical features often are known prior to the catheterization and only specific questions (such as pressures, flows, and resistances) remain to be determined. In selected patients with certain lesions—such as secundum-type atrial septal defect (ASD) and coarctation of the aorta—catheterization is no longer a required or routine step prior to surgery and is performed only when there are unresolved issues following echocardiography.

Since a review of all the congenital cardiac anomalies is beyond the scope of this chapter, the discussion will be limited to the most common nonvalvular congenital defect found in the adult patient—the atrial septal defect.

Atrial Septal Defect

FEATURES. The most reliable echocardiographic feature of an ASD is right ventricular enlargement, a consequence of the increased blood flow through the right side of the heart. A normal-sized right ventricle essentially excludes a hemodynamically significant ASD. On the other hand, the degree of right ventricular enlargement is not a precise guide to the actual size of the left-to-right shunt. The inter-ventricular septum demonstrates normal thickening, but often moves "paradoxically" anteriorly during systole, in contrast to its normal posterior motion. This is the result of posterior displacement of the septum during diastole as a consequence of the right ventricular volume overload.

Direct visualization of the atrial septum is possible with two-dimensional echocardiography. Low-lying defects in the septum in the region of the atrioventricular valves are seen with a primum type ASD (endocardial cushion defect). Associated abnormalities of the atrioventricular valves and ventricular septum may also be seen. Secundum-type ASDs are found in the region of the fossa ovalis, which is so thin normally that it may not be visualized even in a patient without a defect, thus simulating an ASD. Orienting the echocardiographic beam more perpendicularly to the atrial septum (using subcostal portals) increases the reliability of direct visualization of the defect, but ordinarily, apparent holes in the atrial septum near the fossa ovalis should be diagnosed with caution because of the normal "drop-out" of echocardiographic signals in this region (Fig. 2c). Mitral valve prolapse is frequently seen with a secundum ASD.

Contrast echocardiography is often useful in evaluating suspected intracardiac shunts. Large left-to-right shunts at the atrial level frequently produce negative defects in the right atrium when blood from the left atrium without contrast mixes with the contrast-filled right atrial blood. Right-to-left shunting is easily detected by the appearance of contrast in the left side of the heart; this is not seen normally, since the contrast effect is defeated by the lungs. Since most ASDs have a trivial amount of right-to-left shunting, this may be detected by contrast echocardiography, and the diagnosis of an intracardiac shunt confirmed.

DIFFERENTIAL DIAGNOSIS.   Right ventricular volume overload (right ventricular enlargement and abnormal interventricular septal motion) may be found in a variety of conditions besides an ASD, including tricuspid and pulmonary regurgitation; the echocardiographic findings must be interpreted in the clinical setting. Contrast and Doppler echocardiography may be of benefit in equivocal cases.

Defects in the low-lying atrial septum (near the atrioventricular valves) always indicate an ASD. Conversely, one may find an apparent defect in the fossa ovalis normally, due to the thinness of the tissue.

UTILITY OF ECHOCARDIOGRAPHY.   The echocardiographic findings form an important junction in the process of managing a patient with a suspected ASD. A normal study without right ventricular enlargement essentially excludes a hemodynamically significant ASD. Further evaluation is rarely fruitful or indicated. Should there be unusual features that suggest an ASD despite a negative echocardiogram (including contrast echocardiography), a radionuclide angiocardiogram should be obtained. If no shunt is detected, an ASD of significance is excluded (although a "probe patent" foramen ovale is not).

The distinction between a primum and secundum ASD is usually an easy one to make. Associated defects are often apparent. Some patients with uncomplicated secundum ASDs may be sent directly to surgery without cardiac catheterization.

PULSE RECORDINGS

Joshua Wynne

By placing a transducer over the carotid artery, internal jugular vein, and cardiac apex impulse, a tracing may be obtained that displays in graphic form the pressure and volume fluxes of the underlying structures. Although the resultant external recordings are not direct measurements of intraluminal pressure, the morphology of the carotid, jugular, and apex pulse tracings closely mirrors the intracavitary pressure recordings obtained from within the aorta, right atrium, and left ventricle, respectively. In specific pathologic conditions, tracings may be obtained from other locations, such as recording the right ventricular impulse with pressure overload of the right ventricle, or the hepatic pulse with tricuspid regurgitation.

Carotid Pulse

The normal carotid pulse tracing is composed of a rapid upstroke (anacrotic limb) terminating in an initial peak or percussion wave (Fig. 18). The percussion wave is followed by a less prominent, somewhat more rounded tidal wave. The percussion wave appears to be related primarily to the peak aortic flow rate, while the tidal wave is related to peak aortic pressure. Thus, the tidal wave often becomes more prominent with systemic hypertension, following the infusion of a vasoconstrictor, and in elderly patients. The descending limb of the carotid pulse tracing, which normally is less steep than the ascending limb, is interrupted by the incisura or dicrotic notch. This notch is due to aortic valve closure. Although the morphology of the carotid pulse tracing resembles that of an intraaortic pressure recording, it is delayed by approximately 20–50 milliseconds, which is the time it takes the pulse wave to travel from the heart to the neck.

CAROTID PULSE ABNORMALITIES

Atherosclerosis of the carotid artery may produce abnormalities of the carotid pulse tracing; in the absence of local carotid disease, abnormalities of the pulse may be generally categorized as *hyperkinetic* (bounding) or *hypokinetic* (weak) (Table 3). In a variety of disease states, specific abnormalities of the carotid pulse often can be identified.

Aortic Stenosis

This condition typically shows a small hypokinetic pulse with a delayed systolic peak (Fig. 19). An anacrotic shoulder, occurring in the early to mid portion of the ascending limb of the carotid pulse tracing, reflects decreased aortic flow velocity

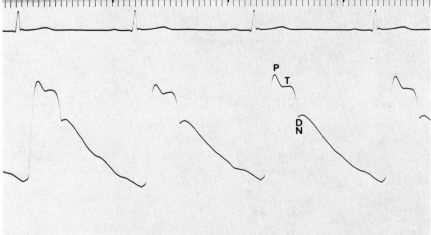

Figure 18 Normal carotid pulse tracing. The percussion wave, P, is more prominent than the subsequent tidal wave, T. DN, dicrotic notch.

secondary to obstruction to left ventricular emptying, as well as turbulent flow. A "shudder" is often noted, also a consequence of turbulent blood flow.

Obstructive Hypertrophic Cardiomyopathy

In contrast to the findings in fixed orifice left ventricular outflow obstruction, in the dynamic obstruction seen with hypertrophic cardiomyopathy, there is a hyperkinetic pulse of large amplitude with a rapid upstroke (Fig. 20). As left ventricular volume decreases during systole, the anterior leaflet of the mitral valve moves towards the septum and narrows the outflow tract. Consequently, there is a sudden decrease in the carotid pulse amplitude, reflecting a sudden fall in ejection rate. A secondary

Table 3. General Causes of Abnormalities of the Carotid Pulse Tracing

Hyperkinetic pulse
 Increased cardiac output states, such as anxiety, fever, exercise, pregnancy, and anemia
 Widened pulse pressure, as with aortic regurgitation, persistent ductus arteriosus, and
  Paget's disease of the bone
 Decreased arterial distensibility
Hypokinetic pulse
 Fixed left ventricular outflow tract obstruction, as with aortic stenosis and discrete
  subaortic stenosis
 Reduced forward stroke volume as with myocardial infarction, cardiomyopathy, and
  severe mitral regurgitation
 Narrow pulse pressure, as with cardiac tamponade, constrictive pericarditis

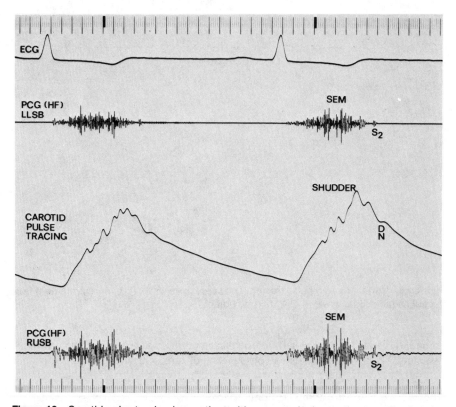

Figure 19 Carotid pulse tracing in a patient with severe valvular aortic stenosis, showing a low anacrotic shoulder and systolic shudder. The phonocardiogram, PCG, demonstrates a mid- to late-peaking systolic ejection murmur, SEM, with soft aortic component of the second heart sound, S_2. DN, dicrotic notch; HF, high frequency; LLSB, left lower sternal border; RUSB, right upper sternal border. (Used with permission from Borow KM, Wynne J. External pulse recordings, systolic time intervals, apexcardiography, and phonocardiography, in Cohn PF, Wynne J, eds: *Diagnostic methods in clinical cardiology.* Boston, Little Brown, 1982, p 144.)

wave is generated until the end of systole, resulting in the characteristic "spike and dome" pulse curve configuration.

Jugular Venous Pulse

The normal jugular venous pulse recording consists of two major peaks (a and v) and two major descents (x and y). (Fig. 21) The a wave is the result of the displacement of blood into the jugular vein by right atrial systole; it is the most prominent positive wave and is absent when effective atrial systole is lacking. Atrial relaxation is associated with the x descent, which continues to the x trough, the most negative wave of the normal jugular pulse recording. The x descent usually is interrupted by the c wave, a small wave resulting from closure of the tricuspid valve. Further accumulation of blood behind the still-closed tricuspid valve results in the v wave, due to passive filling of the right atrium. The y descent is generated by the opening tricuspid valve and flow of blood from the right atrium into the right ventricle.

JUGULAR VENOUS PULSE ABNORMALITIES

A prominent a wave is found when right atrial systole is unusually forceful as a consequence of an impediment to right atrial emptying. This is usually the result of increased stiffness (diminished compliance) of the right ventricle as a consequence of right ventricular hypertrophy of any etiology (chronic obstructive lung disease, mitral valve disease, pulmonary artery hypertension, pulmonic stenosis, etc.).

The x descent is reduced in atrial fibrillation, since atrial relaxation is absent. It is shallow or obliterated in tricuspid insufficiency, since there is active regurgitation of blood into the right atrium. A positive systolic wave (or c-v wave) replaces the x trough in severe tricuspid regurgitation. With severe tricuspid regurgitation, a similar systolic pulsation may often be recorded from over the liver (Fig. 22). In cardiac tamponade, a prominent x descent is noted. Conversely, the x descent is reduced

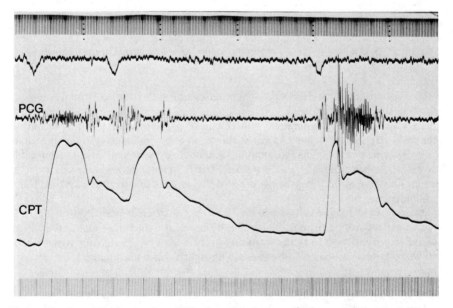

Figure 20 Carotid pulse tracing, CPT, phonocardiogram, PCG, recorded at the left lower sternal border, and electrocardiogram in a patient with provocable dynamic subaortic obstruction due to hypertrophic cardiomyopathy. Recordings made after an atrial premature beat demonstrate precipitation of a spike and dome configuration on CPT and accentuation of the systolic ejection murmur, indicating that dynamic obstruction was provoked. (Used with permission from Borow KM, Wynne J. External pulse recordings, sytolic time intervals, apexcardiography, and phonocardiography, in Cohn PF, Wynne J, eds: *Diagnostic methods in clinical cardiology*. Boston, Little Brown, 1982, p 148.)

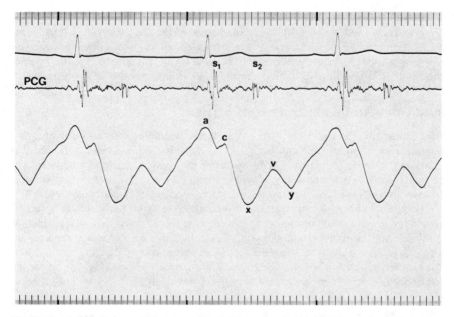

Figure 21   Jugular venous pulse recording from a normal subject. The a wave is the largest positive wave, while the x trough is the more prominent negative wave. The phonocardiogram, PCG, is a low-frequency recording at the lower left sternal border, showing first, S_1, and second, S_2, heart sounds.

with constrictive pericarditis; a prominent x descent in this setting strongly suggests effusoconstrictive disease.

The v wave is more prominent with enhanced passive refilling of the atrium, as seen in an atrial septal defect. As noted above, an early and large systolic regurgitant wave is seen in tricuspid regurgitation. Although by common usage, regurgitant waves have been referred to as v waves, strictly speaking, a v wave is solely the result of passive atrial filling, while the systolic wave is due to active systolic filling of the atrium.

The y descent is unusually rapid and brief in constrictive pericarditis, and ends with an early diastolic plateau. This reflects the small right ventricular end-diastolic volume and restriction to filling, resulting in the so-called square root sign. A deep and sharp y descent may also be found with right ventricular failure.

The Apexcardiogram

The movement of the heart against the chest wall throughout the cardiac cycle results in motion of the left precordial surface, which can be recorded on the apexcardiogram. This closely resembles the left ventricular pressure pulse in morphology (Fig. 23).

The rapid upstroke of the apexcardiogram begins with left ventricular isovolumic systole (c point). The upstroke terminates at the e point, which coincides with the onset of left ventricular ejection. During the second half of left ventricular systole, the curve usually undergoes a gentle decline. At approximately the time of aortic valve closure, the curve begins a sharp decline, correlating with the onset of the ventricular isovolumic relaxation period. This downward deflection terminates near the end of mitral valve opening (end of isovolumic relaxation period), an event that is variably approximated by the 0 point of the apexcardiogram. Vigorous ventricular filling in early diastole produces the rapid filling wave (RFW), which is followed by the less vigorous slow filling wave (SFW). The a wave is the final diastolic wave, and corresponds to the distension of the left ventricle as a consequence of left atrial contraction.

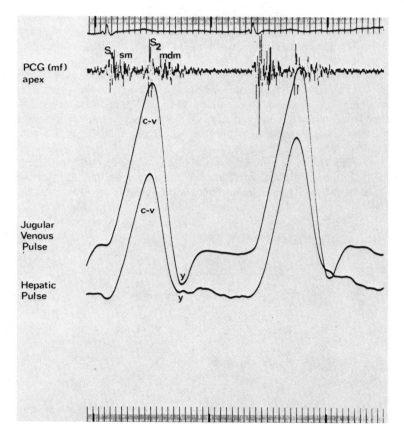

Figure 22 Jugular venous and hepatic pulse tracings in a patient with Ebstein's anomaly and tricuspid regurgitation. A giant c-v systolic wave is noted, with an abrupt y descent. The hepatic pulse recording is similar to the jugular pulse tracing. PCG, phonocardiogram; sm, systolic murmur; mf, midfrequency; mdm, middiastolic murmur. (Used with permission from Borow KM, Wynne J. External pulse recordings, sytolic time intervals, apexcardiography, and phonocardiography, in Cohn PF, Wynne J, eds: *Diagnostic methods in clinical cardiology.* Boston,, Little Brown, 1982, p 131.)

APEXCARDIOGRAPHIC ABNORMALITIES

The a wave is absent in patients with atrial fibrillation, and is increased (greater than 15% of the overall height of the apical pulse tracing) in cases of diminished left ventricular compliance (Fig. 24).

The systolic bulge of the apexcardiogram may be unusually forceful, although typically not sustained, in volume overload of a compensated left ventricle (increased stroke volume). This may be found in mitral or aortic regurgitation, anemia, anxiety, thyrotoxicosis, and so forth. A *sustained* apical impulse, on the other hand, is found with left ventricular pressure overload (aortic stenosis or systemic hypertension), and with left ventricular dysfunction (cardiomyopathy, left ventricular failure, left ventricular aneurysm) (Fig. 24).

An unusual double or bifid apical impulse may be seen with hypertrophic cardiomyopathy with obstruction. Since diminished left ventricular compliance is also often found, the a wave may be quite prominent as well, resulting in a characteristic triple apical impulse.

A prominent rapid filling wave is found in patients with augmented early diastolic filling, often as a result of left ventricular volume overload (mitral regurgitation being the most commonly encountered example). The rapid filling wave is reduced with diminished left ventricular compliance, since the increased stiffness of the ventricle limits its ability to expand in early diastole. The rapid filling wave is blunted and shortened in duration with mitral stenosis.

The apexcardiogram is particularly useful in clarifying the timing of auscultatory events. An ejection sound occurs in relationship to the e point. A mitral valve opening snap is found near the 0 point, while a third heart sound is found later, at the peak of the rapid filling wave. The fourth heart sound is found at the time of the a wave.

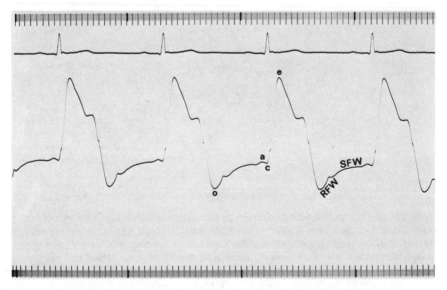
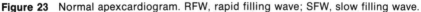

Figure 23 Normal apexcardiogram. RFW, rapid filling wave; SFW, slow filling wave.

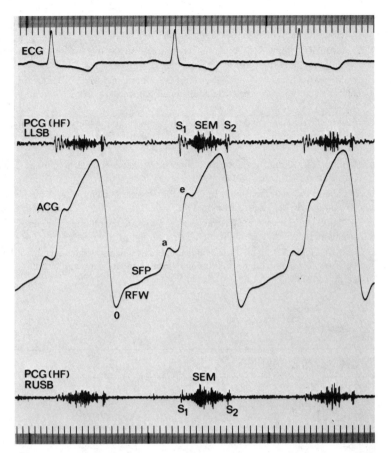

Figure 24 Apexcardiogram ACG, in a patient with severe valvular aortic stenosis. The systolic wave is sustained, with a continued rise throughout ventricular ejection. The a wave is exaggerated. HF, high frequency; LLSB, left lower sternal border; PCG, phonocardiogram; RFW, rapid filling wave; RUSB, right upper sternal border; SEM, systolic ejection murmur; SFP, slow filling phase. (Used with permission from Borow KM, Wynne J. External pulse recordings, systolic time intervals, apexcardiography, and phonocardiography, in Cohn PF, Wynne J, eds: *Diagnostic methods in clinical cardiology*. Boston, Little Brown, 1982, p 145.)

Bibliography for Sections 1 and 2

DeMaria AN, Bommer W, Joye J, et al: Value and limitations of cross-sectional echocardiography of the aortic valve in the diagnosis and quantification of valvular aortic stenosis. *Circulation* 62:304, 1980.

DeMaria AN, King JF, Salel AF, et al: Echography and phonography of acute aortic regurgitation in bacterial endocarditis. *Ann Intern Med* 82:329, 1975.

Falsetti HL, Marcus ML, Kerber RE, et al: Quantification of myocardial ischemia and infarction by left ventricular imaging (editorial). *Circulation* 63:747, 1981.

Fowles RE, Martin RP, Popp RL: Apparent asymmetric septal hypertrophy due to angled interventricular septum. *Am J Cardiol* 46:386, 1980.

Henry WL, DeMaria A, Gramiak R, et al: Report of the American Society of Echocardiography on nomenclature and standards in two-dimensional echocardiography. *Circulation* 62:212, 1980.

Martin RP, Rakowski H, Kleiman J, et al: Reliability and reproducibility of two dimensional echocardiographic measurement of the stenotic mitral valve orifice area. *Am J Cardiol* 43:560, 1979.

Motro M, Neufeld HN: Should patients with pure mitral stenosis undergo cardiac catheterization? (editorial) *Am J Cardiol* 46:515, 1980.

Risser TA, Wynne J: Echocardiography. In Conn PF, Wynne J (eds): *Diagnostic Methods in Clinical Cardiology*. Boston, Little Brown, 1982, p 83.

Steward JA, Silimperi D, Harris P, et al: Echocardiographic documentation of vegetative lesions in infective endocarditis: clinical implications. *Circulation* 61:374, 1980.

Tajik AJ, Seward J, Hagler DJ, et al: Two-dimensional real-time ultrasonic imaging of the heart and great vessels: Technique, image orientation, structure identification and validation. *Mayo Clin Proc* 53:271, 1978.

SECTION 3

SYSTOLIC TIME INTERVALS

Carl E. Orringer
Robert A. Kloner

Systolic time intervals (STIs) are noninvasive measurements used to assess and follow the course of patients with left ventricular dysfunction and/or valvular heart disease. These intervals are calculated using the simultaneous recording of the external carotid pulse, a phonocardiogram, and an electrocardiogram. The three STIs most commonly used are illustrated in Figure 1 and include (1) total electromechanical systole (TS), which is measured from the onset of the Q wave of the electrocardiogram of the first high frequency component of the aortic second heart sound; (2) left ventricular ejection time (LVET), measured from the beginning of the carotid upstroke to the dicrotic notch of the externally recorded carotid pulse tracing; and (3) preejection period (PEP), which is derived by subtracting LVET from TS. While LVET measures the duration of ejection of blood from the left ventricle, the PEP includes both the electromechanical interval and isovolumetric contraction time. In recording STIs, it is crucial that the carotid pulse tracing clearly delineate the onset of left ventricular ejection and the dicrotic notch, the phonocardiogram clearly demonstrate the aortic component of the second heart sound, and the electrocardiographic lead accurately show the onset of electrical depolarization—either a QR or an RS complex. The usual sites to record A_2 of the phonocardiogram are at either the upper right sternal border or at the apex; A_2 is best recorded during expiration.

THE SYSTOLIC TIME INTERVALS

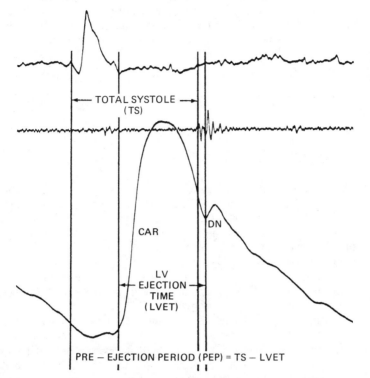

Figure 1 Measurement of systolic time intervals. Top line represents the ECG, middle line the phonocardiogram, and bottom line the carotid, CAR, pulse tracing. LVET, left ventricular ejection time; TS, total systole; DN, dicrotic notch of the carotid pulse tracing.

In the noninvasive laboratory at the Brigham and Women's Hospital, systolic time intervals are performed using a paper speed of 250 millimeters per second. If the patient is in sinus rhythm, the intervals from one complex to the next are usually similar and, in our laboratory, three complexes are tabulated and averaged to arrive at final values. If the patient is in atrial fibrillation, we look for an area of relative regularity of the RR interval, particularly one in which the RR interval exceeds 800 milliseconds, and usually average five complexes. It should be noted that systolic time intervals can also be accurately derived from an echocardiogram.

It is known that heart rate affects the STIs. As heart rate increases, LVET and PEP shorten. In general, the changes in LVET with heart rate are more pronounced than variations which occur in PEP—which are usually minor. Bazett established the following formula which can be used to correct the LVET for heart rate:

$$\text{Corrected value} = \frac{\text{Observed value}}{\text{Square root of preceding RR interval in seconds}}$$

Weissler et al. have developed other equations that correct for heart rate. Other correction factors may be needed in cases of left bundle branch block (LBBB), since this conduction disturbance prolongs the electromechanical coupling time and therefore the PEP. One technique involves the use of the following formula:

PEP corrected for LBBB =

   Observed PEP − (observed QRS duration − "normal" QRS duration [0.08 sec])

Factors Affecting the STIs

Left ventricular ejection time is a function mainly of the status of the aortic valve and the ratio of the left ventricular (LV) stroke volume to the LV end-diastolic volume, although LV contractility, mean arterial pressure, and heart rate are also of some importance. LVET is prolonged in aortic stenosis, aortic insufficiency, and in idiopathic hypertrophic subaortic stenosis (IHSS). Left ventricular failure of virtually any etiology and beta-adrenergic blockade lead to a shortening of the LVET because of a diminished LV stroke volume relative to the LV end-diastolic volume. Digitalis glycosides, beta-adrenergic agonists, and hyperthyroidism, by increasing the velocity of LV ejection, also shorten the LVET.

The PEP is affected by the length of the electromechanical interval as discussed above and also by the length of isovolumic contraction. The isovolumic contraction period is a function of the speed with which the left ventricular pressure exceeds central aortic pressure (the pressure required to open the aortic valve). Thus, factors that enhance the rate of left ventricular pressure rise (interventions that increase left ventricular dP/dt—digitalis glycosides, beta-adrenergic stimulation, hyperthyroidism) shorten PEP. Factors that diminish left ventricular dP/dt (such as left ventricular failure, beta-adrenergic blockade, and hypothyroidism) lengthen PEP. PEP is also affected by the aortic diastolic pressure; as the aortic diastolic pressure falls, PEP shortens. This effect is seen in aortic insufficiency, and may also contribute to the shorter PEP in aortic stenosis and IHSS. Finally, increases in left ventricular end-diastolic volume and in left ventricular stroke volume are associated with a diminution in the isovolumic contraction time and a shortening of PEP (which may be a function of increased LV dP/dt due to increased preload i.e., Starling's law). Hypovolemia exerts the opposite effect; diminished left ventricular end-diastolic preload is associated with a lengthening of PEP.

Use of STIs in Clinical Practice

Normal values for STIs are shown in Table 1. STIs are useful in following left ventricular function over time in patients with chronic myocardial disease and are useful in assessing the severity of aortic and mitral valve disease and concomitant LV function. One of the most useful STI measures for following heart failure is the ratio

Table 1. Normal Values for Systolic Time Intervals[a]

	Seconds
LVETc, corrected for heart rate	0.285–0.340
PEP	0.070–0.110
PEP/LVET	0.28–0.42
T time	Upper limit of normal is .05 sec; greater than .07 is clearly abnormal

[a] As used at Brigham and Women's Hospital.

of PEP/LVET. This ratio is less sensitive to the effects of heart rate than its individual components, and it is used widely in clinical practice. This ratio is normally 0.34 ± 0.08 or less but is increased in left ventricular dysfunction of any cause. Studies by Weissler et al. have shown the PEP/LVET correlated with cardiac output and stroke volume. While patients with class I congestive heart failure typically have a PEP/LVET ratio, which is normal, patients with class III symptoms have ratios between 0.50 to 0.60 and those with class IV symptoms have ratios of 0.60 or more. Studies have shown that PEP/LVET also closely correlated with angiographic ejection fraction. Systolic time intervals have been used in some studies to follow left ventricular function in patients receiving cardiotoxic chemotherapy.

STIs have been helpful in following patients with aortic stenosis. A prolonged LVET (corrected for heart rate) of 0.43 second or greater in conjunction with the clinical findings of aortic stenosis suggest hemodynamically significant obstruction that might require further invasive studies. A prolonged Q-peak murmur duration of 0.240 second or greater and a diminution of the maximal rate of rise of the carotid pulse of less than 400 mm per second also suggest hemodynamically significant aortic stenosis. A T time (the time needed for the carotid pulse tracing to reach ½ its peak amplitude measured from onset of upstroke) of greater than 0.07 second also suggests aortic stenosis. PEP is short in this condition. However, in the later stages of aortic stenosis, LV failure occurs, which tends to shorten the LVET as discussed above and prolong PEP. Thus, patients with aortic stenosis and severe heart failure may have an LVET and PEP in the normal range. Since patients with minimal or no gradient across the aortic valve may also have "normal" STIs, we recommend that the noninvasive evaluation for aortic stenosis also include other studies, such as echocardiography or radionuclide angiography which, by delineating global left ventricular function, improve the predictive accuracy of the STIs.

Aortic insufficiency, like aortic stenosis, is associated with a shortened PEP; the LVET may be prolonged or normal. The development of LV dysfunction is associated with prolongation of the PEP and a shortening of the LVET. The STIs may be especially useful in assessing patients with aortic insufficiency, in that they provide objective noninvasive data that help determine the onset of LV dysfunction.

The presence of the typical spike and dome morphology of the carotid pulse tracing, together with a prolonged LVET, is a helpful indicator of dynamic subaortic obstruction. The STIs can be of major diagnostic importance in exposing the presence of provocable dynamic subaortic obstruction. The Valsalva maneuver and amyl nitrite administration often accentuate left ventricular outflow tract obstruction in this disease and, thus, lead to a prolongation of the LVET.

In mitral regurgitation, the PEP is prolonged and LVET is shortened. Use of the PEP/LVET ratio may aid in separating patients with mitral regurgitation alone from those with mitral regurgitation plus concomitant LV dysfunction. Wanderman et al. showed that a PEP/LVET ratio of up to 0.50 could be explained solely on the basis of the presence of mitral regurgitation; values exceeding 0.50 were found to be consistently associated with LV dysfunction. In mitral stenosis, STIs are usually normal or may show an increased PEP and decreased LVET due to decreased left ventricular filling.

STIs are a technically easy and clinically useful tool especially helpful for serial observations in patients. However, they must be used in conjunction with other means of clinical assessment—both noninvasive and, in some situations, invasive.

Bibliography for Section 3

Baragan J, Fernandez F, Coblence B, et al: Left ventricular dynamics in complete right bundle branch block with left axis deviation of the QRS. *Circulation* 42:797, 1970.

Baragan J, Fernandez-Caamano F, Sozutek Y, et al: Chronic left complete bundle branch block. *Br Heart J* 30:196, 1968.

Bonner AJ Jr, Sacks HN, Tavel ME: Assessing the severity of aortic stenosis by phonocardiography and external carotid pulse recordings. *Circulation* 48:247, 1973.

Bonner AJ Jr, Tavel ME: Systolic time intervals. Use in congestive heart failure due to aortic stenosis. *Arch Intern Med* 132:816, 1973.

Carter WH, Whalen RE, Morris JJ Jr, et al: Carotid pulse tracings in hypertrophic subaortic stenosis. *Am Heart J* 82:180, 1971.

Garrard CL Jr, Weissler AM, Dodge HT: The relationship of alterations in systolic time intervals to ejection fraction in patients with cardiac disease. *Circulation* 42:455, 1970.

Lewis RP, Rittgers SE, Forester WF, et al: A critical review of the systolic time intervals. *Circulation* 56:146, 1977.

Saebra-Gomes R, Sutton R, Parker DJ: Left ventricular function after aortic valve replacement. *Br Heart J* 38:491, 1976.

Tavel ME: *Clinical phonocardiography and external pulse recording*, Chicago, Year Book Medical Publishers, Inc, 1972, p 46.

Wallace AC, Mitchell JH, Skinner NS, et al: Duration of the phases of left ventricular systole. *Circ Res* 12:611, 1963.

Wanderman KL, Goldberg MJ, Stack RS, et al: Left ventricular performance in mitral regurgitation assessed with systolic time intervals and echocardiography. *Am J Cardiol* 38:831, 1976.

Weissler AM, Harris WS, Schoenfeld CD: Systolic time intervals in heart failure in man. *Circulation* 37:149, 1968.

White CW, Simmerman TJ: Prolonged left ventricular ejection time in the post-premature beat. A sensitive sign of idiopathic hypertrophic subaortic stensos. *Circulation* 52:306, 1975.

Zoll PM, Belgard AH, Weintraub MJ, et al: External mechanical cardiac stimulation. *N Engl J Med* 294:1274, 1976.

6

EXERCISE TESTING AND AMBULATORY ELECTRO- CARDIOGRAPHIC MONITORING

Elliott M. Antman
Thomas B. Graboys

Although careful scrutiny of the routine resting 12 lead electrocardiogram (ECG) can provide a wealth of information about myocardial disease, it has a number of well-recognized limitations. Even with advanced coronary artery disease, the myocardial oxygen supply at rest may not be reduced significantly to cause myocardial ischemia reflected on the routine supine electrocardiogram. Furthermore, since the standard electrocardiogram provides, at best, one minute of continuous recording of the ECG signal, it is a low yield procedure for evaluating cardiac arrhythmias. To circumvent these difficulties, the techniques known as *exercise testing* and *ambulatory monitoring* have been widely applied in the clinical practice of cardiology.

Exercise Testing

APPLICATIONS

Since the static resting electrocardiogram provides a sample of information limited in time and limited to a single minimally demanding physiologic state, exercise testing has been developed to increase the myocardial oxygen requirements and unmask a reduced relatively fixed coronary blood flow. In addition, the controlled atmosphere of the exercise testing laboratory provides an excellent opportunity to quantitate cardiovascular performance and detect stress-induced abnormalities, such as cardiac arrhythmias.

The major applications of exercise testing are shown in Table 1. In a recent review of stress testing, Ellestad and coworkers indicated that mortality rates established by a survey of multiple centers range between 1 per 10,000 tests to 1 per 20,000 tests. The infarction rate is approximately 3.6 per 10,000 tests. Thus, the risks appear to be acceptable and are far outweighed by the benefits of the information obtained during a carefully performed exercise testing procedure.

When performing an exercise test for the evaluation of coronary artery disease, one should be aware of certain important statistical factors. As emphasized by Redwood and colleagues, the majority of symptomatic patients with significant coronary artery obstructions can be diagnosed on clinical grounds alone. In addition, according

Table 1. Applications of Exercise Testing

Evaluation of coronary artery disease
  Confirmation of diagnosis of coronary artery disease
  Detection of asymptomatic or subclinical coronary artery disease
  Evaluation of therapy and longitudinal follow-up
  Planning coronary arteriography
Evaluation of arrhythmias
Evaluation of other effort-related symptoms, such as dyspnea, palpitations, and
  syncope
Functional evaluation of patients with noncoronary cardiovascular disease

---

to Bayes' theorem, the predictive value of a test (i.e., the degree of likelihood that a positive result is true) is influenced not only by the sensitivity of the test but, most especially, by the "prior probability" that an individual has the disease which he is being tested for (i.e., the prevalence of the disease in the population being tested). Thus, if one assumes that an exercise test has a sensitivity for ischemic heart disease of 80% and specificity of 90%, then in a population where the prevalence of ischemic heart disease is 50%, it can be estimated that a patient with a positive exercise test would have an 89% probability of having ischemic heart disease. On the other hand, with a disease prevalence of only 3%, the probability that an individual with a positive test has ischemic heart disease falls to only 20%. Rifkin and Hood utilized a Bayesian analysis of the electrocardiographic response to exercise stress testing and cautioned that terms such as *positive* and *negative* may be misleading. Results should be interpreted in terms of a continuum of risk based upon a number of variables examined during the exercise test, including peak heart rate, changes in blood pressure, ST segment shifts, arrhythmias or conduction disturbances provoked, and patient symptomatology.

Thus, with these caveats in mind, the clinician who performs an exercise test for confirmation of the clinical diagnosis of coronary artery disease is hoping to observe the patient during an attack of chest discomfort, determine the degree of stress required to provoke an attack, and record an electrocardiogram during an episode of chest discomfort. The items above represent the rationale of Goldhammer and Scherf when introducing exercise stress testing for coronary artery disease nearly 50 years ago.

Controversy surrounds the use of exercise testing for the detection of asymptomatic or subclinical coronary artery disease. Since the population of patients who are asymptomatic and have a limited number of cardiovascular risk factors is likely to have a low prevalence of coronary artery disease, the chance of a false positive exercise test is increased. Some investigators have argued that people whose jobs involve matters of public safety, such as commercial airline pilots and bus drivers, should routinely undergo serial exercise testing, since their sudden incapacitation could endanger the lives of others. At present, it seems advisable to perform exercise tests in asymptomatic patients in the general public only when a combination of risk factors, such as hypertension, cigarette smoking, positive family history, and hyperlipidemia raises the suspicion of subclinical coronary artery disease.

Another important aspect of the evaluation of patients with coronary artery disease

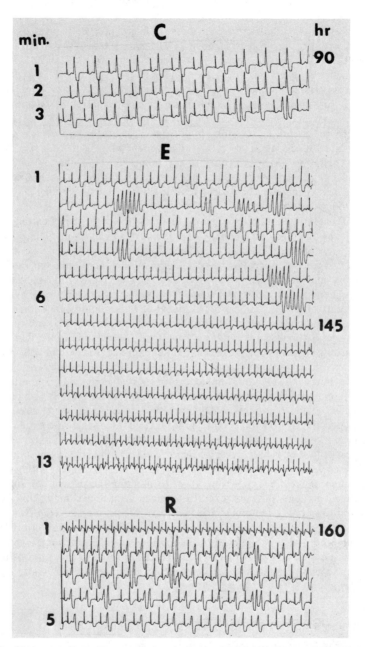

Figure 1 Slow-speed continuous electrocardiographic recording, or trendscription, can be used to record the control (C), exercise (E), and recovery (R) phases of the stress test. In this case ventricular bigeminy and ventricular couplets occurred during control; salvoes of ventricular tachycardia emerged beginning in the second minute of exercise, followed by overdrive suppression as the heart rate accelerated.

is the assessment of medical or surgical therapy. In addition, periodic exercise testing in patients with an established diagnosis of coronary artery disease affords the opportunity to screen for a change in the pattern of myocardial ischemia as suggested by the emergence of exercise-induced hypotension or ventricular arrhythmias. Finally, exercise testing is useful in planning coronary arteriography in patients with coronary artery disease. Thus, individuals who are suspected of having left main coronary obstructions based upon the constellation of findings of profound global ST segment depression and systolic hypotension should be approached more cautiously in the catheterization laboratory. The patient who has a chest pain syndrome typical of angina pectoris but occurring at minimal levels of exertion and who has an equivocal or negative exercise test may be suffering from coronary artery spasm and should be considered for provocative testing with a substance such as ergonovine during coronary arteriography.

A second major application of exercise testing is the exposure of cardiac arrhythmias. Although the arrhythmogenicity of exercise has been acknowledged for many years, only recently has exercise been specifically employed to expose cardiac arrhythmias and assess antiarrhythmic drug efficacy. By increasing sympathetic nervous activity and decreasing parasympathetic nervous activity in association with the development of myocardial ischemia, exercise testing often provokes ventricular ectopic activity. The development of transient left ventricular dysfunction may result in left atrial hypertension and atrial arrhythmias as well. In a large review of exercise testing for the provocation of cardiac arrhythmias, Jelinek and Lown demonstrated that the arrhythmogenicity of isometric (static) exercise is less than that of isotonic (dynamic) exercise. Ventricular arrhythmias during exercise testing can be increased by utilizing maximal symptom-limited protocols and employing a continuous recording system, which allows the identification of all arrhythmias or conduction disturbances. Although patients who exhibit single ventricular premature beats during exercise testing do so with a limited reproducibility, patients who exhibit frequent complex repetitive forms may be expected to do so with less variability than those who exhibit only rare isolated ectopic beats. Since the most common times for the emergence of ventricular premature beats are at peak exercise and within the initial three minutes of recovery, it is important to monitor the patient carefully during those periods. In some patients, exercise-induced arrhythmias may show overdrive suppression as exercise continues and the heart rate accelerates (Fig. 1).

Additional applications of exercise testing include the evaluation of other effort-related symptoms such as dyspnea or palpitations and the functional evaluation of patients with noncoronary cardiovascular disease. By referring to established nomograms, one may quantitate the degree of effort tolerance and use this as a guide to management.

METHODOLOGY OF EXERCISE TESTING

The standards for adult exercise testing laboratories are shown in Table 2. These are summarized from the recent report of the American Heart Association's Subcommittee on Rehabilitation Target Activity Group. The proposed standards indicate the optimal laboratory conditions and minimal requirements for testing and resuscitative equipment. The usual contraindications to exercise testing are summarized in Table 3. It is essential that a careful history and physical examination be performed

Table 2. Standards for Adult Exercise Testing Laboratories

Laboratory
    Temperature: 68–75°F, or 20–23°C
    Humidity: 60%
Staff
    Supervised by at least one physician
    At least two staff members present during test
Testing equipment
    Motorized treadmill or bicycle ergometer for graded exercise testing
    ECG recording instruments
        Conform to AHA standards
        Multiple lead systems: 3, 6, 12
        Continuous oscilloscopic monitoring of at least one lead
    Blood pressure: calibrated aneroid or mercury manometer
Emergency equipment
    Defibrillator: output through 50 ohm load of at least 250 ws
    Drugs: atropine, morphine, $CaCl_2$, epinephrine, lidocaine, sodium bicarbonate, nitroglycerin tablets

prior to administering an exercise test, so as to exclude the existence of one of these conditions.

Shown in Table 4 are the recommended procedures for electrocardiographic recording, choice of exercise load, end points for termination of the exercise test, and evaluation of the patient during the recovery period. Controversy exists regarding the optimal number of electrocardiographic leads to be used during exercise testing. While some investigators favor only a single bipolar lead with the active electrode at V_5, a number of workers feel that some ischemic type ECG responses will be missed if only a single lead is recorded. Although a number of orthogonal lead systems have been proposed, based on current evidence, the recommended choice of exercise ECG leads is the conventional 12 lead set using the torso (Mason-Likar) locations for limb leads. This enables the physician to use a standard three channel ECG recorder employing the same set of leads for control exercise and recovery tracings.

Table 3. Usual Contraindications to Exercise Testing

Acute myocardial infarction
Unstable angina pectoris
Acute myocarditis
Acute pericarditis
Congestive heart failure
Left main coronary stenosis
Rapid atrial and/or ventricular arrhythmias
Advanced atrioventricular block
Severe aortic stenosis
Uncontrolled hypertension

Table 4. Testing Procedures

ECG recording
  Ensure adequate signal by skin preparation
  Small silver–silver chloride disc electrodes mounted in plastic cups with adhesive
    rings
  Obtain 12 lead electrocardiogram and BP supine, standing, and after hyperventilation
    for 30–45 seconds
Work loads: see Table 5
Endpoints
  Achievement of target level
    85% predicted HR for submaximal test
    Peak performance for maximal test
  Indications for termination of test before achievement of target level
    Evidence of hypoperfusion and/or diminishing cardiac reserve: vasoconstriction,
      abnormal cerebral function, dyspnea, undue fatigue
    Evidence of progressive myocardial ischemia: worsening ST segment deviations or
      chest discomfort, drop in blood pressure or heart rate as exercise continues,
      electrical alternans, progressive widening of QRS complex
    Cardiac arrhythmias, unless test specifically being performed for assessment of
      arrhythmias: sustained supraventricular arrhythmias, increasing VPB frequency,
      ventricular tachycardia of 3 or more consecutive beats
Recovery
  Monitor HR, BP, and ECG changes
  Confirm that control levels of all patient functions have been reestablished

---

Additional considerations include the skin electrode interface and frequency response of the electrocardiograph machine. The usual skin resistance of 50,000 to 100,000 ohms may be reduced to 5,000 ohms by rubbing and as low as 1,000 ohms by application of an intermediate speed dental burr. The ECG recording instrument should be capable of adequately reproducing repolarization events, and this is best accomplished by a low frequency cut-off of 0.05 Hz. To eliminate "noise" on the ECG signal, a number of exercise testing laboratories are now employing computer signal averaging techniques to provide a high fidelity QRS complex and ST segment.

Exercise tests may be *maximal* or *submaximal* in design. Maximal tests are limited by symptoms or predetermined signs and attempt to approximate the physiological maximal performance, in which oxygen uptake fails to increase further with increasing work. Submaximal exercise tests are usually guided by a specific target heart rate, often representing 85% of the maximum predicted heart rate for the patient's age and sex.

Stress testing protocols may consist of a single level of exercise but usually involve graded or progressive increases in work load. The exercise modes suitable for graded exercise testing include the variable step, treadmill, and bicycle ergometer. The oxygen requirements for these commonly employed modes are summarized in Table 5. These protocols are oriented to load increments in terms of METs, based on the physician's assessment of the patient's exercise tolerance. (One MET is the energy expenditure at rest equivalent to approximately 3.5 ml of O_2/min/kgm body weight.) The most commonly employed treadmill protocol for routine diagnostic purposes is that described by Bruce. A reduced work load graded exercise test suitable for evaluation of post–myocardial infarction patients and those with a known limited exercise capacity has been developed by DeBusk.

INTERPRETATION OF EXERCISE TESTS

Shown in Table 6 are the five major components of interpretation of an exercise test. The establishment of ECG criteria for a positive ischemic response has been the subject of much investigation. The original criterion developed by Masters for the two step exercise test was 0.5 mm of horizontal or downsloping ST segment depression in the postexercise recording. An excellent summary of more recent experience with exercise electrocardiography has been provided by Sheffield. Exertionally induced ST segment displacement can be classified into three types. The first and most common type consists of J point depression with an ST segment that is entirely flat for the first 80 milliseconds of its duration. The optimal balance between sensitivity and specificity for the detection of myocardial ischemia appears to be served by requiring 0.1 millivolt (1 mm) of flat ST segment displacement in a standard electrocardiographic lead. It should be realized that other types of electrocardiographic leads have sensitivities different from the standard leads and warrant different criteria: for bipolar leads, ST segment displacement of 0.2 millivolts (2 mm) is often used, and for the Frank leads, 0.05 to 0.10 millivolts (0.5 to 1 mm) have been proposed.

The type I ischemic ST segment response is characteristically seen at peak exercise and improves rapidly in recovery (Fig. 2). By contrast, the type II ischemic ST segment response shows progressive negative displacement of the ST segment, which may even become downsloping and be associated with an inverted T wave in the immediate postexercise period. From five to 20 minutes may be required for the repolarization changes to return to normal. Type III is the least common type of ST segment response and consists of ST segment elevation. Once reciprocal changes are accounted for, ST elevation may be due to profound transmural ischemia, perhaps as a result of coronary spasm, or in other cases, it may be related to the presence of scarring and dyskinesis from previous infarction.

More complex ST segment criteria have been proposed in an attempt to improve the diagnostic accuracy of exercise electrocardiography. An example of such a modification is the ST segment index, which is the algebraic sum of the J point depression in millimeters and the ST slope in millivolts per second. A negative index is considered abnormal, assuming that the magnitude of ST segement depression is at least one millimeter and that the index is applied only during exercise or in the immediate recovery period.

McHenry and coworkers have emphasized the need to analyze the ECG for inverted or negative U waves during or after exercise. This may occur in the absence of diagnostic ST segment shifts and when present on a V_5 lead, usually indicates significant stenosis of the left anterior descending coronary artery. A number of investigators have indicated that a normal electrocardiographic response to exercise consists of a decrease in R wave amplitude. The R wave amplitude actually increases in many patients with coronary artery disease, particularly those with significant two or three vessel coronary obstructions. When used in combination with ST segment criteria, R wave amplitude criteria may reduce the number of false positive and false negative exercise tests.

Table 5. Oxygen Requirements for Step, Treadmill, and Bicycle Ergometer[a]

Functional Class	METS	O₂ Requirements (ml O₂/kg/min)	Step Test — Nagle Balke Naughton (2-min stages, 30 steps/min; Step height increased 4 cm q 2 min) Height (cm)	Bruce 3-min stages (mph % gr)	Kattus 3-min stages (mph % gr)	Balke % grade at 3–4 mph	Balke % grade at 3 mph	DeBusk 3-min stages (mph % gr)	Bicycle Ergometer (For 70 kg body weight) kgm/min
	16	56.0				26			
	15	52.5				24			
	14	49.0			4 22	22			
	13	45.5		4.2 16		20			1500
Normal and I	12	42.0	40		4 18	18	22.5		1350

118

Functional class	METs	O2 req. (ml O2/kg/min)	Step test	Treadmill % grade	Treadmill A (mph / % grade)	Treadmill B (mph / % grade)	Treadmill (% grade / mph)	Bicycle ergometer (kg-m/min)
	16							1200
	14							1050
	12							900
	11	38.5	36	20.0		4 / 14	17.5 / 3	
	10	35.0	32	17.5	3.4 / 14		15 / 3	750
	9	31.5	28	15.0			12.5 / 3	
	8	28.0	24	12.5		4 / 10	17.5 / 2	600
	7	24.5	20	10.0	2.5 / 12		14 / 2	
II	6	21.0	16	7.5		3 / 10	10.5 / 2	450
II	5	17.5	12	5.0	1.7 / 10		7 / 2	
III	4	14.0	8	2.5		2 / 10	3.5 / 2	300
III	3	10.5	4	0.0			0 / 2	
	2	7.0						150
IV	1	3.5						

Modified from Ellestad MH et al. standards for adult exercise testing laboratories, American Heart Association Subcommittee on Rehabilitation, Target activity Group. *Circulation* 59:421A, 1979. With permission of American Heart Association.

[a] Oxygen requirements increase with work loads from bottom of chart to top in various exercise tests of the step, treadmill, and bicycle ergometer types.

Table 6. Interpretation of Test

ECG response
ST segment depression
ST segment elevation
Evolution of T wave inversion
U wave inversion
R wave amplitude changes
Symptoms
Character and distribution of chest discomfort
Response to rest, TNG, CSP maneuver
Hemodynamic response
Arrhythmias
Quantitation of exercise tolerance
Functional aerobic capacity
Functional aerobic impairment

Although coronary artery stenoses are the most common cause of the ST segment shifts described above, abnormal pressure overload of the left ventricle due to either arterial hypertension or obstruction to ventricular outflow may produce profound subendocardial ischemia and an abnormal exercise electrocardiographic response. In addition, altered patterns of conduction result in an abnormal activation sequence of the ventricle, with secondary repolarization changes. A number of drugs can modify the significance of an exercise electrocardiographic response. The most common of these is digitalis, which may cause abnormalities of the ST segment at rest and during exercise. Table 7 lists other drugs that may affect the exercise electrocardiographic response and produce a false positive result.

Additional information that can be obtained during the exercise test includes the presence or absence of angina pectoris in association with abnormal ST segment responses. The physician should carefully question the patient and assess the response to interventions. Multivariate analysis has been utilized to improve predictive capacity of stress testing. Important clinical variables that have emerged as markers for underlying severe coronary artery disease include an inappropriate heart rate response (failure of the rate to increase to greater than 120 bpm), an inappropriate

Table 7. Drugs That May Affect Electrocardiographic Exercise Results

Digitalis preparations
Sympathetic nervous system blocking agents: propranolol, guanethidine, methyl-dopa
Diuretics
Nitroglycerin
Quinidine
Procainamide
Atropine
Phenothiazine derivatives
Lithium

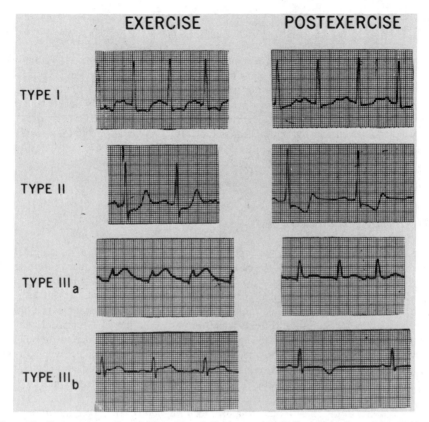

Figure 2 Types of exertional ST-segment displacement. (I) Transient depression during exercise that has virtually disappeared one minute after exercise. (II) Depression during exercise that becomes more pronounced after exercise before belatedly returning to normal. (III_a) ST elevation characteristic of Prinzmetal's angina. (III_b) ST elevation of modest degree usually caused by dyskinesis or scarring of the left ventricle. (Used with permission from Sheffield T. Exercise stress testing, in Braunwald E, ed: *Heart Disease: A Textbook of Cardiovascalar Medicine*. Philadelphia, Saunders, 1980, p 263.)

blood pressure response (failure of the systolic blood pressure to increase to greater than 140 mm of Hg), and complex ventricular arrhythmias emerging at low exercise work loads.

Maximal oxygen uptake refers to the highest level of oxygen uptake that an ambulatory person can achieve by dynamic exercise of a large fraction of the total body muscle mass. Functional capacity may be expressed as the peak estimated oxygen uptake in milliliters per minute per kilogram or equivalent MET units during a symptom-limited maximal test. By reference to a nomogram and knowledge of a patient's age, daily activity status, and duration of exercise, the physician can estimate functional aerobic impairment. This represents the percentage deviation between observed and predictive values for maximal oxygen consumption, assuming that oxygen consumption can be estimated from exercise duration.

New Exercise Procedures

Promising new procedures include scintigraphic studies during exercise. Techniques such as thallium-201 perfusion imaging at rest and during stress and technetium pyrophosphate blood pool scanning are likely to improve the sensitivity and specificity of the exercise stress testing procedure. Such radionuclide studies are particularly helpful when the standard electrocardiogram is confounded by the presence of ventricular hypertrophy, conduction defects, the preexcitation syndrome, and the presence of drugs such as those listed in Table 7. The value of exercise testing in the postinfarction period for predictive and rehabilitative purposes is currently being explored.

Ambulatory Monitoring

The technique known as ambulatory monitoring—also referred to as ambulatory electrocardiography, ambulatory recording, Holter monitoring, Holter recording, or long term electrocardiographic recording is designed to record the electrocardiographic signal over an extended period of time for playback and analysis at a late date. It differs from continuous monitoring (as is found in coronary care units or exercise stress testing laboratories), which provides on-line ECG printouts for immediate analysis. The principles and techniques employed in current ambulatory monitoring procedures were originally devised by Norman J. Holter over 20 years ago. Improvements since the original models were introduced consist of miniaturization of the recording apparatus, greater fidelity of the recorded signal, and improved playback and scanning devices.

The optimal duration of monitoring has been the subject of investigation over the last several years. As summarized in a recent review by Winkle, ambulatory monitoring for greater than a six to 12 hour period not only improves the total yield of ventricular premature beats, but greatly enhances the chance of finding complex or high grade ventricular premature beats (ventricular couplets and salvos of ventricular tachycardia). Thus, recording over a 24 hour period enables the physician to correlate a patient's complaints of palpitations or lightheadedness with disturbances of cardiac rhythm. In addition, one can catalogue the frequency and complexity of ventricular premature beats, which many investigators feel are a marker for sudden cardiac death.

COMPONENTS OF AN AMBULATORY MONITORING SYSTEM

The components of an ambulatory monitoring system are shown in Table 8. As discussed above for exercise electrocardiography, it is necessary to reduce skin impedance by rubbing. Pregelled adhesive electrodes are applied to the torso to provide either single or dual channel recording. The leads monitored correspond most closely to standard precordial lead V_5 for single channel recordings and leads V_5 and V_1 for dual channel recordings. The recording apparatus consists of a lightweight (2 lb) tape recorder, which may be worn on the belt. The electrocardiographic signal may be recorded on a standard cassette or reel to reel system. The most

Table 8. Components of an Ambulatory Monitoring
System

Recording apparatus
Scanner
Data analysis
Quality control

commonly employed apparatus is the continuous recorder, which provides a complete recording of all electrocardiographic activity. A less commonly employed type of recording apparatus is the event recorder. These are of two types. The first may be activated by the patient in response to symptoms such as palpitations or lightheadedness. The second type of event recorder continuously monitors the electrocardiographic signal, but will only record rhythm disturbances outside a previously programmed range.

The system known as trendscription was introduced by Lown and coworkers in 1973. This consists of a radio telemetry transmitter and receiver. The electrocardiographic signal is directly printed on paper attached to a drum that is rotating at slow speed. Either 30 minutes or two hours of direct ECG recording may be obtained. Finally, transtelephonic monitoring can be used for stable outpatients with cardiac arrhythmias and for follow-up of patients with implanted cardiac pacemakers. The ECG signal is transmitted over a standard phone line using leads that can be easily applied in the form of bracelets on the patient's forearms.

Playback scanners operate at 60 or 120 times real time and provide the technician with a superimposed image of QRS complexes. This is coupled to an audio signal. Changes in heart rate or rhythm are manifested as a shift in the visual image or audio signal and a direct ECG printout may be obtained of selected portions of the tape recording. Since a typical 24 hour recording may contain over 100,000 QRS complexes, a method of data analysis is required. A simple approach is to provide a count of all the ventricular premature beats (VPBs) that occurred during a 24 hour period. Since it appears that the risk of sudden cardiac death is related to the frequency of complex VPBs, Lown and Wolff introduced a grading system for VPBs shown in Table 9. Criticisms of this system have been raised, since it does not provide

Table 9. Lown Grading System

Grade	Characteristics
0	No ventricular beats
1a	Occasional, isolated VPBs, less than 30 per hour: less than 1 per minute
1b	Occasional, isolated VPBs, less than 30 per hour: more than 1 per minute
2	Frequent VPBs: more than 30 per hour
3	Multiform VPBs
4a	Repetitive VPBs: couplets
4b	Repetitive VPBs: salvos, or ventricular tachycardia
5	Early VPBs: abutting or interrupting the T wave

either a quantitative assessment of ventricular ectopic activity or reflect the density of VPBs during a given portion of the tape (Michaelson et al, Sami et al). Nevertheless it remains the most commonly employed and clinically useful system at present.

Semiautomated scanning systems are available that report an overall error rate compared to real time of approximately five to 10% in detection of ectopic beat frequency. Fully automated computer based systems are being developed that may reduce the error rate to less than 1%. Introduction of technician editing capabilities improves the accuracy of semiautomated recordings, but at the expense of speed of interpretation.

CLINICAL APPLICATIONS OF AMBULATORY MONITORING

Winkle has recently summarized the results of 11 studies examining the incidence of ventricular arrhythmias during ambulatory recordings on normal subjects. Infrequent VPBs occur commonly but complex ventricular arrhythmias are unusual, particularly in younger patients. A number of epidemiologic studies have indicated an association between frequent and high grade ventricular arrhythmias in patients with coronary artery disease and the risk of sudden cardiac death.

Cardiac arrhythmias are often sporadic events resulting in variability in arrhythmia frequency over a 24-hour period or when two 24-hour periods are compared. Recent sophisticated statistical analyses of the variability of arrhythmia frequency and complexity on serial ambulatory recordings have proposed stringent criteria for the diagnosis of antiarrhythmic drug efficacy. It should be realized that these statistically oriented studies have a number of shortcomings. The number of subjects analyzed is small and the individuals subjected to repeated ambulatory recordings were from selected groups having widely disparate cardiac diagnoses. It is not clear that information gained from such a selected group of patients can be extrapolated to people with a different clinical profile. Patients exhibiting marked variability of ectopic beat frequency often have minimal structural heart disease and may not require antiarrhythmic therapy. However, those patients suffering from malignant ventricular arrhythmias and recurrent cardiac arrests show considerably less variability in ventricular arrhythmias and probably should not be subjected to such rigorous statistical standards. It may be necessary to establish for each individual the degree of arrhythmia variability, utilizing control recordings, before initiating drug therapy.

The major clinical indications for obtaining ambulatory recordings are listed in Table 10. Cardiac arrhythmias are usually suspected when patients complain of light-

Table 10. Major Clinical Indications for Ambulatory Monitoring

---

Diagnosis of suspected cardiac arrhythmias

Diagnosis of suspected myocardial ischemia

Evaluation of therapy
  Antiarrhythmic drugs
  Pacemaker function
  Post–myocardial infarction

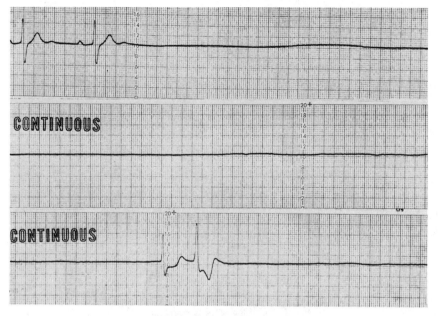

Figure 3 This elderly patient's complaints of lightheadedness were documented on ambulatory monitoring to be caused by profound sinus arrest and ventricular stand still.

headedness, palpitations, or dizziness. These symptoms may be due to bradyarrhythmias, such as profound sinus bradycardia or sinus arrest (Fig. 3) or disturbances of atrioventricular conduction leading to pauses in ventricular activity (Fig. 4). Alternatively, supraventricular arrhythmias with a poorly controlled ventricular response (Fig. 5) or bursts of rapid ventricular tachycardia or ventricular flutter can cause diminished cerebral perfusion and alterations of consciousness (Fig. 6). Widespread application of ambulatory monitoring has yielded dramatic examples of accelerating ventricular tachyarrhythmias in patients out of the CCU setting (Fig. 7). Patients suffering sudden cardiac death during ambulatory recordings have been described in the literature. The majority of these had ventricular fibrillation initiated by early cycle ventricular complexes.

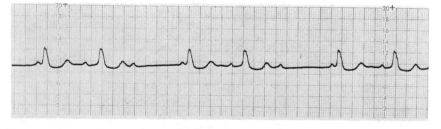

Figure 4 Classical Wenckebach-type second-degree atrioventricular block was found to be the etiology of this patients "irregular pulse" and complaints of "palpitations."

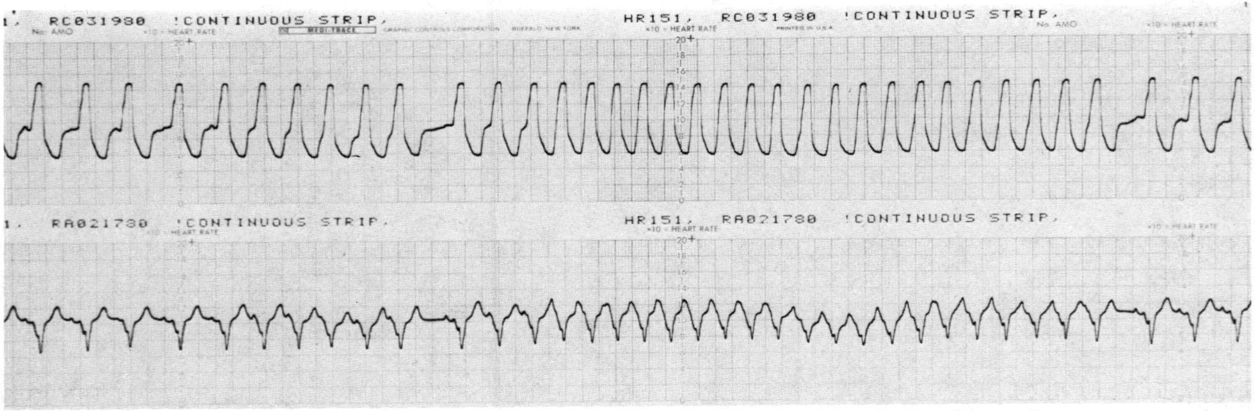

Figure 5 This 16-year-old with familial hypertrophic cardiomyopathy had episodic lightheadedness related to paroxysms of supraventricular tachycardia with a rapid ventricular response. Sinus rhythm is seen at the left, with a wide QRS complex, representing an intraventricular conduction delay and/or conduction over an accessary tract. (Two-channel recording)

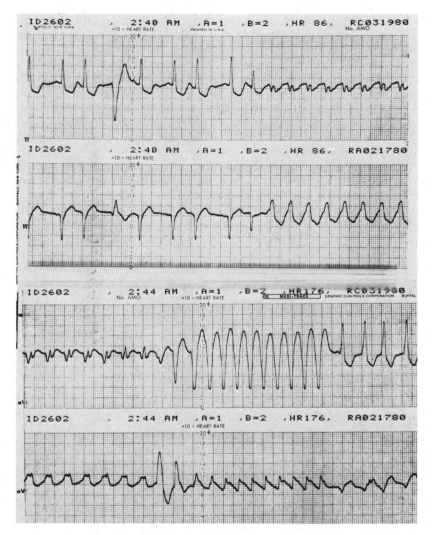

Figure 6 This middle-aged man with severe biventricular failure had repetitive paroxysms of ventricular tachycardia, VT. In this continuous *two-channel recording*, VT is initiated at the right end of the top strip; an R or T beat occurs in the middle of the third strip, causing a shift in axis and acceleration of the rate of VT, which later slows and terminates spontaneously.

Myocardial ischemia is usually suspected when patients complain of effort-related substernal chest discomfort. Ambulatory recordings on such patients give the clinician an opportunity to perform repeated "exercise tests" on patients with coronary disease as they engage in daily activities. Slow speed electrocardiographic recordings by Maseri and coworkers have revealed an unsuspected high frequency of transient ST-T wave shifts in patients with coronary disease. These have been demonstrated to be due to coronary vasospasm, which probably occurs much more frequently than previously recognized. Occasional patients reveal spontaneous ST segment elevation during ambulatory recordings, which may or may not occur in association with chest discomfort. One should be cautious when interpreting ST-T wave shifts on ambulatory recordings because of a number of peculiarities of the ECG pattern obtained by such techniques as compared with the standard electrocardiographic leads. These peculiarities include deeper S waves, notches, or dips before the following T waves; shifts in ST segment position; and T wave lability, probably due to a combination of physiologic changes in the patient as well as alterations of patient position during the recording (e.g., from the supine to standing position).

The last major indication for ambulatory recording is evaluation of therapy.. The efficacy of antiarrhythmic drugs during acute drug testing or more chronic therapy is easily evaluated by ambulatory monitoring. Transtelephonic monitoring and full 24-hour recordings may be used to evaluate characteristic forms of pacemaker malfunction: failure to sense, failure to capture the myocardium, or inappropriate alterations in pacing rate (Fig. 8). Since pacemaker therapy has now become an ex-

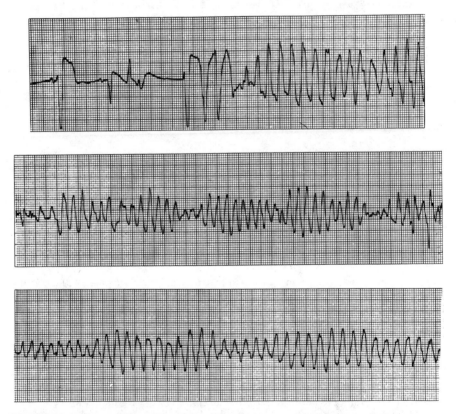

Figure 7 In this continuous recording, rapid repetitive early-cycle VPBs in the middle of the top strip are seen initiating a run of coarse ventricular flutter/fibrillation, with oscillation of the amplitude of QRS complexes.

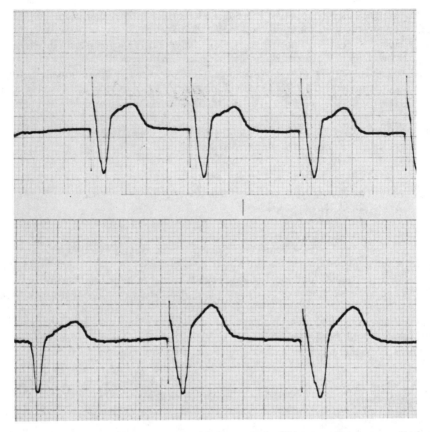

Figure 8 This figure shows two isolated segments of a 24-hour ambulatory monitoring session on a patient with a permanent ventricular demand pacemaker. An apparent inappropriate decrease in pacing rate is seen when one compares the intervals between pacing spikes in the top and bottom strips. This was due in this case to variation in the tape drive speed of the monitoring device—note the difference in QRS width and QT interval in the two strips—rather than pacemaker generator malfunction or appropriate sensing of isoelectric VPBs in the lead being recorded.

traordinarily complex field, the specifications of the particular device implanted in any patient should be reviewed before basing a diagnosis of pacemaker malfunction on ambulatory recordings.

Another useful application of ambulatory monitoring is immediately prior to discharge of a patient recuperating from an acute myocardial infarction, as well as at varying intervals during the first year following an acute myocardial infarction. Since there appears to be a relationship between advanced grades of ventricular arrhythmias found on such recordings and subsequent death (including sudden death), current recommendations are to treat such ventricular arrhythmias aggressively with antiarrhythmic drugs during the initial year following acute myocardial infarction. Preliminary data suggest that abolition of high-grade ventricular premature beats may indicate a greater chance of patient survival. Further studies and more long term follow-up are required for confirmation of this finding.

Ambulatory recordings appear to be superior to the standard treadmill exercise test for the detection of ventricular arrhythmias in patients with coronary heart disease, the mitral valve prolapse syndrome, and hypertrophic cardiomyopathy. However, approximately 10% of patients will demonstrate ventricular arrhythmias only on exercise testing; therefore, the two techniques should be considered complementary. It is recommended that patients at high risk for sudden cardiac death (e.g., history of primary ventricular fibrillation) should be evaluated by both an ambulatory monitoring session and treadmill exercise test.

Future Directions of Exercise Testing and Ambulatory Monitoring

New therapies are actively being investigated for the treatment of angina pectoris and the reduction of myocardial infarct size. The impact of these therapeutic modalities on ventricular function and long term patient survival requires careful scrutiny. Techniques such as exercise testing and ambulatory monitoring are excellent tools for both epidemiologic studies and individual patient considerations. Computer assisted electrocardiographic diagnosis of ischemic ST segment shifts and cardiac arrhythmias hold great promise for the busy clinician but should be viewed as complementary to the judgment and experience of a skilled observer.

Bibliography

Bigger JT, Wenger TL, Heissenbuttel RH: Limitations of the Lown grading system for the study of human ventricular arrhythmias. *Am Heart J* 93:727, 1977.

Bruce RA: Progress in exercise cardiology, in Yu PN, Goodwin JF (eds): *Progress in Cardiology*. Philadelphia, Lea and Febiger, 1974, vol 3, p 113.

Bruce RA, Hornsten TR: Exercise stress testing in evaluation of patients with ischemic heart disease. *Prog Cardiovasc Dis.* 11:371, 1969.

Clarke LJ, Bruce RA: Exercise testing, in Cohn PF (ed): *Diagnosis and Therapy of Coronary Artery Disease*. Boston, Little Brown, 1979, p 81.

Davidson DM, DeBusk RF: Prognostic value of a single exercise test 3 weeks after uncomplicated myocardial infarction. *Circulation* 61:236, 1980.

DeBusk R: The value of exercise stress testing. *J Am Med Assoc* 232:956, 1975.

Ellestad MH, Blomquist CG, Naughton JP: Standards for adult exercise testing laboratories. American Heart Association Subcommittee on Rehabilitation, Target Activity Group. *Circulation* 59:241A, 1979.

Ellestad MH, Cooke BM, Greenberg PS: Stress testing: clinical application and predictive capacity. *Prog Cardiovasc Dis* 16:479, 1974.

Faris JV, McHenry PL, Morris SN: Concepts and applications of treadmill exercise testing and the exercise electrocardiogram. *Am Heart J* 95:102, 1978.

Force T, Graboys TB: Exercise testing and ambulatory monitoring in patients with preexcitation syndrome. *Arch Inter Med* 141:88, 1981.

Froelicher VF, McKirnan MD: Rehabilitation and exercise early after acute myocardial infarction, in Karliner JS, Gregoratos G (eds): *Coronary Care*. New York, Churchill Livingstone, 1981, p 897.

Goldhammer S, Scherf D: Elektrokardiographische untersuchungen bei kranker mit angina pectoris: Ambulatorischer typus. *Zschr Klin Med* 122:134, 1933.

Grayboys TB, Wright RF: Provocation of supraventricular tachycardia during exercise stress testing. *Cardiovasc Rev and Reports* 1:57, 1980.

Grayboys TB: Detection of cardiac arrhythmias and conduction abnormalities in coronary artery disease, in Cohn PF (ed): *Diagnosis and Therapy of Coronary Artery Disease*. Boston, Little Brown, 1979, p 63.

Holter NJ: Radioelectrocardiography: A new technique for cardiovascular studies. *Ann NY Acad Sci* 65:913, 1957.

Jelinek MV, Lown B: Exercise stress testing for exposure of cardiac arrhythmia. *Prog Cardiovasc Dis* 16:497, 1974.

Kennedy HL, Caralis DG: Ambulatory electrocardiography: A clinical perspective. *Ann Int Med* 87:729, 1977.

Lown B, Podrid PJ, DeSilva RA, et al.: Sudden cardiac death: Management of the patient at risk. *Curr Prob Cardiol* 4:7, 1980.

Lown B, Matta RJ, Besser HW: Programmed trendscription: A new approach to electrocardiographic monitoring. *JAMA* 232:39, 1975.

Lown B, Wolf M: Approaches to sudden death from coronary heart disease. *Circulation* 44:130, 1971.

Maseri A, Severi S, Nes MD, et al.: "Variant" angina: One aspect of a continuous spectrum of vasospastic myocardial ischemia: Pathogenic mechanisms, estimated incidence and clinical and coronary arteriographic findings in 138 patients. *Am J Cardiol* 42:1019, 1978.

Master AM: The master two-step test. *Am Heart J* 75:810, 1968.

McHenry PL: The actual prevalence of false positive ST-segment responses to exercise in clinically normal subjects remains undefined. *Circulation* 55:683, 1977.

Michaelson EL, Morganroth J: Spontaneous variability of complex ventricular arrhythmias detected by long-term electrocardiographic recording. *Circulation* 61:690, 1980.

Morganroth J, Michelson EL, Horowitz LN, et al.: Limitations of routine long-term electrocardiographic monitoring to assess ventricular ectopic frequency. *Circulation* 58:408, 1978.

Moss AJ, Davis JH, DeCamilla J, et al.: Ventricular ectopic beats and their relation to sudden and nonsudden cardiac death after myocardial infarction. *Circulation* 60:998, 1979.

Redwood DR, Borer JS, Epstein ST: Whither the ST segment during exercise? *Circulation* 54:703, 1976.

Rifkin RD, Hood WB: Bayesian analysis of electrocardiographic exercise stress testing. *N Engl J Med* 297:681, 1977.

Ruberman W, Weinblatt E, Goldberg J, et al.: Sudden death after myocardial infarction: Runs of ventricular premature beats and R on T as high risk factors. *Am J Cardiol* 45:444, 1980.

Ruberman W, Weinblatt E, Goldberg JD, et al.: Ventricular premature beats and mortality after myocardial infarction. *N Engl J Med* 297:750, 1977.

Sami M, Kraemer H, Harrison DC, et al.: A new method for evaluating antiarrhythmic drug efficacy. *Circulation* 62:1172, 1980.

Schultze RA Jr, Strauss WH, Pitt B: Sudden death in the year following myocardial infarction:

Relation to ventricular premature contractions in the late hospital phase and left ventricular ejection fraction. *Am J Med* 62:192, 1977.

Sheffield LT: Exercise stress testing, in Braunwald E (ed): *A Textbook of Cardiovascular Medicine.* Philadelphia, Saunders, 1980, p 253.

Sheffield LT, Reeves TJ, Blackburn H, et al.: The exercise test in perspective. *Circulation* 55:681, 1977.

Sheffield LT, Rottman D: Stress testing methodology. *Prog Cardiovasc Dis* 19:33, 1976.

Winkle RA: Ambulatory electrocardiography and the diagnosis, evaluation and treatment of chronic ventricular arrhythmias. *Prog Cardiovasc Dis* 23:99, 1980.

Winkle RA: Antiarrhythmic drug effect mimicked by spontaneous variability of ventricular ectopy. *Circulation* 57:116, 1978.

CHAPTER

7

NUCLEAR CARDIOLOGY

Joseph F. Polak
B. Leonard Holman

Over the last decade, a large number of nuclear medicine procedures have become available to the clinician. In the case of the cardiovascular system, continuing changes in the availability of instrumentation and of radiopharmaceuticals have made the selection of appropriately useful diagnostic procedures increasingly difficult, even to the nuclear medicine specialist. Because the best diagnostic test frequently depends on experience and availability, clinicians should confer with their nuclear cardiology consultants prior to ordering the tests described in this chapter.

Only those examinations that are noninvasive, requiring intravenous administration of the radiopharmaceutical, and that use standard imaging and processing instrumentation will be discussed.

Myocardial Imaging

Many radiopharmaceuticals and imaging modalities are available to aid in the assessment of both the functional and metabolic integrity of the heart (Table 1). A number of these techniques have demonstrated their clinical value and have become routine diagnostic procedures. Three specific types of examinations will be discussed:

1. Technetium-99m pyrophosphate imaging for the detection of irreversibly damaged myocardium
2. Thallium-201 imaging for the evaluation of both myocardial perfusion and integrity
3. Cardiac wall motion studies with technetium-99m labeled red blood cells for the assessment of ventricular contraction

TECHNETIUM-99M PYROPHOSPHATE

Technetium-99m pyrophosphate, originally introduced as a bone scanning agent, is but one of many pharmaceuticals that concentrate at the site of recent myocardial necrosis. It is the most commonly used of these tracers because it is readily available and possesses the greatest tracer concentration within the infarct, relative to background.

133

Table 1. Radiopharmaceuticals Presently Available for the Scintigraphic Assessment of the Cardiovascular System

Modalities Available	Principle	Type
Potassium and cationic analogues (cesium, rubidium and thallium)	Uptake; proportional to blood flow	Noninvasive; thallium-201 is available commercially
Metabolic substrates (^{13}N-ammonia, fatty acids, glucose)	Uptake; proportional to local metabolism	Noninvasive; positron emitters ^{13}N, ^{15}O, [11]C
Gases ([85]Kr or ^{133}Xe)	Washout; proportional to blood flow	Invasive; intraarterial injections
Labeled microspheres (^{99m}Tc, ^{111}In)	Uptake; proportional to blood flow	Invasive; intraarterial injections
Immunologic complexes (labeled antibodies to myosin)	Increased uptake in necrosis	Under development
Inflammatory infiltrate (^{67}Ga, leukocytes labeled with ^{111}In)	Increased uptake in inflammation	Under development
[99m]Tc complexes (pyrophosphate, tetracycline), [203]Hg mercurials	Increased uptake in necrosis	[99m]Tc pyrophosphate used extensively
First pass angiocardiography with any ^{99m}Tc complex ^{133}Xe, [113m]In-DPTA, [191]Ir, [178]Ta	Cardiac function	Generally available; most effective with multicrystal camera
Equilibrium ventriculography (^{99m}Tc red blood cells)	Cardiac function	Generally available; computer interfacing necessary

Pathophysiology

The distribution of pyrophosphate uptake parallels the amount of calcium present in the region of recently damaged myocardium. The exact localization of this compound is still a contested point. The myocardial cell mitochondria, the cellular fraction of damaged cells, and the insoluble apatite crystals may account for the uptake of this pharmaceutical. Pyrophosphate deposition is also dependent on persistent perfusion to the site of ischemic damage. Highest myocardial concentration of tracer occurs at 20 to 50% of the normal resting blood flow. Experimentally, the smallest infarct that can be visualized is three grams. In the clinical situation, these factors result in an *optimal* imaging time of 36 to 72 hours after *transmural infarction*. Increased myocardial uptake can be seen as early as four hours after infarction, however.

Imaging Characteristics

A standard gamma camera (Anger type) can be used. Optimal imaging time is at least three hours after the intravenous injection of this pharmaceutical. Early images, if they are obtained, identify the location of the myocardial blood pool and therefore may prove useful if a diffuse pattern of uptake is present.

Patterns of Myocardial Uptake

Various scoring systems have been used in attempts to quantify the amount of pyrophosphate uptake in the myocardium (Fig. 1). In the classification we use, the scintigraphic patterns are divided into the following types:

Normal	Myocardial uptake equal to that over the right hemithorax (no identification of a discrete cardiac silhouette)
Mild diffuse (low probability of acute myocardial infarction)	Myocardial uptake exceeds the uptake over the right hemithorax but is less intense than that over the ribs and is distributed over most or all of the myocardium
Moderate diffuse (indeterminate for the diagnosis of acute infarction)	Myocardial uptake equal to or greater in intensity than the uptake over the ribs but less intense than that over the sternum
Focal	Discrete myocardial uptake
Massive (focal and massive: high probability of acute infarction)	An increase in myocardial uptake involving 50% or more of the cardiac silhouette and is equal to or more intense than the uptake over the sternum

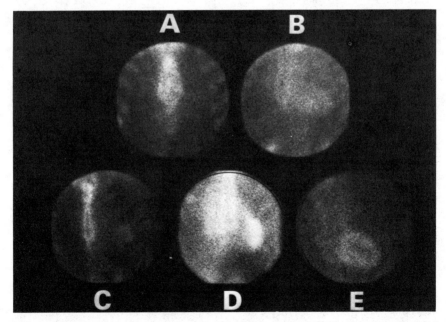

Figure 1   Scintigraphic classification of myocardial uptake of ^{99m}Tc-pyrophosphate. (*a*) Normal. (*b*) Diffuse. (*c,d*) Focal. (*e*) Massive.

When myocardial uptake is focal, it can be localized to one or more segments of the myocardial wall from an analysis of the scintigrams obtained in multiple projections. The inferior and lateral segments of the wall are perpendicular to the detector in the anterior projection, whereas the inferior, true posterior, and anterior segments are perpendicular to the detector in the lateral projection. Frequently, many segments of wall are involved.

THALLIUM-201

This radiopharmaceutical is a potassium analogue. Its administration results in a lower radiation dose and improved spatial resolution when compared to other potassium analogues, such as rubidium and cesium. It is used clinically for the assessment of regional myocardial perfusion.

Pathophysiology

Immediately following an intravenous injection of thallium, the pattern of myocardial uptake reflects regional blood flow. Since the heart is capable of an extraction rate of 80–90% for this cation, approximately 4% of the administered dose is captured by the myocardium.

In a normal subject at rest, local myocardial uptake of this isotope depends on blood flow and is, therefore, homogeneously distributed throughout the left ventricle. With exercise, a proportional increase in regional myocardial perfusion results again in uniform left ventricular distribution of the tracer. With coronary artery disease, thallium uptake is unchanged if regional blood flow is normal. Areas of exercise induced ischemia show decreases in thallium uptake, since regional delivery of the isotope is compromised. Areas of absent thallium uptake can also be seen at rest: these may represent previously damaged myocardium now replaced by fibrous tissue or areas of severely reduced blood flow.

Soon after the intravenous administration of this pharmaceutical, a phenomenon called redistribution occurs and represents a transitional period between thallium distribution, which is flow dependent, and a steady state, in which thallium uptake is proportional to the size of the local potassium pool. Clinically, this transitional period begins soon after the injection. If the tracer injection is performed at the time of exercise, the discrepancies in flow caused by stenosed coronary arteries appear as areas of relative decreased thallium uptake. As the patient stops exercising, the redistribution phase begins and is usually completed in 4 to 6 hours. Areas with persistent thallium defects are thought to represent irreversibly damaged myocardium. In some patients, a true steady state is never reached and a repeat resting study must be performed if the size of the resting metabolically active myocardium is to be assessed.

Imaging Characteristics

A gamma camera (Anger type) with either medium sensitivity or high resolution collimators can be used. Images of the heart are obtained from the anterior and at

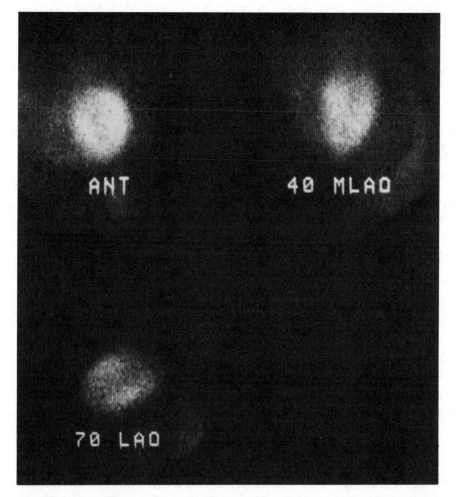

Figure 2 Normal myocardial perfusion scintigraphy. Activity is uniform throughout the left ventricular wall. ANT, anterior; 40 MLAO, 40° modified left anterior oblique; 70 LAO, 70° left anterior oblique.

least two other left anterior oblique (LAO) projections (40° and 70°) so that all the cardiac segments are well visualized (Fig. 2).

When this test is performed during stress or exercise, the patient should reach a maximal exercise point (most commonly, 85% of the maximum predicted heart rate of the Bruce protocol) before being injected. He or she should also continue to exercise for one to two minutes or until the tracer has cleared the blood. For best results, imaging should be carried out immediately or within as short an interval as possible. Images are also obtained at 4 to 6 hours following the injection and, if necessary, a repeat resting study can be ordered over the next week.

Patterns of Myocardial Uptake

A consistent scoring system must be used to describe the results of a thallium scan. A normal study either shows a homogeneous distribution of the isotope in the ventricle walls or a small apical defect, best seen in the anterior and 30° LAO views. This apparent apical thinning is due both to ventricular geometry and motion during the cardiac cycle. Localized areas of decreased uptake can be related to the territories of diseased coronary arteries. Multiple focal defects that fail to conform to these distributions may represent involvement by other processes, such as sarcoidosis. Diffuse decreases in uptake suggest the presence of a cardiomyopathy.

When attempting to diagnose coronary artery disease, indirect evidence of myocardial dysfunction such as ventricular dilatation or increased lung uptake should be reported. Accuracy is increased if proper contrast enhancing schemes are used; decreases in uptake of 10% that affect 20 to 30% of the circumference of the heart are usually considered abnormal.

MYOCARDIAL CONTRACTILITY

Both left and right ventricular function can be assessed with either first pass or gated equilibrium radionuclide angiocardiography. The increasing use of these methods is due to the accuracy, the safety, and, with the increasing availability of computer packages for data processing, the ease with which the blood pool can be labeled using ^{99m}Tc red blood cells.

Pathophysiology

Radionuclide angiocardiography can be used to measure a number of useful indices of ventricular performance. The ejection fraction is a sensitive index of the contractile state of the left ventricle. Regional changes in contractility have also correlated well with the absence of contracting myocardium, either when it is replaced by scar or when ischemia is present.

More recently, exercise radionuclide angiocardiography has been introduced as a potential screening test for coronary artery disease. Patients with hemodynamically significant coronary artery stenoses will usually have changes suggesting decompensation of normal myocardial contractility, global decreases of left ventricular ejection fraction, or the appearance of new wall motion abnormalities.

Imaging Characteristics

Resting studies are more often performed with the patient supine. In a first transit study, a rapid bolus is injected so that the bolus remains compact when it reaches the left ventricle. The multicrystal camera is the instrument of choice for such a study, since it possesses a high count rate capability and permits the extraction of statistically significant information during the short transit time of the injected bolus. Since most of the isotope is in the ventricular cavity during the critical imaging period, there is minimal interference from the small amount distributed to adjacent anatomic structures such as the lungs. The patient can therefore be positioned in the anterior, left anterior oblique, or right anterior oblique position.

The equilibrium radionuclide angiocardiogram requires a greater degree of sophistication. First, the contents of the heart chambers must be labeled and remain so for the duration of the study. Labeling albumin or red blood cells with technetium-99m satisfies this requirement. Second, patient radiation exposure must be kept to a minimum while collecting images with satisfactory statistics. This is achieved by synchronization of individual cardiac beats to the R wave of the electrocardiogram and by summation of many individual cycles into a representative cardiac cycle. This is easily done if the cardiac rhythm is regular and without serious ectopy. Quantitative assessments of ejection fraction are more reproducible when a left anterior oblique projection is used. Minimal overlap of the left ventricle with other cardiac chambers occurs in this position (Fig. 3). Supplementary projections are used for additional qualitative interpretations (anterior, right anterior oblique, left lateral, or left posterior oblique positions).

With exercise, the first pass study can be performed with the patient either supine or upright in either the right anterior oblique, anterior, or left anterior oblique projections. When the predefined exercise level is attained, a repeat injection of radionuclide is given and a study acquired. This approach does not permit evaluation at graded levels of exercise, since each injection contaminates future studies by adding background activity in the heart and surrounding tissues. With equilibrium studies, imaging is commonly performed during several stages of graded supine bicycle exercise. No repeat injections are necessary. The major constraints are patient motion and the short duration of acquisition. A commonly used protocol increases the exercise stage every three minutes, while imaging is conducted in the last two minutes of each stage.

With both modalities, regional wall motion abnormalities are assessed qualitatively during the dynamic display of a reconstructed representative cardiac cycle or with computer processed images of ejection fraction or paradox.

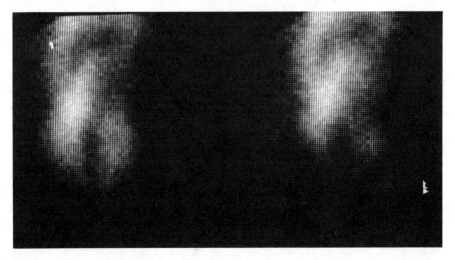

Figure 3 Gated radionuclide angiocardiogram in the left anterior oblique projection. (Left) The diastolic image shows the ventricles maximally dilated. (Right) The systolic image shows strong uniform contraction of the left ventricle.

Patterns of Contractility

The lower limits of ejection fraction for the left ventricle range from 45 to 55%, depending on the laboratory. Similarly, the criteria for an abnormal exercise response vary from laboratory to laboratory. Frequently cited criteria include either a fall of global ejection fraction, a failure to increase by 5%, or the development (or worsening) of regional wall motion abnormalities.

Detection of Coronary Artery Disease

With the proliferation of noninvasive diagnostic tests aimed at evaluating coronary artery disease, it is critically important that the clinician keep very clearly in mind the questions he or she wishes answered and the bases on which the pertinent tests have been validated. The application of decision making theory and, more important, of Bayes' theorem gives us insights into the limitations of these screening procedures. Consider, for example, a patient with a finite pretest likelihood of disease (arrived by integrating all of the available clinical data). If we assume that the outcome of the test is either positive or negative, the patient's posttest likelihood of disease depends on not only the sensitivity and specificity of the procedure, but also the pretest likelihood of disease. If the patient has a high pretest likelihood of disease, it becomes almost impossible to rule out disease with a negative test, while a low pretest likelihood of disease makes it very difficult to rule in disease with a positive test.

If we apply the same logic to standard exercise electrocardiographic testing, there is no doubt that in a group of symptomatic patients the test will do well. In asymptomatic patients, the test is a poor discriminator between the presence or absence of disease.

WHAT IS THE ROLE OF THALLIUM STRESS IMAGING?

If detection of coronary artery disease is the end point, then a set of "sensitive" criteria can be used, in the same way that the presence of resting Q waves on an electrocardiogram adds to the detection sensitivity of an electrocardiographic stress or exercise treadmill test (ETT). When the presence of either a stress-induced or a resting decrease in thallium uptake is used, the sensitivity of an abnormal test is 85%, while the specificity is 81%; disease prevalence is normally 80% in the populations studied (Table 2). For similar population groups, the ETT is 65% sensitive and 85% specific.

More specific criteria can be introduced if the clinical question is the assessment of ongoing ischemia in patients suspected of having significant coronary artery disease. A fair proportion of these patients have resting Q waves or resting thallium defects. The appearance of a new defect or the worsening of a previously present thallium defect on exercise is 73% sensitive and 90% specific for the presence of significant coronary artery disease. (Ritchie et al., McCarthy et al., Botvinick et al.) The appearance of ST segment changes is 77% sensitive and 86% specific in the sample populations when acceptable electrocardiographic exercise tolerance tests are reviewed (Table 2).

Thallium studies play an important role in the assessment of patients with an unsatisfactory electrocardiographic stress test. Resting electrocardiographic abnormalities (left bundle branch block, ST segment depression secondary to digitalis effect) or the inability to reach established exercise end points occur in 5 to 20% of the population groups commonly screened. Under these circumstances, the stress thallium test can be 77% sensitive and 78% specific for the detection of coronary artery disease (Table 2).

WHAT IS THE ROLE OF EXERCISE VENTRICULOGRAPHY?

For the detection of coronary artery disease, sensitive criteria include the presence of a reduced resting ejection fraction, with or without regional wall motion abnormalities; and, with exercise, either appearance of new or worsening of old regional wall motion abnormalities; and/or failure of the ejection fraction to rise by 0.05 resting EF units or 7% of the resting ejection fraction. Sensitivity is over 90%, while specificity is 58%, when this method is used to attempt to pick out those patients with coronary artery disease among those presenting with chest pain. An abnormal response is, however, rarely seen in normal, asymptomatic subjects.

More specific criteria can be introduced if an assessment of the functional status of the left ventricle is desired. These include a failure to increase ejection fraction by the appropriate amount and/or the appearance of new or worsening of old areas of regional wall motion abnormality. Sensitivity is estimated at 84% as compared to 94% when less specific criteria are used (Table 3).

LIMITATIONS OF RADIONUCLIDE METHODS

Right ventricular (RV) involvement secondary to coronary artery disease cannot be assessed by myocardial scintigraphy with thallium, since the RV walls are not normally seen. By inference, resting or exercise defects seen in the inferior wall of the left ventricle may suggest right coronary disease. The sensitivity for detection of abnormal thallium uptake in cases of significant right coronary artery single vessel

Table 2. Value of Exercise Thallium-201 Scintigraphy Compared to Exercise Treadmill Testing (ETT) for the Diagnosis of Coronary Artery Disease

	Thallium-201[a]	Exercise Treadmill Testing (Equivocal Tests Excluded)	Thallium-201 in Patients with Equivocal ETT[b]
Sensitivity	83%	77%	77%
Specificity	81%	86%	78%

[a] Defect at rest or appearing with exercise (Boucher et al; Pohost GM, Boucher CH, Zir LM, et al.).

[b] 20% prevalence of equivocal tests; defect appearing with exercise only (Richie JL, et al.; McCarthy DM, et al.; Botvinick CH, et al.).

Table 3. Comparative Accuracy of Exercise Radionuclide Ventriculography and Thallium-201 Scintigraphy for the Detection of Coronary Artery Disease

Author	% Lumen Diameter Narrowing	Previous MI	Propranolol	Ventriculography[a]		Thallium-201[a]	
				Sens.	Spec.	Sens.	Spec.
Jengo	>75%	21/42	Yes[b]	41/42	16/16	39/42	15/16
Johnstone	>50%	10/39	No	35/39	9/9	30/39	9/9
Caldwell	>50%	15/41	28/41	39/41	6/11[c]	35/41	11/11
TOTAL				115/122 (94%)	(31/36) —	104/122 (85%)	(35/36) —

[a] Resting and/or exercise induced abnormalities

[b] Number of patients not specified

[c] Abnormal resting and/or abnormal response to exercise for global left ventricular ejection fraction only

disease (54 to 63%) or inferior myocardial infarction (88%) is reduced when compared to cases of anterior wall ischemia (71 to 85%) or infarction (100%). Similarly, single vessel disease involving the circumflex is detected less reliably (33 to 44%). Even the use of special imaging devices, such as seven pinhole tomography, does not affect the overall detection accuracy.

Although the overall detection efficiency is quite good, thallium imaging does not offer increased specificity in assessing the extent of significant coronary artery disease. For example, a perfusion defect in the territory of the left anterior descending artery (anterolateral left ventricular wall) is seen in 80% of cases with solitary involvement of this vessel but in only 50% of cases with concomitant involvement of the other coronaries. When specific patterns of uptake are present, it may be possible to identify a group of high risk patients: those with significant left main coronary artery disease or with so-called "left main equivalent" three vessel disease. In these cases, however, thallium imaging must be used conjointly with stress electrocardiography to increase the detection rate from 43 to 69%. When combined, these tests can offer assistance by confirming that a patient is at high risk of myocardial infarction.

The value of thallium uptake as a predictor of operative response to saphenous aortocoronary bypass surgery is still being evaluated. Postoperatively, it does offer a semiqualitative method for assessing graft patency and surgical effectiveness. Its usefulness is limited to the detection of new areas of acute myocardial damage and to the assessment of those areas where perfusion defects were first detected (at rest or exercise) preoperatively.

Radionuclide ventriculography is still in its infancy. Specificity is yet to be reported in large patient groups. Global and regional left ventricular function can be abnormal in patients with valvular disease or cardiomyopathies, thereby requiring a concomitant assessment by another imaging modality, such as echocardiography. The presence of left bundle branch block is also a potential cause of false positives.

The interpretation of exercise ventriculography should take into consideration the distinction between the screening for the presence of coronary artery disease and assessing its physiological importance. The resting study should serve as a first step.

A low ejection fraction and/or regional wall motion abnormalities are suggestive of ischemic heart disease. For global left ventricular function, the reproducibility of the method within the physiologic range of normals and abnormals is critical. For regional wall motion, the reliability of the qualitative and/or quantitative assessments must be well defined and not limited to one projection.

If resting function is abnormal, then the results of the exercise test will more sensitively reflect the physiologic state of the ventricle. For example, patients with previously abnormal ventriculographic responses to exercise often demonstrate a return to normal exercise ejection fraction response in the early postaortocoronary bypass surgery period.

Ideally, the stress tests should be performed 48 hours or more after propranolol has been withdrawn. Propranolol decreases the sensitivity and specificity of both stress thallium imaging and stress radionuclide ventriculography for the detection of coronary artery disease. Nitroglycerin can also reverse areas of decreased thallium uptake or areas of regional dysfunction as detected by ventriculography.

Exercise and resting ventriculography are unreliable when a significant amount of arrhythmias are present. This segment of the population should probably be assessed with thallium scintigraphy. At this time, although radionuclide ventriculography appears to be more sensitive than thallium-201 scintigraphy (Table 3), its specificity is quite low for detecting the presence of coronary artery disease among patients with chest pain (Jones et al.).

Myocardial Infarction

PYROPHOSPHATE: TECHNETIUM-99M

The overall sensitivity for the detection of acute myocardial infarction varies from 51 to 100%, depending on the patient population and the interpretive criteria (Cowley et al., Ahmad et al., Mussie et al., Lyons et al).

When transmural myocardial infarction is suspected, sensitivity approaches 100% in patients imaged sequentially up to six days following the estimated acute event (Wynne, Holman). The criterion for an abnormal scan is an uptake of 2 + or more, that is, uptake distinct from the blood pool activity and equal to or greater in intensity than rib uptake. When a focal pattern (2 + or more in intensity) is required for a scan to be called positive, the sensitivity is 82%; while false positives are due, most often, to previous myocardial infarctions (Table 4). False negative results occur in 6 to 7% of cases (75% of which are inferior infarcts) giving a specificity of 93% to this method of interpretation.

Frequently, subendocardial infarcts present a diagnostic problem. When a focal pattern of uptake is used as the criterion for infarction, the sensitivity decreases to 43%. There is, however, increase in specificity (68%). The clinical significance of a subendocardial infarct with a distinct pattern of focal uptake should probably be considered similar to a comparatively sized transmural infarct.

Pyrophosphate imaging can assist in the clinical problem of documenting recent myocardial damage in a patient presenting with an unreliable electrocardiogram (left bundle branch block) or presenting too late in the clinical course for serial elevation of the cardiospecific enzymes.

Table 4. Causes of Apparent Myocardial Uptake by
^{99m}Tc Pyrophosphate

	Pattern	
Cause	Diffuse	Focal
Acute transmural infarction	+	+ + + +
Acute nontransmural infarction	+ +	+ +
Unstable angina pectoris	+ +	+
Previous myocardial infarction	+	+ +
Postelectric cardioversion	+	+ +
Postcardiac contusion	+	+ +
Cardiac adjacent neoplasms	+	+ +
Congestive cardiomyopathy	+ +	+ +
Left ventricular aneurysm	+	+ +
Calcified valves	+	+ +
Persistent blood pool	+ +	−
Stable angina pectoris	+	+ +
Post chest irradiation	+	+
Skin lesions	−	+
Calcified costal cartilages	−	+
Breast neoplasms/inflammation	+	+
Rib fractures	−	+

Abnormal pyrophosphate uptake occurs in one-third of patients with unstable angina. Even when minimal electrocardiographic changes are present, positive scans have been shown to correlate with myocardial damage as documented by serum creatine kinase (MB-band) elevation in two-thirds of these cases. Of the remaining one-third, close to one-half show uptake at the site of old infarcts. Recent data suggests that subclinical ongoing myocardial necrosis probably accounts for a large proportion of these cases.

Patients presenting with electrocardiographic evidence of inferior myocardial wall infarction have recently been studied by infarct avid scintigraphy. The sensitivity of detecting infarction of this region of the ventricle remains high (94%). ^{99m}Tc pyrophosphate imaging has also been used to delineate any associated extension of the zone of necrosis into the right ventricle. This phenomenon occurs in more than one-third of the cases of inferior infarction and can easily be demonstrated by radionuclide imaging.

In patients with known or suspected coronary artery disease, infarct avid scintigraphy is a sensitive and specific means of establishing whether myocardial infarction occurred in the perioperative period. The addition of a preoperative scan increases the accuracy of the examination, especially in patients undergoing saphenoaortocoronary bypass grafting. Potential false positives (Table 4) are thus identified when the pre and postoperative studies are compared.

The pattern and intensity of pyrophosphate uptake also holds prognostic significance. The amount of pharmaceutical taken up by the infarcted myocardium correlates with mortality and morbidity in the early period following release from hospital. The "doughnut" pattern of uptake is also associated with a high mortality rate (5/6) in the year following acute myocardial infarction. The failure of pyrophosphate uptake either to resolve or to decrease in intensity within 30 days of the first examination identifies patients with an increased death rate in the year following the infarct. A high incidence of concommitant left ventricular dysfunction is seen in this group of patients.

THALLIUM-201

When a patient population with documented myocardial infarction is studied, it becomes apparent that this imaging procedure detects both infarction and regions of periinfarct ischemia. The overall sensitivity in acute (<6 hr) events is 100%; for events occurring between 6 and 24 hours before the imaging period, the sensitivity decreases to 88%. When imaging is carried out at more than 24 hours following the onset of symptoms, the sensitivity decreases to 72% (Wackers et al.). The overall detection rate for transmural events is 88%, while for subendocardial infarctions, sensitivity is 63%. When infarct size is measured using enzymatic criterion, the sensitivity for large infarcts is 94% while for small areas of damage, it is 57%.

For general screening purposes, early (<10 hours following *onset of symptoms*), imaging is nonspecific. False positives occur in patients with angina pectoris (20%), unstable angina (21 to 53%), previous infarcts (38 to 76%), and atypical chest pain (0 to 16%). Using rigid criteria (significant defects seen on three views), the sensitivity is 88% and the specificity is 88%; if a more lax criterion is imposed (a significant defect on *any* of the three views), the sensitivity increases to 100% with a specificity of 65%.

A more careful analysis of the subgroup of patients with unstable angina shows that between 40 to 67% of patients have a positive study when imaging is carried out within 18 hours of the onset of symptoms. Neither the pattern of pharmaceutical uptake, nor discrepancies between the images and other criteria (ECG, enzymatic, history) are of any reliable use in screening those patients that will go on to infarct or to require emergency aortocoronary bypass surgery.

The test can be used to detect the presence of previous myocardial infarction. Blood et al. have reported that the detection rate of a resting thallium study for previous infarction is 54%, while abnormal exercise studies with poor redistribution detect more than 90% of infarctions.

Right ventricular infarction cannot be appreciated on thallium images unless abnormally increased uptake is present in this wall. This will be possible only in patients with hypertrophied right ventricular walls. This is most common in patients with chronic elevations of pulmonary artery pressures.

Thallium imaging is useful in patients after aortocoronary bypass surgery when graft patency is questioned. Exercise and redistribution thallium images are obtained pre and postoperatively. The graft patency rate is over 80% if no new defects are seen on rest/redistribution images or if transient defects are present on the postoperative study. A persistent defect suggests graft occlusion (73%) and, by inference, myocardial damage. In patients with unstable angina or with angina refractory to medical treatment, bypass surgery seems to normalize thallium uptake in those regions showing late redistribution on preoperative scans (77%). Persistent defects represent either new damage in a previously ischemic region or a site of myocardial scarring.

RADIONUCLIDE ANGIOCARDIOGRAPHY (FIRST PASS AND/OR EQUILIBRIUM)

This imaging modality is used to identify alterations in regional and/or global ventricular function seen during and after ischemic damage.

Using the global left ventricular ejection fraction as a criterion, the sensitivity for detection of anterior transmural infarction is high (96 to 100%) while, for inferior myocardial infarctions, the overall sensitivity is 66%. The lack of sensitivity in the latter group can be understood if these patients are divided into two sub-groups, one without ST segment depression on the precordial leads (sensitivity 14%) and one with ST depression (sensitivity 94%).

The early experience with quantitative and qualitative regional ventricular performance in patients with transmural infarction indicates an increased sensitivity in detecting both anterior (13/13) and inferior (16/18) asynergy.

Serial evaluations of both global left ventricular ejection fraction and regional wall motion abnormalities in the postinfarction period have shown that regional and global asynergy improves slowly with little change at two weeks after infarction with more dramatic results at two to four months.

Global left ventricular ejection fraction identifies patients with increased mortality in the postinfarction period; the presence of both low ejection fractions (less than 40%) and complex arrhythmias define a subclass of high-risk patients.

Inferior wall infarction is associated with depressed resting right ventricular ejection fraction in approximately 50% of cases. This concomitant compromise of right ventricular function reflects extension of the infarct zone into the right ventricular wall. The rare case of right-sided congestive failure, low cardiac output, and relatively preserved left-sided function seen with right ventricular infarction can thus be identified by radionuclide angiography, and appropriate therapy with fluids can be instituted.

PREVIOUS MYOCARDIAL INFARCTION

Documentation of previous myocardial infarction can be obtained from thallium or radionuclide ventriculographic studies. Abnormal myocardial uptake of pyrophosphate decreases in intensity in the first two to three weeks following infarction in most patients; while defects on thallium-201 scintigraphy shrink with time after infarction and, by seven months, have disappeared entirely in 25% of patients with previous infarction. The wall motion abnormalities measured by radionuclide angiocardiography do not change significantly in the first four to six weeks following myocardial infarction. A detection rate of greater than 80% can be expected if the results of previous correlative studies with contrast angiography are verified.

Assessment of Miscellaneous Cardiac Disorders

THALLIUM-201

Areas of absent or decreased myocardial uptake may result from any invasive process that replaces cardiac muscle with fibrous tissue, granulomas, or tumor. Thus, focal areas of decreased thallium uptake may be seen in patients with myocardial sarcoidosis, amyloidosis, or other infiltrative processes (as described by Strauss et al.).

In patients with asymmetrical hypertrophic cardiomyopathy, the relative asymmetry of uptake between septum and left ventricular free wall can confirm the presence of this entity. Patients with symmetrical hypertrophy secondary to pressure overload show relatively normal ratios of left ventricular and septal wall uptake.

Right ventricular hypertrophy and concomitant elevations in pulmonary arterial pressures can be estimated by comparing the uptake of the right and left ventricular free walls. Kaaja et al. confirmed the presence of significant pulmonary artery pressure elevations (>30 mm Hg) in 28 of 33 patients when uptake of the right ventricular free wall was comparable to left ventricular free wall uptake. The amount of right ventricular wall uptake also appears to correlate with pulmonary artery pressure elevation and increased pulmonary vascular resistances.

Patients with congestive cardiomyopathy can be expected to have large areas of decreased left ventricular uptake ($>40\%$ circumference) when an underlying ischemic etiology is responsible (sensitivity: 100%). Idiopathic cardiomyopathies more often present with an inhomogeneous diffuse pattern of decreased uptake; large focal areas are less common (incidence: 25%).

VENTRICULOGRAPHY

Pohost et al. demonstrated the feasibility of using gated ventriculography in detecting atrial myxomas: these patients have an area of decreased uptake in the area of the valve plane. The size of these tumors reflect their ease of detection; lesions greater than 80 cm^3 in size were detected when multiple views were taken.

Similarly, left ventricular aneurysms can be detected during either first pass or gated studies. Although no large series are available, differentiation between true and false aneurysm is possible.

Congestive cardiomyopathy can be diagnosed and evaluated using the radionuclide angiocardiogram. Ejection fraction will be decreased at rest ($>40\%$) and the left ventricular cavity will be enlarged. Coronary artery disease is likely to be the etiology if (1) contraction of the basal portions of the left ventricle is the last to be compromised; (2) regional asynergy involves a large contiguous portion of the ventricular contour ($>40\%$); and (3) if the right ventricle is spared. Generalized hypokinesis with occasional areas of dyskinesis is more common in idiopathic cardiomyopathy.

Confirmation of left-sided valvular regurgitation and left ventricular volume overload in the absence of concomitant right-sided valvular regurgitation is possible for cases of significant (regurgitant fraction >0.20) valvular incompetence. The method most frequently used relies on good geometric separation of both ventricles and atria and considers the ratio of left to right ventricular stroke volume counts:

$$\frac{\text{LV stroke volume} - \text{RV stroke volume}}{\text{LV stroke volume}} = \text{Regurgitant fraction}$$

The applicability of this method is now being assessed (Rigo et al.).

Central Circulation

The transit of an intravenously injected bolus of a nondiffusible radiopharmaceutical can be followed and recorded, providing qualitative information about the anatomy of the heart chambers and of the major vessels. This angiocardiogram can also be used to estimate the size of the heart chambers and the patency of the major veins and of the aorta and to detect and quantify physiological shunts.

This technique can be used to provide gross anatomic and functional information in patients with suspected congenital anomalies. Tricuspid atresia and Ebstein's anomaly are identified by a right-to-left shunt through their atrial septal defect. With pulmonary atresia, either a right-to-left shunt is seen through an open ventricular septal defect, or, if this shunt is absent, the bolus persists in the right atrium. The bolus persists in either the right atrium or right ventricle if either tricuspid stenosis or pulmonic stenosis is present. On the left side of the heart, the left atrium is enlarged in the presence of mitral stenosis; in addition, pharmaceutical transit into the left ventricle and aorta is delayed. In severe aortic stenosis at birth or in hypoplastic left heart, a right-to-left shunt via a patent ductus arteriosus may also be detected. In transposition of the great vessels, cardiac activity disappears quickly with only the right heart and aorta being identified.

Right-to-left shunts are measured using either of two techniques. Radioactive particles, such as ^{99m}Tc-labeled macroaggregated albumin (20–50 μm diameter), is injected intravenously; the number of particles impacted in the pulmonary, renal, and cerebral circulations is then measured. Since a small number of particulates (20,000–100,000) is injected, no side effects have been reported. The calculation is made as follows:

$$\% \text{ right-to-left shunt} = \frac{\text{Counts (total body} - \text{lung)}}{\text{Counts (total body)}} \times 100\%$$

Alternatively, the time activity curve (the relationship between time and the quantity of a radioactive tracer in an organ or region of an organ as measured by an external detector) can be analyzed as the bolus passes over the left ventricle:

$$\% \text{ right-to-left shunt} = \frac{\begin{array}{c}\text{Early portion of time-activity curve}\\\text{(extrapolated shunted flow)}\end{array}}{\text{Total curve (total flow)}} \times 100\%$$

For left-to-right shunts, a time activity curve is generated over the lung fields and is mathematically processed to obtain a curve representing the pulmonary circulation and a second curve representing pulmonary recirculation. The difference between these two curves is proportional to systemic flow. The shunt is then calculated as a pulmonary to systemic (QP:QS) flow ratio; ratios greater than 1.2:1 are abnormal. An excellent correlation has been obtained between *oximetry* and this radionuclide method (as described by Parker et al.).

Bibliography

Ahmad M, Dubiel JP, Logan KW, et al: Limited clinical diagnostic specificity of technetium-99m stannous pyrophosphate myocardial imaging in acute myocardial infarction. *Am J Cardiol* 39:50, 1977.

Berman DS, Garcia EV, Maddahi J: Role of thallium-201 imaging in the diagnosis of myocardial ischemia and infarction, in Freeman LM, Weissmann HS (eds): Nuclear Medicine Annual 1980. New York, Raven Press, 1980, p 1.

Blood DK, McCarthy DM, Sciacca RR, et al: Comparison of single dose and double dose thallium-201 myocardial perfusion scintigraphy for the detection of coronary artery disease and prior myocardial infarction. *Circulation* 58:777, 1978.

Borer, JS, Kent KM, Bacharach SL, et al: Sensitivity, specificity and predictive accuracy of radionuclide cineangiography during exercise in patients with coronary artery disease: Comparison with exercise electrocardiography. *Circulation* 60:572, 1979.

Borer JS, Bacharach SL, Green MV, et al: Real time radionuclide cineangiography in the noninvasive evaluation of global and regional left ventricular function at rest and during exercise in patients with coronary artery disease. *N Engl J Med* 296:839, 1977.

Botvinick EH, Taradash MR, Shames DM, et al: Thallium-201 myocardial perfusion scintigraphy for the clinical clarification of normal, abnormal, and equivocal electrocardiographic stress tests. *Am J Cardiol* 41:43, 1978.

Boucher CA, Zir LM, Beller GA, et al: Increased lung uptake of thallium-201 during exercise myocardial imaging: Clinical, hemodynamic and angiographic implications in patients with coronary artery disease. *Am J Cardiol* 46:189, 1980.

Buja LM, Tofe AJ, Kulkarni PV, et al: Sites and mechanisms of localization of technetium-99m phosphorous radiopharmaceuticals in acute myocardial infarcts and other tissues. *J Clin Invest* 60:724, 1977.

Bulkley BH, Hutchins GM, Gailey I, et al: Thallium-201 imaging and gated cardiac blood pool scans in patients with ischemic and idiopathic congestive cardiomyopathy: A clinical and pathologic study. *Circulation* 55:753, 1977.

Caldwell JH, Hamilton GW, Sorensen SG, et al: The detection of coronary artery disease with radionuclide techniques: A comparison of rest-exercise thallium imaging and ejection fraction response. *Circulation* 61:610, 1980.

Cowley MJ, Mantle JA, Rogers WJ, et al: Technetium 99m stannous pyrophosphate myocardial scintigraphy: Reliability and limitations in assessment of acute myocardial infarction. *Circulation* 51:192, 1977.

Fortuin NJ, Weiss JL: Exercise stress testing. *Circulation* 56:699, 1978.

Hellman C, Schmidt DH, Kamath ML, et al: Bypass graft surgery in severe left ventricular dysfunction. *Circulation* 62 (Suppl I):103, 1980.

Herman MV, Heinle RA, Klein MD, et al: Localized disorders in myocardial contraction: Asynergy and its role in congestive heart failure. *N Engl J Med* 277:222, 1967.

Holman BL, Wynne J: Infarct avid (hot spot) myocardial scintigraphy. *Radiol Clin North Am* 18:487, 1980.

Holman BL, Lesch M, Alpert JS: Myocardial scintigraphy with technetium-99m pyrophosphate during the early phase of acute infarction. *Am J Cardiol* 41:39, 1978.

Jengo JA, Freeman R, Brizendine M, et al: Detection of coronary artery disease: Comparison of exercise stress radionuclide angiocardiography and thallium stress perfusion scanning. *Am J Cardiol* 45:535, 1980.

Johnstone DE, Sands MJ, Berger HJ, et al: Comparison of exercise radionuclide angiocardiography and thallium-201 myocardial perfusion imaging in coronary artery disease. *Am J Cardiol* 45:1113, 1980.

Jones RH, McEwan P, Newman GE, et al: Accuracy of diagnosis of coronary artery disease by radionuclide measurement of left ventricular function during rest and exercise. *Circulation* 64:586, 1981.

Kaaja F, Alah M, Goldstein S, et al: Diagnostic value of visualization of the right ventricle using thallium-201 myocardial imaging. *Circulation* 59:182, 1979.

Kolibash AJ, Call TD, Bush CA, et al: Myocardial perfusion as an indicator of graft patency after coronary bypass surgery. *Circulation* 61:882, 1980.

Lyons KP, Olson HG, Aronow WS: Pyrophosphate myocardial imaging. *Semin Nucl Med* 10:168, 1980.

Massie BM, Botvinick EH, Werner JA, et al: Myocardial scintigraphy with technetium-99m stannous pyrophosphate: An insensitive test for nontransmural myocardial infarction. *Am J Cardiol* 43:186, 1979.

McCarthy DM, Blood DK, Sciacca RR, et al: Single dose myocardial perfusion imaging with thallium-201: Application in patients with nondiagnostic electrocardiographic stress tests. *Am J Cardiol* 43:899, 1979.

Parker JA, Treves S: Radionuclide detection, localization and quantitation of intracardiac shunts and shunts between the great arteries, in Holman BL, Sonnenblock DH, Lesch M, (eds), *Principles of cardiovascular nuclear medicine,* New York, Grune and Stratton, 1978, p 189.

Pavel DG, Zimmer AM, Patterson VN: In vivo labeling of red blood cells with ^{99m}Tc: A new approach to blood pool visualization. *J Nucl Med* 18:305, 1977.

Pohost GM, Boucher CA, Zir LM, et al: The thallium stress test: The qualitative approach revisited. *Circulation* 60 (Suppl II):581A, 1979.

Pohost GM, Zir LM, Moore RH, et al: Differentiation of transiently ischemic from infarcted myocardium by serial imaging after a single dose of thallium-201. *Circulation* 55:294, 1977.

Reduto LA, Berger HJ, Cohen LS, et al: Sequential radionuclide assessment of left and right ventricular performance after acute transmural myocardial infarction. *Ann Intern Med* 89:441, 1978.

Rigo P, Alderson PO, Robertson RM, et al: Measurement of aortic and mitral regurgitation by gated cardiac blood pool scans. *Circulation* 60:306, 1979.

Ritchie JL, Zaret BL, Strauss HW, et al: Myocardial imaging with thallium-201: A multicenter study in patients with angina pectoris or acute myocardial infarction. *Am J Cardiol* 42:345, 1978.

Sharpe DN, Botvinick EH, Shames DM, et al: The noninvasive diagnosis of right ventricular infarction. *Circulation* 57:483, 1978.

Strauss HW, McKusick KA, Boucher CA, et al: Of linens and laces: The eighth anniversary of the gated blood pool scan. *Semin Nucl Med* 9:296, 1979.

Strauss HW, Harrison K, Langan JK, et al: Thallium-201 for myocardial imaging: Relation of thallium-201 to regional myocardial perfusion. *Circulation* 51:641, 1975.

Wackers FJTh, Lie KI, Liem KL, et al: Potential value of thallium-201 scintigraphy as a means of selecting patients for the coronary care unit. *Br Heart J* 41:111, 1979.

Weich HF, Strauss HW, Pitt B: The extraction of thallium-201 by the myocardium. *Circulation* 56:188, 1977.

Wynne J, Holman BL: Acute myocardial infarct scintigraphy with infarct-avid radiotracers. *Med Clinics North Am* 64:119, 1980.

Zaret BL, DiCola VC, Donabedian RK, et al: Dual radionuclide study of myocardial infarction: Relationships between myocardial uptake of potassium-43, technetium-99m stannous pyrophosphate, regional myocardial blood flow and creatine phospokinase depletion. *Circulation* 53:422, 1976.

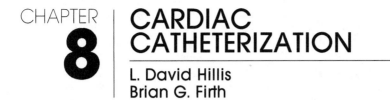

CHAPTER
8
CARDIAC CATHETERIZATION

L. David Hillis
Brian G. Firth

Since its inception in the 1940s, cardiac catheterization has played an important role in the understanding of cardiac and circulatory physiology and pathophysiology and in the diagnosis of assorted cardiac abnormalities. During its early years, catheterization was performed sparingly and with substantial risk. As time has elapsed, however, it has become established throughout the world, and the associated morbidity and mortality have fallen drastically. Therefore, cardiac catheterization now plays a vital role in the diagnostic evaluation of the patient with suspected cardiac disease and can be performed with minimal risk to the patient.

Indications and Contraindications

Cardiac catheterization is appropriate in several clinical circumstances. First, it is indicated to confirm or exclude the presence of a condition already suspected because of findings on physical examination and/or noninvasive evaluation. In such a circumstance, it allows one both to establish the presence and to assess the severity of cardiac disease. Second, catheterization is indicated to clarify a confusing or obscure clinical problem, that is, to arrive at a diagnosis in a patient whose clinical presentation and noninvasive evaluation are inconclusive. Third, with only rare exceptions, catheterization should be performed in all patients for whom corrective cardiac surgery is contemplated, in order to confirm the suspected abnormality and to exclude associated defects that might require the surgeon's attention. Occasionally, cardiac catheterization is performed purely as a research procedure.

Catheterization is absolutely contraindicated if a mentally competent individual does not consent. It is relatively contraindicated if an intercurrent condition exists that, corrected, would improve the safety of the procedure. Examples of such conditions include ventricular irritability, uncontrolled cardiac failure, digitalis toxicity, electrolyte imbalance, high fever, severe anemia, hypovolemia, uncontrolled systemic arterial hypertension, and an uncorrected bleeding diathesis. Catheterization is unwarranted in the patient with a recent myocardial infarction unless immediate surgery is planned.

Techniques of Cardiac Catheterization

The catheterization of the right and left sides of the heart can be accomplished by the introduction of catheters either by direct vision (into the brachial vein and artery)

153

or by percutaneous puncture (of the femoral vein and artery). To use the brachial approach, local anesthetic is introduced into an area 3–4 cm in diameter 1–2 cm above the flexor crease of the arm, after which a transverse cutdown is performed. If both right and left heart catheterization is planned, the incision should be wide (2–3 cm in length) and located over the brachial artery; if only right heart catheterization is contemplated, a small incision can be made directly over a medial vein. Once the skin incision is made, the subcutaneous tissues are separated by blunt dissection with a curved hemostat, and the vein and artery are isolated, separated from adjacent tissues, and tagged. The catheters are introduced under direct vision and are advanced into the great vessels and heart.

Following catheterization by the brachial approach, the catheters are removed, and the vein used for right heart catheterization is ligated. The artery used for left heart catheterization is cleaned and rendered free of thrombi, after which the arteriotomy is repaired. After the arteriotomy has been closed successfully and blood flow has been restored to the distal arm, the wound is flushed with saline, the incision is sutured, and the site of the cutdown is dressed appropriately.

To use the percutaneous femoral approach, local anesthetic is introduced into an area 3–4 cm in diameter 1–2 cm below the inguinal crease. A small incision (about $\frac{1}{2}$ cm long) is made over the vessels to be used for catheter introduction and passage, after which a "tunnel" is constructed with a straight hemostat from the skin incision to the desired femoral vessel. An 18 gauge needle (Seldinger needle) is introduced through the skin incision and tunnel at a 45–60° angle into the lumen of the femoral artery or vein. Once there is free blood flow through the needle, a guide wire is advanced into the lumen of the punctured vessel. The wire is held firmly in place as the needle is removed. Then, with the wire in the vessel, a catheter is threaded onto it and into the vessel lumen, after which the wire is removed.

Following catheterization by this approach, the catheters are removed, and hemostasis is achieved by hand pressure over the puncture site for sufficient time to insure the cessation of bleeding. Hemostasis is generally obtained after pressure has been placed on the femoral vein for 5–10 minutes and on the femoral artery for 15–20 minutes. Subsequently, the patient is required to remain in bed and to immobilize the involved leg for 12–24 hours.

The choice of approach (brachial or femoral) for both venous and arterial catheterization is determined by the preference and experience of the catheterizer and by the anatomic and pathophysiologic abnormalities of the patient. In general, right heart catheterization is easier via the brachial approach in the patient with right ventricular and right atrial dilatation. In contrast, right heart catheterization is performed preferentially via the femoral approach in the patient with a suspected secundum atrial septal defect. Thus, in choosing the route for right heart catheterization, it is necessary to be cognizant of anatomic abnormalities and specific disease entities. In most patients, left heart catheterization can be performed by either the brachial or the femoral approach. Certain conditions make it difficult to perform left heart catheterization by the femoral approach, such as extensive peripheral vascular disease, severe obesity, severe systemic arterial hypertension, bleeding diatheses, and any disorder that causes a markedly augmented arterial pulse pressure (e.g., severe aortic regurgitation or thyrotoxicosis). In turn, the brachial approach for left heart catheterization is relatively contraindicated if there is evidence of severe brachiocephalic arterial disease.

In most catheterization laboratories, the brachial or femoral approach is used in almost all procedures. Occasionally, catheterization of one or more cardiac chambers is necessary via another route. For example, a rare patient with severe left-sided valvular disease may require a direct puncture of the left ventricle to measure left ventricular pressure and to perform a ventriculogram.

Hemodynamic Measurements

CARDIAC OUTPUT

The role of the heart is to deliver an adequate quantity of blood to the body. This flow of blood is known as the cardiac output (CO) and is expressed in liters per minute. Since the magnitude of CO is proportional to body surface area, one person may be compared to another by means of the cardiac index (CI), that is, the CO adjusted for body surface area. The normal CI is 3.1 liters per minute per square meter of body surface (range, 2.8–4.2) (Table 1).

There are two major methods of measuring CO, the Fick method and the indicator dilution technique; the latter can be performed by the injection of indocyanine green or by the thermodilution technique.

Fick Method

The measurement of CO by the Fick method is based on the hypothesis that the uptake or release of a substance by an organ is the product of the blood flow to that organ and the regional arteriovenous (AV) concentration difference of the particular substance. To measure CO in humans, this principle is applied to the lungs, and the substance measured is oxygen (O_2). By measuring the amount of O_2 extracted from inspired air by the lungs and the AV O_2 difference across the lungs, pulmonary blood flow may be calculated. Since pulmonary blood flow equals systemic blood flow in most people, the Fick method allows one to measure systemic blood flow.

The Fick formula for the calculation of CO is:

$$\text{CO (L/min)} = \frac{O_2 \text{ consumption (ml/min)}}{\text{AV } O_2 \text{ difference across the lungs}}$$

The O_2 consumption is determined directly by collecting a timed sample (usually 3–4 minutes) of expired air in a special receptacle called a Douglas bag. The volume of this collection is measured, and the difference in O_2 content between inspired and expired air is calculated. From these data, the person's O_2 consumption (in ml/min) is determined. Determining the AV O_2 difference across the lungs requires that blood from the vessels adjacent to the lungs (i.e., the pulmonary artery and vein) be analyzed for O_2 content. Since the saturation of pulmonary venous blood is similar to that of systemic arterial blood, pulmonary arterial and systemic arterial samples are usually obtained for the Fick determination of CO. The O_2 content of pulmonary and systemic arterial blood may be measured directly or calculated from the O_2

Table 1.   Normal Hemodynamic Values

Flows	
Cardiac index (L/min/m^2)	2.8–4.2
Stroke volume index (ml/m^2)	30–65
Pressures (mm Hg)	
Systemic arterial	
Peak systolic/end diastolic	100–140/60–90
Mean	70–105
Left ventricle	
Peak systolic/end diastolic	100–140/3–12
Left atrium (pcw)	
Mean	1–10
a wave	3–15
v wave	3–15
Pulmonary artery	
Peak systolic/end diastolic	16–30/0–8
Mean	10–16
Right ventricle	
Peak systolic/end diastolic	16–30/0–8
Right atrium	
Mean	0–8
a wave	2–10
v wave	2–10
Resistances	
Systemic vascular resistance	
Dynes-sec-cm^{-5}	770–1500
Resistance units	10–20
Pulmonary vascular resistance	
Dynes-sec-cm^{-5}	20–120
Resistance units	0.25–1.5
Oxygen consumption (L/min/m^2)	110–150
Arteriovenous O$_2$ difference (ml/100 ml)	3.0–4.5

saturation of the blood: O$_2$ content = Hgb (in gm/100 ml) $\times$ 1.39 $\times$ saturation, where 1.39 ml is the maximum O$_2$-carrying capacity of 1 gm of Hgb.

The normal O$_2$ consumption index (O$_2$ consumption/m^2 of body surface) is 110–150 ml/min/m^2 (Table 1). In general, the O$_2$ consumption is higher in young people than in the old. It increases with hyperthyroidism, hyperthermia, and exercise and decreases with hypothyroidism or hypothermia. The normal AV O$_2$ difference is 3.0 to 4.5 volumes percent (ml O$_2$/100 ml of blood).

The following is an example of the Fick calculation of CO: (1) O$_2$ consumption

= 250 ml/min; (2) Hgb = 15 gms/100 ml; (3) systemic arterial O_2 saturation = 0.95 (95%); (4) pulmonary arterial O_2 saturation = 0.70 (70%):

$$CO = \frac{250}{(15)(1.39)(10)(0.95) \; - \; (15)(1.39)(10)(0.70)}$$

$$= \frac{250}{198.1 \; - \; 145.9} = 4.78 \text{ L/minute}$$

The Fick method has several potential sources of error: (1) an incomplete collection of expired air causes an underestimation of O_2 consumption, leading to a falsely low figure for CO. This is the most common source of error. (2) Incorrect timing of the expired air collection leads to a faulty estimate of O_2 consumption. (3) The Douglas bag analysis should be performed soon after its collection, since air diffuses in and out of the bag if there is a substantial delay. (4) The spectrophotometric determination of O_2 saturations in the blood samples may be inaccurate if certain substances, such as indocyanine green, have been introduced into the blood. (5) The mixed venous blood sample (pulmonary arterial) must, indeed, be *mixed venous*. It must be obtained from the pulmonary artery, not from a systemic vein, right atrium, or right ventricle; similarly, it must not be partially contaminated by pulmonary capillary wedge blood.

The average error in determining O_2 consumption is about 6%, and that for AV O_2 difference is 5%. When the AV O_2 difference is small, errors in measurement are particularly likely to occur. Therefore, the Fick method is most accurate in the patient with a low CO and least accurate in one with a high CO.

Indicator Dilution Technique

This technique is based on the principle that the volume of fluid within a container can be measured if one adds a known quantity of indicator to the fluid and then measures the concentration of the indicator after it has been completely mixed with the fluid. The indicator most often used is indocyanine green, an easily detectable, water-soluble, nontoxic substance. To measure CO using indocyanine green, (1) a known concentration of indicator must be injected; (2) there must be complete mixing of the indocyanine green between the sites of injection and sampling; but (3) there must be no metabolism or disappearance of the indicator between the sites of injection and sampling. In most catheterization laboratories, CO is measured by injecting indocyanine green into the pulmonary artery while blood is withdrawn at a constant rate from a systemic artery through an optical densitometer. The lungs, left atrium, and left ventricle act as adequate mixing sites, and there is no degradation of indocyanine green between the pulmonary and systemic arteries.

More recently, cold saline or 5% dextrose-in-water have been used as indicators to measure CO. The catheter used for this measurement is a balloon-tipped, flow-directed, polyvinylchloride catheter with two openings, one at the tip and the other 25–30 cm proximal to the tip. In addition, a small thermistor is located 2–5 cm from the tip. This catheter is inserted into a vein and advanced to the pulmonary artery. Thus, the distal opening is in a large pulmonary artery, and the proximal opening is in the right atrium. Iced fluid is injected into the right atrial opening, and the temporary change in temperature at the thermistor is recorded.

The calculation of CO by the indicator dilution technique is usually done by a minicomputer, which establishes that the downslope of the inscribed curve is exponential and then computes the area under the curve, while excluding the recirculation peak. These calculations can be done manually, but require a clear mathematical separation of the initial circulation peak from that of normal recirculation.

With both indocyanine green and cold saline or dextrose, therefore, CO can be determined by assessing the concentration of an indicator after adequate mixing with blood has occurred. To insure an accurate assessment of CO, great care must be taken, first, to inject an exact amount of indicator; second, to inject the indicator as rapidly as possible (so that, in fact, it is delivered as a bolus); third, to calibrate the densitometer and recorder systems precisely; and fourth, to insure that the withdrawal of blood (in the case of indocyanine green) at the sampling site is uniform and not accompanied by air bubbles. If care is taken to eliminate these sources of error, the indicator dilution technique is a reliable method of measuring CO. This technique is least accurate in the individual with a low CO and most accurate in one with a high CO.

PRESSURE MEASUREMENTS

One of the most important functions of cardiac catheterization is the accurate measurement and recording of intracardiac pressures. Once a catheter has been positioned in the desired cardiac chamber, it is connected either directly or through stiff, fluid-filled tubing to a pressure transducer, which transforms a pressure signal into an electrical signal. The accurate measurement of pressures requires close attention to the details of the catheter-transducer system, including proper transducer balancing as well as removing air bubbles from the catheters and connections. Errors in pressure measurement may occur in several ways: (1) An accurate zero reference is essential. All manometers must be referenced to the same zero level, which must be changed if the patient's position is altered. (2) Pressure transducers must be calibrated frequently, preferably before each pressure recording.

During most catheterizations, pressures are measured directly from each of the cardiac chambers except the left atrium. A direct pressure measurement is obtained with a catheter in the right atrium, right ventricle, pulmonary artery, ascending aorta, and left ventricle. In contrast, the left atrium is seldom entered unless a transseptal catheterization is performed (passage of a catheter from the right atrium across the interatrial septum into the left atrium). The left atrial pressure is generally recorded "indirectly," that is, as the pulmonary capillary wedge pressure. To accomplish this, an end-hole catheter is placed in the pulmonary artery and advanced into the pulmonary arterial tree until it is effectively wedged. If the catheter is wedged adequately, the resultant pressure is left atrial in origin, and the blood withdrawn from it is fully saturated. The demonstration that fully saturated blood can be withdrawn from the catheter confirms that the pressure is indeed left atrial.

In addition to the recording of pressures from each of the cardiac chambers, it is important that the pressures from certain chambers be examined simultaneously to confirm or exclude the presence of valvular lesions. Thus, left ventricular and pulmonary capillary wedge pressures should be recorded simultaneously to ascertain if mitral stenosis is present (Figs. 1 and 2). Likewise, the left ventricular and systemic arterial pressures should be displayed concurrently to evaluate the presence or absence of left ventricular outflow tract obstruction (Figs. 3–5).

Recording intracardiac and peripheral vascular pressures can demonstrate hemodynamic evidence of valvular regurgitation. For instance, large regurgitation waves in the pulmonary capillary wedge tracing are indicative of severe (and usually acute or subacute) mitral regurgitation (Fig. 6). Conversely, a wide peripheral arterial pulse pressure in conjunction with a greatly elevated left ventricular end-diastolic pressure is suggestive of aortic regurgitation (Fig. 7). In short, both the absolute level and the qualitative configuration of the intracardiac and peripheral vascular pressures are important in the diagnosis and quantitation of valvular heart disease.

The normal intracardiac and peripheral vascular flows, pressures, and resistances are listed in Table 1.

RESISTANCES

The resistance of a vascular bed can be described by dividing the pressure gradient across the bed by the mean flow through it. Thus:

Systemic vascular resistance =

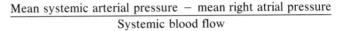

$$\frac{\text{Mean systemic arterial pressure } - \text{ mean right atrial pressure}}{\text{Systemic blood flow}}$$

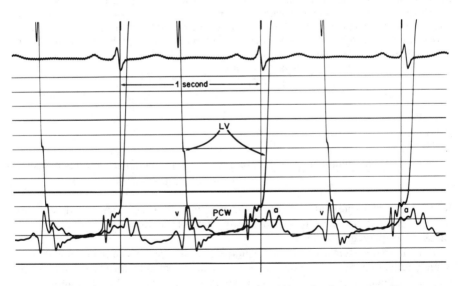

Figure 1 Simultaneous recording of left ventricular, LV, and pulmonary capillary wedge, PCW, pressures in a patient without mitral valve disease. The distance between each horizontal line above the baseline represents 4 mm Hg, and the distance between each vertical line represents 1 sec. The PCW a wave occurs in conjunction with the a wave of the LV pressure trace, and the PCW v wave occurs with the downslope of the LV trace. Note that during diastole the LV and PCW pressures are superimposed; that is, there is no pressure gradient between the PCW and LV.

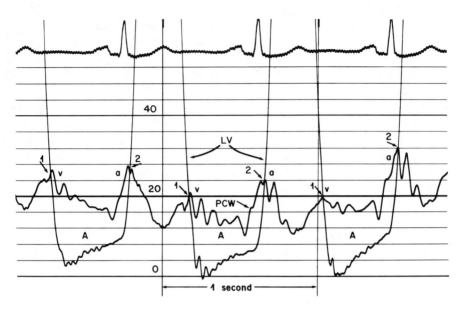

Figure 2 Simultaneous recording of LV and PCW pressures in a patient with mitral stenosis. Throughout diastole, from points 1 to 2, there is a pressure gradient between the PCW and LV pressures. This patient, a 28-year-old woman, had a cardiac output of 3740 ml/min, measured simultaneously with this pressure tracing. The heart rate was 68 beats/min, the mean diastolic filling period was 0.49 sec/beat, and the mean pressure gradient, derived by dividing A by the average gradient duration, was 12.7 mm Hg. Using the Gorlin formula, the mitral valve area was

$$\frac{3740/(68)(0.49)}{(38)(\sqrt{12.7})} = 0.82 \text{ cm}^2$$

Pulmonary vascular resistance =

$$\frac{\text{Mean pulmonary arterial pressure} - \text{mean pulmonary venous pressure}}{\text{Pulmonary blood flow}}$$

Resistances are expressed in either resistance units (mm Hg/L/min) or dynes-sec-cm^{-5} (resistance unit determination × 80). The normal values for vascular resistances are displayed in Table 1.

An increased systemic vascular resistance is usually present in patients with systemic arterial hypertension. It may also be seen in the patient with a reduced forward CO and compensatory arteriolar vasoconstriction. In turn, a reduced systemic vascular resistance may be present in the patient with an inappropriately increased CO, the causes of which include AV fistula, severe anemia, high fever, and thyrotoxicosis. An elevated pulmonary vascular resistance may be present because of severe primary lung disease, Eisenmenger's syndrome (alterations in the pulmonary vasculature in response to increased pulmonary blood flow), and a greatly elevated pulmonary venous pressure due to left-sided myocardial and/or valvular dysfunction.

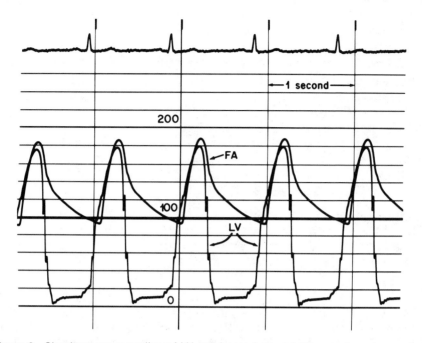

Figure 3 Simultaneous recording of LV and femoral arterial, FA, pressures in a patient without LV outflow tract obstruction. Pressures are indicated in mm Hg on the vertical scale. Note that there is no pressure gradient during systole between LV and FA; in fact, the peak systolic FA pressure is about 5 mm Hg higher than LV. See Fig. 4 for an explanation of this phenomenon.

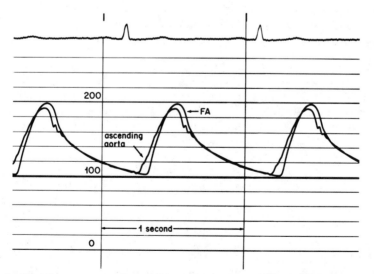

Figure 4 Simultaneous recording of ascending aortic and FA pressures in a normal individual. The peak systolic FA pressure is slightly higher than the peak systolic ascending aortic pressure, due to peripheral amplification of pressure, a normal phenomenon.

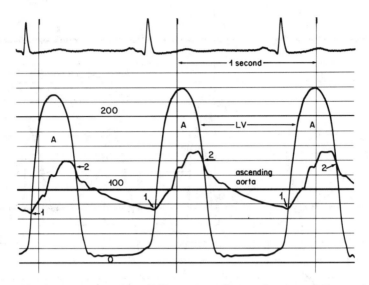

Figure 5 Simultaneous recording of LV and ascending aortic pressures in a patient with severe aortic stenosis. Throughout systole, from points 1 to 2, there is a pressure gradient between LV and aorta. This patient, a 50-year-old man, had a cardiac output of 3350 ml/min, a heart rate of 62 beats/min, a mean systolic ejection time of 0.36 sec/beat, and a mean pressure gradient throughout systole of 83 mm Hg, determined by dividing A by the average duration of the gradient. Thus, the aortic valve area equals

$$\frac{3350/(62)(0.36)}{(44.5)(\sqrt{83})} = 0.37 \ cm^2$$

VALVE AREAS

Through the application of standard fluid dynamic principles, the resistance to blood flow through a stenosed valve can be expressed as a valve orifice area. The data required for the calculation of a valve area may be obtained during cardiac catheterization. Specifically, the pressures on either side of a stenotic valve and the flow across it must be known. The Gorlin equation is then used to calculate the valve area:

$$Valve \ area = \frac{CO/(DFP \ or \ SEP)(heart \ rate)}{(constant)(\sqrt{mean \ pressure \ gradient})}$$

where DFP = diastolic filling period, and SEP = systolic ejection period. If an atrioventricular valve (mitral or tricuspid) is in question, the diastolic filling period is employed; if the aortic or pulmonic valve is involved, the systolic ejection period is used. The constant used is 38 for the mitral valve and 44.5 for the other valves. The mean pressure gradient is the average gradient throughout systole (for aortic and pulmonic valves) or diastole (for mitral or tricuspid valves). Note that the square root of the mean pressure gradient is used in the calculation.

The normal mitral valve is 3–5 cm^2. Substantial stenosis can occur before a pressure gradient appears. A mitral valve with an area of 0–1.0 cm^2 is considered severely stenotic (Fig. 2); 1.0–1.25 cm^2, moderately stenotic; and 1.25–1.50 cm^2, mildly stenotic. A valve area over 1.50 cm^2 is not necessarily normal, but does not usually constitute a hemodynamically significant obstruction to blood flow. The normal aortic valve has a cross-sectional area of 3–3.5 cm^2, but hemodynamically important aortic stenosis does not develop until the valve area falls below 1.1–1.2 cm^2. Specifically, an aortic valve with an area of less than 0.7 cm^2 is severely stenotic (Fig. 5); 0.7 to 1.0 cm^2, moderately stenotic; and 1.0 to 1.2 cm^2, mildly stenotic.

It is essential that all the variables used to calculate a valve area (CO, systolic ejection period or diastolic filling period, heart rate, and pressure gradient) are measured in close temporal proximity to one another and with the patient in a hemodynamically stable state. Great care must be exercised in the acquisition of these data, since the decision for operative intervention is based on the calculated valve area.

SHUNT DETECTION AND MEASUREMENT

The detection and quantitation of an intracardiac shunt can be accomplished by several techniques. (See also Chapter 18.) First, the measurement of O$_2$ content within the cardiac chambers and the peripheral vessels allows one to localize the site of intracardiac shunting and to determine its magnitude. Once the site of intra-

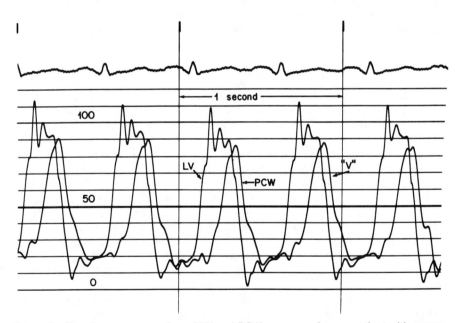

Figure 6 Simultaneous recording of LV and PCW pressures from a patient with severe, acute mitral regurgitation due to an inferior myocardial infarction with resultant papillary muscle rupture. Note that there is no gradient between LV and PCW during diastole. However, the PCW tracing demonstrates large regurgitant v waves as high as 90 mm Hg.

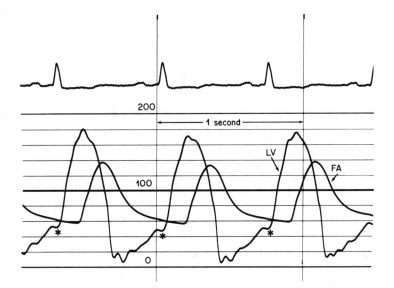

Figure 7 Simultaneous recording of LV and FA pressures from a patient with mixed aortic stenosis and regurgitation. The FA upstroke occurs later than that of the LV, due to the time required for pulse wave transmission from the LV to the FA. There is a systolic gradient between LV and FA of about 40 mm Hg peak to peak. The FA pulse pressure is only minimally widened. During diastole, the LV pressure demonstrates a gradual and steady rise, so that the LV pressure at end-diastole (asterisks) is about 50 mm Hg.

cardiac shunting is determined, one can calculate the blood flow to the pulmonary and systemic circulations. The oximetric determination of intracardiac shunting is highly specific but relatively insensitive for detecting such shunting; that is, an oximetric assessment reliably demonstrates the presence of a large shunt but usually fails to detect a small one.

Second, the presence and magnitude of an intracardiac shunt can be demonstrated and quantitated by indicator dilution injections. By performing the injection of indocyanine green and the simultaneous withdrawal of blood from several sites within the heart and great vessels, one can determine the site and size of the intracardiac shunt (Figs. 8–10). Indocyanine green injections are more sensitive than oximetry for detecting and quantitating small intracardiac shunts. The intravenous injection of hydrogen (dissolved in saline) with simultaneous sensing with a platinum-tipped electrode in the aorta can be used to detect very small right-to-left shunts. This technique is the most sensitive method available for the detection of right-to-left shunts.

Third, angiography can be used to demonstrate an intracardiac shunt, but this technique does not allow one to quantitate the shunt. For example, a ventricular septal defect with shunting from the left to the right ventricle can be demonstrated with a left ventriculogram in a 30–40° left anterior oblique projection. Alternatively, a patent ductus arteriosus with shunting from the aorta to the pulmonary artery can be detected via a proximal aortogram.

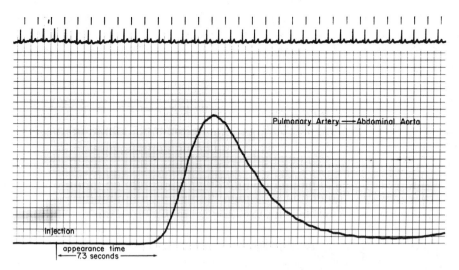

Figure 8 A normal curve following the injection of 5 mg of indocyanine green into the pulmonary artery, with simultaneous withdrawal of blood from the abdominal aorta. The time between injection and first appearance of the indicator is 7.3 sec.

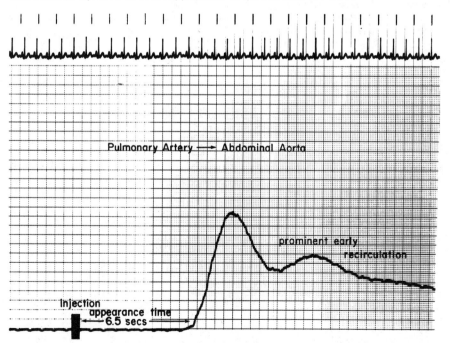

Figure 9 A curve following the injection of 5 mg of indocyanine green into the pulmonary artery, with blood withdrawal from the abdominal aorta, in a patient with a large left-to-right intracardiac shunt, in this case, an atrial septal defect. In comparison to a normal curve (Fig. 8), there is a very prominent early recirculation peak. The appearance time is normal, thus excluding a right-to-left shunt distal to the site of injection.

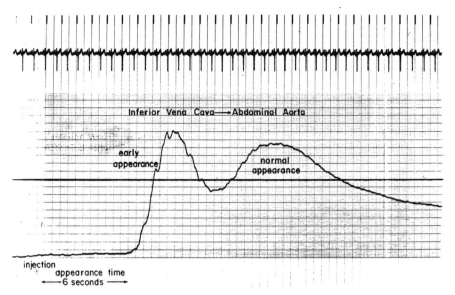

Figure 10 A curve following the injection of 5 mg of indocyanine green into the inferior vena cava, with blood withdrawal from the abdominal aorta, in a patient with a large right-to-left intracardiac shunt, in this case, a large ventricular septal defect with pulmonary infundibular stenosis, or tetralogy of Fallot. The initial peak represents early appearance of indocyanine green in the abdominal aorta, a reflection of the blood being shunted right-to-left through the VSD. The second peak represents normal appearance of indocyanine green.

BALLOON-TIPPED, FLOW-DIRECTED (SWAN-GANZ) CATHETERS

In 1970, the balloon-tipped, flow-directed catheter was introduced for right heart catheterization at the bedside, without the need for fluoroscopy. At present, it is widely used to monitor pulmonary arterial and pulmonary capillary wedge pressures in the critically ill patient in an intensive care unit. The catheter, which has an inflatable balloon at its tip, is made of polyvinylchloride and, therefore, is extremely soft. The standard balloon-tipped catheter has two lumina—the smaller lumen allows inflation of the balloon; the larger lumen allows one to measure pressures and obtain blood specimens.

Before using the balloon-tipped catheter, the balloon should be inflated in a bowl of saline to exclude an air leak, and the catheter lumen should be flushed with saline. The catheter may be inserted at the bedside either percutaneously (via the femoral, internal jugular, or subclavian vein) or by direct exposure of the brachial vein. When it is introduced without the use of fluoroscopy, it should be passed into the vasculature for 10–30 cm (depending on the site of introduction) before the balloon is inflated. The catheter is marked at 10 cm intervals to facilitate this procedure. Before advancing the catheter, blood should be aspirated through it to insure that it is intravascular. Then the balloon is inflated gently with up to 1 ml of air. If there is resistance to balloon inflation, the catheter should be advanced or withdrawn carefully until the balloon can be inflated freely. The catheter is then connected to a pressure transducer to record right atrial pressure. It is also valuable to obtain a blood sample for oximetric analysis in each right heart chamber or vessel where pressures are recorded to exclude left-to-right intracardiac shunting.

Once a blood sample and pressure have been obtained from the right atrium, the catheter is advanced gently with the balloon inflated while pressure and the electrocardiogram are observed. Particular care must be exercised while traversing the right ventricle; if more than 2–3 consecutive ventricular premature beats are provoked, the catheter should be withdrawn quickly. If the catheter does not pass easily from the right ventricle to the pulmonary artery, it should be withdrawn to the right atrium and the procedure repeated. Once it has passed to the pulmonary artery and the pressure has been recorded (Fig. 11), it is advanced gently (with the balloon still inflated) until the waveform changes to that of a pulmonary capillary wedge pressure (Fig. 12). A fully oxygenated blood specimen from this site confirms that the catheter is truly in a wedged position. When the balloon is deflated, the waveform should change to that of pulmonary arterial pressure.

It is occasionally impossible to pass the balloon-tipped catheter without the use of fluoroscopic control, particularly in the patient with a large right atrium, right ventricle, or pulmonary hypertension. In this case, it may be necessary to use a guide wire to stiffen the catheter while it is passed under fluoroscopic visualization. It is generally easier to pass the catheter without the use of fluoroscopy when the site of vascular entry is central (i.e., internal jugular or subclavian vein) rather than peripheral.

The balloon-tipped, flow-directed catheter offers several advantages over the more traditional stiff catheter used for right heart catheterization; at the same time, it has

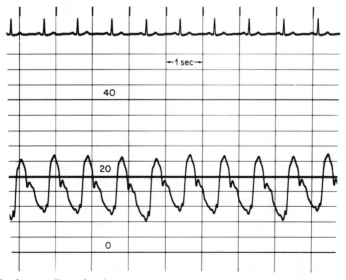

Figure 11 A recording of pulmonary arterial pressure with a Swan-Ganz catheter; the pressure averages about 25/10 mm Hg.

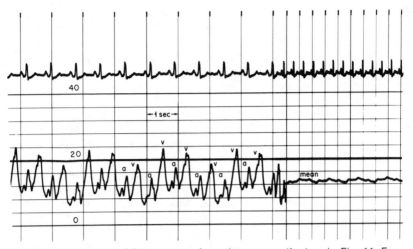

Figure 12 A recording of PCW pressure from the same patient as in Fig. 11. For each QRS complex, there are two pressure waves: a and v. The mean PCW pressure is 13 mm Hg.

certain drawbacks. Since it is unusually soft, perforation of the major vessels and heart is virtually impossible, whereas such perforation occasionally occurs with the use of a stiff catheter. As indicated, the flow-directed catheter can be inserted and advanced without fluoroscopic control, although catheter manipulation is easier with fluoroscopic assistance. Apart from its safety, the balloon-tipped, flow-directed catheter can be equipped with a distal thermistor and a third lumen 25–30 cm from the tip through which iced saline is injected and CO measured by the thermodilution technique.

The major disadvantages of the balloon-tipped, flow-directed catheter stem from the same features that are responsible for its advantages. First, because the catheter is unusually soft, the pressure recordings obtained through it may contain a good deal of "catheter whip," that is, artifact introduced by the movement of the catheter itself within the heart. Second, since the catheter is no larger than 7 French in size and yet contains two or, in the case of a thermodilution catheter, three lumina, the distal lumen is small in size, making blood sampling difficult. Third, since this catheter is advanced in the direction of blood flow, its placement in the pulmonary artery may be impossible if flow within the right heart chambers is bidirectional. For example, advancing a balloon-tipped, flow-directed catheter to the pulmonary artery in a patient with severe tricuspid regurgitation may be impossible, since the jet of regurgitation directs the catheter from the right ventricle back into the right atrium. Despite these limitations, this catheter allows one to measure right and left-sided filling pressures and to make appropriate therapeutic decisions regarding fluid and drug administration.

The risks and complications of the balloon-tipped, flow-directed catheter are similar to those of any catheter used for right-sided catheterization: ventricular irritability during passage through the right ventricle and local inflammation or infection at the site of entrance. In addition, because of its softness, the balloon-tipped catheter is easily knotted. Improper inflation and deflation of the balloon can lead to rupture of a small pulmonary artery or to subsegmental pulmonary infarction. By and large, however, the balloon-tipped, flow-directed catheter is extremely safe. Once it is positioned in the pulmonary artery, it may be left in place for 48–72 hours.

Electrophysiologic Measurements

The normal surface electrocardiogram provides a record of atrial depolarization (P wave), ventricular depolarization (QRS complex), and ventricular repolarization (T wave). The PR interval is the period during which the electrical impulse passes through the atrioventricular node, the bundle of His, and the left and right bundle branches. None of these events is recorded on the surface electrocardiogram. However, an electrical recording may be made directly from the bundle of His using an electrode catheter positioned across the tricuspid valve immediately adjacent to the His bundle. Catheter introduction and manipulation for this recording are most easily performed from the femoral vein. A tripolar electrode catheter is advanced from the right atrium to the right ventricular outflow tract, after which it is withdrawn slowly and rotated until it is positioned midway across the tricuspid valve. This makes possible the recording of discrete signals from the right atrium, His bundle, and right ventricle (Fig. 13). In addition, electrode catheters may be positioned in the right

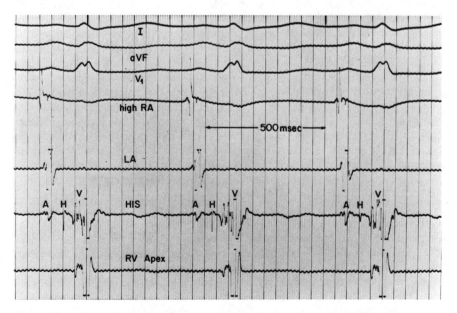

Figure 13 A typical recording from an electrophysiologic study. From top to bottom, impulses are recorded from (1) surface leads 1, aV$_F$, and V$_1$; (2) high RA; (3) LA, catheterized from the RA via a patent foramen ovale; (4) His bundle; and (5) RV apex. The A (atrial), H (His), and V (ventricular) impulses of a normal His bundle recording are labeled accordingly.

atrium, coronary sinus or left atrium (via a patent foramen ovale), and left or right ventricles to allow atrial or ventricular pacing at different rates while intracavitary electrical signals are recorded from the His bundle and other sites (Fig. 13).

His bundle electrocardiography is useful in several clinical situations. (1) It is helpful in determining the origin of impulses with a wide QRS morphology on the surface electrocardiogram, particularly when discrete P waves are absent. In this instance, a His bundle recording allows one to differentiate beats of supraventricular origin with aberrant ventricular conduction from those of ventricular origin. (2) His bundle electrocardiography is often used to define the site of atrioventricular conduction delay, namely, whether such delay is above or below the His bundle. This is of prognostic importance and may help to determine the need for permanent pacemaker implantation. (3) A His bundle electrocardiogram is valuable in determining the site of origin and underlying mechanism of both supraventricular and ventricular tachyarrhythmias. As such, it may allow more rational therapy for these arrhythmias. (Electrophysiologic measurements are also discussed in Chapter 17.)

Angiographic Measurements

LEFT VENTRICULOGRAPHY

The opacification and simultaneous cineangiocardiography of the left ventricle allows one to assess global and segmental left ventricular function, left ventricular volumes and ejection fraction, and the presence and severity of mitral regurgitation. To achieve adequate opacification, a large bolus of radiographic contrast material must be delivered to the left ventricle over a short period of time. In the normal adult, 55–60 ml of contrast material is injected over 3–4 seconds; thus, approximately 13–20 ml are injected per second. As the contrast material is injected into the left ventricle, cineangiocardiography is performed. The filming of the left ventricle may be performed in one projection (single plane) or in two projections (biplane). Single plane left ventriculography is usually performed in a 30° right anterior oblique projection (Fig. 14 and 15). If biplane angiography is available, a 60° left anterior oblique projection (thus, two projections 90° apart in obliquity) is also performed.

A number of different catheters may be used for left ventriculography, but all have certain features in common. (1) The catheter should be of sufficient size so that a high-pressure injection of contrast material does not cause it to recoil, with resultant ventricular irritability. (2) The catheter should be designed so that the jet of injected contrast material exits through a series of side holes rather than through an endhole; as a result, the chance of a high pressure jet of contrast material being injected into the endocardium (so-called endocardial staining) is minimized. (3) Although the angiographic catheter should have multiple side holes for the injection of contrast material, these holes should be confined to the distal 2–3 cm of the catheter, else the contrast material will be injected into both the left ventricle and the proximal ascending aorta.

From the left ventriculogram, left ventricular volumes and ejection fraction may be calculated using a standard area-length formula. End-diastolic and end-systolic volumes are both measured; from these, left ventricular stroke volume is derived

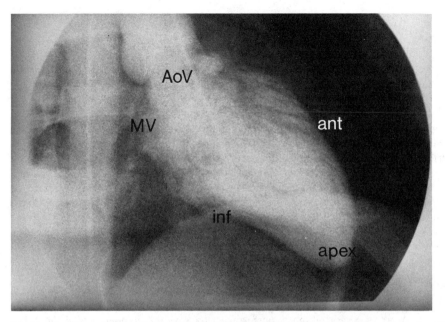

Figure 14 The end-diastolic image from an RAO left ventriculogram in a patient with normal wall motion. AoV, aortic valve; MV, mitral valve; inf, inferior wall; ant, anterior wall; apex, apex of the left ventricle.

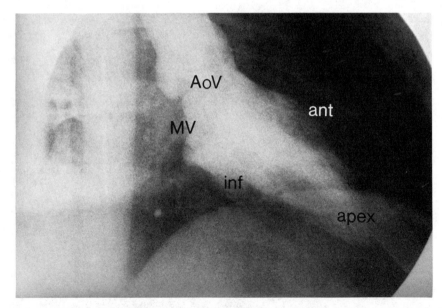

Figure 15 The end-systolic image from a RAO left ventriculogram in the same patient as shown in Fig. 14. Abbreviations are also similar. In comparison to Fig. 14, all segments of the left ventricular wall have contracted normally.

Table 2. Normal Angiographic Values

End-diastolic volume index	50–100 ml/m²
End-systolic volume index	15–35 ml/m²
Stroke volume index	30–65 ml/m²
Ejection fraction	0.55–0.80

(end-diastolic volume minus end-systolic volume), and ejection fraction is calculated (stroke volume divided by end-diastolic volume). The normal values for left ventricular volumes and ejection fraction are displayed in Table 2. In addition to the calculation of left ventricular volumes, segmental wall motion may be assessed. A segment of the left ventricular wall with reduced systolic motion is said to be hypokinetic; a segment that does not move at all during ventricular contraction is akinetic; and one that moves paradoxically during ventricular systole is termed dyskinetic (Figs. 16 and 17). Finally, the presence and severity of mitral regurgitation may be evaluated and quantitated in rough terms (Fig. 18).

AORTOGRAPHY

Aortography is the rapid injection of a large amount of contrast material into the aorta. A proximal aortogram is performed to assess the competency of the aortic valve and to evaluate the anatomy of the proximal aorta and large vessels that supply the head and neck. In turn, a distal aortogram is performed to assess the presence

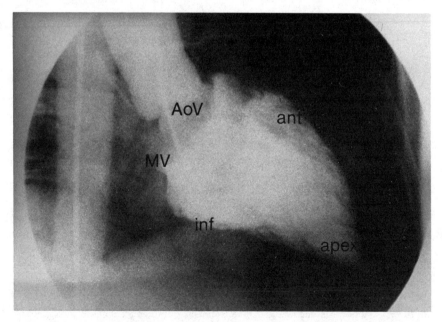

Figure 16 The end-diastolic image from a RAO left ventriculogram in a patient with a previous inferior myocardial infarction. Abbreviations are those used in Fig. 14.

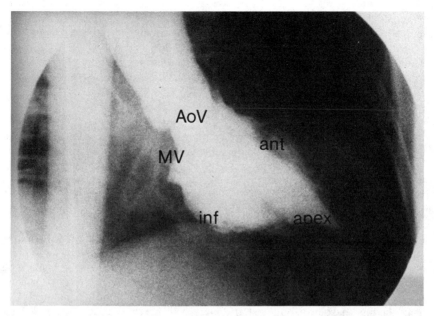

Figure 17   The end-systolic image from a RAO left ventriculogram in the same patient as shown in Fig. 16. Note that the anterior wall (ant) and apex move normally during systole but that the inferior wall (inf) is akinetic; that is, it does not move during systole.

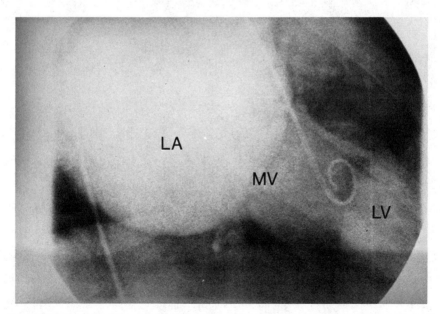

Figure 18   A selected frame from a RAO left ventriculogram in a patient with severe, long-standing mitral regurgitation. Note that the LA is larger than the LV and that it is more densely opacified with contrast material. MV, mitral valve.

of vascular abnormalities (e.g., aneurysm, intraluminal thrombus). The catheters employed for aortography are similar to those used for left ventriculography. For proximal aortography, 50–60 ml of contrast material is injected over 2–2½ seconds and filmed either by cineangiography or rapid cutfilm angiography. The standard proximal aortogram is filmed in a 45–60° left anterior oblique projection (Fig. 19).

PULMONARY ANGIOGRAPHY

Pulmonary angiography is performed primarily to confirm or exclude the presence of pulmonary emboli. A large-bore angiographic catheter is advanced from a systemic vein to the main pulmonary artery and is positioned so that catheter recoil during contrast injection does not cause the catheter tip to fall back into the right ventricle, with resultant ventricular irritability. A large injection of contrast material (55–60 ml) is performed over 2–2½ seconds. During the injection, rapid cut-filming is performed.

If the mainstream injection of the pulmonary artery does not allow a definitive diagnosis, several subselective injections are made into those segments of lung where the suspicion of pulmonary emboli is highest. These injections can be made with either a small power injection through the same angiographic catheter or a hand injection through a balloon-tipped catheter, with simultaneous cut-film angiography.

Once the films have been obtained, they must be interpreted meticulously. Several radiographic signs are diagnostic of pulmonary embolism, including a large intra-

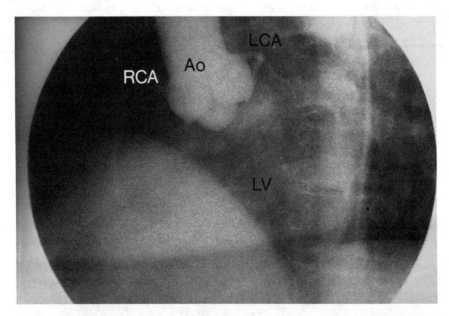

Figure 19 A selected frame from an LAO supravalvular aortogram in a patient without aortic regurgitation, Ao, proximal aorta; RCA, proximal right coronary artery; LCA, proximal left coronary artery; LV, left ventricle. The 3 aortic valve cusps are easily discernible.

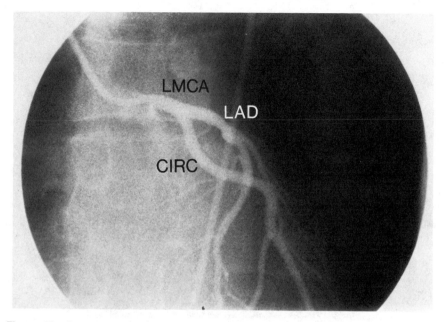

Figure 20   An anteroposterior view of a normal left coronary artery. LMCA, left main coronary artery; LAD, left anterior descending; CIRC, left circumflex.

luminal filling defect or an abrupt pulmonary arterial cutoff. Other radiographic signs, such as localized oligemia and asymmetry of pulmonary blood flow are suggestive but not strictly diagnostic of embolism.

SELECTIVE CORONARY ARTERIOGRAPHY

Selective coronary arteriography is usually performed to determine the presence and severity of fixed, arteriosclerotic coronary artery disease. It is occasionally performed to evaluate the presence of dynamic alterations of coronary arterial tone, that is, coronary arterial spasm. Each coronary arterial ostium is selectively engaged with a catheter, after which injections of contrast material are made by hand. Since arteriosclerotic coronary artery disease is often eccentric within the coronary arterial lumen, injections of each of the two coronary arteries are performed and filmed in several different obliquities (Figs. 20–25).

Several important features about selective coronary arteriography deserve emphasis. (1) Systemic arterial pressure and heart rate should be observed closely during coronary arteriography, since it can induce transient hypotension and/or bradycardia. The latter can be treated with intravenous atropine and, if necessary, placement of a temporary transvenous ventricular pacemaker. (2) Cineangiography of the coronary arteries should be performed with as much image magnification and, at the same time, as little image distortion as possible. (3) With very few exceptions, coronary arteriography should not be performed during an episode of angina. Rather,

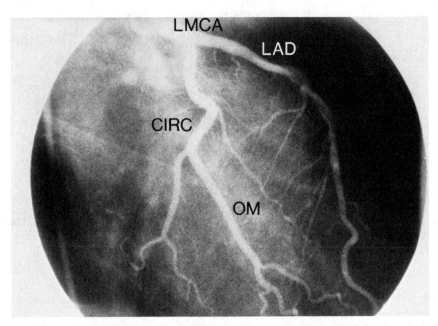

Figure 21 An RAO projection of a normal left coronary artery. Abbreviations are similar to those used in Fig. 20. OM, obtuse marginal branch of the circumflex.

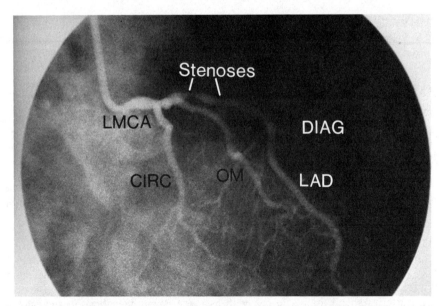

Figure 22 An RAO projection of the left coronary artery in a patient with two stenoses of the proximal LAD, marked appropriately. LMCA, left main coronary artery; CIRC, left circumflex coronary artery; OM, obtuse marginal branch of circumflex coronary artery; LAD, left anterior descending coronary artery; DIAG, diagonal branch of the LAD.

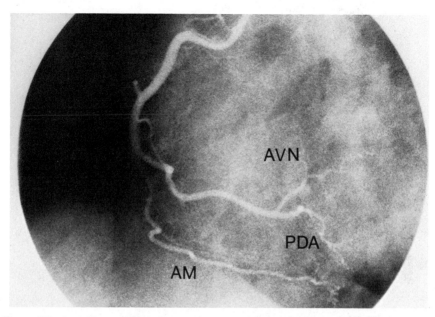

Figure 23 An LAO projection of a normal right coronary artery. AM, acute marginal branch; PDA, posterior descending artery; AVN, atrioventricular nodal artery.

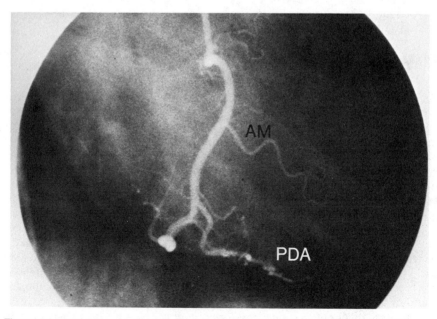

Figure 24 An RAO projection of a normal right coronary artery. Abbreviations are similar to those used in Fig. 23.

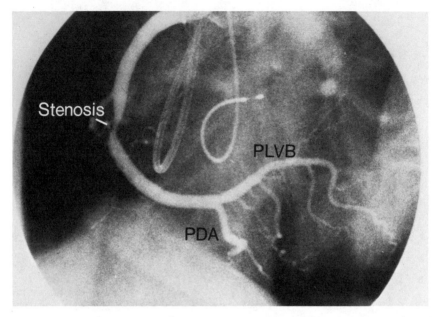

Figure 25   An LAO projection of a right coronary artery with a severe stenosis in its midportion. PDA, posterior descending artery; PLVB, posterior left ventricular branch.

the patient should receive sublingual nitroglycerin, and sufficient time should be allowed for pain to resolve. Then, coronary arteriography may proceed.

Risks and Complications

As cardiac catheterization has become more frequently performed, the incidence of complications has diminished. However, even in the most skilled hands, the procedure is not without risk. The overall incidence of a major complication—death, myocardial infarction (MI), or cerebrovascular accident—during or within 24 hours of catheterization is 0.3–0.6%. Of these major complications, death in the catheterization laboratory or within 24 hours of catheterization occurs in 0.1–0.3% of patients, the majority of whom have extensive cardiac disease. Such deaths may be caused by perforation of the heart or great vessels, cardiac arrhythmias, or acute myocardial infarction with resultant left ventricular dysfunction. Myocardial infarction during or immediately following catheterization occurs in 0.3–0.5% of patients, but most infarctions are small and uncomplicated. Cerebrovascular accidents in the pericatheterization period are either embolic (from the arterial catheter or thrombus in the left ventricle or atrium) or thrombotic (i.e., existence of previous extensive cerebrovascular disease that, in association with the hemodynamic alterations induced by arteriography, leads to inadequate cerebral perfusion).

Numerous minor complications may cause morbidity but have no effect on mortality. (1) Following arterial catheterization by the brachial approach, restoration of blood flow to the arm can be imperfect and the patient require a thrombectomy after catheterization. (2) Hemorrhage and/or hematoma formation can occur at the site of the femoral arterial puncture and, if severe, can require limited surgical exploration. Occasionally a femoral arterial thrombectomy is required following a percutaneous puncture, and a very rare patient may require a lower limb partial amputation. (3) Local infection may occur at the site of catheter entrance and manipulation, but this can usually be treated with meticulous wound care and a short course of antibiotic therapy. (4) The injection of contrast material commonly causes nausea and vomiting as well as a transient fall in systemic arterial pressure. Occasionally such injections are associated with allergic reactions of varying severity, and a rare individual develops anaphylaxis due to contrast material. In addition, the endocardial injection of contrast material during ventriculography can cause ventricular irritability.

Postcatheterization Concerns

During the 24 hours after catheterization, there are several important considerations. The patient should remain at complete bed rest for 8–12 hours if the arterial catheterization was performed by the brachial approach and for 24 hours if it was performed via the femoral approach. The patient should be observed closely after catheterization to insure that heart rate and blood pressure are stable and that the arterial and venous entrance sites do not show evidence of bleeding. Radiographic contrast material is extremely hyperosmolar and, as a result, causes an osmotic diuresis during the 12–24 hours after catheterization. Therefore, sufficient oral and intravenous fluids should be administered to insure that such a diuresis does not induce intravascular volume depletion.

Bibliography

Adams DF, Fraser DB, Abrams HL: The complications of coronary arteriography. *Circulation* 48:609, 1973.

Branthwaite MA, Bradley RD: Measurement of cardiac output by thermal dilution in man. *J Appl Physiol* 24:434, 1968.

Dalen JE, Brooks HL, Johnson LW, et al: Pulmonary angiography in acute pulmonary embolism: indications, techniques, and results in 367 patients. *Am Heart J* 81:175, 1971.

Damato AN, Lau SH, Berkowitz WD, et al: Recordings of specialized conducting fibers (AV nodal, His bundle, and right bundle branch) in man using an electrode catheter technique. *Circulation* 39:435, 1969.

Forrester JS, Ganz W, Diamond G, et al: Thermodilution cardiac output determination with a single flow-directed catheter. *Am Heart J* 83:306, 1972.

Gorlin R, Gorlin SG: Hydraulic formula for calculation of area of stenotic mitral valve, other cardiac valves, and central circulatory shunts. *Am Heart J* 41:1, 1951.

Hamilton WF, Riley RL, Attyah AM, et al: Comparison of the Fick and dye injection methods of measuring the cardiac output in man. *Am J Physiol* 153:309, 1948.

Judkins MP: Percutaneous transfemoral selective coronary arteriography. *Radiol Clin N Amer* 6:467, 1968.

Rackley CE, Dear HD, Baxley WA, et al: Left ventricular chamber volume, mass, and function in severe coronary artery disease. *Circulation* 41:605, 1970.

Sasahara AA, Stein M, Simon M, et al: Pulmonary angiography in the diagnosis of thromboembolic disease. *N Engl J Med* 270:1075, 1964.

Scherlag BJ, Lau SH, Helfant RH, et al: Catheter technique for recording His bundle activity in man. *Circulation* 39:13, 1969.

Seldinger SI: Catheter replacement of the needle in percutaneous arteriography, a new technique. *Acta Radiol* 39:368, 1953.

Sones FM, Shirey EK: Cine coronary arteriography. *Mod Concepts Cardiovasc Dis* 31:735, 1962.

Swan HJC, Ganz W, Forrester J, et al: Catheterization of the heart in man with use of a flow-directed balloon-tipped catheter. *N Engl J Med* 283:447, 1970.

Visscher MB, Johnson JA: The Fick principle: Analysis of potential errors in its conventional application. *J Appl Physiol* 5:635, 1953.

ANGINA PECTORIS

Edward J. Brown, Jr.
Robert A. Kloner

Angina pectoris (an' ji nah; usually, though incorrectly, an-ji' nah) is defined in Stedman's Medical Dictionary as a severe constricting pain, often radiating from the precordium to the left shoulder and down the arm, due to ischemia of the heart muscle and usually caused by coronary artery disease. Coronary artery disease is the number one cause of death in the United States, accounting for 700,000 deaths per year. This number represents more than one-third of all yearly deaths in the United States. Coronary artery disease can present clinically as sudden death, congestive heart failure, an acute myocardial infarction, or angina pectoris. This chapter will deal with angina pectoris, and discuss the diagnosis, evaluation, and treatment of this disorder.

Although we will not deal here with chest pain due to causes other than myocardial ischemia, it is important to consider the differential diagnosis of chest pain, which is shown in Table 1. Even though myocardial ischemia is a common cause of chest pain, it is not the only cause; and it is always important to remember that two or more conditions that cause chest pain can coexist.

Diagnosis and Evaluation of Angina Pectoris

THE CLINICAL HISTORY

Chest pain is a common complaint in emergency rooms, physician's offices, and hospitals. A careful and thorough clinical history can provide important diagnostic clues and often prevent unnecessary, expensive, and often dangerous procedures (Table 2). The location, quality, duration, and radiation of the pain, as well as associated symptoms, all yield important clues that help the clinician determine whether or not angina pectoris is the correct diagnosis. Angina pectoris is often described as a heavy, pressing, burning discomfort or as a feeling of chest constriction. If a physician uses the word *pain* in reference to the complaint, the patient will often correct him or her and substitute a more accurate description.

Usually, angina pectoris is located in the anterior chest with or without radiation to other parts of the body. Angina pectoris presenting as arm or jaw pain without associated chest discomfort is unusual (Sampson and Cheitlin). Most often, the patient will locate chest symptoms better with the hands than with words, and the discomfort will be described as diffuse and deep within the precordium in the area of the sternum. Specific localization with finger pointing suggests chest pain that is not related to myocardial ischemia. Clenching of the fist over the sternum is very suggestive that the pain is related to myocardial ischemia (Levine's sign).

Table 1. Conditions That Cause Chest Pain

Noncardiovascular disorders
  Neuromuscular
    Costochondritis and other chest wall syndromes
    Radicular syndromes
    Inflammatory syndromes of the shoulder joint
  Gastrointestinal
    Esophageal disease and hiatal hernia
    Peptic ulcer or gastritis
    Gallbladder disease
  Psychologic
    Psychoneuroses
    Psychosomatic complaints
Cardiovascular and pulmonary disorders
  Coronary artery disease (atherosclerotic versus nonatherosclerotic diseases)
  Aortic valve disease
  Idiopathic hypertrophic subaortic stenosis
  Primary myocardial disease
  Pericarditis
  Dissecting aortic aneurysm
  Mitral valve prolapse syndrome
  Pulmonary embolus-infarction
  Pulmonary hypertension and/or right ventricle strain
  Pneumothorax
  Pleuritis
  Intrathoracic tumor
Disorders of unknown cause
  Chest pain with normal coronary arteriograms

From Cohn PF: *Diagnosis and Therapy of Coronary Artery Disease.* Boston: Little, Brown & Co., p. 53, 1979.

The duration of the chest symptoms is important. Discomfort secondary to myocardial ischemia usually builds over seconds and lasts for less than 15 minutes. Pains that are constant, lasting hours to days, or pains that last only 5–15 seconds and are described as sharp and well localized are rarely secondary to myocardial ischemia.

Radiation of chest pain due to myocardial ischemia is a common complaint. The upper and lower arms, the neck, and the jaw are the most common sites of radiation (Sampson and Cheitlin). Occasionally, patients will consult dentists with jaw pain that is actually radiation of pain secondary to angina pectoris.

Precipitating factors can provide useful clues to help include or exclude angina pectoris. Chest pain or discomfort brought on by exertion is the most common presentation. Coronary artery stenoses, which allow only a limited amount of oxygen rich blood to pass, coupled with the increased oxygen requirements of the myocardium during exercise can result in a myocardial oxygen demand and supply imbalance. This condition causes myocardial ischemia and angina pectoris. Chest pain following meals is often due to myocardial ischemia, although the reason for this is not clear (Goldstein et al.). Another common precipitating factor is cold. Frequently, an habitual activity such as walking a set distance to catch a bus, will be accompanied by chest pain only during cold weather (Freedberg et al., Epstein et al.). Mudge, et al. explained this phenomenon by demonstrating an increase in coronary vascular resistance precipitated by cold. This results in a decrease in coronary artery blood supply for any given level of exercise.

It is important to note that angina pectoris can occur in the absence of exertion. This form of myocardial ischemia can be due to coronary artery spasm (Prinzmetal's angina) that results in an episodic decrease in coronary blood flow (covered in detail in Chapter 10). Other factors can precipitate angina pectoris at rest, including severe

Table 2.   Typical Features of Angina Pectoris

Clinical History

Description

  Heavy, pressing, squeezing or burning chest discomfort

Location

  Diffuse anterior chest with or without radiation

Duration

  >15 seconds <15 minutes

Radiation

  Jaw, arms (left > right) back, epigastrium, neck

Precipitating factors

  Cold, exertion, anxiety, meals

Associated symptoms

  Breathlessness, fatigue, nausea, palpitations, diaphoresis

Pain relief

  Resting in a standing or sitting position, nitroglycerin, usually takes 1–5 minutes

Associated risk factors

  Age, sex, cigarette smoking, hypertension, hypercholesterolemia, positive family history for atherosclerotic heart disease, diabetes mellitus

Physical Examination

Physical findings present chronically

  Xanthelasma and xanthomas, carotid or femoral bruits, hypertension

Physical findings present during active ischemia

  Cold and clammy skin, diaphoresis, transient S_4 gallops, transient mitral regurgitation murmur, pulsus alternans, transient precordial bulge, tachycardia, transient hypertension, paradoxical splitting of S_2

Physical findings that suggest chest pain is not due to angina pectoris

  Tender precordium, systolic murmur consistent with mitral valve prolapse, a marfanoid body habitus, which increases the likelihood that chest pain is due to aortic dissection

---

anemia, which results in a decreased blood oxygen carrying capacity; fever; arrhythmias, especially tachycardia; hyperthyroidism; drugs, such as digoxin and the catecholamines, which increase myocardial oxygen consumption at rest; and cigarette smoking, which decreases blood oxygen capacity by addition of carbon monoxide to the blood. Also, cigarette smoking increases myocardial oxygen demand through a nicotine related increase in heart rate and blood pressure (Aranow).

Symptoms associated with chest pain or discomfort can provide important diagnostic clues. Breathlessness, fatigue, feelings of uneasiness or doom, palpitations (unusual), and diaphoresis associated with chest pain suggest the diagnosis is angina pectoris. Such symptoms are attributed to transient cardiac failure, ischemia related arrhythmias, and a sudden reduction of cardiac output.

Clues concerning the etiology of chest pain can be obtained from the manner in which pain relief is achieved. Angina pectoris precipitated by exertion is generally relieved after one to five minutes in a standing or sitting position. Supine position may aggravate angina pectoris because it is associated with increased venous return. This results in increased wall stress, a major determinant of myocardial oxygen consumption. The response to nitroglycerin can be a helpful signal, as angina pectoris often abates within $\frac{1}{2}$ to 2 minutes after the nitroglycerin dissolves. However, esophageal spasm, a condition that can result in chest pain, can also be regularly relieved by the administration of nitroglycerin. Pain relieved when the patient leans forward or decreases his or her respiratory excursion is generally not due to angina pectoris but is more characteristic of pericarditis.

In addition to chest pain characteristics, an evaluation of risk factors can be helpful. Age is of definite importance. Angina pectoris as a cause of chest pain is very unlikely in patients in their 20s, while it is more likely an explanation for chest pain in patients in their 60s. Similarly, a positive family history of heart disease or a diagnosis of diabetes mellitus, hyperlipidemia, hypertension, and cigarette smoking increase the chances that a patient with chest pain is suffering from angina pectoris. Recently, Stadel demonstrated that young women who smoke cigarettes and use oral contraceptives have an increased risk of ischemic heart disease and; therefore, in this group of patients with chest pain, the diagnosis of angina pectoris or myocardial infarction should be seriously considered. (Also see Chapters 23 and 26 for discussion of risk factors.)

THE PHYSICAL EXAMINATION

A careful physical examination can sometimes provide information that can help exclude angina pectoris (Table 2). In the absence of active chest pain there are physical findings that aid in differentiating chest pain due to ischemic heart disease from chest pain due to other causes. Xanthomas, if present, suggest hyperlipidemia and increase the likelihood that the patient has coronary artery disease. Carotid or femoral bruits suggest the presence of peripheral vascular ⌐ ase; and if the peripheral arteries have atherosclerotic lesions, it is likely that the coronary arteries are also involved. The presence of hypertension during active chest pain can be due to anxiety and is not helpful. However, chronic hypertension is a risk factor for coronary artery disease and increases the likelihood that a patient has coronary artery disease. During an attack of chest pain, transient physical findings can occur that are helpful in diagnosing angina pectoris. Patients' skin may be cold and clammy and patients are often diaphoretic. S_3 (uncommon) and S_4 (common) diastolic gallops are sometimes heard during an attack of angina pectoris (Cohn et al, 1971). A transient systolic murmur, which can result from ischemic papillary muscle dysfunction, is helpful if present (Martin et al.).

Other physical findings that suggest chest pain secondary to ischemia are pulsus alternans, a precordial bulge (best appreciated if the patient is in the left lateral position), elevated blood pressure and heart rate (Proudfit et al.), and a paradoxically split second heart sound. Although these physical findings are not always present during angina pectoris, their presence during an episode of chest pain are diagnostically very helpful.

During the physical examination of patients with chest pain there are physical signs that, if present, suggest the diagnosis is not angina pectoris. A tender area over the precordium suggests pain of musculoskeletal origin. A typical systolic murmur and delayed carotid upstroke suggest significant aortic stenosis, which can cause chest pain. A cardiac murmur should raise the possibility of idiopathic hypertrophic subaortic stenosis or mitral valve prolapse, two conditions that can result in chest pain mimicking angina pectoris. In idiopathic hypertrophic subaortic stenosis, the systolic murmur decreases with maneuvers that increase preload or increase afterload; the characteristic murmur of mitral valve prolapse is a late systolic murmur preceded by a midsystolic click. A marfanoid body habitus should raise the suspicion that aortic dissection is the cause of an episode of chest pain. The presence of these physical findings are only helpful in determining the etiology of chest pain; and it should be remembered that coronary artery disease as a cause of chest pain can present concomitantly with any of the disorders above.

INITIAL DIAGNOSIS AND EVALUATION OF ANGINA PECTORIS

Most patients evaluated for chest pain are seen initially in a physician's office, an emergency room, or perhaps in a hospital for other reasons (Fig. 1). Following the history and physical examination, a decision as to additional evaluation and therapy must be made. The information gathered from the history and physical examination may allow the physician to exclude the diagnosis of angina pectoris with no further investigation. For example, the chest pain may clearly be due to a recently acquired chest wall bruise. A second possible decision is that the chest pain *may* be due to angina pectoris; in this case, further diagnostic inquiry is necessary. A third possibility is that the chest pain is definitely angina pectoris. In this case, the next step is to classify the condition as either chronic stable (mild or severe) angina pectoris or unstable angina pectoris. Chronic stable angina pectoris is present in patients whose chest pain has remained unchanged in terms of severity, frequency, and duration over a period of several weeks to several months. Mild angina pectoris describes those patients who have attacks only after unusual exertion and who, in general, do not have to alter their lifestyles to prevent chest pain. Severe chronic stable angina pectoris describes patients who experience frequent attacks and who must modify their usual daily routine to exclude strenous activities. Those patients with mild chronic stable angina pectoris, when seen for the first time, usually do not require hospitalization and evaluation and treatment can be performed on an outpatient basis. Patients with severe chronic stable angina pectoris, when seen for the

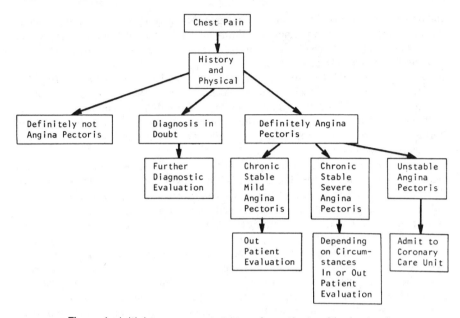

Figure 1   Initial management strategy for patients with chest pain.

first time, may or may not require hospitalization for evaluation and treatment. Whether or not to hospitalize patients in this group depends on the severity of their disease, and decisions must be made on an individual basis. Certainly, patients having 5–10 daily episodes of angina pectoris precipitated by very minimal exertion can be most safely evaluated in the hospital.

Patients categorized from the history and physical examination as having unstable angina pectoris should be hospitalized. The precise definition of unstable angina pectoris is controversial and different physicians define the term differently. Included among the many definitions of this syndrome are intermediate coronary syndrome, acute coronary insufficiency, impending myocardial infarction, preinfarction syndrome, crescendo angina, and accelerated angina. All definitions have a common concern; the state of blood supply to the myocardium is tenuous and myocardial infarction is likely to follow if no treatment is instituted. Features common to all definitions of unstable angina pectoris include new onset angina pectoris, more severe or prolonged angina pectoris superimposed on chronic stable angina pectoris, and angina pectoris occurring at rest.

Differentiating chest pain due to myocardial ischemia and myocardial infarction from chest pain due to other causes remains one of the most difficult and challenging problems in clinical medicine. Because the number of patients complaining of chest pain is large, it is impractical to admit all such patients to coronary care units for further cardiac evaluation. However, to send home a patient suffering from a myocardial infarction or unstable angina with an incorrrect diagnosis of chest pain of noncardiac origin can be a mistake fatal to the patient. Thus, one must have a low threshold to admit patients when there is any reasonable doubt as to the correct diagnosis. An important point to remember is that patients with an acute myocardial infarction often have a vague feeling of uneasiness that is difficult for them to describe. For most people an emergency visit is not a regular event, and the fact that they felt worried enough to come to an emergency room is itself an important sign that something is very wrong, whether or not the problem is well stated.

LIMITATIONS OF THE HISTORY AND PHYSICAL EXAMINATION

Many important decisions about the evaluation and treatment of patients with angina pectoris are made on the basis of the initial history and physical exam. For this reason, it is important to be aware of how accurately these tools can reflect the presence and degree of coronary artery disease. Proudfit et al., Cohn, and Banks et al. have demonstrated that even the most skillfully and carefully conducted clinical history has limitations. In a series of 188 patients classified as having unstable angina pectoris, Alison et al. found that 10.6% of patients had normal coronary arteries when coronary angiography was performed. Similar numbers of patients with normal coronary arteries have been found in other series of patients with the diagnosis of unstable angina pectoris (Fischl et al.; Conti et al.).

Equally distressing is that group of patients with severe coronary artery disease or myocardial ischemia who have no symptoms. Cohn calls this phenomenon "silent myocardial ischemia." Although this syndrome is not well understood, it occurs in 2–3% of asymptomatic and presumably healthy adult men (Erikssen et al.).

Thus, classification of patients with angina pectoris from the history and physical examination may lead to inaccuracies in some cases. Certain patients will undergo expensive diagnostic tests only to find that the history was misleading and that they do not have coronary artery disease. Likewise, some patients will miss the advantages of modern cardiac diagnosis and treatment because of histories that appear to exclude coronary artery disease. However, in spite of their deficiencies, the history and physical examination remain the most frequently used screening tests in cardiac diagnosis and, when properly done, are accurate tools in diagnosing and staging most patients with angina pectoris.

FURTHER DIAGNOSIS AND EVALUATION OF ANGINA PECTORIS

Patients classified as having angina pectoris should undergo further studies to confirm the diagnosis and to stage the extent of their disease (Fig. 2). Modern cardiology now offers the physician a great many noninvasive and invasive cardiac diagnostic procedures that allow accurate diagnosis and staging of the extent of coronary artery disease. A proper understanding of the information that can be obtained from each of the available procedures and the limitations of each is necessary if the physician is to choose the proper test or combination of tests for each patient. As shown in Figure 2, angina pectoris begins with a decrease in coronary blood supply usually caused by a stenotic lesion. Coronary arteriography allows visualization of the coronary artery and the amount of coronary artery stenosis can be directly seen. Thallium-201 imaging is a measure of the amount of blood passing through a stenotic lesion, relative to blood passing through the remainder of the heart. Occasionally, regions of myocardium perfused by severely stenosed coronary arteries can have

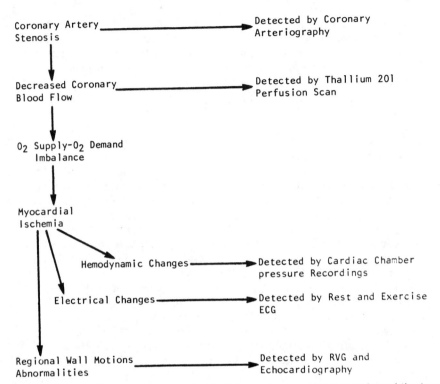

Figure 2 Schematic showing the pathophysiology of myocardial ischemia and the type of information recorded by the various cardiac diagnostic techniques.

normal perfusion—perhaps because enough blood is passing through the stenosis to meet the regional cardiac myocardial oxygen demands, or perhaps because blood is reaching the area through collateral vessels. Thallium-201 imaging will detect the adequacy of perfusion to a region. If myocardial oxygen demand exceeds the supply, myocardial ischemia will result. Electrocardiography detects the electrical events associated with myocardial ischemia, which appear as ST segment depression or elevation. Regional wall motion abnormalities that occur when myocardial tissue becomes ischemic can be detected and measured by M-mode and two-dimensional echocardiography and radionuclide ventriculography. Thus, the many tests available to the physician provide diagnostic and quantitative information in different forms.

Because cardiology diagnostic studies are expensive and, in some cases, associated with risk to the patient, care and skill must be used when choosing the most appropriate means of evaluating each patient.

Resting Electrocardiogram

The resting electrocardiogram should be a part of the evaluation of any patient with suspected or proven angina pectoris. The presence of Q waves indicate an old myocardial infarction, which is usually, although not always, secondary to coronary artery disease. (Emboli or trauma can also result in myocardial infarction). Other abnormalities, such as intraventricular conduction delays, atrial or ventricular arrhythmias, or nonspecific ST-T wave changes are not specific and are frequently related to conditions other than coronary artery disease; but in the presence of chest pain, they increase the suspicion that the pain is related to myocardial ischemia. Often during an attack of angina pectoris, there will be ST segment depression which resolves when the pain resolves. This is a very specific finding for myocardial ischemia and a good reason for obtaining an electrocardiogram during chest pain in patients in whom the etiology of chest pain is not known. A normal electrocardiogram is not very helpful and can be seen frequently in patients with angina pectoris.

Exercise Stress Testing

Patients categorized as having suspected or known stable coronary artery disease should undergo exercise stress testing as a part of their evaluation. Exercise stress testing has many purposes. In patients with chest pain of uncertain etiology, the exercise stress test is used as as diagnostic tool. This test relies on indirect signs of ischemia to detect coronary artery disease; and it is important here, too, to understand the strengths and limitations of this technique in order to best utilize the information obtained.

An exercise stress test must be interpreted in the context of the information obtained from the history and physical examination, because its predictive value varies with the population being studied. In a population with a statistically low incidence of coronary artery disease, such as premenopausal nonsmoking women with chest pain, the predictive ability is very low (Rifkin and Hood). However, in studies of patients with a high likelihood of coronary artery disease, such as men over the age of 60 with multiple risk factors, the predictive value is higher. Thus, in the latter group, a positive stress test is likely to be associated with the presence of coronary artery disease, while a negative test is likely to reflect the absence of coronary artery disease. The explanation for this variation in predictive value involves Bayes' theorem, which is also discussed in Chapter 6.

The role of exercise stress testing in patients with known coronary artery disease is to provide prognostic information and to give the physician an indication of the severity of the disease present. Strongly positive exercise tests with greater than 1 mm of ST depression occurring at a low level of exercise indicate a likelihood of multivessel disease (Goldman et al.) or left main coronary artery disease (Cheitlin et al., Lavine et al.). In addition to prognostic information, exercise stress testing is useful in planning medical or surgical therapy. Rehabilitation programs can be prescribed from results of exercise stress testing.

In addition to the objective results obtained from such testing—such as a degree of ST depression, duration of exercise testing, and blood pressure response—useful subjective information can be obtained when the physician observes the test. It is possible to gain a picture of how fatigued a patient is when ischemia results and how the maximum level of activity during exercise stress relates to the patient's daily lifestyle.

Thallium-201 Myocardial Perfusion Scintigraphy

Thallium-201 perfusion imaging is usually done in conjunction with exercise stress testing. (See also Chapter 7.) While exercise electrocardiograms depend on ischemia related electrical changes, thallium-201 images depend on differences in myocardial perfusion. Areas of the myocardium supplied by stenotic vessels do not receive as much blood as surrounding normally perfused areas and appear as nonthallium containing perfusion defects. Although underperfused areas are usually ischemic areas or scar tissue, abnormal images do not always depend on the presence or absence of ischemia.

Pitt and Strauss have shown that thallium-201 stress imaging has a sensitivity of 85–90% and a specificity of 65–70% for the detection of significant coronary artery disease. Exercise testing without thallium-201 is generally reported to have a somewhat lower sensitivity and a lower specificity. The value of combining diagnostic techniques was demonstrated in a multicenter study that evaluated thallium-201 imaging and exercise electrocardiography. Ritchie et al. demonstrated that in a group of 190 patients, 148 of whom had significant coronary artery disease, exercise electrocardiography detected 73% of the patients with significant coronary artery disease and thallium-201 imaging detected 76% of those with significant coronary artery disease. Thus, sensitivities were similar. Specificity was also found to be similar: 86% for exercise electrocardiography and 88% for thallium-201 imaging. However, when the two studies were combined, sensitivity was significantly improved to 91%, better than either test alone. Specificity was not improved when combining the two techniques.

Due to the extra cost of adding thallium-201 imaging to an exercise stress test, it should not be routinely ordered whenever an exercise test is performed. If a patient has a strongly positive exercise electrocardiogram, thallium-201 imaging, although reassuring when positive, adds little diagnostic information. Likewise, in a clearly negative exercise electrocardiogram, thallium-201 imaging will add little to the care of a patient. One of the most common indications for thallium-201 perfusion imaging is the evaluation of patients with an abnormal resting electrocardiogram. In the presence of abnormal resting ST segments due to left bundle branch block, left ventricular hypertrophy, digoxin, and so forth, the diagnostic value of exercise electrocardiography is greatly decreased and thallium-201 imaging should be included when exercise testing is done.

Thallium-201 imaging is also indicated in patients undergoing evaluation for chest pain and who have equivocal electrocardiographic changes with exercise. A negative thallium-201 image can allow the clinician and patient to avoid coronary angiography, while a positive thallium-201 scan under the same circumstances makes significant coronary artery disease more likely and can lead to further appropriate diagnostic and therapeutic measures.

There are also indications for thallium-201 imaging in patients with angina pectoris and known coronary artery disease. In patients with severe coronary artery disease, it is generally believed that resting coronary blood flow is normal in the absence of angina pectoris or an acute myocardial infarction. However, Gerwitz et al. and Wackers et al., using thallium-201 imaging, have demonstrated that this may not be true. In patients with severe coronary artery disease, some defects that appear on initial images following injections at rest fill in on delayed images, suggesting decreased perfusion at rest. Although it is not clear what the best course is for patients with resting perfusion abnormalities, it is likely that they will benefit most from intensive medical therapy and should be strongly considered for revascularization surgery.

Patients with very severe left ventricular dysfunction and congestive heart failure due to diffuse coronary artery disease generally are not recommended for coronary artery bypass surgery because of the high mortality. This is particularly true in the absence of angina pectoris. Coronary angiography and left ventriculography usually reveal severe three vessel coronary artery disease with diffuse hypokinesis and/or akinesis. However, how much of the left ventricular dysfunction is due to scar and how much to reversible ischemia is difficult to determine. Thallium-201 perfusion imaging that demonstrates perfusion defects that fill in over time suggests reversibly ischemic tissue. If extensive areas of reversibly ischemic tissue can be demonstrated in this group of very ill patients, Atkins et al. have suggested that coronary artery bypass surgery may result in clinical improvement.

Thallium-201 perfusion imaging can be useful in the evaluation of a stenosis of uncertain hemodynamic significance noted on coronary angiography. A lesion of 40–60% may or may not limit flow with exercise. A corresponding thallium-201 perfusion defect with exercise would support the hemodynamic significance of the lesion, while a negative scan would be good evidence that the lesion was not responsible for flow limitations or, by inference, ischemia.

Radionuclide Ventriculography and Echocardiography

These two noninvasive cardiac techniques are covered together because they both depend on ischemia produced regional myocardial dysfunction for the detection of coronary artery disease. Regional wall motion abnormalities are sensitive markers of myocardial ischemia and appear with flow reductions of only 10–20% (Vatner). The indications for these studies are expanding rapidly as newer and more quantitative techniques are being developed to analyze the data obtained. The potential advantage of both techniques is the possibility of quantitating the amount of ischemic myocardium and this information may allow more rational decision making concerning medical versus surgical therapies.

Cardiac Catheterization

If the history, physical exam, and the results of noninvasive studies are properly conducted and interpreted, few cardiac catheterizations will be necessary for diagnostic purposes. Indeed, most cardiac catheterizations are done to stage and localize coronary artery disease and to evaluate the desirability of coronary artery bypass surgery. Coronary arteriography gives anatomic information about the location of coronary artery stenosis. Interpretation of the results is subject to inter- and intraobserver variation. As with any other cardiac examination, it is important to interpret the results of coronary arteriography in the context of other information gathered about the patient. The coronary angiogram does not identify decreased perfusion or ischemia and cannot reveal what the functional status of a stenosis is. Thus, a good history and good noninvasive studies are necessary to understand the significance of coronary artery stenoses identified during coronary arteriography.

Natural History and Pathophysiology of Angina Pectoris

NATURAL HISTORY OF PATIENTS WITH ANGINA PECTORIS

The goals of therapy for angina pectoris are to relieve symptoms and to prolong life. To evaluate the effect of therapy on longevity, one must know the natural history of untreated angina pectoris. If coronary arteriography has been performed, natural history studies of patients with angina pectoris (carried out prior to widespread use of current medical or surgical therapies) that are based on coronary anatomy can be useful when dealing with individual patients. Patients with one vessel disease had an annual mortality rate of less than 4%. In patients with two vessel disease, this figure increased to 7–10% and in those with three vessel disease, to 10–12%. Patients with left main coronary artery obstructions had a yearly mortality of 15–25% (Humphries). Left ventricular dysfunction worsens the prognosis. Often patients with angina pectoris are managed without knowledge of the coronary anatomy. In such patients, natural history studies based on the clinical history or noninvasive criteria can be helpful. An example of one subset of patients based on clinical findings are patients with unstable angina pectoris. Using a definition of unstable angina pectoris that includes both accelerating symptoms and ST segment changes during chest pain, Mulcahy et al. followed 101 patients treated with only bed rest and sublingual nitrates for recurrent pain, and found a 9% rate of nonfatal myocardial infarction and a 4% incidence of death within the first 28 days. At the end of one year, the incidence of nonfatal myocardial infarction was 12% and the incidence of cardiovascular death was 10%. Natural history studies such as this are helpful as guidelines when making diagnostic and therapeutic decisions for patients presenting with unstable angina pectoris and unknown coronary anatomy.

PATHOPHYSIOLOGY OF ANGINA PECTORIS

When one has obtained information that allows accurate diagnosis and staging of coronary artery disease, the next step is to attempt to alleviate symptoms and favorably alter the natural history of the disease. To choose among the many possible treatment modalities, one must understand the factors that influence myocardial oxygen supply and those that influence myocardial oxygen demand.

Factors That Influence Myocardial Oxygen Supply

Delivery of oxygen to the myocardium depends on both the amount of blood flowing through the coronary arteries and the ability of the myocardial cells to extract oxygen from the blood. Unlike other organs of the body, the heart has the unique property of nearly maximal oxygen extraction at rest; thus, there is little reserve capability for increasing myocardial oxygen supply by increasing myocardial oxygen extraction. Myocardial oxygen supply can be adjusted to meet oxygen demands by changing coronary blood flow, which can and does fluctuate depending on the needs of the myocardium.

The amount of blood flowing through the coronary arteries depends on both the perfusion pressure and the resistance across the coronary vascular bed:

$$CBF = \frac{AO\ pressure - RA\ pressure}{Coronary\ vascular\ resistance}$$

where AO = aortic, RA = right atrial, and CBF = coronary blood flow. Because of the high intramural pressures during systole, resistance to flow is high and relatively little blood is delivered to the left ventricular myocardium during systole. Most flow occurs during diastole; therefore, aortic diastolic pressure and the duration of diastole are important determinants of myocardial blood flow. Factors that increase the aortic diastolic pressure or prolong the time spent in diastole will, therefore, increase the blood supply to the myocardium. Conversely, factors that reduce diastolic pressure or factors, such as tachycardia, that shorten the time the ventricle spends in diastole reduce the blood supply to the myocardium.

In addition to the pressure, the resistance to coronary blood flow is an important determinant of myocardial oxygen supply. The coronary arteries are not rigid pipes, but flexible tubes that exist in a state of tone. Relaxation of the vessels will decrease resistance to flow and increase coronary blood flow, while contraction (or spasm) of the vessels will increase resistance and decrease coronary blood flow. The factors that control coronary vascular resistance are incompletely understood. External compression of the vessels is important, particularly during systole when the high intramyocardial pressures increase resistance almost to the point of stopping flow. During diastole the end-diastolic ventricular pressure, if elevated, can increase intramyocardial pressure and, therefore, increase resistance and decrease flow through the coronary arteries.

Other influences that control coronary vascular resistance include neural, hormonal, and local metabolic factors. Present and future investigations should increase our knowledge of the mechanism and relative contributions of these factors and lead to therapeutic interventions aimed at reducing coronary vascular resistance and increasing coronary blood flow.

Factors That Influence Myocardial Oxygen Demand

Unlike the skeletal muscles, the heart depends almost exclusively on aerobic metabolism for its energy. The myocardial oxygen consumption is, therefore, almost identical to the total metabolic requirements of the heart. There are three major determinants of myocardial oxygen consumption (Braunwald et al.) (Fig. 3). The first is systolic wall tension development which, when increased, increases myocardial oxygen demand. Systolic wall tension is directly related to systolic arterial pressure and intraventricular radius and indirectly related to wall thickness. The second factor is heart rate, which, when faster, increases myocardial oxygen demand. The third major factor is contractility. Increased contractility leads to increased myocardial oxygen demand. A frequently used noninvasive index of myocardial oxygen demand is the "double product," which is obtained by multiplying the heart rate and the systolic blood pressure. Inaccuracies arise when using this index because it does not consider contractility, intraventricular volume, or wall thickness.

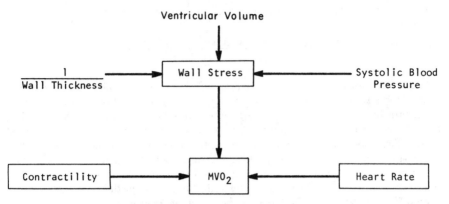

Figure 3   Major determinants of myocardial oxygen demand, MVO_2.

Treatment of Angina Pectoris

The goal of any treatment program is to relieve or, ideally, to eradicate symptoms and to favorably alter the natural history of a disease process. When planning a treatment program, it is important to consider the factors that influence myocardial oxygen supply and those that influence myocardial oxygen demand. The ideal therapeutic regimen will maximize myocardial oxygen supply, minimize myocardial oxygen demand and be devoid of any adverse side effects.

When considering treatment for a patient with angina pectoris, it is helpful to think of various options arranged as a pyramid, as shown in Figure 4. At the base of the pyramid are basic treatment measures, which should form the foundation of any treatment regimen. Next in order are the nitrates (sublingual, oral, cutaneous), which should be considered for patients with angina pectoris unresponsive to general treatment measures. Nitrates have few side effects and are inexpensive; and, on a prn basis, patient compliance is excellent. If patients do not respond to these treatments, other forms of treatment can be added. As one moves up the pyramid, treatments become increasingly costly, both financially and in terms of side effects and complications. Thus, for the relief of symptoms, one should choose a treatment plan that begins at the bottom of the pyramid and includes as little intervention as possible. Treatment regimens designed to prolong life and prevent heart attacks are more controversial and will be considered below.

GENERAL TREATMENT MEASURES See Table 3.

In all patients presenting with angina pectoris, there are some general measures that should be instituted. Although the efficacy of altering risk factors is controversial, such measures should be recommended to all patients. A low-cholesterol, low–saturated fat diet should be provided, particularly for those patients with elevated serum lipids. Although beginning such a diet when a patient presents with symptomatic coronary artery disease may be futile, the goal is to slow the progress of the disease.

Hypertension, if present, should be controlled. There are two reasons to correct an abnormal blood pressure: first, to alter a risk factor and to slow the progress of coronary artery disease; second, to decrease myocardial oxygen demand, which is dependent in part on the systolic blood pressure. Control becomes particularly important in severely hypertensive patients presenting with unstable angina pectoris.

Patients who smoke cigarettes should be encouraged to stop. It is now clear that cigarette smoking leads to an increased incidence of atherosclerotic heart disease (United States Department of Health, Education and Welfare). Thus, one reason to encourage patients to discontinue smoking is to reverse or at least slow the progress of atherosclerosis. A second reason is to halt the acute adverse effects of cigarette smoking on the heart. Nicotine released in cigarette smoke causes a release of endogenous catecholamines. Thus, myocardial oxygen demand is increased due to the catecholamine related increase in heart rate, blood pressure, and myocardial contractility. Catecholamines can also decrease coronary blood supply by stimulation of coronary artery alpha receptors, which results in coronary artery vasoconstriction. An additional adverse effect of nicotine related catecholamine release is increased platelet aggregation. Carbon monoxide, abundant in cigarette smoke, increases blood levels of carboxyhemoglobin and decreases the capacity of the blood to deliver oxygen to myocardial tissue. Thus, it is not surprising that cigarette smoking leads to decreased exercise tolerance measured by exercise treadmill testing (Aranow). Additional reasons to discontinue smoking include its adverse effect on the lungs and other organs and the possible health hazzards and certain annoyance factors suffered by nearby nonsmokers.

The effects of exercise on patients with angina pectoris remains a controversial

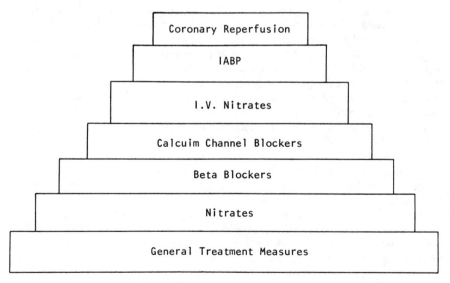

Figure 4 Treatment options for patients with angina pectoris. Basic treatment measures at the base of the pyramid progress upward to more complex treatment measures, which, although often more effective, are also associated with more side effects and complications.

Table 3. General Treatment Measures for
Patients with Angina Pectoris

Alter risk factors
   Lower cholesterol intake
   Control hypertension
   Discontinue smoking
   Weight loss
   Control diabetes mellitus
   Less stressful lifestyle
Avoid activity that precipitates angina pectoris
Exercises
Treat severe anemia
Treat hyperthyroidism

---

issue. Certainly, exercise that precipitates angina pectoris should be discouraged. Patients with unstable angina pectoris should not exercise at all but should be restricted to bed rest. Exercise increases myocardial oxygen demand, which may exceed myocardial oxygen supply and, thus, precipitate angina pectoris in patients with coronary artery disease. Although it is agreed that a long-term exercise program can improve a patient's sense of well-being, its ability to slow or reverse atherosclerosis or to improve collateral blood supply to the myocardium remains unknown. A recent and very interesting study by Kramsch et al. demonstrated a reduction in coronary atherosclerosis in exercised monkeys fed an atherogenic diet compared to sedentary monkeys also fed an atherogenic diet. Redwood et al. have shown that patients with chronic stable angina participating in exercise programs can exercise for a longer period of time prior to developing angina pectoris. In part, this effect is due to the ability of the heart to maintain peripheral muscle oxygenation at a lower myocardial oxygen demand. This effect may be due to a decrease in systemic vascular resistance secondary to exercise and the ability of trained muscles to increase their oxygen extraction efficiency. The improved exercise tolerance following exercise training may also be due to an increase in collateral flow and, thus, an increase in oxygen supply (Redwood et al., Sim and Neill).

At the present time, exercise can be prescribed to patients at minimal risk with the promise that at the very least, it can increase their sense of well-being. Future studies should demonstrate whether or not exercise has an effect on collateral development and atherogenesis in humans.

The risk that exercise will precipitate sudden death or an MI is minimal. Ellestad et al., Irving and Bruce, and Doyle and Kinch have reported a generally safe experience with exercise treadmill testing that supports this view. Therefore, particularly in cooperative patients, an exercise program can be an important component of a treatment program for angina pectoris.

Although it is difficult to alter patients' lifestyles, it is helpful to suggest that patients avoid stressful situations, particularly if such situations regularly precipitate angina pectoris.

Systemic conditions such as severe anemia and hyperthyroidism can worsen angina pectoris and should be treated if present.

Nitrates

Nitrates have been and continue to be the mainstay of pharmacologic treatment for angina pectoris. They are relatively inexpensive and are associated with very few side effects. Nitrates are prescribed in patients with angina to relieve symptoms and not to prolong life. Therefore, there is little reason to prescribe long acting nitrates in asymptomatic patients unless they are experiencing episodes of silent myocardial ischemia. Nitrates can be used prophylactically prior to activities that usually precipitate episodes of angina pectoris.

The administration of nitrates produces a transient decrease in myocardial oxygen demand by reducing venous tone and, therefore, preload. With lower filling pressures, the heart size is decreased and myocardial wall stress, a major determinant of myocardial oxygen demand, is reduced. To a lesser extent, nitrates reduce arterial tone and, therefore, afterload, which also reduces wall stress.

In some patients, nitrates can have a detrimental effect. Decreased arterial tone, while beneficial for myocardial oxygen demand, can decrease coronary artery perfusion and, thus, myocardial oxygen supply. Therefore, caution should be observed when administering nitrates to patients with low blood pressure. Similarly, in patients with low filling pressures or preload, nitrates can further lower pressures and can cause a dangerous decrease in cardiac output.

The effect of nitrates on the coronary vessels is less well understood than their effects on the peripheral vasculature. Cohn et al. (1977) have shown that nitrates can increase flow to myocardium supplied by stenotic coronary arteries if the areas are also supplied by well-developed collateral vessels. The clinical importance of this increased flow, however, is not known. If coronary artery spasm contributes to atherosclerotic-related angina pectoris, nitrates may be helpful in relieving this spasm.

It is important to stress to patients that nitrates are not analgesics. Patients must be reassured that they will not develop a tolerance to the pain relieving effects and they should be encouraged to take nitrates whenever they experience angina pectoris. Shown in Table 4 are the various forms of nitrates available, the routes of administration, and the usual doses.

Nitroglycerin Sublingual

The least expensive nitrate preparation and the drug of choice for an acute attack of angina pectoris is nitroglycerin sublingual. The usual dose if 0.3–0.4 mg. Patients with angina pectoris should be instructed to carry nitroglycerin with them at all times and to take the medication as soon as angina pectoris occurs. The onset of action is usually in 1–3 minutes, with a duration of action of 10–15 minutes. If the angina is not relieved, the dose may be repeated one or two times at five minute intervals. For more prolonged or unresponsive pain, patients should be instructed to seek medical attention. Nitroglycerin can also be taken prior to regular activities known to precipitate angina pectoris. Because nitroglycerin decreases blood pressure, patients should be instructed to sit down when taking the medication, in order to avoid

Table 4. Nitrates: Dosage and Formulation

Preparation	Usual Dosage	Onset of Effect	Duration of Action
Nitroglycerin tablets (SL)	0.3–0.4 mg prn	1–3 min	10–15 min
Isosorbide dinitrate (SL)	5.0–10 mg q 2–3 hr	15–30 min	2–3 hr
Isosorbide dinitrate (oral)	5.0–30 mg* q 3–4 hr	30 min	2–3 hr
Nitroglycerin ointment 2% (topical)	½–3 in q 4–6 hr	15–30 min	3–4 hrs
Nitroglycerin patches (transdermal)	a	30 min	24 hr
Nitroglycerin intravenous	10–800 µg/min[b]	Immediate	As long as drip is continued

[a] Varies depending on manufacturer

[b] High dose sometimes necessary when using polyvinylchloride infusion systems that absorb large amounts of nitroglycerin.

* Isosorbide dinitrate also comes in an oral sustained-release form-40 mg q 12 hrs.

syncope. Nitroglycerin is light sensitive and should be stored in dark containers. It is wise to replace the tablets with new ones every six months.

Isosorbide Dinitrate
This long-acting preparation comes in sublingual, oral, and chewable forms. Although there are few studies documenting the efficacy of these agents, in general, their onset of action is longer than that of nitroglycerin—approximately 15–30 minutes. Their duration of action is generally 2–3 hours. The indication for this medication is frequent angina pectoris and doses should be given every 3–4 hours for an adequate therapeutic response. Because their onset of action is so prolonged, they should not be prescribed for acute attacks of angina pectoris.

Nitroglycerin Ointment
Like isosorbide dinitrate, nitroglycerin ointment should be used to prevent angina; its onset of action is too slow to treat an acute attack of angina pectoris. Whether or not the duration of action is longer than that of isosorbide dinitrate has not been well-documented. The drug is effective for nocturnal angina. A second advantage is that if the patient becomes hypotensive, the remaining medication can be wiped off. It is, however, messy and not a good medication to prescribe to ambulatory patients.

Nitroglycerin Patches (Transdermal Nitroglycerin)
This is the newest form of nitroglycerin delivery. The drug is applied to a patch, which manufacturers claim delivers nitroglycerin over a 24 hour period. Like other long-acting nitroglycerin preparations, this form of medication should not be used for acute attacks, but to prevent attacks in patients with frequent episodes of angina pectoris. Further clinical trials and experience with this medication are needed to define its role in relationship to other available therapies.

Intravenous Nitroglycerin

Intravenous nitroglycerin administration should be considered in patients with unstable angina pectoris that fails to respond to other nitrate preparations and beta-blocking drugs. It has the advantage of rapid onset of action and certain absorption; the dose can be tailored to the needs of the particular patient to assure that blood pressure is not too severely lowered and that excessive reflex tachycardia does not occur. For acute ischemia, patients can be given a bolus of 50–100 μg and then be started on a continuous infusion of 10–15 μg/min. The continuous infusion can be increased by 5–10 μg per minute every 3–5 minutes until the angina fades, headache occurs, or the mean arterial blood pressure drops by more than 20 mm Hg.

Until recently, pharmacists have prepared intravenous nitroglycerin by dissolving nitroglycerin tablets in sterile dextrose solution and passing the resulting solution through a millipore filter. There are now a number of pharmaceutical companies that sell nitroglycerin solutions. Because the nitroglycerin is in part absorbed by polyvinylchloride (PVC) administration sets, some manufacturers have offered non-PVC infusion sets made of less pliable polyethylene. The problem with administering the latter has been the inability of some automatic infusion pumps to fully occlude the less pliant polyethylene tubing and this causes excessive flow or, in some cases, when the instrument is stopped the nitroglycerin solution continues to flow freely by gravity. One solution is to use PVC tubing and to put up with infusion system absorption, controlling the dose of nitroglycerin by following hemodynamic parameters.

Side Effects

Headache, flushing, and hypotension are the most common side effects and can often be relieved by lowering the dose of nitrate and, in the case of sublingual nitroglycerin, instructing the patient to sit when taking the medication. Severe hypotension can be deleterious because of a lowered coronary perfusion pressure and decreased coronary blood supply. For these reasons, these medications should be used with caution in hypotensive patients. Reflex tachycardia increases oxygen demand, and therefore, excessive tachycardia should be avoided. Beta blocking drugs can be helpful in abolishing the reflex tachycardia.

BETA BLOCKADE

When patients with angina pectoris do not respond to control of hypertension, discontinuance of cigarette smoking, avoidance of precipitating activities, and the use of nitrates, the addition of beta-blockade therapy should next be considered.

The beta-blocking drugs work by competing with endogenous catecholamines for beta-adrenergic receptor sites. The beta receptors are subdivided into two types; $beta_1$ and $beta_2$. $Beta_1$ receptors, when stimulated, result in increased heart rate, increased contractility, and accelerated atrioventricular conduction. Other noncardiac effects include increased insulin release and increased muscle glycogenolysis. $Beta_2$ receptors, when stimulated, cause bronchodilation, dilation of peripheral blood vessels, and uterine smooth muscle relaxation.

Beta-blocking drugs affect the factors that determine both oxygen supply and oxygen demand and not all their effects are beneficial. Propranolol can actually decrease myocardial oxygen supply by blocking the vasodilating $beta_2$ receptors located in the walls of the coronary arteries, thereby increasing coronary vascular resistance and decreasing coronary blood flow. The hypotensive effect of beta blockers can contribute to a reduction of coronary blood flow by reducing aortic pressure. Another potentially adverse effect is an increase in ventricular volume, which results in increased wall tension and, therefore, increased myocardial oxygen demand.

Beneficial effects of beta blockade include a decrease in heart rate and a decrease in contractility, factors that lead to a decrease in myocardial oxygen demand. Schrumpf et al. have demonstrated that beta-blocking drugs shift the oxygen-hemoglobin curve to the right, resulting in an increased delivery of oxygen to the myocardium. Back et al. have shown that they may also have a beneficial effect on coronary blood flow in ischemic areas by redistributing blood flow from subepicardium to subendocardium. Overall, the effect of beta blockade in most patients is favorable. Only in the failing or near-failing heart does beta blockade sometimes have a detrimental effect. In such patients, increases in left ventricular size and wall tension lead to an increase in myocardial oxygen demand and can also increase the duration and severity of angina pectoris.

In addition to relieving angina pectoris, beta blockers have also been shown to reduce the morbidity and mortality in patients with coronary artery disease if administered following an acute myocardial infarction. Timolol was the beta-blocking drug used by the Norwegian Multicenter Study Group, and it was begun 7–28 days after the onset of myocardial infarction. Follow-up of 945 timolol–treated patients and 939 placebo—treated patients for a mean of 17 months demonstrated a reduction in both mortality and reinfarction in the timolol-treated patients compared to the placebo-treated patients. In a similar study by the National Heart, Lung, and Blood Institute (BHAT), propranolol or placebo was administered to 3,837 patients 5–21 days post acute myocardial infarction. The propranolol-treated group had a reduced mortality compared to the placebo group.

Whether patients with coronary artery disease and a remote myocardial infarction or no history of a myocardial infarction will benefit with decreased mortality and a decreased incidence of reinfarction if given beta blockers is not known. Because some patients receiving beta blockers will suffer from side effects, it is probably not correct to administer beta blockers to patients with coronary artery disease and mild or no angina pectoris, who have not had a recent myocardial infarction. Rather, in this group of patients, beta blockade should be reserved to treat symptoms when patients do not respond to other, simpler methods of treatment.

Currently there are six beta-blocking drugs available in the United States (Table 5). Propranolol was the first beta blocker available in this country. It can be effectively administered twice daily in doses ranging from 40–320 mg per day, although some patients will respond favorably to total daily doses as high as 1000 mg. Timolol has been recently used to prevent death following an acute myocardial infarction. Like propranolol, twice daily administration is effective. Nadolol, which has been released for the treatment of angina pectoris, has a long half-life, which allows a single daily dose to be prescribed. Also, it is hydrophilic, unlike propranolol, which is lipophilic. Hydrophilic substances do not easily penetrate the central nervous system, so nadolol should be associated with a decreased incidence of central nervous system side effects, and decreased severity when these side effects occur. Metoprolol is a selective beta blocker released for the treatment of hypertension. Like nadolol, this drug is hydrophilic. Metoprolol at low doses blocks primarily beta$_1$

Table 5. Beta Blockers

	Frequency of Administration	Daily Dosage
Propranolol	bid	40–320 mg
Nadolol	qd	40–240 mg
Timolol	bid	20–60 mg
Metoprolol	bid	100–450 mg
Atenolol	qd	50–100 mg
Pindolol	bid to tid	20–60 mg

receptors. However, in doses above 100 mg/day some degree of $beta_2$ receptor blockade is also present in most patients. The fifth beta blocker available in the United States is atenolol. This drug blocks primarily $beta_1$ receptors, has been released for the treatment of hypertension, has a long half-life, and can be given once daily. Pindolol is a beta-adrenergic receptor blocker with intrinsic sympathomimetric activity. It has been released for treatment of hypertension.

When administering beta blockers, the heart rates at rest should be in the 50s or 60s and should not go over 90–110 beats per minute with moderate exercise. Increased doses of beta blockers after these heart rate goals are achieved can be beneficial because, although the negative chronotropic or heart rate slowing effect may not increase with increasing doses, the negative inotropic effect does continue to increase with increased doses.

The side effects of beta-blocking drugs are shown in Table 6. The negative inotropic effects which can lead to congestive heart failure in the failing or near failing ventricle

Table 6. Adverse Effects of Beta-Blockade Therapy

Cardiac
   Increase in ventricular volume resulting in congestive heart failure
   Excessive heart rate slowing
   Propranolol withdrawal syndrome
Noncardiac
   Fatigue
   Mental depression
   Insomnia
   Hallucinations
   Bad dreams
   Gastrointestinal upset
   Raynaud's phenomenon
   Bronchoconstriction
   Worsening of insulin-induced hypoglycemia
   Sexual dysfunction
   Further renal function deterioration in patients with renal disease

have been covered. In some patients, mild congestive heart failure precipitated by beta blocking drugs can be reversed with digitalis. Thus, the addition of digitalis may allow the continuance of beta blockade, and such patients can benefit with improved exercise tolerance and reduced angina pectoris. Excessive heart rate slowing can be a serious problem with beta blocker administration. In some patients, probably those with intrinsic sinus node disease, rates at rest will fall to the 40s, 30s and even lower. In such patients, either the beta-blocking drug must be discontinued or in some instances the rate can be supported with permanent cardiac pacing.

The propranolol withdrawal syndrome has been described in several reports. It has been suggested that the abrupt discontinuance of beta blockers can precipitate acute myocardial ischemia. The basis for this phenomenon is unclear, and different theories have been proposed. First, progression of the underlying coronary atherosclerosis may have occurred during the time the patient was on the drug. Second, the patient may have increased his level of activity and not appropriately reduced it when the drug was stopped. Third, there may be a physiologic rebound effect involving increased sympathetic stimulation soon after the drug is stopped. It is certainly wise to discontinue beta blockade gradually, especially if the patient is an outpatient. In hospitalized patients with chronic stable angina pectoris, administering one-half the usual dose for 24 hours and discontinuing it on day two is a safe approach. In patients with unstable angina pectoris, beta blockade should not be discontinued without compelling reasons.

Other noncardiac adverse effects, shown in Table 6, can sometimes be avoided by changing from one beta-blocking drug to another. Now, with several drugs available, with similar but not identical pharmacologic properties, most patients who can benefit from beta blockade should be able to take one that will not lead to noncardiac adverse effects.

CALCIUM CHANNEL BLOCKING AGENTS

Calcium channel blocking drugs have been in clinical use in Europe for more than 15 years. Three such agents are now available in the United States: nifedipine, verapamil, and diltiazem. These agents decrease the influx of calcium ions into smooth muscle and myocardial cells. This results in an increase in coronary blood flow and a decrease in peripheral vascular resistance. Although originally these agents were used for the treatment of coronary artery spasm or variant angina pectoris, it is now clear that they are effective for the treatment of classical effort-induced angina pectoris and unstable angina pectoris. Calcium channel blockers have been shown to be as effective as nitrates and beta blockers in the treatment of chronic stable angina pectoris. Whether or not they are more effective in certain patients, and what their role is in combination with other antianginal therapy is not known, although current investigations should soon answer these questions. An important difference between calcium channel blocking agents and other antianginal therapy is in side effects. For example, patients with chronic obstructive pulmonary disease, asthma, or peripheral vascular disease unable to take beta blockers, should be able safely to take a calcium channel blocking agent. Currently, in the treatment of patients with classical exertion related angina pectoris and unstable angina pectoris, calcium channel blocking agents should be reserved for those who do not adequately respond to nitrates and beta blockers. The usual starting dose of nifedipine is 10 mg three times a day. The usual effective dose is 10–20 mg three times a day, which can be increased to 20–30 mg three to four times a day, if necessary. More than 180 mg daily is not recommended. The usual starting dose of verapamil is 80 mg three times a day. The usual effective dose is 320–480 mg per day. The medication should be given either three or four times a day. More than 480 mg per day is not recommended. Although differences between nifedipine and verapamil are not completely understood, nifedipine decreases contractility less, slows AV conduction less, and decreases peripheral vascular resistance more than verapamil. Diltiazem has recently been released in this country. The initial dose is 30 mg 4 times a day which is gradually increased to 240 mg daily (given in divided doses 3 or 4 times a day).

INTRAAORTIC BALLOON COUNTERPULSATION

For patients with severe unstable angina pectoris not responding to the measures discussed above, intraaortic balloon counterpulsation can often be effective in relieving ischemia (Weintraub et al.). Intraaortic balloon counterpulsation relieves angina pectoris by decreasing systolic blood pressure and, therefore, myocardial oxygen demand; at the same time it increases diastolic blood pressure and, therefore, increases coronary perfusion pressure and myocardial oxygen supply.

The problems with this technique are the frequent complications, most of which are due to vascular damage and thrombosis. More serious complications include perforation of the aortic wall and ischemia distal to the site of insertion in the femoral artery. Severe peripheral vascular disease, aortic aneurysms, aortic insufficiency, and uncontrollable arrhythmias are all relative contraindications to use of intraaortic balloon counterpulsation. This technique should be reserved for patients who continue to have angina pectoris in spite of other measures discussed. Because the longer the balloon is in place the more likely complications will occur, insertion of the balloon should include plans for coronary angiography and possible coronary artery bypass surgery soon afterward.

PERCUTANEOUS TRANSLUMINAL CORONARY ANGIOPLASTY (PTCA)

An effective method to increase coronary blood flow beyond stenotic lesions was recently introduced by Gruntzig by dilating the stenotic area mechanically. This is done by passing an arterial catheter into the stenosis and inflating a balloon on the tip of the catheter, which compresses the arterial plaque against the arterial wall and widens the coronary lumen. The technique is now mainly applicable to proximal subtotal stenoses that permit passage of the angioplasty catheter. An international registry established by the National Heart, Lung, and Blood Institute has reported a success rate of 59% in a series of over 800 patients from 40 contributing centers. Successful angioplasty is associated with symptomatic improvement and objective improvement in exercise tolerance measured by treadmill exercise testing.

Not all patients with coronary artery disease are candidates for angioplasty. Hamby and Katz estimate that 5–10% of patients who have indications for coronary bypass surgery may be suitable candidates for PTCA. Lesions most suitable for angioplasty should be proximal, concentric, and noncalcified. Very severely narrowed areas of stenosis (>95%) may not permit the dilating catheter to cross. The risk in PTCA increases when more than one vessel is involved because of a potential disruption in collateral flow while a stenosis is being dilated. Stenoses of the left anterior descending coronary artery are more accessible than lesions of the right coronary or left circumflex coronary arteries. The left main coronary artery is the most accessible area, but due to a high incidence of late deaths in the small number of patients who have had dilations of the left main coronary artery, such lesions are generally now being avoided. The experience with dilating lesions in saphenous vein bypass grafts is limited, but such dilations can be performed.

Complications include 6–8% of patients developing sudden occlusions at the site of the attempted dilation, resulting in persistent pain or impending infarction and requiring immediate coronary bypass surgery.

Although initial follow-up results are encouraging, the late course of patients undergoing PCTA is unknown. The mechanism of successful PTCA is not completely understood. The role of atheromatous plaque compression versus plaque disruption needs further study, as does the natural history of dilatated areas of stenosis over time.

Improved techniques and further understanding of this exciting procedure should lead to an increase in the indications and application of percutaneous transluminal angioplasty.

CORONARY ARTERY BYPASS SURGERY

The most direct way to treat angina pectoris is to increase the amount of oxygen rich blood flowing into the ischemic myocardium; currently, coronary artery bypass graft surgery (CABG) is the most popular way to achieve this. As with any other treatment, CABG must be evaluated first for its ability to relieve symptoms and second, for its ability to alter the natural history of coronary artery disease and prolong the life of patients. The decision to recommend coronary artery surgery to a patient is a major one, both because of the risk of the procedure and its expense. The issue of expense and how many CABG operations our health care system can afford has not yet been satisfactorily dealt with.

There is no question that CABG surgery relieves angina pectoris. In prospective random sample studies, 76–90% of patients have less angina pectoris following CABG surgery, while 33–55% of patients become asymptomatic (Rahimtoola). Patients should be considered for CABG surgery for symptomatic relief of angina pectoris only after they have failed rigorous medical therapy. Individual patient lifestyles should also be considered. Patients who have been inactive and who are on medical therapy with only rare episodes of angina pectoris should not be sent for CABG surgery for the purpose of symptom relief. Conversely, patients with frequent angina pectoris, particularly those unable to perform their usual daily activities and who are not responding to maximal medical therapy, are appropriate candidates.

To recommend CABG surgery to patients for the purpose of altering the natural history of the disease is a more complex decision. The survival data from the many nonrandomized studies is difficult to interpret, although in general the survival of patients undergoing CABG surgery is very good, in spite of their known severe coronary artery disease. Because patients with coronary artery disease are not a homogeneous population, randomized trials must be large to assure inclusion of all subsets of patients suffering from it. Patients with left main disease and left ventricular dysfunction cannot be compared to patients with distal right coronary artery disease and normal left ventricular function. Three large randomized studies that have provided useful survival information are the VA Cooperative Study (Murphy et al.) the European Cooperative Surgery Study Group, and the Coronary Artery Surgery Study (CASS). Results from the first two studies suggested that subgroups of patients with three vessel coronary artery disease and left main coronary artery disease are more likely to survive with CABG surgery than they are with medical therapy. Generally, this group of patients will also have severe angina pectoris, and CABG surgery is indicated for symptom relief as well as for improved survival. However, the more recent CASS study showed that patients with mild to moderate angina and single, double, or triple vessel disease had a prognosis which was similar whether they received medical (1.6% annual mortality) or surgical (1.1% annual mortality) therapy. Patients with minimal or no angina pectoris and left main coronary artery disease present difficult problem. If, as a group, these patients can benefit with improved survival from CABG surgery, the problem of detecting them becomes important. Noninvasive studies have many limitations and routine screening coronary angiography is clearly not the solution. At present, there is no good method for screening and detecting such patients, although a strongly positive exercise stress test with marked ST depression at a low level of exercise can be very strong evidence for the presence of severe coronary artery disease. At the present time, patients with one and two vessel disease and angina pectoris should, in general, be referred for CABG surgery only for the relief of symptoms. The occasional patient who undergoes coronary arteriography in spite of only minimal or no angina pectoris and is found to have single or double vessel disease, but lesions that are very severe and proximal (for example, a tight proximal left anterior descending lesion), presents a problem. Whether or not such a patient should undergo CABG surgery is controversial and recommendation for surgery must be individualized for the particular patient under consideration.

For CABG surgery itself, the risks are not great. Operative mortality is 1.3%, with a range of nearly 0% in patients with single vessel disease and normal left ventricular function to 3.5% in patients with three vessel disease and left ventricular dysfunction (Rahimtoola). With constantly improving surgical technique, 70–86% of grafts can be expected to be patent at 6 to 12 months post CABG surgery. Grafts that remain open for more than one year are unlikely to occlude. If graft failure does occur during the first 6 months, it is likely to be secondary to thrombosis, while graft failure occurring beyond 1 year is most likely due to fibrosis or atherosclerosis developing in the bypass vein.

Bibliography

Alison HW, Russel RO Jr, Mantle JA, et al: Coronary anatomy and arteriography in patients with unstable angina pectoris. *Am J Cardiol* 41:204, 1978.

Aranow WS: Smoking, carbon monoxide, and coronary heart disease. *Circulation* 48:1169, 1973.

Atkins GW, Pohost GM, DeSanctis RW, et al: Selection of angina-free patients with severe left ventricular dysfunction for myocardial revascularization. *Am J Cardiol* 46:697, 1980.

Back JD, Gross GJ, Warltier DC, et al: Comparative effects of cardioselective versus noncardioselective beta blockade on subendocardial blood flow and contractile function in ischemic myocardium. *Am J Cardiol* 44:647, 1979.

Banks DC, Raftery ED, Oram S: Clinical significance of the coronary arteriogram *Br Heart J* 33:863, 1971.

Braunwald E, Ross J Jr, Sonnenblick EH: Myocardial energetics, in Braunwald E, Ross J Jr, Sonnenblick EH (eds): *Mechanisms of Contraction of the Normal and Failing Heart.* Boston, Little Brown, 1976, p 171.

CASS Principal Investigators and their Associates; Coronary artery surgery study (CASS); a randomized trial of coronary artery bypass surgery. Survival data. *Circulation* 68:939, 1983.

Cheitlin MD, Davia JE, deCastro CM, et al: Correlations of "critical" left coronary artery lesions with positive submaximal exercise tests in patients with chest pain. *Am Heart J* 89:305, 1975.

Cohn PF: Severe asymptomatic coronary artery disease. A diagnostic, prognostic and therapeutic puzzle. *Am J Med* 62:565, 1977.

Cohn PF: Diagnosis and therapy of coronary artery disease. Boston, Little Brown, 1979, p 311.

Cohn PF, Maddox DE, Holman BL, et al: Effect of sublingually administered nitroglycerin on regional myocardial blood flow in patients with coronary artery disease. *Am J Cardiol* 39:672, 1977.

Cohn PF, Vokonas PS, Williams RA, et al.: Diastolic heart sounds and filling waves in coronary artery disease. *Circulation* 44:196, 1971.

Conti CR, Brawley RK, Griffith LS, et al.: Unstable angina pectoris. Morbidity and mortality in 57 consecutive patients evaluated angiographically. *Am J Cardiol* 32:745, 1973.

Doyle JT, Kinch SH: The prognosis of an abnormal electrocardiographic stress test. *Circulation* 41:54, 1970.

Ellestad MH, Allen W, Wan MC, et al.: Maximal treadmill stress testing for cardiovascular evaluation. *Circulation* 39:517, 1969.

Epstein SE, Stampfer M, Beiser GD, et al.: Effect of a reduction in environment temperature on the circulatory response to exercise in man. Implications concerning angina pectoris. *N Engl J Med* 280:7, 1969.

Erikssen J, Enge I, Forfand K, et al.: False positive diagnostic tests and coronary angiographic findings in 105 presumably healthy males. *Circulation* 54:371, 1976.

European Coronary Surgery Study Group: Coronary artery bypass surgery in stable angina pectoris: Survival at two years. *Lancet* 1:889, 1979.

Fischl SJ, Herman MV, Gorlin R: The intermediate coronary syndrome: clinical, angiographic and therapeutic aspects. *N Engl J Med* 228:1193, 1973.

Freedberg AS, Spiegel ED, Riseman JEF: Effect of external heat and cold on patients with angina pectoris: Evidence for the existence of a reflex factor. *Am Heart J* 27:611, 1941.

Gerstenblith G, Ouyang P, Achuff SC, et al.: Nifedipine in unstable angina: A double blind, randomized trial. *N Engl J Med* 306:885, 1982.

Gerwitz H, Beller GA, Strauss WH, et al: Transient defects of resting thallium scans in patients with coronary artery disease. *Circulation* 59:707, 1979.

Goldman S, Tselos S, Cohn K: Marked depth of ST-segment depression during treadmill exercise testing: Indicator of severe coronary artery disease. *Chest* 69:729, 1976.

Goldstein RE, Redwood DR, Rosing DR, et al: Alterations in the circulatory response to exercise following a meal and their relationship in postprandial angina pectoris. *Circulation* 44:90, 1971.

Gruntzig A: Transluminal dilatation of coronary artery stenosis. *Lancet* 1:263, 1978.

Hamby RI, Katz S: Percutaneous transluminal coronary angioplasty: Its potential impact on surgery for coronary artery disease. *Am J Cardiol* 45:1161, 1980.

Humphries JO: Expected course of patients with coronary artery disease, in Rahimtoola SH (ed): *Coronary bypass surgery.* Philadelphia, FA Davis Company, 1977, p 48.

Irving JB, Bruce RA: Exertional hypotension and postexertional ventricular fibrillation in stress testing. *Am J Cardiol* 39:849, 1977.

Kent KM, Bonow RO, Rosing DR, et al: Improved myocardial function during exercise after successful transluminal coronary angioplasty. *N Engl J Med* 306:441, 1982.

Kent K, et al: Percutaneous transluminal coronary angioplasty (PTCA): Update from NHLBI Registry. *Circulation* 62 (Suppl III):160, 1980.

Kramsch DM, Aspen AJ, Abramowitz BM, et al: Reduction of coronary atherosclerosis by moderate conditioning exercise in monkeys on an atherogenic diet. *N Engl J Med* 305:1483, 1981.

Lavine P, Kimbiris D, Segal BL, et al: Left main coronary artery disease: Clinical, arteriographic, and hemodynamic appraisal. *Am J Cardiol* 30:791, 1972.

Martin CE, Shaver JA, Leonard JJ: Physical signs, apexcardiography, phonocardiography, and systolic time intervals in angina pectoris. *Circulation* 46:1098, 1972.

Mudge GH Jr, Grossman W, Mills RM Jr, et al: Reflex increase in coronary vascular resistance in patients with ischemic heart disease. *N Engl J Med* 295:1333, 1976.

Mulcahy R, Daly L, Graham I, et al: Unstable angina: Natural history and determinants of prognosis. *Am J Cardiol* 48:525, 1981.

Murphy ML, Hultgren HN, Detre K, et al: Treatment of chronic stable angina: A preliminary report of survival data of the randomized veteran's administration cooperative study. *N Engl J Med* 297:621, 1977.

National Heart, Lung, and Blood Institute: Cooperative Trial. Preliminary report. The beta-blocker heart attack trial. *JAMA* 246:2073, 1981.

Pitt B, Strauss HW: Clinical application of myocardial imaging with thallium. In Strauss HW, Pitt B (ed): *Cardiovascular Nuclear Medicine,* ed 2. London, C.V. Mosby Company, 1979, p 243.

Proudfit WL, Hodgman JR: Physical signs during angina pectoris. *Prog Cardiovas Dis* 10:283, 1968.

Proudfit WL, Shirey EK, Sheldon WC, et al: Certain clinical characteristics correlated with extent of obstructive lesions demonstrated by selective cinecoronary arteriography. *Circulation* 38:947, 1968.

Rahimtoola SH: Coronary bypass surgery for chronic angina—1981: A perspective. *Circulation* 65:225, 1982.

Redwood DR, Rosing DR, Epstein SE: Circulatory and symptomatic effects of physical training in patients with coronary artery disease and angina pectoris. *N Engl J Med* 286:959, 1972.

Rifkin RD, Hood WB Jr: Bayesian analysis of electrocardiographic exercise stress testing. *N Engl J Med* 297:681, 1977.

Ritchie JL, Zaret BL, Strauss HW, et al: Myocardial imaging with thallium-201: A multicenter study in patients with angina pectoris or acute myocardial infarction. *Am J Cardiol* 42:345, 1978.

Sampson JJ, Cheitlin MD: Pathophysiology and differential diagnosis of cardiac pain. *Prog Cardiovas Dis* 13:507, 1971.

Schrumpf JD, Sleps DS, Wolfson S, et al.: Altered hemoglobin-oxygen affinity with long-term propranolol therapy in patients with coronary artery disease. *Am J Cardiol* 40:76, 1977.

Sim DN, Neill WA: Investigation of the physiological basis for increased exercise threshold after physical conditioning. *J Clin Invest* 54:763, 1974.

Stadel BV: Oral contraceptives and cardiovascular disease. *N Engl J Med* 305:612, 1981.

Stedman's Medical Dictionary, ed 21. Baltimore, Williams and Wilkins, 1966.

The Norwegian Multicenter Study Group: Timolol-induced reduction in mortality and reinfarction in patients surviving acute myocardial infarction. *N Engl J Med* 304:801, 1981.

United States Department of Health, Education and Welfare: *The health consequences of smoking*. Washington, D.C., Government Printing Office, 1975.

Vatner SF: Correlation between acute reduction in myocardial blood flow and function in conscious dogs. *Circ Res* 47:201, 1980.

Wackers FJ, Lie KL, Liem KL, et al: Thallium-201 scintigraphy in unstable angina pectoris. *Circulation* 57:738, 1978.

Weintraub RM, Voukydis PC, Aroestry JM, et al: Treatment of preinfarction angina with intraaortic balloon counterpulsation and surgery. *Am J Cardiol* 34:809, 1974.

DYNAMIC CORONARY OBSTRUCTION: CORONARY SPASM AND VASOCONSTRICTION

James E. Muller

It is now recognized that *fixed* atherosclerotic blockages may be only partially responsible for ischemic injury in patients with various forms of angina pectoris. Many develop myocardial ischemia as a result of *dynamic* obstruction to coronary blood flow, which may result from one of two processes: the rare form, in which a portion of a coronary artery temporarily narrows beyond physiologic limits is called *coronary spasm*. The common form of dynamic obstruction is that which results from physiologic changes in *coronary vasomotor tone*. Under normal circumstances such changes in vasomotor tone cause no harm; however, when combined with partial fixed obstruction produced by coronary atherosclerosis they may be sufficient to produce myocardial ischemic injury.

The spectrum of combinations of *fixed* and *dynamic* coronary obstruction sufficient to cause myocardial ischemia is portrayed in Figure 1. In the combination indicated at the left of the figure, severe fixed blockage is present, and only a small amount of dynamic obstruction in the form of coronary vasoconstriction will produce ischemia. A situation in which the artery is relatively free of fixed obstruction but afflicted with coronary artery spasm is depicted on the right of the figure. The actual distribution of patients with ischemic heart disease along this spectrum is unknown. It is likely that, in many instances, ischemia is produced by significant degrees of both fixed and dynamic coronary artery obstruction.

An appreciation of the possible dual nature of coronary obstruction is essential for rational design of therapy. Significant fixed obstruction is best treated with coronary artery bypass surgery or agents that decrease myocardial oxygen demand, such as the beta blocking agents. Dynamic obstruction is best treated with coronary vasodilators, such as nitrate preparations or calcium channel blocking agents. The effectiveness of the latter in dilating the coronary arteries makes awareness of the possible presence of dynamic obstruction very important.

Prinzmetal's Angina

The consequences and therapy of dynamic coronary obstruction are most clearly visible in this unusual disorder. The diagnosis refers to patients who demonstrate reversible ST segment elevation during an anginal attack (Fig. 2). It has recently

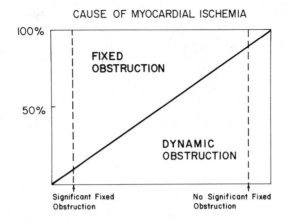

CAUSE OF MYOCARDIAL ISCHEMIA

Figure 1 A diagram indicating that variable mixtures of fixed and dynamic coronary obstruction may produce myocardial ischemia. The dashed line on the left represents a case in which fixed obstruction is the major cause of ischemia. The dashed line on the right depicts a situation in which dynamic obstruction predominates.

ECG SIGNS OF CORONARY SPASM

(A) BEFORE PAIN

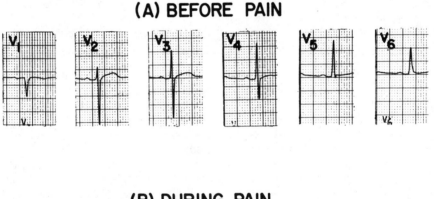

(B) DURING PAIN

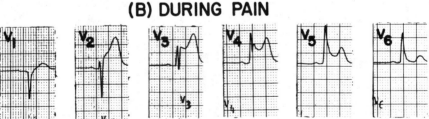

Figure 2 (A) An ECG before an episode of dynamic obstruction. Only nonspecific T wave changes are present. (B) The ECG during an episode of dynamic obstruction. The ST segments are now markedly elevated in V_2–V_6. Five minutes after nitroglycerin was administered, the ECG returned to its baseline appearance.

been recognized that the disorder may occur with or without rest angina, with or without exertion induced angina, and with or without significant fixed coronary atherosclerosis. Although Prinzmetal's angina is rare, the condition has recently attracted interest because of the possible role of dynamic coronary obstruction in the more common condition of classic angina pectoris.

PATHOGENESIS

The episodic anginal pain and ST segment elevation that characterize Prinzmetal's angina are caused by transmural ischemia of a major portion of the myocardium. The ischemia, in turn, may result from a combination of fixed and dynamic coronary obstruction.

The cause of local coronary spasm that can occlude an artery without significant atherosclerotic obstruction is unknown. It is possible that minor intimal damage caused by nonobstructive atherosclerosis may prompt local platelet aggregation and formation of thromboxane A_2, an extremely potent coronary vasoconstrictor. Thromboxane A_2 is highly unstable and is rapidly transformed into the chemically stable but inactive thromboxane B_2. The level of thromboxane B_2 in venous blood of patients with Prinzmetal's angina has been found to be markedly elevated; but this may be the consequence rather than the cause of the spasm, as shown by Leroy et al.

The coronary vessels are richly innervated with sympathetic and parasympathetic fibers, which may also cause focal spasm. However, these fibers cannot be the only cause for the abnormal contraction, since coronary artery spasm has been found to occur in some patients with cardiac transplants whose hearts are totally denervated (Clark et al.).

In patients *with* significant coronary atherosclerosis, a normal increase in vasomotor tone may be sufficient to occlude the coronary lumen, as previously discussed.

DIAGNOSIS AND EVALUATION

The single most common clue to the presence of this life-threatening illness is the occurrence of angina *at rest* with preservation of exercise capacity. The patient will usually experience numerous brief unprovoked attacks of angina that resolve spontaneously or following sublingual nitroglycerin. The onset of the problem may be quite sudden. The illness may start on a single day with numerous attacks of severe transient chest pain. The attacks may be associated with syncopal episodes. In a few patients, other disorders of smooth muscle tone, such as Raynaud's phenomenon or esophageal spasm, may be present. The disorder occurs with equal frequency in men and women; the average age of the patients is five to ten years less than that of patients with classic angina. Recognition of the disease is of great importance because without therapy it is associated with a significant mortality, presumably from ischemia-induced arrhythmias.

For patients with such a history, every effort should be made to obtain an ECG during an attack of pain. If the chest pain is being caused by Prinzmetal's angina, the ECG during pain will show changes similar to those seen during the very early stages of an acute myocardial infarction (Fig. 2). The ST segment rises above the baseline, the R wave increases in height, and the S wave disappears. These ECG changes begin to resolve as the patient's chest pain diminishes. Within minutes the

QRS complex and ST segment return to normal, but T wave changes often persist for a longer period. These changes generally occur in several of the anterior or the inferior leads, reflecting events in the distribution of a major coronary artery. Ventricular arrhythmias and atrioventricular conduction disturbances occur in over 30% of patients. There is no doubt that these ECG changes reflect the sudden onset and resolution of severe transmural myocardial ischemia. An identical sequence of ECG changes can be produced in the experimental animal by the temporary occlusion of a major coronary artery.

If the attacks occur at the rate of at least once every three to four days, admission to a coronary care unit is generally the best method to obtain an ECG during pain. In patients with less frequent attacks, Holter monitoring may reveal episodic elevation of the ST segment. ST segment elevation may, in some instances, occur without chest pain. When both the chest pain and ECG changes can be observed, it will be found that the ECG changes generally *precede* the onset of chest pain. The patient should be evaluated for the presence of complete heart block or ventricular tachycardia with Holter monitoring and ECG recordings during pain.

It is the general practice to perform coronary arteriography in all patients with Prinzmetal's angina to determine the presence or absence of fixed coronary obstruction. This knowledge is of therapeutic value, since coronary artery bypass grafting and beta blockade should be considered only for patients with fixed obstructive lesions.

The intravenous injection of ergonovine maleate produces focal spasm in the coronary arteries of patients with Prinzmetal's angina, but causes only a diffuse narrowing in patients without the condition. The test has been used frequently in patients with chest pain syndromes to establish or exclude the diagnosis of Prinzmetal's angina. The patient is given gradually increasing doses of ergonovine and observed for evidence of an attack. A coronary arteriogram is then obtained to determine the presence or absence of coronary spasm. There is a growing awareness that this test may be more dangerous than originally thought and that its use for clinical purposes should be more limited (Buston et al.). Certainly, patients known to have rest pain with documented reversible ST segment elevation need not be subjected to ergonovine provocation. In patients whose pain is likely to be from dynamic obstruction, a therapeutic trial of nitrates or nifedipine should be started to determine whether or not the symptoms can be controlled. If it is less certain that the patient's symptoms are caused by coronary spasm, the ergonovine test may be of value. A negative response will prevent a patient from receiving needless therapy for coronary spasm. The test is most safely performed during cardiac catheterization when intracoronary nitroglycerin may be given if intense spasm develops. A calcium channel blocking agent should also be available for emergency use.

The ergonovine test has been used for research purposes to study the course of patients with Prinzmetal's angina. It has been found that sensitivity to ergonovine, which presumably reflects the intensity of the tendency to spasm, varies markedly over time.

THERAPY

The complications of Prinzmetal's angina determine the urgency of treatment and the degree of control that is necessary. If the attacks occur with great frequency or are associated with life-threatening arrhythmias, rapid and complete control must be sought. Prolonged attacks of spasm may lead to myocardial infarction and should be treated aggresively. However, if the attacks end spontaneously without arrhythmia and occur rarely, attempts at control need not be as vigorous.

Sublingual Nitroglycerin

As a first step, the patient should be instructed to take a nitroglycerin tablet (0.3 mg) sublingually at the beginning of an attack. Another tablet may be taken three to five minutes later if pain persists. This maneuver may prevent spasm from becoming severe and may accelerate the spontaneous resolution of an attack.

Long Acting Nitrates

Oral isosorbide dinitrate and nitroglycerin paste are often effective in preventing attacks. Isosorbide dinitrate can be started in a dosage of 10 mg every six hours and gradually increased to 20 mg every four hours or higher if attacks persist and side effects of significant hypotension and headache do not occur.

Calcium Channel Blocking Agents

The most promising new development in the control of Prinzmetal's angina has been the recent availability of agents that block the slow channel calcium current. The smooth muscle cells in walls of the coronary arteries that produce dynamic obstruction are particularly sensitive to these agents. This sensitivity results from the dependence of these cells on the slow calcium channel for the generation of their action potential and from a relatively specific effect of the blocking agents on cells in this location. Among these agents, nifedipine and verapamil have been the most widely used and diltiazem recently has been approved. Nifedipine is a coronary vasodilator that can produce coronary flow equal to reactive hyperemia. It was originally developed in 1971 as a coronary vasodilator for use in patients with classic angina pectoris. In preliminary observations, it has also been found to be extremely useful in the management of Prinzmetal's angina. The collective experience in the United States with its use for Prinzmetal's angina has recently been summarized by Antman et al. (1980).

Data were available from 127 patients. All patients had chest pain at rest with reversible ST segment elevation or coronary artery spasm visualized during catheterization. Most patients had failed to respond to conventional therapy with nitrates. The average number of attacks per week fell markedly from 16 per week prior to nifedipine to two per week after nifedipine. Complete elimination of attacks was achieved in 63% of the patients, while only 7% showed less than a 10% decrease in the number of attacks.

Only minor reversible side effects such as mild hypotension, flushing, and dysesthesias were noted. In some patients pedal edema unrelated to heart failure occurred. This lack of serious side effects is in accord with more extensive experience in Europe and Japan, where nifedipine has been widely used for several years in patients with classic angina.

The usual starting dose for nifedipine is 10 mg every six hours; it can be increased to 20 mg every four hours if necessary. It is contraindicated in women of childbearing potential because of possible teratogenic effects. The most commonly encountered side effects, which are mild and reversible, are headache, flushing, and ankle edema.

Verapamil is a similar agent, which has also been useful for the treatment of Prinzmetal's angina, but is more likely to produce atrioventricular block and depress myocardial contractility than is nifedipine. Diltiazem is a recently developed calcium channel blocking agent that has been approved for general use. Although experience with diltiazem is limited, it appears to be as effective as nifedipine or verapamil for the treatment of Prinzmetal's angina. Details of the pharmacology of the calcium channel blockers are presented in Table I.

Beta-Adrenergic Blockade

In general, agents such as propranolol are not as effective in patients with Prinzmetal's angina as in patients with classic angina. In patients with classic angina, propranolol is effective in suppressing the periodic *increase in oxygen demand,* which causes pain; in Prinzmetal's angina, control of increases in oxygen demand has little effect, since the primary problem is a periodic *decrease in oxygen supply.* Furthermore, it is theoretically possible that blockade of the beta-sympathetic receptors, which dilate the coronary arteries, could actually enhance spasm. It is likely that beta blockers may be most effective in patients with Prinzmetal's angina who have severe fixed obstructive disease. Many clinicians begin a therapeutic trial of a beta blocker in patients who have continued attacks on maximal nitrate therapy. Beta blockers should be avoided in patients whose attacks are complicated by heart block.

Antiarrhythmic Agents

The highest priority in the treatment of Prinzmetal's angina complicated by arrhythmia should be given to prevent coronary spasm and recurrent ischemia. Antiarrhythmic agents, such as procainamide or quinidine, should be used only in the small number of patients in whom prevention of attacks of ischemia cannot be accomplished.

Coronary Artery Bypass Grafting

In most instances, attempts to bypass areas of focal spasm in patients without significant coronary atherosclerosis have not been successful. Failure apparently results from intrinsic abnormality of the entire artery. In one patient, a major section of the epicardial portion of a coronary artery was seen to constrict into a cordlike structure at the time of thoracotomy. Vessels with such abnormal reactivity are likely to constrict at sites distal, as well as proximal, to the site of anastomosis of a saphenous vein bypass graft.

Even when severe fixed obstruction is present, bypass grafting is not as successful in patients with Prinzmetal's angina as in patients with classic angina. Bypass grafting is most likely to relieve symptoms in those patients in whom the transient ischemia results from normal changes in coronary vasomotor tone superimposed on a signif-

Table 1. Calcium Channel Blockers

Drug	Oral Dose	Absorption	Onset of Action	Peak Effect	Plasma Half-Life	Metabolism and Elimination	Side Effects
Nifedipine	10–30 mg/4–8 hr	>90%	<20 min	1–2 hr	4 hr	Extensively metabolized to inert products; 80% excreted via kidney	Headache, hypotension, flushing, digital dysesthesias, leg edema
Verapamil	80–160 mg/8 hr	>90%	2 hr	5 hr	3 to 7 hr	Extensively metabolized in liver; 85% first pass hepatic elimination after oral administration; 75% excreted via kidney	Constipation, headahce, vertigo, hypotension, AV conduction disturbances
Diltiazem	30 mg 4 times daily increasing to 240 mg /day divided in 3–4 doses	>90%	<15 min	30 min	4 hr	Extensively metabolized; 60% excreted via liver; 35% excreted via kidney	Headache, dizziness, flushing, AV conduction disturbances

icant fixed lesion. Thus, surgery should be considered for patients with severe fixed stenosis and attacks of ischemia that cannot be controlled medically. Surgery for patients with stenosis who become asymptomatic on medical therapy is as controversial as surgery for patients with classic angina who become asymptomatic with medical therapy.

Duration of Therapy

With the use of long-acting nitrates and calcium channel blockers, it is possible to prevent virtually all attacks of Prinzmetal's angina in the majority of patients. After patients are asymptomatic for six months or more, the issue of discontinuation of one or all of the medications arises. In principle, discontinuation may be justified because the natural history of the disorder includes spontaneous disappearance of the stimulus for spasm. The agents must be gradually withdrawn, however, because the withdrawal of long-acting nitrates or nifedipine over a 48 hour period has led to prolonged coronary artery spasm, causing myocardial infarction. Tapering of dosage should, therefore, be done in gradual steps over a period of weeks rather than days. During this period, the patient should be instructed to take sublingual nitroglycerin at the first sign of an attack and to reinstitute the previous level of preventive therapy. Since patients frequently miss doses of medication while on chronic therapy, the physician may gain useful information by inquiring about the occurrence of attacks during the period without therapy. Patients who once had over 20 attacks of Prinzmetal's angina per day may be found to be completely free of attacks off all medications a year later.

Classic Angina

Although the presence of dynamic obstruction is most frequently recognized in cases of Prinzmetal's angina, its greatest importance may be the role it plays in the pathogenesis of the far more common condition of classic angina. A number of recent observations in patients with classic angina have expanded our understanding of the pathogenesis of the disorder.

Patients with stable angina have been shown to have temporary inappropriate increases in coronary artery resistance with certain circumstances. Mudge et al. demonstrated that immersion of the arm in ice water (the cold pressor stimulus) produced increases in coronary resistance at a time when myocardial work actually increased as a consequence of increased arterial pressure. In some patients, the increase in coronary resistance was associated with production of lactate by the myocardium and the occurrence of angina pectoris.

Patients without significant coronary atherosclerosis did not show an increase in coronary vascular resistance. It is likely that the vasoconstriction of the large coronary arteries produced by the cold stimulus can produce ischemia in patients with significant fixed obstruction.

A study was conducted to determine if nifedipine could block this inappropriate coronary vasoconstriction in classic angina, since the agent had been found to be so effective against dynamic obstruction in Prinzmetal's angina. Fifteen patients with classic angina pectoris were given the cold pressor challenge while coronary flow was being measured with a coronary sinus thermodilution catheter. With the cold pressor challenge, systemic arterial pressure increased, producing an increase in myocardial oxygen demand that could be met by a decrease in coronary vascular resistance. However, coronary resistance actually increased (from 0.80 ± 0.12 to 0.94 ± 0.20 [SD] resistance units). Three of the patients developed chest pain and lactate production. Following recovery from the first cold pressor challenge, ten of the patients were given 10 mg of nifedipine, which was chewed for buccal absorption. The cold pressor challenge was then repeated. In the presence of nifedipine, none of the patients developed an increase in coronary vascular resistance. The mean coronary resistance fell (from 0.85 ± 0.16 to 0.76 ± 0.16), as was appropriate for the increase in systemic arterial pressure. None of the patients developed angina pectoris or net lactate production by the myocardium. These studies provide evidence that coronary vasoconstriction can play a role in the production of classic angina pectoris and that such vasoconstriction can be selectively blocked by nifedipine. It is likely that verapamil or diltiazem could also block such vasoconstriction.

Evidence for the presence of dynamic obstruction in patients with classic angina has also been obtained with the use of psychologic stress. Schiffer et al. found that ST changes and angina produced by a stressful quiz occurred at lower rate-pressure products than angina produced by physical exertion. The rate-pressure product reflects myocardial oxygen demand. The occurrence of angina at a lower demand implies that oxygen supply is diminished, presumably secondary to dynamic coronary obstruction.

RECOGNITION OF DYNAMIC OBSTRUCTION IN PATIENTS WITH CLASSIC ANGINA

Although reliable methods for the identification of dynamic obstruction in patients with classic angina are yet to be developed, there are a number of clinical clues that suggest its presence. The research findings mentioned above suggest that patients whose angina is precipitated by cold exposure or psychologic stress may have such a mechanism. Maseri has pointed out that patients with a variable threshold for angina are likely to have a primary change in oxygen supply. Fixed blockages cannot explain situations in which a patient develops angina during mild exertion one day yet performs strenuous exercise a day later without developing angina. Other clues to the presence of dynamic obstruction may be the presence of abnormal vasoreactivity in other vessels, as observed in patients with Raynaud's syndrome or migraine headaches.

Therapy

Nitrate preparations and calcium channel blockers are the agents of choice for the treatment of dynamic coronary obstruction. Since beta-adrenergic blocking agents block receptors that mediate coronary vasodilation, giving such agents to a patient whose primary problem is dynamic obstruction can theoretically increase dynamic obstruction and angina. However, since the prevalence of fixed obstruction is so high in patients with classic angina, the beneficial effect of beta blockade in decreasing oxygen demand generally outweighs any detrimental effect produced by an increase in the tendency toward dynamic obstruction.

It is important to know that nitrates and calcium channel blockers may also decrease myocardial oxygen consumption. The nitrates reduce both preload and afterload; the calcium blockers reduce afterload and, in higher doses, may have a mild negative inotropic effect. These properties, together with their well-known effectiveness against dynamic obstruction, account for their antianginal effect in a group of unselected patients. It is likely that, in such a group with classic angina, there will be some patients whose response to coronary vasodilation will be far greater than their response to beta-blockade. Specific recommendations for the relative roles of coronary vasodilators and beta blockers in the treatment of classic angina must await refinement of methods to identify patients in whom dynamic obstruction is the primary underlying pathophysiologic process.

THE ROLE OF DYNAMIC CORONARY OBSTRUCTION IN UNSTABLE ANGINA PECTORIS, MYOCARDIAL INFARCTION AND SUDDEN DEATH

The role dynamic obstruction plays in these disorders is currently a subject of great interest with many unresolved issues. The severity and frequency of these three conditions plus the availability of effective therapy against dynamic coronary obstruction combine to make this an important area of ongoing research.

Unstable Angina Pectoris

As previously discussed, unstable angina accompanied by ST segment elevation (Prinzmetal's angina) is generally caused by dynamic obstruction and responds extremely well to coronary vasodilators with a calcium channel blocking agent. Maseri and other investigators have obtained evidence that patients with unstable angina without ST segment elevation may also suffer from dynamic obstruction. In some patients, continuous hemodynamic monitoring has revealed that increases in heart rate and arterial pressure (changes indicating an increase in oxygen demand) follow, rather than precede, the onset of ischemic ST segment changes and chest pain. In some cases, dynamic obstruction has been documented with coronary angiograms obtained during an attack of pain.

These observations, plus the results of several pilot studies, have led to the initiation of studies to compare nifedipine with conventional therapy for the treatment of unstable angina (Moses et al.). These studies will also test the clinical impression that patients who fail to respond to conventional therapy will often respond to nifedipine, thereby avoiding the need for intraaortic balloon counterpulsation or emergency surgery.

Acute Myocardial Infarction

For years clinicians have suspected that coronary spasm might cause myocardial infarction in certain instances. Infarctions that began suddenly after an emotional shock or occurred in patients who were subsequently found to be free of coronary atherosclerosis suggested such a mechanism. Oliva and Breckenridge provided evidence for such a possibility by demonstrating that the intracoronary administration of nitroglycerin could open occluded arteries in some patients with acute myocardial infarction.

Recent studies in which the intracoronary administration of a thrombolytic agent has been preceded by administration of nifedipine or nitroglycerin have also demonstrated reflow following the administration of the vasodilator (Mathey et al.). However this phenomenon has been less frequently encountered in the recent studies than in the experience of Oliva. It is possible that dynamic obstruction initiates the ischemia but in many cases is rapidly followed by thrombosis, which cannot be reversed with a vasodilator alone.

Sudden Cardiac Death

The role of dynamic obstruction in this condition is difficult to evaluate because most patients die without medical observation. It is certain that patients with Prinzmetal's angina, who are known to have dynamic obstruction, often exhibit high-grade ventricular arrhythmias including ventricular fibrillation. It is possible but yet to be proven that dynamic obstruction may be the underlying pathophysiologic process in a substantial proportion of the many patients who suffer sudden cardiac death.

Bibliography

Antman E, Muller J, Goldberg, S, et al: Nifedipine therapy for coronary artery spasm: Experience in 127 patients. *N Engl J Med* 302:1269, 1980.

Antman EM, Stone PH, Muller JE, et al: Calcium channel blocking agents in the treatment of cardiovascular disorders. Part One: Basic and clinical electrophysiologic effects. *Ann Int Med* 93:875, 1980.

Buston A, Goldberg S, Hirshfeld JW, et al: Refractory ergonovine induced coronary vasospasm: importance of intracoronary nitroglycerin. *Am J Cardiol* 46:329, 1980.

Clark DA, Quint RA, Mitchell RL, et al: Coronary artery spasm: Medical management, surgical denervation, and autotransplantation. *J Thorac Cardiovasc Surg* 73:332, 1977.

Conti CR, Curry RC, Christi LG, et al: Clinical use of provocative pharmacoangiography in patients with chest pain. *Adv Cardiol* 26:44, 1979.

Gunther S, Green L, Muller JE, et al: Prevention by nifedipine of abnormal coronary vasoconstriction in patients with coronary artery disease. *Circulation* 63:849, 1981.

Leroy RI Weiner L, Smith JB et al: Comparison of plasma concentrations of thromboxane B_2 in Prinzmetal's variant angina and classical angina pectoris. *Clin Cardiol* 2:404, 1979.

MacAlpin RN, Kattus AK, Alvaro AB: Angina pectoris at rest with preservation of exercise capacity: Prinzmetal's variant. *Circulation* 47:946, 1973.

Maseri A: Variant angina and coronary vasospasm: clues to a broader understanding of angina pectoris. *Cardiovas Med* 4:647, 1979.

Mathey DG, Kuck K-H, Tilsner V, et al: Nonsurgical coronary artery recanalization in acute transmural myocardial infarction. *Circulation* 63:489, 1981.

Moses JW, Wertheimer JH, Bodenheimer MM, et al: Efficacy of nifedipine in rest angina refractory to propranolol and nitrates in patients with obstructive coronary disease. *Ann Int Med* 94:425, 1981.

Mudge GH, Grossman W, Mills RM, et al: Reflex increase in coronary vascular resistance in patients with ischemic heart disease. *N Engl J Med* 295:1333, 1976.

Muller JE, Braunwald E: Prinzmetal's angina. *Harrison's Principle of Internal Medicine,* Update I. New York, McGraw-Hill Book Company, 1981, p 107.

Muller JE, Gunther SJ: Nifedipine therapy for Prinzmetal's angina. *Circulation* 57:137, 1978.

Oliva PB, Breckinridge JC: Arteriographic evidence of coronary arterial spasm in acute myocardial infarction. *Circulation* 56:366, 1977.

Oliva PB, Potts DE, Pluss RG: Coronary arterial spasm in Prinzmetal's angina: documentation by coronary arteriography. *N Engl J Med* 288:745, 1973.

Prinzmetal M, Kennamer R, Merliss R, et al: Angina pectoris. I. A variant form of angina pectoris. *Am J Med* 27:375, 1959.

Schiffer F, Hartley LH, Schulman CL, et al: The quiz electrocardiogram: A new diagnostic and research technique for evaluating the relation between emotional stress and ischemic heart disease. *Am J Cardiol* 37:41, 1976.

Stone PH, Antman E, Muller JE, et al: Calcium channel blocking agents in the treatment of cardiovascular disorders. Part Two: Hemodynamic effects and clinical applications of the calcium channel blocking agents. *Ann Int Med* 93:886, 1980.

Theroux P, Waters D, Affaki G, et al: Provocative testing and ergonovine to evaluate the efficacy of treatment with calcium antagonists in variant angina. *Circulation* 60:504, 1979.

CHAPTER 11 | ACUTE MYOCARDIAL INFARCTION

Robert A. Kloner

Myocardial infarction (MI) is one of the most common serious health problems of contemporary Western society. In this country alone, approximately 1,300,000 patients develop myocardial infarction and approximately 650,000 die from complications of this disease each year. *Myocardial infarction* implies histologic myocardial necrosis, which occurs secondary to myocardial ischemia. *Myocardial ischemia* is the condition in which coronary blood flow is not adequate to meet the oxygen demand of the heart, resulting in anaerobic metabolism. Myocardial infarction is usually related to severe atherosclerotic narrowing of the coronary arteries with a reduction in O_2 supply/demand ratio. Transmural myocardial infarctions are probably the result of a total occlusion of a coronary artery. This may be secondary to (1) thrombus in a coronary artery overlying an atherosclerotic plaque; (2) hemorrhage into or rupture of an atherosclerotic plaque; (3) coronary spasm; or (4) dissection of the coronary artery. Recent studies, in which patients with acute transmural infarctions received intracoronary injections of fibrinolytic agents with relief of their obstruction documented by coronary angiography, suggest that most transmural infarctions are in fact due to thrombus overlying a narrowed segment of the coronary artery. Platelet aggregability has been shown to be increased in patients with acute myocardial infarction. Thromboxane A_2 may play a role in this platelet aggregability as well as increasing coronary arterial tone. Emboli may cause myocardial infarctions without preexisting coronary disease. Subendocardial myocardial infarctions may not be associated with a total occlusion of a vessel, but often severe narrowing of the coronary arteries is present in the setting of increased O_2 demand. Sudden death secondary to arrhythmia may occur due to a myocardial ischemic event before any histologic evidence of necrosis develops. These patients often have severe narrowing, but total coronary occlusions are less common. Myocardial infarctions may extend, indicating increased amount of necrosis, or expand, indicating thinning and dilatation of the ventricular wall without new necrosis (Hutchins and Bulkley).

Diagnosis of Myocardial Infarction

HISTORY

The typical history is one of severe substernal chest pain, described as crushing or severe pressure. The pain may occur at rest and is usually more severe and of longer duration than the pain of angina pectoris, lasting longer than 20–30 minutes. The pain often radiates down the left arm and shoulder but may also radiate to the lower jaw or epigastrium. It is associated with diaphoresis, weakness, and anxiety. While the pain of angina is usually relieved by rest, the pain of acute myocardial infarction is not, and patients cannot find a comfortable position. In addition, while the pain of angina is relieved by nitroglycerin, the pain of myocardial infarction usually is not, although the pain may become less severe. Some patients describe a sense of impending doom. Vagal symptoms are common in patients with inferior and posterior wall myocardial infarctions but may occur with anterior wall myocardial infarctions as well and include nausea, vomiting, diarrhea, and abdominal cramps. Some patients may experience nonspecific symptoms such as "indigestion." In approximately 20% of patients, the myocardial infarction is silent; that is, not associated with symptoms definitely related to the heart. Diabetics with autonomic dysfunction may be more likely to have silent myocardial infarctions. If congestive heart failure is present, patients complain of dyspnea and orthopnea. With right ventricular infarction, patients may complain of right upper quadrant pain, nausea, vomiting, and diarrhea. With severe right ventricular failure and decreased forward cardiac output, patients feel weak, lethargic, and have altered mentation.

PHYSICAL EXAMINATION

Typically, patients appear anxious, restless, and diaphoretic. The skin may be cool and clammy. Patients with strong vagal reactions have reduced heart rate. With severe pump failure, hypotension and tachycardia are present. The pulse may be irregular if arrhythmias are present. Low-grade fever is common during the first few days of myocardial infarction and examination of the lungs reveals rales in the setting of congestive heart failure. The cardiac impulse feels dyskinetic when a large portion of the anterior left ventricular wall undergoes paradoxical systolic bulging. Auscultation reveals an S_4 in most cases. If congestive heart failure is present, an S_3 also is heard. With right ventricular infarction, signs of right ventricular failure may be present with jugular venous distension, tender enlarged liver, peripheral edema and in severe cases signs of low forward output with hypotension and decreased mentation. The murmur of tricuspid regurgitation may be heard if the right ventricle is severely dilated.

ELECTROCARDIOGRAPHIC FINDINGS

Transmural Myocardial Infarction

The initial feature may be hyperacute T waves with R waves taller than normal. This is followed by J point and ST segment elevation, or so-called current of injury (Fig. 1). ST elevation implies that ischemia is transmural. As myocardial cells begin to die, R wave voltage is lost and pathologic Q waves develop. Pathologic Q waves are defined as being at least 0.04 second wide and having an amplitude of at least 25% of the QRS complex. Eventually the R waves are lost and deep QS complexes remain. The T waves invert at a time when ST segment elevation is still present. This is in contrast to pericarditis, in which the ST segment returns to baseline before the T waves invert. Eventually the ST segment returns to baseline except in cases of ventricular aneurysm, in which it remains elevated indefinitely. The T waves may remain inverted for months. Months to years after the infarction there may be late diminishing, and in some cases disappearance of, the Q waves. This is especially common with inferior wall myocardial infarction.

LOCALIZATION OF MI

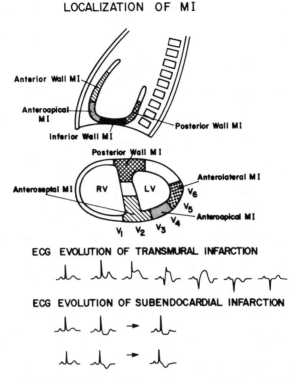

Figure 1 Nomenclature for the localization of myocardial infarction. ECG evolution of transmural infarction showing development of Q waves. ECG evolution of subendocardial infarction showing persistent ST-T wave abnormalities.

It has recently been recognized by combined electrocardiographic and nuclear studies that ST changes previously thought to represent reciprocal changes may actually represent ischemia in other areas of the heart. In one study, moderate or severe anterior precordial ST depression in patients with acute inferior infarction was found to be a sensitive and specific indicator of extensive damage involving the posterolateral region of the heart. Patients with new ECG changes far from the site of the acute infarct may have a higher mortality. (Electrocardiographic findings are also discussed in Chapter 3.)

Subendocardial Myocardial Infarction

In subendocardial infarction (myocardial cell necrosis confined to the subendocardial wall), ST segment depression or symmetrically inverted T waves are present and persist for 48 hours or more in the setting of ischemic pain, usually without the development of Q waves. However, one recent study suggested that subendocardial infarction cannot always be distinguished from transmural infarction on the basis of the presence or absence of QRS changes.

The ECG localization of acute myocardial infarction depends upon which leads the infarction pattern appears in and is shown in Table 1.

SERUM ENZYMES, LABORATORY TESTS

Serum enzymes are released by damaged myocardial cells and are an important part of the diagnosis of myocardial infarction.

1. CK (creatine kinase) rises within 6–8 hours after the onset of infarction and peaks within 24 hours; its duration of elevation is 2–4 days. Other causes for elevation are skeletal muscle damage, trauma, IM injection, rhabdomyolysis, hypothyroidism, and stroke. Serial CK measurements may be useful in estimating the size of the myocardial infarction.
2. GOT (glutamic-oxaloacetic transaminase) rises within 8–12 hours after the onset of infarction, peaks day 2–3, and has a duration of elevation of 3–5 days. Other causes for elevation are hepatic disorders and skeletal muscle damage.
3. LDH (Lactic dehydrogenase) rises within 24–48 hours after onset of infarction, peaks day 4–6, and has a duration of elevation of 10–12 days. Other causes for elevation of LDH include hepatic disorders, hemolysis, and pulmonary infarction.
4. Cardiac isoenzymes help to rule out noncardiac causes that may elevate routine enzymes. The creatine kinase isoenzyme MB-CK has been especially helpful in this regard since it is more specific for myocardial necrosis than CK alone. MB-CK is not elevated following IM injection, noncardiac surgery, exercise, or uncomplicated cardiac catheterization. MB-CK appears between 4–6 hours after the onset of myocardial infarction and peaks between 18–24 hours afterwards. Its duration of elevation is 2–4 days. MB-CK greater than 4% of total CK is suggestive of myocardial cellular damage (Roberts and Sobel).

There are some conditions other than myocardial infarction in which the MB-CK is elevated. These include hypothyroidism, muscular dystrophy, multiple electrical countershocks, polymyositis, widespread muscle destruction or inflammation, cardiac surgery, myocarditis, in patients on chronic hemodialysis, and occasionally in

Table 1. The ECG Localization of Myocardial Infarction[a]

ECG Leads Showing the Infarct Pattern	Localization of the MI
V₁, V₂	Anteroseptal
V₂, V₃	Anteroapical
V₄–V₆, I, aV_L	Anterolateral
V₁–V₆	Extensive anterior
I, aV_L	High lateral
II, III, aV_F	Inferior (diaphragmatic)
V₁, V₂ showing mirror image of typical findings: tall R waves, ST depression, tall T waves	Posterior wall MI

[a] See Figure 1.

an apparently normal individual. Elevated LDH 1 isoenzyme is more specific for cardiac injury than LDH but may also be elevated with hemolysis.

Several studies have shown that serum myoglobin is increased early during the course of acute myocardial infarction. Its advantage over MB-CK has yet to be determined.

Leukocytosis and elevated erythrocyte sedimentation rate also occur in MI.

CHEST X-RAY

The chest x-ray film may be entirely normal or show cardiomegaly. When the pulmonary capillary wedge pressure is 15 mm Hg or greater, pulmonary vascular redistribution may be observed on the x-ray film. When the wedge pressure is greater than 20–25 mm Hg, further signs of congestive heart failure appear with interstitial pulmonary edema (blurring of the pulmonary vasculature, perihilar haze, Kerley B pattern, lattice pattern) and pleural effusions. There may be a lag of 12–24 hours between the time the pulmonary capillary wedge pressure is elevated and chest x-ray findings of congestive heart failure are seen. Similarly, following therapy for congestive heart failure, the chest x-ray findings may not clear until 12–24 hours after the wedge pressure falls.

RADIONUCLIDE SCANS

Radioactive technetium pyrophosphate is taken up by acutely damaged myocardial cells, resulting in a hot spot image. Technetium pyrophosphate scans become positive within the first 12 to 36 hours of myocardial infarction and remain positive for 6–10 days. These scans are most helpful when ECG patterns are obscured by conduction abnormalities, such as bundle branch blocks or when the enzyme results are not entirely characteristic of infarction. Thallium-201 scans result in a cold spot image in which the isotope is taken up by perfused myocardium but not by unperfused tissue in the region of the infarct. Thallium scans cannot differentiate a new infarct from an old infarct or zone of severe ischemia and are more useful when followed serially.

Radionuclide ventrigulograms can be used to locate abnormal wall motion and determine ejection fraction, thus helping to define cardiac function. They will not differentiate old infarcts from new infarcts. Abnormal right ventricular wall motion may be helpful in diagnosing right ventricular infarction.

ECHOCARDIOGRAPHY

Echocardiograms may be helpful for diagnosing various complications of myocardial infarction, such as ruptured papillary muscle, ventricular septal defect (VSD), and pericardial effusion. Two-dimensional echocardiography may offer a basis for quantifying the extent of myocardial damage by allowing one to assess the degree of regional wall motion abnormalities. It is also helpful in diagnosing ventricular aneurysm, right ventricular infarction, and ventricular thrombosis (Parisi et al).

SWAN-GANZ CATHETERIZATION

See Congestive Heart Failure and Cardiogenic Shock sections of this chapter.

Table 2. Disease Entities That May Be Confused with Myocardial Infarction

Disease Entity	Distinguishing Features
Angina	With angina, pain is of shorter duration, less than 20 minutes, and may be less severe; pain is more likely to be relieved with rest and nitroglycerin
Aortic dissection	Pain is sharp, tearing in nature, with radiation to the back; missing pulses; stroke; widened mediastinum on chest x-ray film; ECG or enzyme findings suggestive of MI may be present if dissection into a coronary artery occurs
Pulmonary embolism	Dyspnea, pleuritic chest pain, tachycardia, hypoxia; if pulmonary embolism is massive, right-sided heart failure occurs; LDH may be elevated but CK is not; ECG signs of pulmonary embolism may be present; positive lung scan, positive pulmonary angiogram
Pericarditis	Pain is sharp and positional with pleuritic component; pericardial rub; ECG shows ST elevation that is diffuse; no pathologic Q waves; CK may increase in concomitant myocarditis but usually is normal; responds to antiinflammatory agents
Myocarditis	Often associated with systemic viral or bacterial infection; pain may be vague; CK may be elevated with presence of MB isoenzyme; usually no Q waves on ECG
Chest wall pain	Pain is usually not typical of the substernal pressure type pain of angina or MI; pain may be simulated by chest wall palpation or arm movement; negative ECG findings
Neurologic disorder	Osteoarthritis of cervical vertebrae may result in compression on cervical dorsal root nerves with pain in the upper thorax and arm; negative ECG findings; cervical spine abnormalities on x-ray film may show narrowed foramina; herpes zoster can also mimic MI; diagnosis is made by finding the characteristic skin lesions over the thorax
Gastrointestinal disorders	Reflux esophagitis and esophageal spasm may cause pain with swallowing and lying down after meals; history of food regurgitation may occur with reflux esophagitis; pain often is relieved by antacids; esophageal spasm may be relieved by nitroglycerin; peptic ulcer disease—pain radiates to back; symptoms relieved by food, antacids, cimetidine; endoscopy, upper GI series, and esophageal manometry may be necessary to make diagnosis; gall bladder disease and pancreatitis may on occasion mimic MI; abdominal tenderness is present, amylase increased with pancreatitis; cholecystograms or abdominal ultrasonography for diagnosis of gall bladder disease
Spontaneous pneumothorax	Sudden onset of dyspnea, pleuritic chest pain, absent breath sounds; chest x-ray confirms diagnosis
Pleuritis	Pain is sharp in nature and increases with inspiration; associated pulmonary infection; absence of ECG or enzyme findings

DIFFERENTIAL DIAGNOSIS

Several disease entities may be confused with myocardial infarction and are listed with their distinguishing features in Table 2.

Therapy for Myocardial Infarction

THE CORONARY CARE UNIT

The key to successful initial therapy is transfering the patient to the coronary care unit (CCU). A significant percentage of patients *should* be admitted to the CCU with the diagnosis of suspected myocardial infarction or "rule out" myocardial infarction who in fact do not have the disease.

Patients should be transfered to the CCU as soon as myocardial infarction is suspected. Since the advent of the CCU, considerably fewer in-hospital deaths from infarctions due to arrhythmia have occurred. The main advantage of the CCU is that cardiac rhythm can be monitored continuously and arrhythmias treated promptly. Hemodynamic monitoring in subclasses of patients (see below) allows a more rational approach to therapy. The coronary care unit is staffed by specially trained nurses who are adept in recognition of arrhythmia and in some hospitals will initiate therapy for arrhythmias.

If the patient is initially seen in the emergency ward when the diagnosis of myocardial infarction is considered, it is mandatory that (1) an IV line be inserted; (2) nasal 0_2 (2–4 L/min) be instituted, no more than 2 L/min initially if the patient's ventilation depends on hypoxic drive, as occurs with chronic lung disease; and (3) the patient be accompanied to the CCU by a physician and nurse, a portable cardiac monitor and defibrillator, and a portable oxygen tank, with IV lidocaine, atropine, epinephrine, and sodium bicarbonate available on the stretcher. In some institutions, a bolus of 75–100 mg of IV lidocaine is administered prophylactically prior to transfer followed by an intravenous infusion (1–4 mg/min). If the patient is having severe chest pain and/or is highly anxious, small doses of morphine sulfate 2–4 mg IV can be administered while the patient is still in the emergency ward, especially if there is any delay in transfer to the coronary care unit.

Once in the CCU, the patient is initially kept at bed rest and given nothing by mouth (npo). The timetable for increasing activity and eating must be tailored to each individual patient and depends largely on the patient's progress and the development of complications.

The following are suggested initial CCU protocol:

1. The patient is admitted to the CCU with "rule out MI," suspected MI, or acute MI and is placed on the seriously ill list.
2. Activity: Day 1, bed rest; if the patient is stable, some physicians allow bedside commode privileges; a bedpan may be more uncomfortable and anxiety provoking than a bedside commode. Days 2–3, bed rest is continued but the patient sits in a chair for 15–20 minutes a few times during the day as tolerated.

3. Frequent vital signs, every 30–60 min, during the first 6 hours. Thereafter, every 2 hours for 24 hours and then every 4 hours.

4. Daily weights. Total fluid intake and output.

5. Diet: The patient should be npo for the first 6–24 hours. If the patient remains stable, he or she may be started on a no-salt-added, low-cholesterol, 1,500-calorie diet. Oral fluid should be restricted to 1,000 cc/8 hours, but fluid intake must be tailored to the need of each patient.

6. IVs: If the patient is able to take po fluid and food, IV may be 5% dextrose in water, to keep open. If not, the patient should receive approximately 1,000 cc IV fluid/8 hours. Potassium supplements may be needed. Hypokalemia should be avoided, because of its propensity to cause arrhythmias. Again, IV therapy must be tailored to the volume needs of the patient.

7. Continuous cardiac rhythm monitoring.

8. Suggested laboratory studies: (a) ECGs every day for 3 days. (b) CK every 4–8 hours during the first 24 hours. If the CK is elevated and there are other possible causes for the elevation or if the diagnosis is still not clear CK isoenzymes should be ordered. LDH, SGOT should be ordered on admission and every day for 4 days. (c) Other lab tests on admission are electrolytes, complete blood count, BUN, creatinine, glucose, chest x-ray daily for 2–3 days, urinalysis, stool guaiacs obtained on first stool specimen rather than rectal examination at the time of admission. Rectal examination probably should be avoided during the first 3 days of hospitalization unless lower GI bleeding is suspected.

9. Suggested medications: (a) The patient should receive nasal O_2, 2–4 L/min; if the patient has chronic obstructive lung disease, use 2 rather than 4 L/min initially and check arterial blood gases for PO_2 and evidence of CO_2 retention. (b) Intravenous morphine sulfate is the best agent to use for the chest pain of myocardial infarction; it is not only a potent analgesic but also decreases anxiety and has the added benefit of peripheral venous vasodilation, thus acting as a mild preload reducer. Morphine sulfate usually is administered in 2–5 mg IV doses. The dose may be repeated every 20 minutes until pain is relieved. Rarely should more than 10–12 mg be given, but the total dose will vary depending upon the size of the patient, severity of pain, and sensitivity of the patient to narcotics. In patients with inferior wall MI, the parasympathomimetic effects of morphine can increase vagal discharge; thus some physicians prefer IV meperidine (Demerol) 25–50 mg IV given slowly. (c) Tranquilizers, used to diminish anxiety, a factor which can increase the oxygen requirements of the heart; diazepam 5 mg or chlordiazepoxide 5–25 mg may be used. (d) Patients should receive a stool softener to prevent straining at stool (Valsalva maneuver); the most commonly used ones are dioctyl calcium sulfosuccinate, 240 mg po qd, and milk of magnesia, 30 cc po qhs as needed. (e) The use of full anticoagulation and the use of antiplatelet agents (aspirin) in uncomplicated myocardial infarction remain controversial and are covered in more detail in Chapter 12. Minidose heparin, 5,000 units subcutaneously every 8 hours, may decrease the incidence of thrombophlebitis and subsequent pulmonary emboli in patients with myocardial infarction at bed rest. Early ambulation also may decrease the incidence of thrombophlebitis and pulmonary emboli.

MOBILIZATION AFTER DAY 3

There has been a trend toward early mobilization following uncomplicated myocardial infarction, which presumably decreases the complications of prolonged bed rest, such as thrombophlebitis and pulmonary embolism. Most patients remain hospitalized between 10 to 21 days following uncomplicated infarction, with a mean stay of approximately 12 to 14 days. A study by Baughman et al. showed that there was no difference in long-term survival in patients hospitalized for 2 versus 3 weeks for treatment of myocardial infarction. The duration of hospital stay and progression of ambulation depends on each patient's course and development of complications.

DAYS 4 TO 8

If the patient is stable, he or she may be transferred to an intermediate cardiac unit. These units usually have cardiac monitoring if needed and specialized nursing care. They provide a transition phase between the intensive care setting and the regular hospital ward. Here, the patient's blood pressure is checked lying and standing for orthostatic changes. Standing and gradual ambulation are begun between days 4–8. The patient may walk to the bathroom if it is in the patient's hospital room or nearby.

DAYS 8 TO 14

The patient may be transferred to the ward. The patient may walk in the hall 2–3 times a day but only on his or her own floor of the hospital and not more than 30 minutes at a time initially.

LAST FEW HOSPITAL DAYS

The patient may walk as he or she wishes. It is often helpful for the patient to walk up one flight of stairs with his or her physician just before hospital discharge. This gives both patient and physician an idea of the patient's physical capabilities. Many centers perform Holtor monitoring at this time to check for late ventricular ectopic activity. Some centers also perform a submaximal exercise test prior to discharge. Several studies have shown that submaximal exercise testing within three weeks of acute myocardial infarction is safe and identifies patients at greater risk of further cardiac events. Patients who have a positive modified exercise test with ST depression and chest pain are more likely to develop postinfarction angina, have multivessel coronary artery disease, and have a higher mortality. Inappropriately high heart rates and early fatigue and dyspnea during the test suggest left ventricular dysfunction. Exercise induced ventricular ectopy raises the concern of increased risk of sudden death. Patients who are identified to be at increased risk should be considered for more aggressive medical and surgical therapy. Patients who do well are at lower risk and may have less restriction of physical activity (Fuller et al).

AMBULATION FOLLOWING DISCHARGE FROM THE HOSPITAL

During the first two weeks following discharge, the patient should only engage in moderate activity around the house. The patient should not engage in strenuous activity, lifting heavy objects, or automobile driving. Sexual activity is usually resumed within the first few weeks. At three to four weeks, the patient gradually increases the amount of walking and may walk outside the house. By the end of this period, if the patient is doing well he or she may walk up to $\frac{1}{4}$ to $\frac{1}{2}$ mile a day. By 8–12 weeks most patients return to work. If an exercise tolerance test is negative at this point, the patient enters a medically supervised exercise program (see Chapter 32).

Complications of Myocardial Infarction

The complications of myocardial infarction may be arrhythmic or nonarrhythmic. Both types are discussed below, and arrhythmic complications are further treated in Chapters 16 and 17.

ARRHYTHMIC COMPLICATIONS

Ventricular Ectopic Beats

Ventricular ectopic beats (VPBs) are due to the premature discharge of an ectopic ventricular focus. They occur in 90–95% of all patients during the first few days of myocardial infarction and are important because they often are precursors to more serious ventricular arrhythmias: ventricular tachycardia and ventricular fibrillation.

VPBs can be recognized by (1) wide, bizarre QRS; (2) premature discharge, occurring earlier than the next anticipated beat; (3) ST-T segment abnormality, often with depressed ST and T wave direction opposite to QRS; (4) usually constant coupling interval between ectopic beat and preceeding beat (fixed coupling); and (5) compensatory pause, a pause following the extrasystolic beat that compensates exactly for the ectopic beat's prematurity, with the sum of the pre- and postectopic interval exactly equal to the sum of two consecutive sinus intervals. (See also Chapter 16.)

Correctable causes include (1) electrolyte abnormalities, especially hypokalemia; (2) digitalis toxicity; (3) congestive heart failure; (4) hypoxia; and (5) intracardiac catheters.

Ventricular premature beats during the early phase of infarction should be treated (1) when they are present with a frequency of five or more per minute, including ventricular bigeminy; (2) when they are multifocal; and (3) when they occur in salvoes of two or three consecutive beats. Two consecutive VPBs are referred to as ''couplets''; three consecutive VPBs are often referred to as ''three-beat ventricular tachycardia''. Although there is controversy concerning the significance of the R on T phenomenon in the development of ventricular tachycardia or fibrillation, many physicians prefer to treat these early VPBs.

Therapy
LIDOCAINE. An initial bolus of 50–100 mg IV lidocaine is administered followed by a constant infusion drip of 1–4 mg/min, usually 2 mg/min. Following an IV bolus injection, the drug rapidly distributes and thus there is an initial rapid wash-out from the circulation. The half-life of this first phase of wash-out is very rapid (20 minutes)

while the second phase of washout has a half-life of about two hours. If an infusion drip is not begun shortly after the bolus or if arrhythmias recur, a second bolus (50–75 mg) may be necessary in order to achieve therapeutic drug levels. Since lidocaine is metabolized in the liver, the dose should be smaller in patients with hepatic congestion secondary to congestive heart failure or hepatic failure—50 mg bolus followed by 0.7–1.0 mg/min drip. Since lidocaine's metabolites are execreted in the kidney, the dose also may have to be reduced in renal failure. The overall half-life of lidocaine is 90 minutes; its therapeutic level is 1.2–5 µg/ml. Toxic and side effects include seizures; respiratory depression; and behavioral abnormalities including disorientation, drowsiness, and frank pshychosis. Heart block may occur in patients with underlying conduction abnormalities.

PROCAINAMIDE.   The initial loading dose for procainamide is 50–100 mg IV given slowly every 5 minute to a total of 500 mg to 1 gm, but before the QRS interval widens more than 30% of baseline or hypotension develops. The drug is then continued at an IV infusion rate of 1–4 mg/min. If the patient is stable, procainamide may then be given po 250–375 mg every 3–4 hours. Its half-life is 3–4 hours and therapeutic level is 4–8 µg/ml. The therapeutic level of its active metabolite, N acetyl procainamide, is 2.0–30 µg/ml, but this largely depends on the laboratory in which the assay is run. Elimination of the drug is mainly renal (60%); a smaller component is metabolized in the liver. Toxic and side effects include prolonged conduction, AV block, hypotension, and a lupus-like syndrome. A sustained release form of procainamide is available, in 250 mg and 500 mg tablets, and can be administered at longer intervals (six hours). Dosage should be adjusted to surpress VPBs and maintain a therapeutic drug level.

QUINIDINE.   The dose is 200–300 mg quinidine sulfate every six hours, po. (Note, IV quinidine is not generally used, because of its tendency to produce hypotension. The intramuscular (IM) route may be used, but it may cause hypotension and elevate CK by muscle trauma.) Quinidine's half-life is 4–7 hours and the therapeutic level depends upon the assay technique. In many centers, therapeutic levels are 2.3–5 µg/ml. Quinidine is metabolized by the liver. Cardiovascular toxicity and side effects of the drug include prolongation of QRS and QT intervals, AV block, myocardial depression, and hypotension. Quinidine may increase digoxin levels by decreasing excretion of digoxin and displacing digoxin from binding sites; therefore, the digoxin dose must be decreased when starting quinidine. Gastrointestinal side effects include diarrhea and nausea. The drug may also cause rash, fever, tinnitus, thrombocytopenia, hemolytic anemia, and hepatic toxicity. Quinidine gluconate (324 mg po tid) may cause less gastrointestinal upset.

PHENYTOIN.   This is mainly a second-line drug for treatment of VPBs. It is especially useful in the setting of digitalis toxicity. The dose is 100 mg IV given slowly every five minutes up to 500–1,000 mg. IM administration is painful and poorly absorbed. The po dose is 300–500 mg per day. Phenytoin's half-life is up to 24 hours, and its therapeutic levels are 10–18 µg/ml. Its metabolism is hepatic. Toxic and side effects include nystagmus, ataxia, confusion; nausea; bone marrow suppression; gingival hypertrophy; hypotension; respiratory depression; arrhythmias including idioventricular rhythm, ventricular fibrillation, asystole, and decreased AV block with atrial flutter (1:1 conduction).

PROPRANOLOL. This drug should be used only when other agents have failed. An initial intravenous test dose of 0.25–0.5 mg is administered. Then 1 mg IV every five minutes up to 0.1 mg/kg (no more than 10 mg for a 70 kg person) is administered. The po dose is variable, from 40–480 mg per day. Propranolol's half-life is 3–4.5 hours and therapeutic levels are 40–85 µg/ml. The heart rate is the best therapeutic guide to dosage; one should aim for a sinus rhythm with a rate approximately 60–65/min. Propranolol is metabolized by the liver. Contraindications include congestive heart failure, bronchospasm, heart block, and bradycardia. Toxic and side effects are myocardial depression, bronchospasm, bradycardia, prolonged AV conduction, and central nervous system (CNS) effects—fatigue, lethargy, and nightmares. Other beta blockers for treatment of arrhythmias are described in Chapter 16.

DISOPYRAMIDE (NORPACE). In patients with adequate ventricular function and renal function, an initial 300 mg loading dose is given, followed by 150 mg every six hours to a total of 400–800 mg per day. With renal disease, a lower dose is administered. The half-life of disopyramide is 6.7 hours and its therapeutic level is 2–4 µg/ml. Excretion is 50% renal, 20% in the urine as metabolites, and 10% fecally. Toxic and side effects include anticholinergic symptoms (urinary retention, GI cramps, blurred vision, dry mouth), heart failure, exacerbation of conduction abnormalities, and hypotension. Disopyramide is one of the most negative inotropic agents of the standard available antiarrhythmics; therefore, careful monitoring for increasing signs of congestive heart failure is important.

Ventricular Tachycardia

Ventricular Tachycardia (VT) is characterized by three or more consecutive ventricular ectopic beats with a rate of 100–250 beats/min. The rhythm may degenerate into fatal ventricular fibrillation. VT occurs in 10–40% of transmural myocardial infarctions and it should be promptly treated. If the patient is hemodynamically stable, administer 50–100 mg bolus of IV lidocaine followed by a lidocaine drip. If the VT is not abolished, repeat this dose in two minutes. If VT still persists, electrical cardioversion should be instituted. Bretylium tosylate may be effective in refractory cases (see below). If the patient is not hemodynamically stable (hypotension, heart failure) or is experiencing chest pain, electrical cardioversion is the initial treatment. Begin with 10 watt-sec; if that is unsuccessful, 50 to 100 watt-sec are usually effective. The other pharmacologic agents listed above may decrease the incidence of VT.

Ventricular Fibrillation

Ventricular fibrillation (VF) is fatal unless promptly treated with electrical countershock (175–400 watt-sec). If there is no response, institute cardiopulmonary resuscitation, then repeat defibrillation. Bretylium tosylate may be tried when VF is refractory to electrical defibrillation. The dose is 5 mg/kg IV initially and then 10 mg/kg at 15–30 minutes intervals to a total dose of 30 mg/kg. If the patient remains in VF, electrical defibrillation should be repeated once the patient has received bretylium tosylate. (Also see Chapter 33.)

Because ventricular fibrillation can occur during the early phase of myocardial infarction without being preceded by warning arrhythmias (more than 5 VPBs per minute, multifocal VPBs, ventricular couplets, or brief runs of VT), many centers administer phophylactic lidocaine during the first one or two days of admission. In one study 21% of cases of primary VF (not preceded by ventricular warning arrhythmias) occurred within the first nine hours of acute infarction.

Treatment of Ventricular Arrhythmias Late in the Hospital Course

There is agreement that treatment of frequent and complex ventricular premature beats during the early phase (first few days) of infarction reduces the risk of ventricular fibrillation. However, ventricular arrhythmias occurring in the first 48 hours of infarction do not correlate with long-term survival. Ventricular arrhythmias occurring later in the hospital stay (second or third postinfarction week) correlate with an increased risk of sudden death 4–24 months post infarction, presumably secondary to VF. Patients with acute myocardial infarction should be monitored for arrhythmias for six to 24 hours during the second or third postinfarction week. Although it is unclear whether antiarrhythmic therapy prevents sudden death in the posthospital phase, most cardiologists agree that on-going antiarrhythmic therapy (6–12 months or more) should be administered to patients with late hospital complex ventricular arrhythmias (especially runs of VT of three beats or more) and many treat frequent VPBs, multiform VPBs, ventricular couplets, and VPBs with the R on T phenomenon, as well. Therapy can be assessed by pretreatment and posttreatment Holter monitoring, exercise tests, trendscription, and electrophysiologic testing. (See also Chapter 16.)

Accelerated Idioventricular Rhythm

Accelerated idioventricular rhythm (AIVR) is recognized by three or more widened QRS complexes at a rate similar to the sinus rate. It is often called *slow VT* and tends to alternate with the previous sinus rhythm. Approximately half of the episodes of AIVR are the manifestation of an escape rhythm due to slowing of the basic cardiac rhythm; the other half of episodes are initiated by a ventricular premature beat. It is usually a benign rhythm and occurs in 10–30% of myocardial infarctions; but may be associated with ventricular premature beats and/or ventricular tachycardia. Often treatment is not necessary. If the sinus rate is very slow, treat with atropine 0.6 to 1.0 mg IV. If there is hemodynamic compromise, which occurs rarely, or associated ventricular premature beats, treat with lidocaine, 50–100 mg bolus IV, followed by 2–4 mg/min.

Sinus Tachycardia

In sinus tachycardia, the heart rate is 100 to 150 beats per minute, usually secondary to pump failure, chest pain, infection, fever, pericarditis, hypoxia, or hypovolemia.

Therapy consists of correcting the underlying cause. If there is difficulty distinguishing between congestive failure and hypovolemia, a right-sided heart catheterization with monitoring of the pulmonary capillary wedge pressure will resolve the question and aid in managing the patient's fluid status. If the pulmonary capillary wedge pressure is normal and no other cause for tachycardia is evident, very small doses of propranolol po or IV are often helpful.

Sinus Bradycardia

Sinus bradycardia is present in 15% of myocardial infarctions and is defined as a heart rate of less than 60 beats per minute. It is often seen during the early phase of inferior wall myocardial infarction secondary to vagal discharge. If the patient is not symptomatic and the blood pressure is maintained with no evidence of peripheral hypoperfusion, observation alone may suffice; if the heart rate is less than 50 beats per minute with hypotension, hypoperfusion, or chest pain, administer atropine 0.6–1 mg IV. This dose may be repeated within 4–5 minutes. If the patient is symptomatic and bradycardia persists despite atropine, a temporary transvenous pacemaker should be inserted.

Premature Atrial Beats

In general, premature atrial beats are not important, but sometimes they are a forerunner of other atrial tachyarrhythmias. They occur in up to 60% of myocardial infarctions.

Atrial Fibrillation

Atrial fibrillation is recognized by fibrillatory waves and a variable conduction to the ventricles resulting in an "irregularly-irregular" rhythm. With loss of atrial contraction, there may be decreased diastolic filling of the left ventricle and decreased stroke volume with a fall in cardiac output. If the ventricular rate is rapid, the decrease in diastolic filling also may contribute to the fall in cardiac output. Atrial fibrillation occurs in 10% of patients with myocardial infarction. Therapy includes treating secondary causes such as hypoxia, electrolyte abnormalities, pulmonary embolism, and hyperthyroidism. If the ventricular rate is fast with hemodynamic embarrassment (hypotension, pulmonary edema, or chest pain) cardioversion with 50–200 watt-sec is the treatment of choice. Potassium level should be normal; and if the patient has been on digitalis, a 75–100 mg IV bolus of lidocaine may be given to help prevent ventricular ectopy during cardioversion. If the patient has a fast ventricular rate without chest pain, hypotension, or heart failure, IV digoxin may be administered to slow the rate (0.25 mg q 3–4 hours until rate is 70–80, followed by digoxin maintenance). Occasionally, small doses of propranolol may be given to help slow the rate (10–20 mg po; 0.5–1.0 mg IV), if not contraindicated.

Atrial Flutter

Atrial flutter is recognized by the saw-tooth configuration of atrial flutter waves. The atrial rate is 250–350 beats per minute with variable atrioventricular block. The

AV block is often 2:1 with a ventricular rate of approximately 150. Atrial flutter occurs in 5% of myocardial infarctions. The therapy is electrical cardioversion with 25–50 watt-sec. In general, flutter is very responsive to electrical cardioversion.

Paroxysmal Atrial Tachycardia

In paroxysmal atrial tachycardia (PAT), the atrial rate is approximately 140–230 beats/minute. The QRS complex is narrow, and the ventricular response is quite regular. The fast ventricular rate increases myocardial oxygen consumption and may exacerbate ischemia. Therapy includes carotid sinus massage. If this fails, IV verapamil (5–10 mg) may be administered over a period of 2–3 minutes.

Verapamil's antiarrhythmic effect appears to be due to its effect on inhibiting calcium and possibly sodium flux through slow channels in the cells of the conducting system. It slows AV conduction, prolongs the effective refractory period within the AV node, and interrupts reentry within the AV node. Following IV injection, the drug has an early distribution phase (half-life of about four minutes) followed by a slower elimination phase (half-life of 2.5 hours). Seventy percent of the administered dose is excreted in the urine. Approximately 60–80% of patients with paroxysmal atrial tachycardia convert to sinus rhythm following verapamil. There are several contraindications relevant to patients with suspected myocardial infarction. These include cardiogenic shock or severe hypotension (verapamil reduces both afterload and myocardial contractility), second or third degree AV block, sick sinus syndrome, severe congestive heart failure (unless the heart failure is due to the rapid rate), and finally, for those patients receiving IV beta-blocking agents in whom the addition of IV verapamil may severely depress myocardial contractility and AV conduction. Verapamil must be administered cautiously in patients with bradycardia, heart failure, and hepatic and renal failure.

If carotid sinus massage or verapamil fail to result in sinus rhythm, electrical cardioversion with 50–75 watt-sec should be instituted. Edrophonium and Valsalva maneuver should be avoided as treatment in myocardial infarction patients. If the PAT is recurrent, treat with digoxin or quinidine. If PAT is present with atrioventricular block, one should suspect digitalis toxicity and digitalis should be withheld.

Junctional Rhythms

In junctional rhythms, the QRS configuration is narrow. There may be no P waves, a short PR interval, or inverted P waves. If the heart rate is 40–60 beats per minute, the junctional mechanism may be an escape rhythm from a slower sinus rate and no treatment may be necessary. If the heart rate is very slow with hypotension, give atropine, 0.6–1 mg IV; if there is no response, insert a pacemaker. Treat the underlying cause, such as electrolyte abnormality, congestive heart failure, hypoxia, and digitalis toxicity. Accelerated junctional rhythm is present when the rate is 70–130/min. For fast rates, treat accelerated junctional rhythm as if treating PAT.

Heart Blocks

The type and significance of heart block depends largely on the location of the myocardial infarction. Heart block occurs in 6–17% of myocardial infarctions. In inferior and posterior wall myocardial infarction, heart block may be secondary to increased vagal tone and localized edema in the area of the AV node, which decreases AV conduction. With inferior or posterior infarction, the heart block is often transient and is commonly first-degree AV block (prolonged PR interval) or Mobitz type I second-degree heart block (Wenckebach, with a progressively longer PR interval until QRS is dropped).

Mobitz type I second-degree heart block usually does not require therapy. If the heart rate is very low with hemodynamic embarrassment, 0.6–1 mg IV atropine may be given. Pacemaker therapy is usually not required. Mobitz II second-degree heart block (QRS dropped without progressively prolonged PR interval) and complete heart block (atria and ventricles contract independently and P's and QRSs have no relationship to each other) are uncommon in inferior wall myocardial infarction.

In anterior wall myocardial infarction, heart block is usually secondary to an extensive infarction with damage to the bundle branches. Accompanying pump failure is common, as is a high mortality. Mobitz II second-degree heart block and complete heart block (third-degree heart block) are more common. The ventricular escape focus in complete heart block is usually slow, with a wide QRS and a rate of approximately 40/min. Both Mobitz II block and complete heart block usually require a temporary transvenous pacemaker.

Indications for Transvenous Pacing in the Setting of Acute Myocardial Infarction
The following are indications for transvenous pacing in acute MI:

1. Sinus bradycardia resistant to atropine, with a heart rate less than 50/min and signs of hypoperfusion: decreased blood pressure, decreased urine output, cold and clammy skin, decreased mentation, or increased chest pain or ventricular arrhythmias.

2. Mobitz type II second-degree AV block. Mobitz type I second-degree AV block, or Wenckebach phenomenon, is usually not an indication for pacing, as it is often a transient phenomenon without hemodynamic compromise.

3. Complete heart block with slow ventricular escape rate and broad QRS.

4. Junctional rhythm with slow ventricular rate and signs of hypoperfusion.

5. Controversy still exists as to whether patients with new bundle branch blocks or hemiblocks should have prophylactic pacing wires inserted. One argument is that the prognosis is often poor when these intraventricular conduction defects develop due to the large extent of the infarction and not the conduction abnormality itself. However, many physicians believe that when new bundle branch blocks develop in the setting of acute infarction, a transvenous pacing wire should be inserted. Some series report an improved hospital mortality from 0 to 30% when pacing is instituted in patients with anterior infarcts and new fascicular blocks. According to Escher, the combination of right bundle branch block with left posterior hemiblock is the most threatening to progress to complete AV block, but right bundle branch block alone, right bundle branch block plus left anterior hemiblock, left bundle branch block, and finally, left anterior hemiblock may also progress to complete heart block. She believes that if the appropriate facilities are available patients developing new bundle branch block should receive a temporary wire whether the infarcts are anterior or inferior, although there is probably less of a rush in patients with inferior infarction who are he-

modynamically stable. She also states that patients with new left anterior hemiblocks in the setting of anterior infarcts should receive pacing wires, although many physicians will monitor these patients without prophylactic insertion of pacemaker wires.

6. There is still controversy concerning the question of whether patients with bundle branch block who experienced transient high-degree block (Mobitz II second-degree or complete heart block) during infarction should have permanent pacing. One study suggested lower mortality in patients who received permanent pacemakers. There is also controversy concerning how to manage patients who had transient heart block during infarction without residual abnormalities in conduction. Permanent pacing is indicated in all patients who develop and remain in third-degree, and in some cases second-degree, heart block.

Transvenous Pacmaker Insertion

One method for introducing transvenous pacemaker wires is the Seldinger technique. A seldinger needle is inserted percutaneously into the vessel at an angle no steeper than 45°. When blood return confirms that the needle is in the lumen of the vessel, a flexible-tipped guidewire is inserted into the vessel through the lumen of the needle. The needle then is withdrawn. A sheath is then inserted into the vessel over the guidewire. The guidewire is removed and the sheath is then present within the vessel lumen. The pacemaker wire is then inserted through the sheath.

Another technique is by direct needle puncture, using a needle with an external plastic sheath. Once the sheath is in the vessel, the needle is removed, and the pacing wire is inserted through the sheath. The cutdown approach to veins is seldom used, but in difficult cases in which access is a problem, it may be necessary. The preferred transvenous routes for pacemaker insertion in order of preference are subclavian, jugular (external and internal), femoral, and brachial. The advantage of using jugular or subclavian veins rather than the femoral or brachial approach is that they allow arm and leg motion, the wire is less prone to pacemaker displacement, and chances of thrombus or infection are reduced. Optimally, the pacemaker wire is positioned under fluoroscopic control into the right ventricular apical endocardium. If fluoroscopic control is not available, the wire may be inserted under electrocardiographic control; a No. 4 French pacemaker wire with an inflatable balloon has been devised, which may help guide the pacing wire in this situation.

Following insertion of the pacing lead, the threshold for successful pacing is determined and should be below 0.5 mA to 1.0 mA. If the threshold is higher than this, then the position of the wire should be readjusted. The threshold should be rechecked daily and maintenance output is left at a higher mA than threshold (usually 2–5 mA). The desired heart rate is set and in most cases the pacemaker is set in a demand rather than asynchronous mode. A full discussion of temporary pacemakers is found in Escher (1980).

NONARRHYTHMIC COMPLICATIONS

Pericarditis

The pericarditis of myocardial infarction can occur early, 1 to 3 days after onset of infarction, or late, two weeks to three months after infarction. The latter is known as Dressler's syndrome.

Early Pericarditis

Early pericarditis in the setting of transmural myocardial infarction is associated with typical features of acute pericarditis. The patient complains of sharp chest pain that is worse with inspiration and often with certain positions. The pain tends to be worse lying down and is lessened by sitting up. It is important to differentiate this pain from that of ischemic pain. The patient is usually febrile and a pericardial rub may be present. The rub tends to be evanescent; it is not uncommon for one examiner to hear it and a second examiner not to, shortly thereafter. The ECG shows tachycardia, ST segment elevation, and the QRS voltage may be low. With time the ST segments return to baseline and T waves invert. The cardiac silhouette on chest x-ray film is usually unchanged or slightly increased in size. Large pericardial effusions are unusual. Therapy consists of aspirin (ASA 650 mg qid). Although indomethacin (25–50 mg tid) has been given, some studies show that this agent increases coronary vascular resistance, increases infarct size, and thins the scars of experimental infarcts. Anticoagulation should be avoided if possible because of the possibility of hemopericardium.

Dressler's Syndrome

This syndrome occurs two weeks to three months after infarction and is associated with fever, pericardial pain, pleuritis, and sometimes pneumonitis. The incidence of this syndrome may be declining. Physical exam reveals fever, pleural effusions, tachycardia, and pericardial rub. On chest x-ray film, the cardiac silhouette is usually normal, but may be enlarged. Pleural effusions and pulmonary infiltrates may be present. Heart specific antibodies have been detected in the blood of patients with Dressler's syndrome, and an immunologic etiology is likely. Therapy is similar to that of pericarditis in the early stage of infarction. If aspirin and indomethacin fail, steroids have been used; but multiple doses may impede healing of the infarction.

Papillary Muscle Rupture

This complication usually occurs within the first to second week after the onset of infarction. The patient experiences the onset of sudden dyspnea and may complain of symptoms of decreased forward output including lethargy and light-headedness. If the entire papillary muscle is ruptured, hypotension and rapid hemodynamic deterioration occurs and survival is usually brief. If only a few bellies of the papillary muscle rupture, the hemodynamic deterioration is slower. Rupture of papillary muscles is more common with inferior or posterior wall infarctions and occurs in the setting of a first infarction. The degree of associated myocardial damage is variable but is often less than 25% of the left ventricular mass.

The physical examination reveals signs of congestive heart failure and pulmonary edema. The apical cardiac impulse may be hyperkinetic. S_1 is soft, with a widely split S_2 due to earlier closure of the aortic valve; a pathologic S_3 is present, and there is a loud holosystolic apical murmur due to mitral regurgitation. Chest x-ray film reveals pulmonary vascular redistribution and pulmonary edema. The cardiac silhouette may be normal or increased. Swan-Ganz catheterization of the right heart is useful for both diagnosis and therapy. High left atrial pressures are reflected in a high pulmonary capillary wedge pressure (>12 mm Hg is abnormal; but with acute ruptured papillary muscle, values are likely to be quite high: >20–25 mm Hg). Tall regurgitant systolic (v) waves are present and reflect the increase in left atrial pressure during systole, when blood regurgitates from the left ventricle to the left atrium. There is no increase in right ventricular O_2 saturation; hence, this entity can be differentiated from a ventricular septal defect.

The therapy depends on the severity of the mitral regurgitation. If the signs and symptoms are mild, suggesting only a partial rupture, the patient can be managed with diuretics and digitalis. If the degree of mitral regurgitation is severe, with pulmonary edema and pulmonary capillary wedge pressures of greater than 20–25 mm Hg, more aggressive therapy is needed. If a patient's blood pressure is normal, an afterload reducing agent, such as nitroprusside 15–200 μg/min, should be given. The dose should be titrated so that systolic blood pressure is not less than 100 mm Hg. If systolic blood pressure is less than 100 mm Hg, start dopamine 5–50 μg/kg/min or dobutamine intravenously. Nitroprusside can be added to dopamine, but, again, systolic blood pressure should not fall below 90–100 mm Hg. In severe cases, the intraaortic balloon may be used as well. In general, surgical repair is best performed when the patient is stable—preferably at least six weeks after the rupture, when the infarct is largely scar tissue. In very severe cases, however, when the patient remains unstable despite adequate medical management, surgical intervention with mitral valve replacement is necessary. Optimally, this should be preceded by cardiac catheterization, with coronary angiography for consideration of coronary artery bypass grafting as well. A recent study suggested that since the mitral anulus is seldom necrotic, early mitral valve replacement may be initiated if the patient develops cardiogenic shock.

Papillary Muscle Dysfunction

This complication has a variable time of appearance in relationship to onset of myocardial infarction. The symptoms and signs are those of congestive heart failure. The second heart sound may be widely split and an S_3 present. A systolic apical murmur is heard, usually radiating to the axilla. When the mitral regurgitation is severe and prolonged, the chest x-ray film shows an enlarged left ventricle and left atrium. There may be an associated ventricular aneurysm seen on the film, with evidence of pulmonary vascular redistribution and edema. Swan-Ganz catheterization reveals an elevated pulmonary capillary wedge pressure with tall regurgitant v waves if the papillary muscle dysfunction is acute or subacute. If the papillary muscle dysfunction is chronic, with an enlarged left atrium, the left atrial pressure may not be severely elevated.

The therapy depends largely on the severity of the mitral regurgitation. If the patient's symptoms are mild and physical exam suggests only mild mitral regurgitation, then medical treatment with diuretics, digoxin, and afterload reducers is indicated. If symptoms and signs of mitral regurgitation are severe, mitral valve replacement may be needed. Again, surgery should be delayed for at least six weeks after the onset of infarction if the patient can be successfully managed with medical therapy.

Ventricular Septal Defect

Ventricular septal defect is most likely to occur within the first two weeks of the onset of the myocardial infarction and is due to the development of a necrotic rent in the ventricular septum. Ventricular septal defect is more common in anteroapical myocardial infarction. The patient may experience dyspnea and, in severe cases with low cardiac output, lethargy and decreased mentation. Physical examination reveals signs of congestive failure and a loud systolic murmur over the lower or mid-left sternal border, which may be accompanied by a thrill. Chest x-ray film shows cardiomegaly with an enlarged left ventricle. Pulmonary vascular redistribution and interstitial or alveolar edema may be present. Radionuclide angiography can quantitate the degree of left-to-right shunting. Swan-Ganz catheterization may be necessary to help make the diagnosis and guide the appropriate therapy. The key finding is an O_2 step-up from the right atrium to the right ventricle or pulmonary artery. An O_2 step-up is not found in ruptured papillary muscle, a condition that may mimic ventricular septal defect. The pulmonary capillary wedge pressure is increased, and v waves may be tall. The pulmonary arterial, right ventricular, and right atrial pressures may be elevated. The size of the left-to-right shunt can be determined (Chapters 7 and 8).

Therapy largely depends on the size of the shunt. If the left-to-right shunt is greater than 2:1, surgical correction should be considered. Surgery should be delayed for six weeks after the onset of myocardial infarction if the patient is stable. Cardiac catheterization with coronary angiography should precede surgery so that coronary bypass surgery can be considered. Medical therapy is the same as that discussed above for ruptured papillary muscle.

Cardiac Rupture

Cardiac rupture occurs within the first week of myocardial infarction, a time when the necrotic myocardial wall is the weakest. Cardiac rupture is more common in hypertensive patients, in women, and in patients with early exercise. The symptoms and signs are those of cardiovascular collapse with sudden onset of cardiac tamponade. The ECG complexes are initially preserved in the face of an absent cardiac output (electrical-mechanical dissociation). Chest x-ray film shows an enlarged globular shaped cardiac silhouette due to the hemopericardium. This complication is usually fatal, unless the patient survives long enough to receive a pericardiocentesis and emergency cardiac surgery.

Myocardial Infarct Expansion and Extension

Infarct expansion refers to disproportionate thinning and dilatation of the necrotic zone prior to the development of a well-healed scar. Clinical symptoms and signs of expansion include increased congestive heart failure and chest pain without enzyme or electrocardiographic evidence of further infarction. Expansion occurs in the first week of acute infarction, often after an initial period during which the patient appears stable. Expansion can be detected by two-dimensional echocardiography and may lead to cardiac rupture (Eaton, Weiss, and Bulkley).

Myocardial infarct extension refers to further progression of tissue necrosis, with increasing cardiac enzymes and ECG signs of infarction. In one study, myocardial infarct extension was defined as the reappearance of MB-CK 48 hours after initial symptoms, was found to occur in 14% of cases, and was associated with a high mortality rate. In another study, infarct extension was more common with subendocardial infarctions.

Arterial Embolism

Thrombus may form over the endocardial surface of the nonmoving infarcted ventricle. It may later break off from the site of infarction, usually within the first three weeks of infarction, with resultant arterial embolism. The symptoms and signs depend on the site to which the embolism travels and include those of stroke, renal infarction, and mesenteric infarction. Cold painful extremities and absent pulses occur when the embolism travels to an extremity. Chest x-ray film may be normal or show evidence of a left ventricular aneurysm. Treatment consists of systemic heparinization, followed by oral anticoagulants. Peripheral emboli may require surgical embolectomy. In patients who are at high risk of embolism due to ventricular aneurysm, thrombophlebitis, marked obesity, and low cardiac output, full anticoagulation with heparin should be undertaken if there are no contraindications.

Pulmonary Embolism

Since the initiation of early ambulation for myocardial infarctions and the use of minidose heparin for patients with heart failure, pulmonary embolism has become a less common complication. It may occur any time during the course of myocardial infarction and is more likely to occur in patients with congestive heart failure and prolonged bed rest. Minidose heparin 5000 units subcutaneously every 8–12 hours may prevent pulmonary emboli in patients with mild failure or prolonged bed rest. (See Chapter 25 for further discussion of pulmonary embolism.)

Ventricular Aneurysm

This complication occurs weeks to months following acute myocardial infarction and is associated with worsening congestive heart failure, arrhythmia (especially ventricular), and arterial emboli. Ventricular aneurysm is more common in men and in patients with a history of hypertension. Physical examination reveals a dyskinetic precordial bulge, with or without signs of congestive heart failure. S_4 and S_3 are often present. The murmur of mitral regurgitation occurs when there is associated papillary muscle dysfunction. The ECG shows persistent ST elevation in the region of the infarction. Chest x-ray film may be normal or demonstrate cardiomegaly, with an abnormal bulge or angulation at the site of the left ventricular aneurysm. Calcification is frequently seen in the aneurysmal wall. Radionuclide ventriculography may aid in localizing and assessing the size of the aneurysm. If the patient is asymptomatic and heart size is stable, then the patient's clinical course may be followed. Congestive failure, if mild, may be treated with medical therapy and anticoagulation. If congestive failure or arrhythmias due to the aneurysm are refractory to medical therapy, surgical excision is considered.

Congestive Heart Failure

Congestive heart failure complicating myocardial infarction may be left-sided, right-sided, or both. Left-sided failure occurs due to the decreased pumping ability of the left ventricle. Right-sided failure in the setting of infarction is likely to be secondary to a right ventricular infarction (more likely to accompany an inferior or posterior left ventricular infarction) or secondary to prolonged dysfunction of the left ventricle.

Left-sided Congestive Heart Failure

This complication is likely to occur within hours to days of the acute infarction. Patients complain of dyspnea, orthopnea, and paroxysmal nocturnal dyspnea. Symptoms of low forward cardiac output include fatigue, weakness, and lethargy. On physical examination, findings include pulmonary rales, dullness at the lung bases due to pleural effusions, tachypnea, tachycardia, cardiomegaly, S_3, S_4, and in some cases associated murmurs of mitral insufficiency. The findings of papillary muscle dysfunction or rupture, ventricular septal defect, left ventricular aneurysm, anemia, thyrotoxicosis, and hypertension should all be sought, as these may cause or exacerbate congestive failure. During the initial phases of congestive failure, the cardiac size may appear normal on chest x-ray film, but eventually enlarges with increased left ventricular and left atrial sizes. Chest x-ray also shows pulmonary vascular redistribution, interstitial or alveolar edema, pleural effusions, and Kerley B lines. There may be a lag phase of 12–24 hours between elevated pulmonary capillary wedge pressure and findings in the lung fields. Swan-Ganz catheterization reveals an elevated pulmonary capillary wedge pressure, often greater than 20–25 mm Hg (upper limit of normal is 10–12 mm Hg), and cardiac output may be reduced.

Therapy for congestive heart failure during myocardial infarction includes bed rest, 0_2, low-salt diet, and diuretics. Furosemide, 10 mg–20 mg, may initially be given intravenously, followed by oral therapy. The use of digoxin in the setting of acute infarction remains somewhat controversial, but most cardiologists will prescribe it when the heart size is enlarged and heart failure cannot be controlled by diuretics alone. If the patient remains in heart failure with a pulmonary capillary wedge pressure of $>$ 20 mm Hg, despite the above measures, vasodilator therapy is instituted with careful monitoring of arterial pressure to avoid systolic arterial pressure of less than 100 mm Hg. Nitroglycerin paste (primarily reduces preload) $\frac{1}{2}$ to 2 inches every 4–6 hours may be used; nitroprusside 0.5 to 10 μg/kg/min is a powerful afterload reducing agent. However, the use of nitroprusside in the setting of acute infarction with the complication of congestive heart failure alone remains controversial, since this drug may cause a coronary steal phenomenon, with reduced blood flow to the ischemic bed. Intravenous nitroglycerin 10–100 μg/min is another alternative and, like nitroprusside, usually requires monitoring of both systemic arterial and pulmonary capillary wedge pressures. Dopamine (3–30 μg/kg/min) and dobutamine (2–4 μg/kg/min up to 30 μg/kg/min) are two positive inotropic agents useful in the setting of severe congestive failure. Dobutamine has the advantage of having a positive inotropic action similar to dopamine, but has minimal chronotropic effect. Both these drugs usually require hemodynamic monitoring.

Right-sided Heart Failure Due to Right Ventricular
Infarction

If right-sided failure occurs in the setting of inferior or posterior left ventricular infarction without signs of left-sided failure, then the suspicion of right ventricular infarct should be raised. A study by Nixon showed that one-third of all inferior wall myocardial infarctions have some right ventricular involvement. The symptoms of right-sided failure may occur hours to days after the onset of infarction and include right upper quadrant pain, gastrointestinal symptoms, anorexia, peripheral edema, and in severe cases with reduced forward cardiac output fatigue, lethargy, and reduced mentation. Physical findings include distended neck veins, peripheral edema, ascites, tender enlarged liver, and in severe cases hypotension. A right ventricular lift and the murmur of tricuspid regurgitation may be present. Chest x-ray film reveals an enlarged right atrium and ventricle; the azygous vein and inferior vena cava are enlarged. ST segment elevation may be present in right precordial leads of the ECG. Swan-Ganz catheterization reveals elevated right ventricular end diastolic pressure and right atrial pressures, while the pulmonary capillary wedge pressure is normal or only moderately elevated. The right ventricular systolic pressure is reduced and, in severe cases, so is cardiac output. If a right ventricular infarction is suspected and there is a low cardiac output state with hypotension, volume expanders should be used while monitoring the pulmonary capillary wedge and right atrial pressures. If severe right-sided failure is present with good forward output, mild diuretics can be used. Concomitant left-sided failure should be treated. If left-sided heart failure is severe, right-sided heart failure may eventually develop without right ventricular infarction.

Hypertension Accompanying Myocardial Infarction

Episodes of chest pain may be associated with hypertension and the anxiety of admission to a hospital for "heart attack" may also contribute to hypertension. If hypertension persists, it should be treated, since increased afterload increases myocardial oxygen demand. Therapy includes a trial of an intravenous diuretic (furosemide 10 mg IV: may repeat dose) followed by the use of long acting nitrates; alpha methyldopa; or, if no contraindication, a beta blocker. In some patients, more potent agents such as intravenous nitroprusside or nitroglycerin may be needed, and this necessitates intraarterial lines for monitoring of blood pressure.

Postinfarction Angina

If angina occurs in the immediate post myocardial infarction setting it means that there is still myocardium subject to ischemia and perhaps infarction and should be treated aggressively. These patients often have two or three vessel coronary artery disease, and a recent study suggested that recurrent ischemic pain occurring for the first time after 24 hours in the coronary care unit was a predictor of later readmission to the coronary unit. Therapy includes: nitroglycerin, isosorbide dinitrate or nitroglycerin ointment, beta blockers, and calcium antagonists. If these agents fail to control pain at rest, a trial of intravenous nitroglycerin or intraaortic balloon counterpulsation should be initiated, with consideration of cardiac catheterization and coronary artery bypass surgery. Intraaortic balloon counterpulsation is discussed in Chapter 12.

Cardiogenic Shock

Cardiogenic shock is the state in which the heart can no longer pump sufficient blood to maintain organ perfusion. If organ perfusion remains depressed, organ function fails and, eventually, irreversible organ damage and subsequent death occur. Cardiogenic shock occurs in massive myocardial infarctions when 40% or more of the left ventricle is necrotic. The symptoms and signs are those of decreased perfusion to the organs and include restlessness, lethargy, decreased mentation (hypoperfusion to the brain), and dyspnea due to pulmonary congestion. Signs include dulled senses, cool and clammy skin, hypotension with the systolic blood pressure less than 90 mm Hg, signs of congestive heart failure, diffusely diminished pulse volumes, tachycardia, and a variety of arrhythmias. Urine output is less than 20–30 cc/hr and the chest x-ray film may reveal signs of congestive failure. There are several other shock syndromes that should be differentiated from cardiogenic shock (Table 3) due to myocardial infarction.

Therapy is guided by the results of hemodynamic monitoring. Patients should receive Swan-Ganz catheterization, plus an arterial line for monitoring blood pressure and arterial blood gases. In most cases, the cardiac index is decreased, usually less than 2.2 L/min/m^2. The pulmonary capillary wedge pressure may be low, normal, or elevated. If the wedge pressure is less than 14–18 mm Hg in the setting of shock, then the initial treatment is volume (albumin, dextran, plasma) until the wedge pressure is 18. If the pulmonary capillary wedge pressure is greater than 18 mm Hg in the setting of shock, then dopamine 2–5 μg/kg/min up to 20–50 μg/kg/min or dobutamine in a starting dose of 2–5 μg/kg/min and increased up to 30 μg/kg/min is administered intravenously.

Dopamine has both beta and some alpha-adrenergic activity. It is a positive inotropic and chronotropic drug with vasopressor activity. In low doses (< 5 μg/kg/min) it is also a renal artery vasodilator. Dopamine may cause tachycardia and exacerbate other tachyarrhythmias.

Dobutamine also has beta and alpha-adrenergic activity. At equivalent inotropic doses, dobutamine has weaker beta-2 action than dopmaine. In contrast to dopamine, dobutamine has little effect on heart rate and aortic pressure and lowers left ventricular filling pressure. Dobutamine does not alter renal flow. Other vasopressors include norepinephrine (4 mg in 1 liter of 5% dextrose; infuse the smallest dose to maintain a systolic blood pressure between 90–100 mm Hg, up to a maximum of 15 μg/min) and phenylephine, an alpha-adrenergic agent (0.1–0.5 mg IV).

If the patient has a pulmonary capillary wedge pressure of greater than 20–25 mm Hg with a systolic pressure not less than 90–100 mm Hg, intravenous nitroglycerin or nitroprusside should be added to a positive inotropic agent, such as dopamine or dobutamine. Cautious use of diuretic, such as furosemide (20–40 mg IV), may be undertaken when the pulmonary capillary wedge pressure is this high. The use of digitalis when the more potent inotropic agent dopamine is available for patients in cardiogenic shock is controversial.

All patients in cardiogenic shock should receive oxygen. Flow charts should be kept of vital signs, hemodynamic measurements, fluid intake and output, electrolyte status, blood gas data, and administration of drugs.

If these measures fail, intraaortic balloon counterpulsation is considered. The details of intraaortic balloon couterpulsation are reviewed in Chapter 12. In some patients, emergency cardiac catheterization and coronary artery bypass surgery have been performed, but results usually have been poor.

Recently, there have been several promising new approaches to treating acute myocardial infarctions, including coronary reperfusion by intracoronary streptokinase infusions and reduction of infarct size by pharmacologic agents. In addition, several studies suggest that long-term beta blockade following myocardial infarction reduces mortality. These studies are discussed in more detail in Chapter 12.

Table 3. Shock Syndromes

Cardiogenic shock
  Due to acute MI: loss of contractile mass
  Due to impaired myocardial function in the setting of end-stage cardiomyopathy
  Due to mechanical factors
    Obstruction of flow
      Valvular stenosis: mitral, aortic
      Atrial thrombus or myxoma
      Hypertrophic cardiomyopathy with outflow obstruction
      Cardiac tamponade
    Regurgitation of flow: may occur in setting of MI
      Papillary muscle rupture
      Rupture of interventricular septum
      Large ventricular aneurysm, serves as a reservoir for "regurgitation"
Hemorrhagic shock
Nonhemorrhagic oligemic shock
  Effective vascular volume reduced by sequestration of fluid in a "third space": hemorrhagic pancreatitis, burns, surgical wounds, skeletal muscle trauma, intestinal obstruction
  Effective vascular volume reduced through GI or renal losses: salt wasting, nephritis, excessive diuresis, fluid loss from GI tract (secondary to vomiting, diarrhea)
Distributive shock: vascular volume is maldistributed due to inappropriate regional vasodilation, with reduced arterial pressure and compromise of vital organs
  Septic shock
  Neurogenic shock: subdural hematoma, cerebral arterial occlusion, intracerebral hemorrhage, subarachnoid hemorrhage, spinal cord injury, metabolic, toxic, and drug depression of the central nervous system
  Anaphylactic shock
  Toxic, metabolic and endocrine factors: drug overdose; heavy metal poisoning; severe pulmonary, renal, or hepatic failure; uncontrolled diabetes; addisonian crisis; hypothyroidism; hyperparathyroidism
Pulmonary embolism
Miscellaneous: malignant hyperthermia, angioneurotic and periodic edema, dengue fever

Prognosis in Myocardial Infarction

Approximately 50–60% of all fatal myocardial infarctions occur secondary to arrhythmia outside the hospital. Overall in-hospital mortality is 10–15%. Annual mortality following discharge from the hospital is 5% per year. In-hospital mortality can be predicted from the clinical presentation of the patient or from the hemodynamic classification, as determined by data from right heart catheterization. These are shown in Tables 4 and 5.

Over the last three years, several studies have assessed other prognostic indicators

Table 4. Prognosis from Clinical Presentation of the Patient

Class	Clinical Presentation	In-Hospital Mortality
I	No pulmonary congestion or peripheral hypoperfusion	1%
II	Pulmonary congestion without hypoperfusion	11%
III	Peripheral hypoperfusion without pulmonary congestion	18%
IV	Both hypoperfusion and pulmonary congestion	60%

Adapted from Forrester JS, Diamond G, Chatterjee K, and Swan HJC: Medical therapy of acute myocardial infarction by application of hemodynamic subsets. *N Engl J Med* 295:1361, 1976.

following myocardial infarctions. The following factors have been associated with poorer prognosis following acute myocardial infarction: (1) low left ventricular ejection fraction (< 40%); (2) multivessel coronary artery disease; (3) congestive heart failure; (4) high ventricular premature depolarization rate—in one study patients with ≥ 10 VPBs/hr were 2.6 times as likely to die within a year than patients with a lower frequency—complex ventricular premature beats, and ventricular tachycardia in the late phase of hospitalization; (5) angina, ST depression, short exercise duration, and ventricular ectopy during a submaximal postinfarction exercise test; (6) cardiogenic shock; (7) atrioventricular block; (8) old age; (9) large infarct size as assessed by biochemical markers; (10) presence of a previous infarct; and (11) increased cardiothoracic ratio on chest x-ray film. Some but not all studies have suggested a poorer prognosis for anterior wall infarcts compared to inferior or posterior wall infarcts. Patients who develop ventricular fibrillation during the first 48 hours of admission to the hospital have a lower in-hospital and chronic case fatality rate than those with late ventricular fibrillation.

A study by Schroeder et al. showed that patients hospitalized with acute ischemic chest pain without evolving myocardial infarction have a six to 24 month prognosis, similar to that of patients hospitalized with acute infarction. Another study showed that patients admitted to coronary care units without acute infarction but who had transient ST shifts on their electrocardiogram were at high risk for subsequent nonfatal acute myocardial infarction and/or cardiovascular death.

Table 5. Prognosis from Hemodynamic Classification

Class	Pulmonary Congestion (PCW > 18 mmHg)	Hypoperfusion Cardiac Index (<2.2 L/min/m$_2$)	In-Hospital Mortality
I	−	−	3%
II	+	−	9%
III	−	+	23%
IV	+	+	51%

Adapted from Forrester JS, Diamond G, Chatterjee K, Swann HJC: Medical therapy of acute myocardial infarction by application of hemodynamic subsets. *N Engl J Med* 295:1361, 1976.

Psychologic Aspects of Myocardial Infarction

Patients suffering myocardial infarction may undergo several phases of psychological problems. Anxiety and then denial occur early during hospitalization for myocardial infarction—within the first few days. This is followed by a period of depression, which peaks on the third hospital day. When the patient leaves the coronary unit and enters a step-down unit, there may be a second period of anxiety. The treatment of anxiety and depression includes reassurance with explanation and education of the process and healing of infarctions. An attitude of enlightened optimism is important. Anxiety can be treated with a minor tranquilizer (see suggested CCU protocol). If anxiety and depression are severe, psychiatric counseling should be obtained. Depression in the rehabilitative phases is also helped by a program of physical conditioning if medically feasible. Some denial during the early phase of infarction may be associated with a better prognosis. Patients who deny their fear can relax in the coronary care unit situation and may do better. If denial interferes with patient management either during hospitalization or during rehabilitation, psychiatric evaluation may be needed.

Bibliography

Alpert JS, Braunwald E: Pathological and clinical manifestations of acute myocardial infarction, in Braunwald E (ed): *Heart Disease: A Textbook of Cardiovascular Medicine*. Philadelphia, Saunders, 1980, p 1309.

Asinger RW, Mikell FL, Elsperger J, et al: Incidence of left-ventricular thrombosis after acute transmural myocardial infarction: Serial evaluation by two dimensional echocardiography. *N Engl J Med* 305:297, 1981.

Baker JT, Bramlet DA, Lester RM, et al: Myocardial infarct extension: Incidence and relationship to survival. *Circulation* 65:918, 1982.

Baughman KL, Hutter AM Jr, DeSanctis RW, et al: Early discharge following acute myocardial infarction: Long-term follow-up of randomized patients. *Arch Intern Med* 142:875, 1982.

Bigger JT Jr, Dresdale RJ, Heissenbuttel RH, et al: Ventricular arrhythmias in ischemic heart disease: Mechanism, prevalence, significance and management. *Prog Cardiovasc Dis* 19:255, 1977.

Bigger JT Jr, Weld RM, Rolnitzky LM: Prevalence, characteristics and significance of ventricular tachycardia (three or more complexes) detected with ambulatory electrocardiographic recording in the late hospital phase of acute myocardial infarction. *Am J Cardiol* 48:815, 1981.

Bigger JT Jr, Weld FM, Rolnitzky LM: Which postinfarction ventricular arrhythmias should be treated? *Am Heart J* 103 (4Pt 1):660, 1982.

Carabello B, Cohn PF, Alpert JS: Hemodynamic monitoring of patients with hypotension after myocardial infarction. *Chest* 74:5, 1978.

Chandler AB: Relationship of coronary thrombosis to myocardial infarction. *Mod Concepts Cardiovasc Dis* 44:1, 1975.

Chapman I: Editorial: The cause-effect relationship between recent coronary artery occlusion and acute myocardial infarction. *Am Heart J* 87:267, 1974.

Chou TC, Vander Bel-Kahn J, Allen J, et al: Electrocardiographic diagnosis of right ventricular infarction. *Am J Med* 70:1175, 1981.

Coronary Drug Project Research Group: Prognostic importance of premature beats following myocardial infarction. Experience in the coronary drug project. *JAMA* 233:1116, 1973.

D'Arcy B, Nanda NC: Two-dimensional echocardiographic features of right ventricular infarction. *Circulation* 65:167, 1982.

Dhurandhar RW, MacMillan RL, Brown WG: Primary ventricular fibrillation complicating acute myocardial infarction. *Am J Cardiol* 27:347, 1971.

Dressler W: The post-myocardial infarction syndrome: a report of forty-four cases. *Arch Intern Med* 103:28, 1959.

Eaton LW, Weiss JL, Bulkley BH, et al: Regional cardiac dilatation after acute myocardial infarction: Recognition by two-dimensional echocardiography. *N Engl J Med* 300:57, 1979.

Escher DJW: The use of cardiac pacemakers, in Braunwald E (ed): *Heart Disease: A Textbook of Cardiovascular Medicine.* Philadelphia, Saunders, 1980, p 774.

Fein SA, Klein NA, Frishman WH; Exercise testing soon after uncomplicated myocardial infarction: Prognostic value and safety. *JAMA* 245:1863, 1981.

Forrester JS, Diamond G, Chatterjee K, et al: Medical therapy of acute myocardial infarction by application of hemodynamic subsets. *N Eng J Med* 295:1356 and 1404, 1976.

Freeman AP, Fatches KR, Carter IW, et al. Comparison of serum myoglobin and creatine kinase MB isoenzyme in early diagnosis of acute myocardial infarction. *Br Heart J* 45:389, 1981.

Fuller CM, Raizner AE, Verani MS, et al: Early post-myocardial infarction treadmill stress testing: An accurate predictor of multivessel coronary disease and subsequent cardiac events. *Ann Intern Med* 94:734, 1981.

Ganz W, Buchbinder N, Marcus H, et al: Intracoronary thrombolysis in evolving myocardial infarction. *Am Heart J* 101:4, 1981.

Goldberg R, Szklo M, Tonascia J, et al: Length of time between hospital admission and ventricular fibrillation or cardiac arrest complicating acute myocardial infarction: Effect on prognosis. *Johns Hopkins Med J* 145:187, 1979.

Goldberg HL, Borer JS, Jacobstein JG, et al: Anterior ST segment depression in acute myocardial infarction: Indicator of posterolateral infarction. *Am J Cardiol* 48:1009, 1981.

Hillis LD, Braunwald E: Coronary artery spasm. *N Engl J Med* 299:695, 1978.

Horowitz RS, Morganroth J. Immediate detection of early high-risk patients with acute myocardial infarction using two-dimensional echocardiographic evaluation of left ventricular regional wall motion abnormalities. *Am Heart J* 103:814, 1982.

Hutchins GM, Bulkley BH: Infarct expansion versus extension: Two different complications of acute myocardial infarction. *Am J Cardiol* 41:1127, 1978.

Isner JM, Roberts WC: Right ventricular infarction complicating left ventricular infarction secondary to coronary heart disease. *Am J Cardiol* 42:885, 1978.

Kennedy HL, Goldberg RJ, Szklo M, et al: The prognosis of anterior myocardial infarction revisited: A community-wide study. *Clin Cardiol* 6:455, 1979.

Killip T, Kimball JT: Treatment of myocardial infarction in a coronary care unit: A two-year experience with 250 patients. *Am J Cardiol* 20:457, 1967.

Leinbach RC, Gold HK: Coronary angiography during acute myocardial infarction: A search for spasm. *Am Heart J* 103 (4 Pt 2):768, 1982.

Lie KI, Wellens HJ, Van Capelle FJ, et al: Lidocaine in the prevention of primary ventricular fibrillation: A double-blind randomized study of 212 consecutive patients. *N Engl J Med* 291:1324, 1974.

Lindvall K, Kaijser L: Early exercise tests after uncomplicated acute myocardial infarction before early discharge from hospital. *Acta Med Scand* 210:257, 1981.

Lorell B, Leinbach RC, Pohost GM, et al: Right ventricular infarction. *Am J Cardiol* 43:465, 1979.

Lown B, Wolf M: Approaches to sudden death from coronary heart disease. *Circulation* 44:130, 1971.

Luz P, Weil MA, Shubin H: Current concepts on the mechanisms and treatment of cardiogenic shock. *Am Heart J* 92:103, 1976.

Ma KW, Brown DC, Steele BW, et al: Serum creatine kinase MB isoenzyme activity in long-term hemodialysis patients. *Arch Intern Med* 141:164, 1981.

MacCannell KL, McNay JL, Meyer BM, et al: Dopamine in the treatment of hypotension and shock. *N Engl J Med* 275:1389, 1966.

Madsen EB, Rasmussen S, Svendsen TI: Short term prognostic index in acute myocardial infarction: Multivariate analysis by Cox model. *Eur J Cardiol* 10:359, 1979.

Marmor A, Sobel BE, Roberts R: Factors presaging early recurrent myocardial infarction ("extension"). *Am J Cardiol* 48:603, 1981.

Maroko PR, Braunwald E: Modification of myocardial infarction size after coronary occlusion. *Ann Int Med* 79:720, 1973.

Maseri A, Liabbate A, Baroldi G, et al: Coronary vasopasm as a possible cause of myocardial infarction. *N Eng J Med* 23:1271, 1978.

Meister SG, Helfant RH: Rapid bedside differentiation of ruptured interventricular septum from acute mitral insufficiency. *N Engl J Med* 287:1024, 1972.

Midwall J, Ambrose J, Pichard A, et al: Angina pectoris before and after myocardial infarction: Angiographic correlations. *Chest* 81:681, 1982.

Moss AJ, Davis HT, Decamilla J, et al: Ventricular ectopic beats and their relation to sudden and nonsudden cardiac death after myocardial infarction. *Circulation* 60:998, 1979.

Niemela K, Takkunen JT, Juustila H, et al: Feasibility of early mobilization after acute myocardial infarction. *Ann Clin Res* 10:328, 1978.

Nixon JV: Right ventricular myocardial infarction. *Arch Intern Med* 142:945, 1982.

Nordlander R, Nyquist O: Patients treated in a coronary care unit without acute myocardial infarction: Identification of high risk subgroup for subsequent myocardial infarction and/or cardiovascular death. *Br Heart J* 41:647, 1979.

Oliva PB. Pathophysiology of acute myocardial infarction. *Ann Intern Med* 94:236, 1981.

Palmeri ST, Harrison DG, Cobb FR, et al: A QRS scoring system for assessing left ventricular function after myocardial infarction. *N Engl J Med* 306:4, 1982.

Parisi AF, Moynihan PF, Folland ED, et al: Echocardiography in acute and remote myocardial infarction. *Am J Cardiol* 46:1205, 1980.

Parkey RW, Bonte FJ, Meyer SL, et al: A new method of radionuclide imaging of acute myocardial infarction in humans. *Circulation* 50:540, 1974.

Rackley CE, Russell RO Jr., Mantle JA et al: Modern approach to the patient with acute myocardial infarction. *Curr Probl Cardiol* 1:49, 1979.

Raunio H, Rissanen V, Romppaneu T, et al: Changes in the QRS complex and ST segment in transmural and subendocardial myocardial infarctions: A clinicopathologic study. *Am Heart J* 98:176, 1979.

Roberts R, Sobel BE: Isoenzymes of creatine phosphokinase and diagnosis of myocardial infarction. *Ann Intern Med* 79:741, 1973.

Roberts R, Sobel BE: CPK Isoenzymes. *Hosp Prac* 55–62, Jan. 1976.

Roberts R, Sobel BE: Creatine kinase isoenzymes in the assessment of heart disease. *Am Heart J* 95:521, 1978.

Roberts WC: Coronary arteries in fatal acute myocardial infarction. *Circulation* 45:215, 1972.

Rose G: Early mobilization and discharge after myocardial infarction. *Mod Concepts Cardiovasc Dis* 41:59, 1977.

Sanz G, Castaner A, Betriu A, et al: Determinants of prognosis in survivors of myocardial infarction: A prospective clinical angiographic study. *N Engl J Med* 306:1065, 1982.

Schroeder JS, Lamb IH, Hu M: Do patients in whom myocardial infarction has been ruled out have a better prognosis after hospitalization than those surviving infarction? *N Engl J Med* 303:1, 1980.

Schuster EH, Bulkley BH: Expansion of transmural myocardial infarction: A pathophysiologic factor in cardiac rupture. *Circulation* 60:1532, 1979.

Schuster EH, Bulkley BH: Early post-infarction angina: Ischemia at a distance and ischemia in the infarct zone. *N Engl J Med* 305:1101, 1981.

Singer DE, Mulley AG, Thibault GE, et al: Unexpected readmissions to the coronary care unit during recovery from acute myocardial infarction. *N Engl J Med* 304:625, 1981.

Sivarajan ES, Bruce RA, Almes MJ, et al: In-hospital exercise after myocardial infarction does not improve treadmill performance. *N Engl J Med* 305:357, 1981.

Sobel BE, Braunwald E: Coronary artery disease: Management of acute myocardial infarction, in Braunwald E (ed): *Heart Disease: A Textbook of Cardiovascular Medicine*. Philadelphia, Saunders, 1980, p 1353.

Sobel BE: Cardiac and noncardiac forms of acute circulatory collapse (shock), in Braunwald E (ed): *Heart Disease: A Textbook of Cardiovascular Medicine*. Philadelphia, Saunders, 1980, p 590.

Swan HJC, Forrester JS, Diamond G, et al: Hemodynamic spectrum of myocardial infarction and cardiogenic shock. *Circulation* 45:1097, 1972.

Taylor GL, Humphries JO, Mellitis ED, et al: Predictors of clinical course, coronary anatomy, and left ventricular function after recovery from acute myocardial infarction. *Circulation* 62:960, 1980.

Vismara LA, Anderson EA, Mason DT: Relation of ventricular arrhythmias in the late hospital phase of acute myocardial infarction to sudden death after hospital discharge. *Am J Med* 59:6, 1975.

Vlodaner Z, Edwards JE: Rupture of ventricular septum or papillary muscle complicating myocardial infarction. *Circulation* 55:815, 1977.

Wei JY, Hutchins GM, Bulkley BH: Papillary muscle rupture in fatal acute myocardial infarction: A potentially treatable form of cardiogenic shock. *Ann Intern Med* 90:149, 1979.

Weld FM, Chu KL, Bigger JT, et al: Risk stratification with low-level exercise testing two weeks after acute myocardial infarction. *Circulation* 64:306, 1981.

Winkle RA, Glantz SA, Harrison DC: Pharmacologic therapy of ventricular arrhythmias. *Am J Cardiol* 36:629.

Wolf MA: Ventricular premature beats: To treat or not? *J Cardiovasc Med* 5:133, 1980.

CHAPTER 12

NEWER MODES OF THERAPY FOR ACUTE MYOCARDIAL INFARCTION

John D. Rutherford
Robert A. Kloner

The Concept of Limiting Myocardial Infarct Size

The main factor altering the therapeutic approach to acute myocardial infarction (MI) in the last decade is the observation that the mass of myocardium undergoing necrosis is an important determinant of ultimate prognosis. At one extreme are patients with cardiogenic shock who exhibit 40–50% necrosis of left ventricular myocardium, marginal extension of recent areas of infarction, and who have a mortality of greater than 80% in spite of therapy. At the other extreme are patients with small infarctions and no hemodynamic deficit who carry a mortality of around 2%. There is a relationship between infarct size and mortality, which is most obvious during the patient's hospital course and the first six months after the acute episode. Late mortality rates among survivors become similar for patients with either small or large infarcts. The incidence of ventricular arrhythmia is also directly related to the size of the infarction in the early and late postinfarct periods. Since the ultimate size of the evolving myocardial infarct is only partially determined by the extent and severity of coronary artery disease, it should be emphasized that careful attention to physiologic variables during the phase of evolution can improve the balance between myocardial oxygen supply and demand. The aim of the clinician is either to augment oxygen supply or reduce demand.

By treating pain effectively and promptly and caring for the patient in a quiet calm atmosphere, heart rate, a major determinant of myocardial oxygen consumption, may be lowered. All forms of tachyarrhythmias should be treated promptly and effectively. Since clinical and experimental evidence suggests that increased oxygen in the inspired air protects ischemic myocardium in patients who are hypoxemic, oxygen should be administered to patients with MI and arterial hypoxemia.

There has been recent widespread interest in the concept of directly limiting the size of MI's by either administration of pharmacologic agents or coronary artery reperfusion (intracoronary streptokinase or coronary bypass surgery). There are several potential mechanisms by which infarct size could be reduced (see Table 1). These include improvement of the myocardial oxygen supply-demand ratio by (1) decreasing myocardial oxygen requirements (such as beta-adrenergic blockade); (2) increas-

Table 1. Interventions That Potentially
Reduce Myocardial Injury After Coronary
Artery Occlusion

Decrease myocardial oxygen requirements
    Beta-adrenergic blockade
    Counterpulsation: intraaortic balloon, external
    Decreasing afterload in patients with hypertension
Increase myocardial oxygen supply
    Coronary artery reperfusion; thrombolytic agents,
    coronary artery bypass surgery
    Through collateral vessels
        Intraaortic balloon counterpulsation
        Hyaluronidase
        Nitroglycerin
    Elevating arterial oxygen tension
Augment anaerobic metabolism
    Glucose-insulin-potassium
Protect against autolytic and heterolytic processes
    Corticosteroid

---

ing myocardial oxygen supply (such as coronary reperfusion or improvement in collateral flow); (3) augmentation of anaerobic metabolism (glucose-insulin-potassium); (4) stabilization of cell membranes (corticosteroids); and (5) reduction in cell swelling (mannitol).

Conversely, some pharmacologic agents, such as isoproterenol, may actually increase the size of infarction.

Interventions That May Have a Beneficial Effect on Infarction Patients

Agents being studied currently that may have a salutary effect during infarction are discussed below.

HYALURONIDASE

Bovine testicular hyaluronidase (BTH) has been shown to reduce ischemic myocardial necrosis in several animal models. In a prospective randomized trial involving 31 patients with anterior MI, hyaluronidase diminished development of Q waves and loss of R waves in ischemic areas of myocardium. This study suggested that some degree of protection was provided and that evolution of infarction in certain zones of myocardium was limited. The mechanism for the protective effect is unknown, but it has been suggested that this enzyme depolymerizes myocardial hyaluronic acid and thus improves interstitial transport.

BETA-ADRENERGIC RECEPTOR BLOCKADE

The place of beta-adrenergic receptor blocking agents in the treatment of acute MI has been debated for 15 years. A problem with early clinical trials of therapy with oral agents was that therapeutic blood levels were unlikely to have been achieved during the time that infarct size should have been modified. Some studies in animals have indicated that either pretreatment with propranolol or administration of systemic propranolol after the onset of infarction will reduce infarct size. Improvement in myocardial oxygen balance due to a reduction in heart rate and contractility has also been shown in patients with acute infarction treated with propranolol (Fig. 1). A preliminary study in humans has suggested that threatened MI can in some cases be prevented by early beta-adrenergic receptor blockade. Since acute MI is frequently associated with increased sympathetic activity, and reductions in heart rate and contractility exert favorable effects on myocardial oxygen demand, beta-adrenergic blockade appears promising. It has been established that intravenous propranolol can be safely administered initially in acute MI, provided heart rate and arterial pressure are monitored and provided the agent is not administered in the presence of bradycardia, hypotension, left ventricular failure, bronchospasm or atrioventricular (AV) block. Favorable reductions have been demonstrated in the rate of myocardial lactate production, in the frequency of ventricular arrhythmias, and in the release of cardiac enzymes. In addition, propranolol has been shown to be

REDUCTION OF INJURY WITH PROPRANOLOL

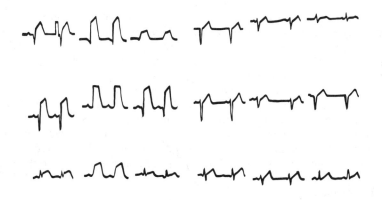

CONTROL (7:18)   AFTER PROPRANOLOL (7:29)

Figure 1 The effect of propranolol administered to a patient with acute myocardial infarction on ST segment elevation. Nine precordial leads are depicted from the V_1, V_3, and V_5 positions (middle panel) and the corresponding sites one intercostal space above and below the standard positions. There is a marked reduction in ST segment elevations after propranolol administration. (From Gold HK et al.: Propranolol-induced reduction of signs of ischemic injury during acute myocardial infarction. *Am J Cardiol* 38:692, 1976.)

effective treatment of patients with hyperdynamic states, early tachyarrhythmias refractory to lidocaine and procainamide, and infarction complicated by refractory, recurrent ischemic pain. Currently, a large multicenter investigation of the limitation of infarct size is in progress in the United States to assess whether propranolol has a favorable effect on indicators of infarct size, arrhythmias, and mortality.

Over the last few years, there have been several studies suggesting that chronic beta blocker therapy post-MI reduces mortality. In a study involving timolol, patients were randomly assigned to timolol therapy (10 mg bid) or placebo, beginning seven to 28 days after MI. Over a follow-up period of 17 months, the cummulative total mortality rate was reduced by 39.3% and cumulative sudden death rate by 44.6% in the timolol-treated group. In the recent Beta Blocker Heart Attack Trial (BHAT), patients treated with 180 to 240 mg of propranolol a day beginning 5–21 days post infarction had a 26% reduction in total mortality compared to patients receiving placebo, over a 25 month follow-up period. In a study with metoprolol, in which patients received the drug (15 mg IV followed by 100 mg orally bid) shortly after hospital admission and continued for 90 days, there was both a reduction in myocardial infarct size and a 36% reduction in death rate compared to a placebo-treated group. Although the mechanism of this protective effect of beta blockade is not yet understood, the results are conclusive enough now to warrant the routine administration of a beta blocker to patients who have suffered an infarction and who have no contraindications to such therapy.

NITRATES

The use of nitrates in patients with acute MI continues to be a controversial issue. Since nitroglycerin reduces systemic arterial pressure with a concomitant reflex increase in heart rate, it can be potentially harmful to patients with acute MI if not given in appropriate dosage associated with hemodynamic monitoring. In experimental animals, administration of IV nitroglycerin in appropriate dosage has been shown to reduce the magnitude and extent of ischemic injury following coronary occlusion, to elicit small reductions in total coronary vascular resistance, and to improve the ratio of endo to epicardial flow in ischemic zones of myocardium. Nitroglycerin does not appear to produce a coronary steal. Provided inappropriate tachycardia and hypotension are avoided and the drug is administered to patients with adequate filling pressures of the ventricles, IV nitroglycerin is useful in acute MI as a vasodilator in patients with left ventricular failure and for the relief of persistent ischemic pain.

VASODILATOR THERAPY

Vasodilator therapy may be useful in the treatment of severe ventricular failure in patients with acute MI. When this therapy is initiated, hemodynamic monitoring of systemic arterial pressure, cardiac output, and pulmonary capillary wedge pressure is important, since the primary aim of vasodilator therapy, that is, reduction of afterload, may lead to excessive systemic diastolic hypotension or an inappropriate fall in ventricular filling pressures. With appropriate use of vasodilator therapy the impedance to ventricular ejection may be reduced, with a concomittant increase in stroke volume and a reduction in myocardial oxygen consumption. This particularly applies to patients with MI complicated by severe left ventricular failure, mitral regurgitation, ventricular septal defect, or systemic hypertension. It should be noted that nitroprusside may potentially cause a coronary steal by dilating coronary vessels in nonischemic regions of myocardium, thus diminishing the perfusion pressure of compromised regions of myocardium. Nitroglycerin does not cause a coronary steal and some physicians prefer to use it in this situation.

DOPAMINE AND DOBUTAMINE

Dopamine, the precursor of norepinephrine, stimulates myocardial contractility by direct myocardial beta-1 adrenergic stimulation and indirectly releases norepinephrine from sympathetic nerve terminals, which in turn stimulate beta-1 receptors also. In patients with reduced cardiac output, increased left ventricular filling pressure, pulmonary vascular congestion, and hypotension, dopamine can be very effective. With infusion rates of 2–5 μg/kg/min, this agent increases cardiac contractility, cardiac output, and renal blood flow with little change in heart rate and either a reduction or no change in total peripheral resistance. The dose can be increased in stepwise manner up to 30 μg/kg/min in order to reduce pulmonary capillary wedge pressure to approximately 20 mm Hg and elevate cardiac index. At high doses, dopamine exhibits alpha-adrenergic vasoconstrictor effects as well as beta-1 effects. Therefore, heart rate, arterial pressure, and peripheral resistance may increase with a fall in renal blood flow. In addition, large doses of dopamine may cause an increase in coronary artery resistance. Therefore, in patients with heart failure, dopamine can exert important beneficial hemodynamic and renal effects; the dose must be adjusted carefully to prevent excessive tachycardia, increases in contractility, and increases in peripheral resistance, which will increase myocardial oxygen demand and intensify myocardial ischemia. Dobutamine, a synthetic cardioactive sympathomimetic amine that stimulates beta-1, beta-2, and alpha-adrenergic receptors, has little vasoconstrictor activity and has less positive chronotropic effects than dopamine.

DIGITALIS

Currently, it is felt that the administration of digitalis to patients with acute MI in the absence of heart failure may lead to an increase in infarct size. In experimental animals following coronary occlusion, digitalis increases infarct size if heart failure is not present. In addition, some investigators feel that digitalis glycosides may increase cardiac arrhythmias soon after an MI, particularly if hypokalemia is present. Conversely, when heart failure is present, the diminution of heart size and wall tension associated with digitalis therapy frequently results in a net reduction of myocardial oxygen requirements, and the severity of ischemia occurring in the presence of experimentally induced congestive heart failure is reduced. In general, the use of digitalis is reserved for control of ventricular rate with arrhythmias, such as atrial flutter and fibrillation and for the treatment of heart failure that persists despite treatment with diuretics. Digitalis does not appear to influence the adverse outcome of cardiogenic shock.

INTRAAORTIC BALLOON COUNTERPULSATION (IABP)

It has become obvious that IABP is a useful adjunct to medical and surgical therapy of acute MI. The IAB is advanced from the femoral artery to the descending thoracic aorta and is timed in a cyclical manner to inflate and deflate with helium, a low viscosity inert gas that allows rapid gas movement. This displaces a volume of blood from a thoracic aorta equal to the balloon volume. By timing the balloon to inflate at the moment of aortic valve closure (using the ECG and arterial pressure pulse), aortic diastolic pressure can be increased by 10–15 mm Hg. Deflation of the balloon occurs just prior to aortic valve opening so that during systole left ventricular pressure work diminishes (Fig. 2). Therefore, the balloon acts to reduce oxygen demand and increase oxygen supply. If flow in the coronary arteries is pressure dependent, that is, in the presence of coronary artery stenosis, IABP will augment diastolic coronary blood flow. If cardiac output is diminished, due to either left ventricular failure or severe myocardial ischemia, than IABP will increase cardiac output by reducing afterload. In the presence of ischemia, the increased diastolic perfusion pressure of the coronary bed will improve myocardial oxygenation, if coronary artery flow is pressure dependent, and will tend to increase cardiac output.

In experimental animals, IABP decreases afterload, preload, and myocardial oxygen consumption and increases coronary blood flow with an improvement in cardiac performance. IABP appears to protect ischemic myocardium in experimental animals, based on analysis of myocardial CK depletion, analysis of ST segment ele-

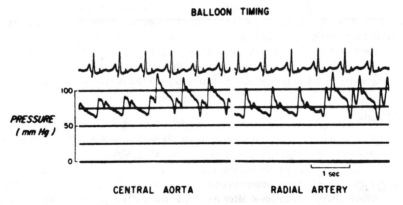

BALLOON TIMING

PRESSURE (mm Hg)

100

50

0

1 sec

CENTRAL AORTA   RADIAL ARTERY

Figure 2 The effect of initiation of intraaortic balloon pumping (IABP) on central aortic pressure (left panel) and radial artery pressure (right panel). The electrocardiogram shows balloon timing markers in the PR and ST segments. In the left panel the upstroke of the balloon pulse is timed to coincide with the central aortic dicrotic notch; however, this timing requires slightly earlier balloon inflation, as judged from the radial artery pressure measurement. The minimal diastolic radial arterial pressure during IABP is approximately 5–10 mm Hg below the diastolic radial pressure prior to IABP. (From Leinbach RC, Gold HK: Intraaortic balloon pumping: Use in treatment of cardiogenic shock and acute myocardial ischemia. In Karliner JS, Gregoratos G, eds: *Coronary Care.* London, Churchill Livingstone, 1981.)

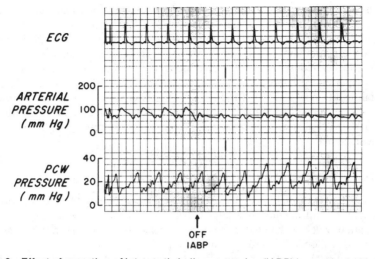

Figure 3 Effect of cessation of intraaortic balloon pumping (IABP) in a patient with severe mitral regurgitation and cardiogenic shock due to a ruptured papillary muscle. With cessation of IABP, arterial pressure is markedly reduced and the mean pulmonary capillary wedge (PCW) pressure rises from 19 mm Hg to 25 mm Hg. Large regurgitant waves are noted in the PCW pressure trace. (From Leinbach RC, Gold HK: Intraaortic balloon pumping: Use in treatment of cardiogenic shock and acute myocardial ischemia. In Karliner JS, Gregoratos, G, eds: *Coronary Care*, London, Churchill Livingstone, 1981.)

vations, and histochemical and histological criteria of necrosis. There is no data suggesting that IABP alters the prognosis in patients with uncomplicated MI; and, indeed, it is likely the risks of IABP would outweigh potential benefits. IABP has a definite role in stabilizing patients with severe unstable angina in whom maximal medical therapy has failed to control recurrent ischemia; in patients with acute MI in one area of myocardium who exhibit symptomatic, ECG, and hemodynamic evidence of threatening large areas of myocardium in another location; and in patients exhibiting intermittent global ischemia who require stabilization prior to coronary angiography and possible myocardial revascularization.

IABP should be considered in MI complicated by a ventricular septal defect or severe mitral regurgitation and in cardiogenic shock. In these situations, increased coronary diastolic perfusion pressure and a reduction in afterload will exert a favorable influence. With mitral regurgitation, IABP will often lower the wedge pressure below the range of pulmonary edema and will allow evaluation of residual ventricular function and coronary anatomy to proceed if surgical repair is contemplated (Fig. 3). If a ventricular septal defect is present, the balloon will augment systemic output with little change in pulmonary flow and a favorable reduction in the pulmonary to systemic flow ratio will result. Since medical treatment of ventricular septal defect complicating acute MI carries a high mortality, the use of IABP will allow both ventricular function and coronary anatomy to be assessed under relatively stable circumstances, and the possibility of surgery can be evaluated. For obvious reasons, the use of IABP is contraindicated in the presence of aortic regurgitation or aneurysms of the ascending aorta. Tachycardia is a relative contraindication, since augmentation by the balloon may be impossible at rapid ventricular rates. The IAB can be inserted by direct exposure of the femoral artery or percutaneously. Both procedures carry the risk of arterial injury, aortic dissection, loss of distal pulses in the leg, or infection and perforation of the aorta. Because of these risks, the use of IABP is only advised in centers with an experienced cardiovascular surgical service. Even in experienced hands, the risks of percutaneous IABP are no less than conventional insertion of IAB, and the ease of insertion alone should not be grounds for liberalizing the indications for IABP in patients who can be managed without it. Use of IABP has made no substantial change in the extremely high mortality of cardiogenic shock.

CORONARY REVASCULARIZATION

If irreversible myocardial injury has already occurred, the performance of coronary bypass surgery will not improve left ventricular performance following acute MI, and the patient will be subjected to the risks of a major operation. However, if surgery is performed while viable tissue is still present, it is possible that this tissue will be salvaged from necrosis. In a recent study by Phillips et al., patients with acute MI received emergency coronary bypass surgery on an average of 6.5 hours after the onset of chest pain. Patients who had been revascularized showed improved left ventricular hemodynamics on repeat cardiac catheterization. Operative mortality was 1.3% and late mortality was 2.8%. Further trials are needed before emergency coronary bypass surgery can be considered routine therapy for acute infarction, but these and other studies suggest that it is feasible for patients with acute infarction to undergo this procedure.

There are some situations in which emergency coronary bypass surgery in the setting of infarction seems warranted. If, during cardiac catheterization, patients appear to be acutely evolving an infarction or if they exhibit global ischemia, emergency operation should be considered and may be effective. Similarly, if a patient with known coronary anatomy awaiting surgery presents in an early acute phase, it may be feasible to perform the bypass operation, particularly if facilities are available for circulatory support by IABP while arrangements for emergency surgery proceed. In patients with nontransmural infarction who threaten other large areas of myocardium by exhibiting postinfarction pain, ECG evidence of ischemia and hemodynamic compromise unresponsive to aggressive medical therapy, IABP, urgent coronary arteriography, and possible surgery should be considered. In these circumstances, an assessment must be made of both right and left ventricular function, which is often most easily accomplished by radionuclide ventriculography. If there is evidence of severe cardiac dysfunction and absence of contractile reserve, conservative, nonsurgical therapy is usually attempted in order to allow the recovery, if possible, from the acute period of infarction.

STREPTOKINASE INFUSIONS

Recently, several groups of investigators have reported results of intracoronary streptokinase infusions in patients with acute ischemic syndromes and acute MI. Streptokinase is a plasminogen activator and can dissolve blood clots. The enthusiasm for investigating the use of this type of therapy in patients with acute infarction has been heightened by recent reports indicating that, during the early hours of transmural infarction, thrombus formation or coronary spasm may be important in the evolution of infarction. It seems that in the first 12 to 24 hours of acute infarction, a dynamic process occurs and intervention may be possible. Platelet aggregation with thrombus formation and the possibility of lysis of clot may be important determinants of the eventual outcome of an acute episode. Initial reports suggest that intracoronary streptokinase infused into the vessel supplying the acute infarct results in clot lysis in approximately 75–80% of patients and restoration of coronary flow with significant relief of ischemic chest pain and salvage of myocardium. Residual coronary stenosis may be present in some patients who then have required bypass surgery.

Several studies have shown improved left ventricular function prior to patient discharge. Some other studies, however, have not found an immediate postreperfusion improvement of left ventricular function. The complications attributed to the procedure are mainly due to heparinization, or bleeding from the puncture site, but otherwise patients appear to tolerate the procedure surprisingly well. Such aggressive investigations are only performed in centers with the potential for emergency coronary revascularization, which is necessary in some instances. Randomized, controlled studies are in progress to evaluate the impact of this technique. If it proves to be beneficial, the technical and economic considerations may still make it an impractical treatment.

Infarct patients in a trial of intravenous streptokinase infusion in one study showed reduced mortality at six months compared to those who received glucose infusion. Preliminary studies suggest that clot lysis may occur in a significant percentage of patients receiving intravenous streptokinase therapy.

PROPHYLACTIC USE OF AGENTS THAT MIGHT PREVENT PLATELET AGGREGATION AND THROMBUS

Since there is considerable evidence that platelet aggregation and platelet induced thrombosis may play a role in the pathogenesis of MI, several trials have been undertaken to evaluate the efficacy of antiplatelet agents in preventing the recurrence of MI. Based on the results of randomized controlled trials, it is currently difficult to state that aspirin, Persantine (dipyridamole), or sulfinpyrazone will reduce the mortality in patients who have survived an MI.

The results of the Aspirin Myocardial Infarction Study Research Group indicate that the regular administration of aspirin in a dose of 1 gm/day does not reduce three-year mortality rates in patients who have survived MI, and the conclusion of the study was that aspirin is not recommended for use in such patients.

However, a recent Veterans' Administration Cooperative Study did show that in men with unstable angina, treatment with 324 mg of aspirin daily reduced the incidence of acute MI as well as death.

In the Persantine-Aspirin Reinfarction Study Research Group, in which patients were chosen at random for treatment with Persantine plus aspirin, aspirin alone, or placebo, there was a suggestion that over a 41 month follow-up period, the total mortality appeared lower in the treated than in the placebo groups. These differences were not statistically significant by the study criterion. Patients who were entered into the study within six months of the qualifying MI, and thus received active treatment earlier, showed the most favorable results.

The results of the Anturane Reinfarction Trial Research Group have been vigorously debated in the recent medical literature. This was a randomized double-blind multicenter trial comparing sulfinpyrazone (200 mg qid) and placebo in the prevention of cardiac mortality over a 16 month period of follow-up. The therapy was commenced within 25 to 35 days after a documented MI. The initial report of the study indicated that sulfinpyrazone reduced the incidence of sudden cardiac death by 43% in postinfarction patients at 24 months and 74% during the two to seven months after infarction. Samples of the case records were subsequently reviewed by the FDA and assignment of the causes of death were questioned. The FDA review group initially stated that the results showing effect on total cardiac mortality were not convincing because they depended heavily on retrospective exclusion from analysis of certain patients who died while receiving the drug. Further reevaluation, however, suggested that the drug probably was effective.

Currently, the evidence suggesting that aspirin, and dipyridamole, with or without

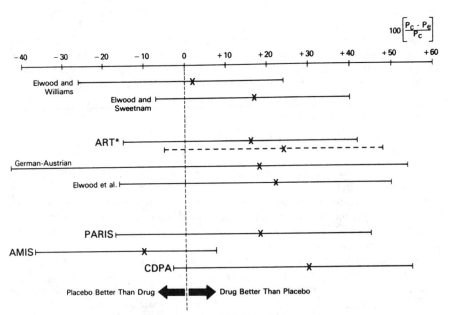

*Solid line denotes all randomised patients, broken line all "eligible" patients

Figure 4   Estimates (X) with 95% confidence intervals of the relative difference in all-cause mortality between placebo (P_c) and platelet-active drug (P_e) in eight trials of post-myocardial infarction patients. These studies are listed in order of increasing time between the qualifying myocardial infarction and patient enrollment into each study. None of the studies has a beneficial effect at the 0.05 level because all 95% confidence intervals include zero. (Reproduced by permission of American Heart Association from *Circulation* 62 (Suppl V), V-114, 1980.)

aspirin, favorably affect mortality rates following MI remains controversial. Sulfinpyrazone may have a favorable effect. It has been pointed out that a possible flaw in these studies relates to the fact that treatment was delayed too long after the initial infarction (Fig. 4). Men with unstable angina do appear to have a lower incidence of infarction and death when treated with aspirin.

Bibliography

Archibald DG, Steinke WE, Smitherman TC, et al: Protective effects of 324 mg aspirin daily in men with unstable angina: Results of a Veteran's Administration Cooperative Study. *Circulation* 66: Supp. II; 11–17, 1982.

Beta Blocker Heart Attack Trial Research Group. A randomized trial of propranolol in patients with acute myocardial infarction. I. Mortality results *JAMA* 247:1707, 1982

Cohn NJ, Franciosa JA, Francis GS, et al: Effect of short-term infusion of sodium nitroprusside on mortality rate in acute myocardial infarction complicated by left ventricular failure: Results of a Veterans' Administration Cooperative Study. *N Engl J Med* 306:1129, 1982.

Durrer JE, Kong II, van Capelle FJL: Effect of sodium nutroprusside on mortality in acute myocardial infarction. *N Engl J Med* 306:1121, 1982.

Elwood PC, Sweetnam PM: Aspirin and secondary mortality after myocardial infarction. *Circulation* 62:53, 1980.

European cooperative study group for streptokinase treatment in acute myocardial infarction. Streptokinase in acute myocardial infarction. *N Engl J Med* 301:797, 1979.

Forrester JS, Diamond G, Chatterjee MB, et al: Medical therapy of acute myocardial infarction by the application of hemodynamic subsets. *N Engl J Med* 295:1356, 1976.

Frishman NH, Ribner HS: Anticoagulation in myocardial infarction: Modern approach to an old problem. *Am J Cardiol* 43:1207, 1979.

Ganz W, Nihomiya K, Hashida J, et al: Intracoronary thrombolysis in acute myocardial infarction: Experimental background and clinical experience. *Am Heart J* 102:1145, 1981.

Grande P, Hanse BF, Christiansen C, et al: Estimation of acute myocardial infarct size in man by serum CK-MB measurements. *Circulation* 65:756, 1982.

Hill NS, Antman E, Green LH, et al: Intravenous nitroglycerin: A review of pharmacology, indications, therapeutic effects and complications. *Chest* 79:69, 1981.

Hirsch J: Selection and results of antiplatelet therapy in the prevention of stroke and myocardial infarction. *Arch Intern Med* 141:311, 1981.

Hjalmarson A, Herlitz J, Malek I, et al: Effect on mortality of metoprolol in acute myocardial infarction: A double-blind randomized trial. *Lancet* 87:823, 1981.

Hood WB: More on sulfinpyrazone after myocardial infarction. *N Engl J Med* 306:988, 1982.

Julian DG, Prescott RJ, Jackson FS, et al: Controlled trial of sotalol for one year after myocardial infarction. *Lancet* (1) 828:1142, 1982.

Kloner, RA, Braunwald E: Observations of experimental myocardial ischemia. *Cardiovasc Res* 14:371, 1980.

Levine FH, Gold HK, Leinbach RC, et al: Safe early revascularization for continuing ischemia after acute myocardial infarction. *Circulation* 60:5, 1979.

Madias JE, Hood WB Jr: Effects of methylprednisolone on the ischemic damage in patients with acute myocardial infarction. *Circulation* 65:1106, 1982.

Marcus FL: Editorial: Use of digitalis in acute myocardial infarction. *Circulation* 62:17, 1980.

Markis JE, Malagold M, Parker JA, et al: Myocardial salvage after intracoronary thrombolysis with streptokinase in acute myocardial infarction. *N Engl J Med* 305:777, 1981.

Maroko PR, Hillis LD, Muller JE, et al: Favorable effects of hyaluronidase on electrocardiographic evidence of necrosis in patients with acute myocardial infarction. *N Engl J Med* 296:898, 1977.

Maroko PR, Kjekshus JK, Sobel BE, et al: Factors influencing infarct size following experimental coronary artery occlusions. *Circulation* 43:67, 1971.

Mathey, DG, Rodewald G, Rentrop P, et al: Intracoronary streptokinase thrombolytic recanalization and subsequent surgical bypass of remaining atherosclerotic stenosis in acute myocardial infarction: Complementary combined approach effecting reduced infarct size, preventing reinfarction, and improving left ventricular function. *Am Heart J* 102:1194, 1981.

Morrison J, Coromilas J, Robbins M, et al: Digitalis and myocardial infarction in man. *Circulation* 62:8, 1980.

Norris RM, Sammel NL, Clarke ED, et al: Protective effect of propranolol in threatened myocardial infarction. *Lancet* 907, 1978.

O'Rourke MF, Norris RM, Campbell TS, et al: Randomized controlled trial in intraaortic balloon counterpulsation in early myocardial infarction with acute heart failure. *Am J Cardiol* 47:815, 1981.

Palmeri ST, Harrison DG, Cobb FR, et al: A QRS scoring system for assessing left ventricular function after myocardial infarction. *N Engl J Med* 306:4, 1982.

Phillips SJ, Kongtahworn C, Zeff RH, et al: Emergency coronary artery revascularization: A possible therapy for acute myocardial infarction. *Circulation* 60:241, 1979.

Reduto LA, Smalling RW, Freund GC, et al: Intracoronary infusion of streptokinase in patients with acute myocardial infarction: Effects of reperfusion on left ventricular performance. *Am J Cardiol* 48:403, 1981.

Relman AS, Hood WB: More on sulfinpyrazone after myocardial infarction. *N Engl J Med* 306:988, 1982.

Rentrop P, Blanke H, Karsch KR, et al: Changes in left ventricular function after intracoronary streptokinase infusion in clinically evolving myocardial infarction. *Am Heart J* 102:1188, 1981.

Rentrop P, Blanke H, Karsch KR: Effects of nonsurgical coronary reperfusion on the left ventricle in human subjects compared with conventional treatment: Study of 18 patients with acute myocardial infarction treated with intracoronary infusion of streptokinase. *Am J Cardiol* 49:1, 1982.

Rentrop P, Blanke H, Karsch KR, et al: Selective intracoronary thrombolysis in acute myocardial infarction and unstable angina pectoris. *Circulation* 63:307, 1981.

Selinger SL, Berg R Jr, Leonard JL, et al: Surgical treatment of acute evolving anterior myocardial infarction. *Circulation* 64:28, 1981.

Swan HJC, Forrester JS, Diamond G, et al: Hemodynamic spectrum of myocardial infarction and cardiogenic shock. *Circulation* 45:1097, 1972.

Taylor SH, Silke B, Ebbutt A, et al: A long-term prevention study with oxprenolol in coronary heart disease. *N Engl J Med* 307:1293, 1982.

The Anturare Reinfarction Trial Research Group. Sulfinpyrazone in the prevention of sudden death after myocardial infarction *N Engl J Med* 302:250, 1980.

The Norwegian Multicenter Study Group. Timolol-induced reduction in mortality and reinfarction in patients surviving acute myocardial infarction. *N Engl J Med* 304:801, 1981.

The Persantine-Aspirin Reinfarction Study (Paris) Research group. The Persantine-aspirin reinfarction Study. *Circulation* 62:V85, 1980.

Yim YI, Williams JF Jr: Large dose sublingual nitroglycerin in acute myocardial infarction: Relief of chest pain and reduction of Q wave evolution. *Am J Cardiol* 49:842, 1982.

Yusuf S, Ramsdale D, Peto R, et al: Early intravenous atenolol treatment in suspected acute myocardial infarction: Preliminary report of a randomized trial. *Lancet* 2:272, 1980.

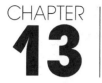

CHAPTER 13 | VALVULAR HEART DISEASE

Robert A. Kloner

Rheumatic Fever

Rheumatic heart disease remains a major cause of valvular heart disease, although its incidence is diminishing. It begins when a patient with rheumatic fever develops carditis with subsequent progressive valvular damage occurring over many years.

Rheumatic fever is a general inflammatory disease which occurs 10 to 21 days after infection with a group A beta hemolytic streptococcus. The disease tends to affect young people 5–15 years of age and, in general, is uncommon in adults. The cardiac injury may be immunologically mediated due to an antigen-antibody complex. The modified Jones criteria for diagnosing rheumatic fever includes the presence of two major criteria or one major plus two minor criteria as suggestive of the disease (Table I).

Symptoms include fever, chills, migratory polyarthritis, fatigue, weakness, irritability, and epistaxis. The incidence of carditis in patients with an initial attack of rheumatic fever varies from 40–60%. Cardiac complaints include dyspnea, pericardial pain, edema, palpitations, and fatigue.

Cardiac examination reveals a tachycardia out of proportion to the fever and persists during sleep, displacement of the cardiac impulse to the left, soft heart sounds, and gallop rhythms. Frequently, a holosystolic murmur at the apex with radiation to the axilla and a low pitched, middiastolic murmur (Carey-Coombs murmur) are heard, both due to mitral valve involvement. The murmur of aortic insufficiency, a pericardial friction rub, and signs of both left and right-sided heart failure may be present.

Electrocardiographic findings include tachycardia, prolonged PR interval (first degree heart block), and second and third degree heart block. Both supraventricular and ventricular arrhythmias occur. The QRS complexes may have diminished voltage and a prolonged QT interval. With pericarditis the ST segments are elevated, but with myocarditis alone nonspecific ST-T wave abnormalities are common.

Chest x-ray film is either normal or may reveal an enlarged cardiac silhouette due to ventricular dilatation or pericardial effusion. Pulmonary vascular redistribution, pulmonary interstitial or alveolar edema, Kerley B lines, and pleural effusions reflect left ventricular failure.

Therapy for acute rheumatic fever includes rest, salt restriction for carditis, and penicillin for eradication of streptococcal infections (600,000 units of benzathine penicillin G IM for children under 27 kg; 1.2 million units for children over 27 kg and adults; or oral penicillin G, 250,000 units qid for 10 days) or in patients who are allergic to pencillin, erythromycin 250 mg po qid for 10 days. Five to eight grams of buffered acetylsalicyclic acid (aspirin) per day in divided doses (q 4–6 hours) are

265

Table 1. Jones Criteria (revised)

Major Manifestations	Minor Manifestations
Carditis	Fever
Polyarthritis	Arthralgia
Chorea	Previous rheumatic fever or rheumatic heart disease
Erythema marginatum	Elevated ESR or positive CRP; leukocytosis
Subcutaneous nodules	Prolonged PR interval

Plus supporting evidence of preceding streptococcal infection: history of recent scarlet fever; positive throat culture for group A streptococcus; increased ASO titer or other streptococcal antibodies.

SOURCE: From Jones Criteria (revised) for guidance in the diagnosis of rheumatic fever. *Circulation* 32:664, 1965, by permission of the American Heart Association, Inc.

ESR = erythrocyte sedimentation rate; CRP = C-reactive protein; ASO = antistreptolysin-O

administered to achieve salicylate levels of 25–35 mg/100 ml; occasionally prednisone 40–80 mg/day is given to patients with marked cardiac dysfunction. Salicylates and steroids reduce the symptoms of rheumatic fever but do not shorten the course of the disease and do not prevent the development of residual heart disease. Patients with congestive heart failure should be treated with salt restriction (no added salt), digitalis, and diuretics. Long-term rheumatic fever prophylaxis should begin, since recurrent episodes may result in further cardiac damage (benzathine penicillin, 1.2 million units IM every month; or oral penicillin 250,000 units qd; or oral erythromycin 250 mg bid; or oral sulfadiazine 0.5 g qd for patients weighing less than 27 kg and 1 g qd for patients weighing more than 27 kg).

The mean duration of a rheumatic attack is approximately three months; with severe carditis, the attack may persist for six months. The eventual development of rheumatic heart disease is largely dependent upon whether carditis was present during an initial attack of rheumatic fever and whether recurrences of rheumatic carditis are prevented. Patients in the United Kingdom–United States Cooperative Study who did not have carditis during the acute attack of rheumatic fever did not develop late rheumatic heart disease. Seventy percent of patients with mild carditis (defined as the presence of mitral regurgitation) had normal hearts at 10 years; only 40% of patients with severe carditis with congestive heart failure during the initial attack had normal hearts at 10 years. Hence, rheumatic heart disease is more likely to develop in those patients with severe carditis during their initial attack of rheumatic fever.

The valvular lesions of rheumatic disease may take years to develop after the initial carditis of rheumatic fever, as there is gradual scaring and thickening of the valve. Clinical valve disease becomes manifest 10–30 years following acute rheumatic fever. In rheumatic heart disease, the mitral valve is involved in approximately 85% of cases; the aortic valve in 44%; the tricuspid valve in 10–16%; the pulmonary valve is rarely involved. When the aortic valve is involved, the mitral valve is usually involved as well. Patients may present with the valvular lesions of rheumatic heart disease and, in a high percentage of cases, cannot give an antecedent clinical history for rheumatic fever.

Left-Sided Valvular Heart Disease

SPECIFIC VALVE LESIONS*

Mitral Stenosis

The etiology of mitral stenosis (MS) is almost always rheumatic heart disease (Fig. 1). Rarely is it due to a congenital anomaly. Stenosis of the mitral valve results in increased left atrial pressure, which leads to increased pulmonary capillary pressure. When pulmonary capillary hydrostatic pressure is greater than plasma oncotic pressure, transudation of fluid occurs into the pulmonary interstitium and alveoli. Over time, pulmonary arteriolar vasoconstriction occurs and acts as a secondary obstruction to blood flow. Subsequently, the right ventricle hypertrophies, dilates, and eventually fails. The left atrium, when severely dilated, often develops atrial fibrillation, with the loss of an effective atrial contraction to aid left ventricular filling. When the ventricular rate is fast, there is also a reduction in the time during which the ventricle can fill resulting in a further fall in cardiac output.

Some studies have shown abnormalities in left ventricular function in patients with mitral stenosis. Studies using echocardiography have shown that the normal velocity of the intraventricular septum and maximum systolic and diastolic endocardial velocities are reduced. Abnormalities of left ventricular contractility are important, especially in the early postoperative period, since pulmonary congestion may occur despite the relief of the mitral stenosis.

The normal mitral valve area is 3–5 cm². The degree of symptomatology of mitral stenosis depends largely on the extent by which the valve orifice is reduced. When the valve is 2.1 to 2.5 cm², patients may be symptomatic with extreme exertion; when the valve is reduced to 1.6 to 2.0 cm² patients are symptomatic with moderate exertion; when the valve size is less than 1.0 cm², the stenosis is said to be critical and symptoms occur with minimal exertion or at rest. Mitral stenosis is more common in women than in men. Symptoms often first appear when patients are in their 30s and may be precipitated by atrial fibrillation and pregnancy. Initially, symptoms reflect elevated pulmonary capillary wedge pressures and include dyspnea, orthop-

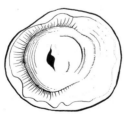

MITRAL STENOSIS
"Fish-mouth" mitral valve

Figure 1 Looking down into the left atrium at a stenotic mitral valve. The mitral leaflets have thickened, the commissures fused, and the mitral orifice has a narrowed "fish-mouth" appearance.

---

* Illustrative examples of chest x-ray film, echocardiography, pulse tracings, and catheterization results of specific valve lesions are found in Chapters 4, 5, and 8.

nea, paroxysmal nocturnal dyspnea, fatigue, weakness, lethargy, and hemoptysis. When pulmonary vascular resistance increases, there may be a transient period during which left-sided symptoms diminish and right-sided symptoms increase. Signs of right ventricular failure include gastrointestinal complaints due to hepatic and mesenteric congestion (nausea, diarrhea, anorexia, right upper quadrant tenderness), peripheral edema, ascites, and marked fatigue with low forward cardiac output. During the late stages of the disease, weight loss (cardiac cachexia) is present and dyspnea returns.

Physical examination reveals a pulse that is irregularly irregular if the patient is in atrial fibrillation. The patient may be thin; the cheeks are frequently ruddy (mitral facies). Rales are heard depending on the degree of interstitial and alveolar edema. The jugular veins are distended if right ventricular failure is present. Palpation of the precordium reveals a normal or small left ventricular impulse, while a right ventricular lift often is felt. With severe pulmonary hypertension, P_2 may be palpated. Auscultation characteristically reveals a loud S_1, a loud P_2 if pulmonary hypertension is present, an opening snap that occurs after S_2; a low-pitched diastolic rumble that begins with the opening snap and becomes louder just before S_1 (presystolic accentuation) if the patient is in sinus rhythm. The murmur is heard best at the apex with the bell of the stethoscope when the patient is in the left lateral decubitus position. If the opening snap is close to S_2 (< 0.07 s) due to left atrial hypertension then the severity of mitral stenosis is worse. Associated murmurs include that of tricuspid regurgitation with severe right heart failure and pulmonary regurgitation (Graham Steell's murmur) with pulmonary hypertension.

With right ventricular failure, examination of the abdomen reveals a tender enlarged liver, which may be pulsatile if there is associated tricuspid regurgitation. Peripheral edema is often present with right ventricular failure. Differential diagnosis is shown in Table 2.

The ECG is remarkable for left atrial enlargement (p mitrale), right axis deviation, and right ventricular hypertrophy. Atrial fibrillation may be present. If the patient is on digitalis for control of ventricular rate, ST-T wave changes characteristic of digitalis effect are seen.

Chest x-ray film reveals an enlarged left atrium as manifested by an elevated left mainstem bronchus, double cardiac density, and straight left heart border. The right ventricle is enlarged, with anterior encroachment on the retrosternal space on the lateral view. Calcification of the mitral valve may be seen on chest x-ray film. Elevated pulmonary capillary wedge pressure is manifested as pulmonary vascular redistribution, interstitial edema, Kerley B lines; pleural effusion may also be present.

Echocardiography is an extremely useful tool for determining the presence of mitral stenosis. The valve leaflets are thickened with a diminished E to F slope and diminished leaflet separation. Calcification of the valve leaflets can sometimes be appreciated. There is concordant motion of the anterior and posterior leaflets, instead of the motion away from each other during diastole. The left atrium is enlarged and left atrial thrombus may be seen. The right ventricle may be enlarged as well. The echocardiogram can distinguish mitral stenosis from a left atrial myxoma or ball valve thrombus, conditions that may mimic mitral stenosis.

Several echocardiographic studies have attempted to determine which parameters are most helpful in noninvasively assessing the severity of mitral stenosis. Fisher et

Table 2. Differential Diagnosis of Mitral Stenosis

Disease Entity	Differentiating Features
Left atrial myxoma (symptoms and signs, especially diastolic murmur, mimic mitral stenosis)	Auscultatory findings change with body position; signs of systemic illness (weight loss, anemia, fever, emboli); usually no opening snap; tumor plop, characteristic echocardiographic findings
Atrial septal defect (increased flow across tricuspid valve causes diastolic flow murmur).	Fixed splitting of the S_2; absence of left atrial enlargement; absence of Kerley B lines; echocardiography reveals normal mitral valve and large right ventricle; left-to-right shunt by catheterization study
High flow states, such as hyperthyroidism (diastolic flow rumbles across AV valves due to increased amount of blood transversing these values)	Hyperactive cardiac state; signs of hyperthyroidism; echocardiogram shows normal mitral valve, hyperkinetic left ventricular motion
Mitral regurgitation (with large amounts of blood flowing across the mitral valve during diastole, a diastolic rumble may be present)	Holosystolic murmur of mitral regurgitation (although mitral regurgitation and mitral stenosis may coexist); concomitant S_3, signs of left ventricular enlargment
Cor triatriatum (uncommon congenital malformation consisting of a fibromuscular membrane that divides the left atrium and impedes flow from pulmonary veins to left ventricle)	Murmurs (both systolic and diastolic) are not typical of mitral stenosis; normal mitral valve by echo with characteristic echo in left atrium; left atrial angiography may visualize membrane
Congenital stenosis of pulmonary veins (unusual congenital entity resulting in signs of pulmonary hypertension, pulmonary venous congestion, and right ventricular failure)	No distinctive murmurs; mitral valve normal by echo
Primary pulmonary hypertension (signs of right ventricular failure; more common in women).	No opening snap or diastolic rumble; no left atrial enlargement or elevated pulmonary artery wedge pressure
Large mitral vegetations from endocarditis	Vegetations may be visualized by echocardiography
Ball-valve thrombus formation in the left atrium	Auscultatory findings change with body position; two-dimensional echocardiography may be helpful

al. compared mitral valve area determined by cardiac catheterization to M-mode echocardiographic measurements. The rate of diastolic closure (E–F slope) was not useful in predicting severity of mitral stenosis, while the maximal diastolic separation of anterior and posterior leaflets was more closely correlated. Narrow separation was associated with severe mitral stenosis; wide separation was associated with mild stenosis. Intermediate separation, however, was not of predictive value.

Phonocardiography may be helpful in assessing the severity of the mitral stenosis. The S_2 to opening snap interval is of shorter duration in severe mitral stensosis (<0.06–0.07 sec) and of longer duration in mild to moderate mitral stenosis (>0.08–0.09 sec). The Q-1 interval (measured from the onset of the Q wave of the ECG to the beginning of the mitral component of the first heart sound) is also useful. If the Q-1 interval is greater than 0.07 seconds, significant mitral stenosis is present; if 0.1 second or longer, the stenosis may be severe.

Cardiac catheterization reveals a left atrial to left ventricular diastolic gradient and an elevated left atrial pressure. The pulmonary capillary wedge pressure is elevated (often greater than 20–25 mm Hg). Pulmonary artery pressures may be elevated; and with the development of right ventricular failure, right ventricular and right atrial pressures are also elevated. Tricuspid regurgitation secondary to right ventricular dilatation may be present with tall regurgitant waves on the atrial pressure tracing. Valve area calculations are discussed in Chapter 8. Fluoroscopy may reveal calcified, poorly moving cusps of the mitral valve.

Digitalis is given for control of heart rate in patients with atrial fibrillation. Dosage ranges from 0.125 to 0.375 mg a day. Digitalis is not beneficial in patients with pure mitral stenosis who are in normal sinus rhythm.

Propranolol in small doses (10–20 mg qid) may help control ventricular rate in patients in whom digitalis alone is not efficacious or in patients who require high doses of digitalis for rate control. Propranolol may also benefit patients with pure mitral stenosis in sinus rhythm who have no cardiac failure but whose symptoms occur during reversible conditions characterized by an increase in heart rate or cardiac output or both (as in exercise). Propranolol may actually reduce the pulmonary capillary wedge pressure and mitral valve gradient in these patients.

Quinidine sulfate (200–300 mg po qid) is used to maintain sinus rhythm in patients previously in atrial fibrillation.

Diuretics (hydrochlorothiazide 50–100 mg po qd or furosemide 20–80 mg po qd) are beneficial in treating the symptoms due to pulmonary congestion. These drugs must be administered cautiously, since reduced ventricular filling may lead to reduced cardiac output with increased symptoms of fatigue. Along the same lines, restriction in sodium intake is indicated, and the patient is placed on a no added salt diet.

Oral anticoagulation with warfarin is indicated in patients with atrial fibrillation to reduce embolic complications. Patients who have had embolic complications, either arterial or venous, should be placed on oral anticoagulants.

Antibiotic prophylaxis for dental and surgical procedures is essential (see Chapter 21 for suggested antibiotic regimen). Long-term, antibiotic therapy as prophylaxis against recurrent episodes of rheumatic fever is advised in patients who have had episodes of acute rheumatic fever. Some physicians favor therapy until age 40; others favor therapy for life.

Surgery consists of mitral commissurotomy or mitral valve replacement, and should be considered once the patient becomes limited by symptoms in spite of salt restriction, diuretics, and digitalis. In patients with severe class III and IV symptoms, surgery is indicated. In patients with class II symptoms with moderate to severe stenosis (valve area <1.0–1.2 cm^2), surgery is recommended; it may be deferred with a valve orifice size of >1.0 cm^2. Patients with systemic embolism inspite of anticoagulation should be operated upon.

Commissurotomy is often the initial operative procedure of choice for pure mitral stenosis. The adhesions and fibrosis causing the narrowed valve are lysed and the valve leaflets are mechanically separated. The procedure has a low operative mortality, with the advantage that no thrombogenic foreign material is implanted, and patients may not need a repeat surgical procedure for eight to 10 years. If the mitral valve is calcified, has concommitant mitral regurgitation, or is nonpliable, commissurotomy is not indicated; the patient should receive a mitral valve replacement.

The prosthetic mitral valves most commonly used include the caged-ball, tilting disc, and porcine heterograft. The caged ball prosthesis has considerable thromboembolic potential; however, the use of the cloth covered valve in addition to anticoagulation with warfarin has diminished the incidence of this complication. The tilting disc prosthesis may be superior to the more bulky caged ball in patients with a small left ventricular cavity or small mitral valve anulus, but it also has considerable thromboembolic potential. The use of the porcine heterograft has reduced the need for anticoagulation; but if the patient is in atrial fibrillation with a large left atrium, long term anticoagulation should be continued even with a porcine valve in the mitral position. Overall, operative mortality for mitral valve replacement is approximately 5% or less.

Mitral Regurgitation

Mitral regurgitation can be acute or chronic and can result from several different etiologies. The etiologies are shown in Table 3.

In mitral regurgitation, the left ventricle ejects blood not only into the aorta but into the left atrium as well. During ventricular systole, tall regurgitant systolic waves (also termed regurgitant v waves or regurgitant cv waves) are recorded in the left atrium or pulmonary capillary wedge pressure tracing. The extra blood is returned to the left ventricle, resulting in left ventricular volume overload with dilatation of the ventricular and left atrial cavities. In acute mitral regurgitation, the left atrium initially is small with high left atrial pressures resulting in pulmonary congestion; forward output may be normal. In chronic mitral regurgitation the left atrium is large

Table 3. Etiologies of Mitral Regurgitation

Acute	Chronic
Ruptured chordae tendineae	Rheumatic heart disease
Papillary muscle rupture	Papillary muscle dysfunction
Endocarditis	Mitral valve prolapse (click-murmur syndrome, Barlow's syndrome, floppy mitral valve)
Trauma	Endocarditis
	Calcification of the mitral valve anulus
	Accompanying IHSS
	Congenital endocardial cushion defect, corrected transposition, endocardial fibroelastosis
	Severe left ventricular dilatation

and dilated; left atrial pressures are not as high and pulmonary congestion may be less. As the left ventricle dilates and eventually fails, forward cardiac output falls. As the left atrial fibers are stretched, the chances that atrial fibrillation will develop increase. This rhythm may also contribute to a falling cardiac output.

The patients' histories are different, depending largely on whether the mitral regurgitation is acute or chronic. In chronic forms, such as that associated with rheumatic heart disease, there may be a long asymptomatic period of 20–30 years followed by the symptoms of dyspnea on exertion, orthopnea, paroxysmal nocturnal dyspnea, weakness, fatigue, and palpitations. If the mitral regurgitation is severe or chronic, symptoms of right ventricular failure may be present. If the mitral regurgitation is due to rheumatic valvular disease, symptoms and signs of concomitant mitral stenosis should be sought. If the left atrium is dilated, systemic emboli may occur, although the frequency of this complication is not as great as with mitral stenosis. In acute mitral regurgitation symptoms of pulmonary congestion occur early.

Physical examination in mitral regurgitation may reveal sinus rhythm; but if mitral regurgitation is chronic, atrial fibrillation may be present. When pulmonary vascular congestion is present, rales are heard. The left ventricular impulse is hyperdynamic and if the left atrium is large and the patient is in sinus rhythm, a late systolic parasternal lift may be palpated. The S_1 tends to be soft, S_2 is widely split, and an S_3 is often present. The typical murmur of rheumatic mitral regurgitation is holosystolic, heard best at the cardiac apex with radiation to the axilla. With acute rupture of chordae tendineae, the murmur may be holosystolic, early, or midsystolic with a crescendo-decrescendo quality.

Several maneuvers may alter the murmur of mitral regurgitation and thus aid in the diagnosis. With mitral regurgitation of rheumatic heart disease, the murmur increases with sudden squatting and decreases with amyl nitrite.

Associated physical findings depend on the etiology of mitral regurgitation. For example, the findings of mitral stenosis or aortic valve disease may coexist with mitral regurgitation when the etiology is rheumatic. The murmur of idiopathic hypertrophic subaortic stenosis (IHSS) and signs of endocarditis should be sought. If mitral regurgitation is long standing, signs of right ventricular failure are present. Differential diagnosis is shown in Table 4.

With chronic mitral regurgitation, the chest x-ray film shows an enlarged left atrium and left ventricle with signs of pulmonary vascular redistribution and often congestive heart failure. The right ventricle may be increased in size. With acute mitral regurgitation, the left atrium initially is not enlarged, pulmonary vascular redistribution is present, and in severe cases, pulmonary edema is present as well. Calcification of the mitral and aortic valve suggests rheumatic heart disease as the etiology of the mitral regurgitation. Mitral valve anulus calcification may be seen and is an important cause of mitral regurgitation in the elderly.

With longstanding mitral regurgitation, the ECG shows left atrial enlargement, left axis deviation, left ventricular hypertrophy, and atrial fibrillation. Right ventricular hypertrophy appears late.

In chronic mitral regurgitation, the echocardiogram reveals left atrial enlargement with systolic expansion, and a dilated and actively contracting left ventricle. If the mitral valve disease is due to rheumatic heart disease, the valve leaflets may appear thickened. If papillary muscle dysfunction is the cause of mitral regurgitation, abnormal regional wall motion may be detected. When vegetations are large, they may

Table 4. Differential Diagnosis of Mitral Valve Regurgitation

Disease Entities	Differentiating Features
Ventricular septal defect (murmur may be confused with mitral regurgitation)	Murmur localized over lower left sternal border. Radionuclide studies confirm left-to-right shunt. Cardiac catheterization reveals O_2 step up from right atrium to ventricle.
Hypertrophic obstructive cardiomyopathy (or Idiopathic hypertrophic subaortic stenosis–IHSS)	Associated mitral regurgitation murmur may be present. However, outflow murmur typical of IHSS is present as well, which increases with Valsalva maneuver and amyl nitrite and decreases with squatting, hand grip. Typical echocardiographic features of IHSS.
Aortic stenosis (murmur may be confused with mitral regurgitation)	The murmur is systolic ejection in quality. Confusion occurs when mitral regurgitation is due to prolapse of posterior papillary muscle or rupture of posterior chordae tendineae with radiation of the murmur to the aortic area. In some patients the murmur of aortic stenosis is loudest at the apex. With aortic stenosis carotid upstroke is delayed, S_2 is single or absent, echocardiographic features of aortic stenosis and calcification of the aortic valve are present.

be seen with endocarditis. The echocardiogram is extremely helpful in diagnosing mitral valve prolapse. Ruptured chordae tendineae may be identified as extraneous echoes, which "flip" in and out of the left atrium and ventricle.

Other noninvasive tests that are sometimes useful include systolic time intervals (see Chapter 5). Newer radionuclide studies may help to quantitate the degree of mitral regurgitation. Gated radionuclide angiography is a noninvasive technique that can be used to estimate the regurgitant fraction. The ratio of left to right ventricular stroke volume is determined by measuring the total number of counts ejected from the right and left ventricles. In normal patients, this ratio is approximately 1. The ratio is increased in patients with mitral or aortic regurgitation in direct proportion to the degree of volume overload of the left ventricle. The technique is not valid if there are intracardiac shunts or right-sided valvular regurgitant lesions. Several studies using this technique have shown good correlation of the extent of mitral or aortic regurgitation with determinations made at cardiac catheterization. The technique can also be used to follow serially patients receiving therapeutic interventions and valve surgery.

The use of pulsed Doppler ultrasound can detect mitral and aortic regurgitation. Studies have compared this noninvasive technique to left ventricular angiographic studies. The sensitivity for moderate to severe mitral regurgitation was 100% in one study but was less in patients with mild mitral regurgitation. Overall, sensitivity in one study was 94%, the specificity of the technique was 89%, and accuracy was 90%. The degree of mitral regurgitation could not be quantitated.

Cardiac catheterization in acute mitral regurgitation reveals a pulmonary capillary wedge pressure that is elevated and may demonstrate tall regurgitant systolic waves.

With chronic mitral regurgitation, the wedge pressure may not be as high and v waves may be normal or only moderately enlarged. Large v waves can be seen in other conditions such as ventricular septal defect, congestive heart failure, and mitral obstruction; hence, tall v waves are not specific for mitral regurgitation.

Increased left ventricular end-diastolic pressure occurs as the left ventricle fails. Long standing mitral regurgitation is associated with elevated pulmonary artery pressures and eventually high right-sided pressures due to right ventricular failure. Left ventricular angiography allows visualization of the regurgitant stream and the severity of mitral regurgitation can be estimated. Left ventricular ejection fraction is variable, depending upon the etiology and duration of the mitral regurgitation. During the early phases, it is often increased; as the left ventricle fails, the left ventricular ejection fraction decreases.

A left ventricular regurgitant fraction can be calculated from the following formula:

$$\frac{\text{Angiographic cardiac output } - \text{ Fick cardiac output}}{\text{Angiographic cardiac output}}$$

If the regurgitant fraction is greater than 60%, severe mitral regurgitation is likely.

Therapy for mitral regurgitation depends upon the etiology, severity, and duration of the regurgitation. If the patient is symptomatic, initial medical therapy includes a low salt diet, diuretic therapy (hydrochlorothiazide 50–100 mg po qd, furosemide 20–80 mg po qd, or ethacrynic acid 50 mg po qd) and digitalis. K^+ supplements may be needed. If the patient is acutely ill, afterload reduction (IV nitroprusside or intra-aortic ballon counterpulsation) should be considered. In chronic mitral regurgitation, afterload reduction by agents such as hydralazine (20–400 mg daily) may be useful. Surgery should be considered when the patient is symptomatic at rest or with usual activity inspite of medical treatment, or when the patient is symptomatic with heavy exertion on medical treatment and has cardiomegaly with an elevated end-systolic volume (>30 ml/m^2). Left ventricular end-systolic volume <30 ml/m^2 predicts normal left ventricular function postoperatively and end systolic volumes of greater than 90 ml/m^2 predicts residual left ventricular dysfunction. Surgery includes mitral valve replacement and, in some centers, mitral valve reconstruction. The types of prosthetic valves used for mitral valve replacement are discussed under the section on mitral stenosis. Antibiotic prophylaxis against bacterial endocarditis is prescribed for all patients with mitral regurgitation (see Chapter 21 for dosage schedule).

Anticoagulation with long term warfarin is indicated in patients with enlarged left atria and atrial fibrillation. If atrial fibrillation is new, a trial of cardioversion (either electrical or with drugs) should be attempted. If this fails, digitalis is administered for control of ventricular rate.

Mitral Valve Prolapse Syndrome

Mitral valve prolapse is a commonly recognized syndrome found in 6–17% of healthy young women and 7% of healthy young men. It is associated with a redundant mitral leaflet apparatus and often myxomatous degeneration of the valves. Associated tricuspid valve prolapse is common. Some studies have shown a very prominent zona spongiosa (mucinous layer) within the valve leaflets. Although in most cases, the

Table 5. Conditions With Which Mitral Valve Prolapse (MVP) Has Been Associated

---

Marfan's syndrome

Ehlers-Danlos syndrome

Duchenne muscular dystrophy

Collagen-vascular diseases: lupus erythematosis, polyarteritis nodosa

Thoracic deformities: straight back syndrome, pectus excavatum

Asthenic habitus (narrow anteroposterior chest diameter, long arm span)

Wolff-Parkinson–White syndrome

Prolonged QT interval

Ischemic heart disease

Rheumatic heart disease

Hypertrophic Obstructive Cardiomyopathy

Post-valve surgery or trauma

Congenital heart disease (secundum atrial septal defects)

Willebrand's syndrome (von Willebrand's disease)

Coronary artery spasm

Abnormalities in platelet coagulant activities

? Cardiomyopathy

Prolapse of tricuspid valve (from 3–50% of patients with MVP) and/or aortic valve (in up to 20% of patients with MVP)

Anxiety neurosis (panic disorders)

Dysautonomia (with abnormal responses of heart rate and blood pressure to Valsalva maneuver)

---

syndrome of mitral valve prolapse is idiopathic, there are familial occurrences (thought to be inherited as an autosomal dominant) and the syndrome has been associated with a large number of other conditions as shown in Table 5. In a recent study, 7% of newborn baby girls were found to have mitral valve prolapse by echocardiography.

The majority of patients with mitral valve prolapse are either asymptomatic or have minimal symptoms. The clinical course is usually benign. The symptoms include palpitations, chest pain (not necessarily associated with exertion), fatigue, dyspnea, dizziness, and syncope. One recent study suggested that the chest pain was, in some cases, due to coronary spasm. Less commonly, mitral prolapse results in transient ischemic attacks or strokes thought to be embolic in nature; neuropsychiatric problems; atrial or ventricular arrhythmias, including rare cases of sudden death; and infective endocarditis. While in most cases, hemodynamically significant mitral regurgitation is not present, occasional patients develop severe mitral regurgitation requiring surgical repair or mitral valve replacement. The signs of endocarditis may be more subtle in mitral prolapse than in other forms, but endocarditis in this setting usually responds to appropriate antibiotic therapy. Progressive valvular dysfunction may be a sequela.

There has been some debate in the literature as to whether idiopathic mitral prolapse is associated with cardiomyopathy. Some studies have reported abnormalities in left ventricular function during exercise in patients with mitral prolapse but without significant mitral regurgitation. Other studies have not demonstrated abnormal ventricular function and have suggested that exercise induced abnormalities of ventricular function in patients with prolapse without significant mitral regurgitation are related to the presence of coronary artery disease. However, a study by Malcolm et al. found histochemical abnormalities of ventricular biopsies in patients with mitral valve prolapse, chest pain, and normal coronary arteries.

Mitral valve prolapse is thought to be a risk factor for cerebrovascular events. In patients under 45 years old with strokes or transient ischemic attacks, mitral valve prolapse was detected in 24% of cases. In older patients, the incidence of prolapse was 6%. A study by Hanson et al. described 24 patients with mitral prolapse ranging from 20 to 63 years old who experienced a cerebrovascular event, including bland cerebral infarction, transient ischemic attack; cerebellar infarctions; parenchymatous and subarachnoid hemorrhage; seizures; and retinal artery occlusion. Other significant risk factors for strokes were lacking in these patients. The authors recommended echocardiography for patients with cerebral ischemic events who lack other clear, recognized risk factors for strokes. Episodes of light headedness, dizziness, and syncope may be due to orthostatic hypotension as well as arrhythmias in some of these patients.

Kavey et al. showed that potentially serious ventricular arrhythmias were common in pediatric patients with mitral valve prolapse and suggested ambulatory ECG monitoring and treadmill exercise testing. Supraventricular arrhythmias have been reported in as many as 55% of patients with mitral valve prolapse, ventricular arrhythmias in 45%, and bradyarrhythmias in 29%.

The characteristic physical findings of mitral valve prolapse include a midsystolic click or clicks, often followed by a mid to late systolic murmur. The murmur may radiate toward the sternum or aortic area if the posterior leaflet prolapses; if the anterior leaflet prolapses, the murmur may radiate posteriorly toward the back and spine. The clicks and onset of the murmur occur earlier with maneuvers that decrease left ventricular cavity size, such as standing, taking amyl nitrite, and during Valsalva maneuver. Squatting results in a later onset of the click and the murmur decreases in intensity.

ECG reveals ST-T wave abnormalities in leads 2, 3, aV_F, V_4–V_6 and the QT interval may be prolonged. Atrial and/or ventricular arrhythmias may be present. By echocardiography, the mitral valve typically prolapses in mid to late systole and the onset of prolapse can be timed with clicks on a simultaneous phonocardiogram. In some cases, the prolapse occurs throughout systole. Other laboratory findings may include elevated blood glucose and 24 hour urinary epinephrine and norepinephrine levels.

Most patients with mitral valve prolapse do not have hemodynamically significant mitral valve regurgitation and require follow-up examinations every few years. These patients should receive antibiotic prophylaxis for dental and surgical procedures. Propranolol is useful for atypical chest pain and the ventricular arrhythmias. In about 15% of patients with mitral valve prolapse, there is progressive mitral regurgitation with signs and symptoms of congestive heart failure. These patients should be treated like other patients with severe mitral regurgitation; some may require valve replacement. Patients with embolic events should be considered for antiplatelet or anticoagulant therapy.

Mitral Anular Calcification

Calcification of the mitral anulus is frequently idiopathic and is a cause of mitral regurgitation in the elderly. Although considered a degenerative change, it appears to be hastened by certain conditions including hypertension, aortic stenosis, diabetes, Marfan's and Hurler's syndromes, and has been associated with hypertrophic obstructive cardiomyopathy. There may be associated calcification of the aortic valve cusps as well. Typical chest x-ray film shows "C" shaped calcification of the mitral valve anulus. The anular calcification can be diagnosed by echocardiography. In one echocardiographic study, anular calcification equal to or greater than 5 mm in thickness was associated with clinical implications of significant mitral regurgitation and congestive heart failure. If the calcium extends into the conduction system, AV or intraventricular conduction defects may develop. Nair et al. recently reported a high prevalence of mitral anular calcification (87%) in patients with symptomatic bradyarrhythmias, including complete AV block, atrial fibrillation with a slow ventricular response, and intermittent sinus arrest. Pacemaker therapy was required in these patients. In patients with massive mitral anular calcification, functional mitral stenosis has been reported.

Aortic Stenosis

There are three major etiologies for adult valvular aortic stenosis: rheumatic; senile-calcific or degenerative aortic stenosis; and congenital bicuspic aortic valve with secondary calcification (Fig. 2). In rheumatic aortic stenosis, the major pathologic feature is fusion of the commissures with thickening and fibrosis of the valve leaflets. Patients may have a murmur in their 20s and 30s, but symptoms may not occur until

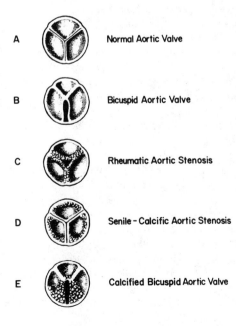

A   Normal Aortic Valve

B   Bicuspid Aortic Valve

C   Rheumatic Aortic Stenosis

D   Senile - Calcific Aortic Stenosis

E   Calcified Bicuspid Aortic Valve

Figure 2 Pathology of aortic stenosis. (*a*) Normal tricuspid aortic valve. (*b*) Bicuspid aortic valve. (*c*) Rheumatic aortic stenosis. The commissiones are fused and the valve leaflets thickened. (*d*) Senile-calcific aortic stenosis. Calcium deposits are present within the cusps of the aortic valve without primarily affecting the commissures. (*e*) Calcified bicuspid aortic valve. (Adapted from Brandenburg RO, Fuster V, and Giuliani E: Valvular heart disease. When should the patient be referred? *Pract Cardiol* 5:50, Aug. 1979, Fig. 1 and Fuster V, Brandenburg RO, and Giuliani et al. Clinical approach and management of acquired valvular heart disease. in *Office Cardiology*. Cardiovascular Clinics 10-3, 126, 1980.)

ages 50–60. With senile-calcific or degenerative aortic stenosis, calcium accumulates in the pockets of the aortic cusps with evential fibrosis. Symptoms typically occur at ages 60–70. With congenital bicuspid valve, calcific changes occur earlier in life, presumably secondary to increased turbulence. There is progressive narrowing of the valves over time and symptoms are present at ages 40–50. Congenital aortic stenosis, in which the aortic valve is dome-shaped, results in symptoms early in life. Isolated aortic stenosis in the adult is unlikely to be secondary to rheumatic disease and likely to be secondary to the congenital bicuspid or senile-calcific variety.

Obstruction to flow between the left ventricle and aorta may be due to hypertrophic obstructive cardiomyopathy, subvalvular aortic stenosis due to an abnormal membrane below the aortic valve, aortic valvular stenosis, or supravalvular stenosis due to an abnormal membrane or narrowing above the valve. Supravalvular stenosis has been associated with hypercalcemia and mental retardation. There is an association between aortic stenosis and GI bleeding. In one study, aortic stenosis was significantly more prevalent among patients with idiopathic GI tract bleeding in comparison to its association with bleeding from a known source.

Aortic stenosis results in increased resistance to flow from the left ventricle. The left ventricle compensates by developing hypertrophy in order to maintain cardiac output. The hypertrophied muscle has diminished compliance, which results in a rise in left ventricular end-diastolic pressure. Left atrial contraction thus becomes important for filling the left ventricle. Hence, patients with significant aortic stenosis often become more symptomatic when they develop atrial fibrillation and lose their "atrial kick." Myocardial oxygen consumption is increased, largely due to increased left ventricular wall tension (due to increased intracavitary left ventricular pressure), while subendocardial coronary blood flow is compromised because of high subendocardial intramural pressure. Hence, patients may exhibit symptoms and signs of ischemia without having coronary artery disease.

Recent studies have shown that progressive stenosis of the aortic valve can occur in adults with isolated aortic stenosis. Significant reductions in valve areas were found to develop over as short a time as 27–29 months.

The classic triad of symptoms with aortic stenosis include (1) the symptoms of congestive heart failure with dyspnea on exertion, orthopnea, paroxysmal nocturnal dyspnea, fatigue, weakness; (2) angina; and (3) syncope or near syncope. Natural history studies of untreated aortic stenosis showed that once these three symptoms developed, death occurred within two to five years (Fig. 3). Angina may occur with or without concomitant coronary artery disease. Patients with angina and aortic stenosis have a 50–64% prevalence of significant coronary artery disease; patients with aortic stenosis and no angina are less likely to have coronary artery disease. Syncope may be exertional and due to peripheral vasodilatation in exercising muscles in the setting of a fixed cardiac output or secondary to atrial or ventricular arrhythmias.

Physical examination reveals a delayed carotid upstroke with an anacrotic notch. There may be a shuddering quality to the carotid pulse and auscultation over the carotids reveals the radiated aortic murmur. If congestive heart failure is present, rales may be heard upon auscultation of the lungs. The left ventricular apical impulse is forceful and prolonged. A palpable a wave is often present. As the left ventricle fails, the apical impulse is displaced downward and to the left. A systolic thrill may be felt along the upper right sternal border. Auscultation reveals an S_2 that may be

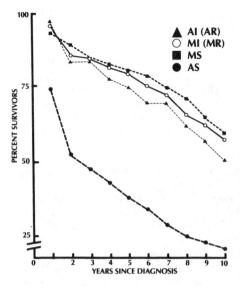

Figure 3 Survival of patients with valvular heart disease treated medically. Note the poor prognosis of patients with aortic stenosis (AS) contrasted with that of aortic insufficiency (AI), mitral insufficiency (MI), and mitral stenosis (MS). (Reprinted from Rapaport E: Natural history of aortic and mitral valve disease. *Am J Cardiol* 35:221–227, 1975, with permission.)

paradoxically split (due to delayed left ventricular emptying), or single due to absence of A_2, suggesting that the valve is very stiff and stenosis severe. An S_4 is usually present if the patient is in sinus rhythm. Early systolic ejection clicks may be present, especially if the aortic stenosis is due to congenitally bicuspid valve. If the patient is in congestive heart failure, an S_3 is present as well. The murmur of aortic stenosis is a systolic-ejection murmur (crescendo-decrescendo), which begins shortly after S_1 and ends just before A_2. It is rasping or rough in quality. As the aortic stenosis becomes more severe, the peak of the ejection murmur occurs later during systole. The murmur is heard best at the aortic area with radiation to the carotids; occasionally it is best heard at the apex. Signs of right ventricular failure are present in late stages of aortic stenosis. Differential diagnosis is shown in Table 6.

The initial chest x-ray film may be normal. Since the left ventricle develops concentric hypertrophy, the overall cardiac silhouette initially does not demonstrate cardiomegaly. Eventually, left ventricular prominence is seen. The ascending aorta is dilated due to poststenotic dilatation and calcification of the aortic valve may be present. With left ventricular failure, the left ventricle appears dilated and pulmonary vascular redistribution is seen, with or without signs of pulmonary edema.

The characteristic electrocardiographic features of aortic stenosis include left axis deviation, left atrial enlargement, and left ventricular hypertrophy with strain. In late phases the QRS complex may be widened with an intraventricular conduction delay or frank left bundle branch block. With severe aortic stenosis, atrial fibrillation may develop, often associated with hemodynamic deterioration due to loss of atrial contraction.

Siegel and Roberts, in a study, showed that the ECG was a useful noninvasive tool for determining the aortic pressure gradient. They showed that the 12 lead QRS amplitude in mm was similar to left ventricular systolic pressure in mm Hg in most patients. They found that subtraction of the indirect systemic arterial systolic pres-

Table 6. Differential Diagnosis of Aortic Stenosis

Disease Entities	Differentiating Features
Aortic valve sclerosis of the elderly, without stenosis (systolic murmur may mimic that of aortic stenosis)	Systolic murmur does not peak late. Carotids do not have delayed upstrokes. No LVH by ECG. Echocardiographic visualization of excursion of valve leaflets usually normal or mildly reduced, but valves may not be visualized. No hemodynamically significant aortic valve gradient by cardiac catheterization.
Hypertrophic obstructive cardiomyopathy (IHSS; systolic murmur may be confused with that of aortic stenosis)	Brisk bifed carotid upstrokes. Murmur usually does not radiate into neck. Characteristic change in murmur with various maneuvers. Pseudoinfarct pattern (large septal Qs) on ECG. Characteristic echocardiographic features.
Mitral regurgitation (systolic murmur may be confused with that of aortic stenosis)	Murmur is holosystolic and radiates to axilla and not carotids. Carotid upstroke may be normal. Dilated left ventricle. Aortic valve normal on echocardiogram unless there is associated aortic valve disease.
Pulmonic stenosis (systolic murmur may be confused with that of aortic stenosis)	Murmur does not radiate into neck; loudest along the left sternal border. Physical exam, chest x-ray film, and ECG may reveal enlarged right ventricle. M-mode echocardiogram reveals right ventricular enlargement and hypertrophy and two-dimensional echocardiography may visualize valve stenosis.

sure in mm Hg from the 12 lead QRS amplitude (mm) provided a reasonable predictor of the peak systolic pressure gradient in patients with moderate to severe aortic stenosis.

Echocardiographic features of aortic stenosis include decreased excursion of aortic leaflets or, with severe aortic stenosis, inability to clearly visualize leaflet excursion, with multiple dense echoes within the aortic root due to thickening and calcification of the valve. Left atrial enlargement and left ventricular hypertrophy are present; eventually left ventricular dilatation is seen. By two-dimensional echocardiography, the size of the valve orifice can be determined in many patients. Echocardiography is especially useful in assessing left ventricular function in these patients.

Other noninvasive techniques may be helpful in diagnosing aortic stenosis. Carotid pulse tracings reveal a prolonged upstroke and an anacrotic notch with prolonged left ventricular ejection time and t time (see Chapter 5). Apexcardiogram is characterized by a prolonged and increased left ventricular systolic impulse with a prominent a wave. Radionuclide ventriculograms are helpful in assessing left ventricular function and determining the ejection fraction.

Cardiac catheterization reveals a gradient in pressure during systole between the left ventricle and aorta. If this gradient is greater than 50 mm Hg in the setting of normal cardiac output, the gradient is considered to be severe. The left ventricular systolic, end-diastolic, and left atrial pressures are elevated. The aortic valve area is determined from the Gorlin formula as discussed in Chapter 8. Normal aortic valve area is 3.0 to 3.5 cm^2. Severe or critical aortic stenosis occurs when the valve area is less than 0.5 cm^2; moderately severe aortic stenosis when the valve area is between 0.5–0.7 cm^2; moderate stenosis when the valve area is 0.7–1.0 cm^2; and mild aortic stenosis when the valve area is 1.0 cm^2–1.2 cm^2. Left ventricular angiography allows assessment of left ventricular function; coronary angiography is performed as well, especially if the patient has a history of angina. Aortic root angiography is useful for determining the presence of concomitant aortic regurgitation.

Initial medical therapy for congestive failure includes the use of digoxin and, in some cases, cautious use of diuretics. Atrial fibrillation should be promptly treated. However, once the patient becomes symptomatic, diagnostic catheterization should be considered, and if significant aortic stenosis is present, the aortic valve should be replaced. The age of the patient per se is not a contraindication to surgery. Several studies have shown that elderly patients in general do well following aortic valve replacement, but that emergency surgery carries a high risk in this age group. Unless left ventricular ejection fraction is very severely depressed, with ejection fractions less than 20%, surgery should be strongly considered. A recent study by Thompson et al. showed that poor left ventricular function (ejection fraction less than 45%) did not increase the risk of aortic valve replacement and that improvement in left ventricular function can be expected in the majority of patients. Other studies have shown similar findings. Endocarditis prophylaxis for dental and surgical procedures are indicated in patients with aortic valve disease (Chapter 21).

Aortic valve replacement includes use of glutaraldehyde-fixed porcine heterographs, caged ball prostheses, and tilting disc prostheses. Caged ball prostheses have the advantage of being durable but the disadvantages of thromboembolic complications and hemolysis. Disc valves have a lower thromboembolic complication rate, excellent hemodynamic properties, and are relatively durable. Porcine heterografts have a low thromboembolic rate and, unlike the other two types, usually do not require long term anticoagulation when in the aortic position. Their durability is still under study; one recent study suggests that they are not more durable than the mechanical valves. Other studies have shown that, in general, they are durable for over six years. Porcine valves may result in a significant aortic valve gradient, especially when implanted in small aortic roots.

There have been cases of endocarditis of porcine heterografts. The infection develops in the fibrin layers that cover the cusps, may involve the collagen within the leaflets, and is rarely associated with abscess of the valve ring. Late failure of porcine heterografts in children occurs in up to 20% of patients, due to extensive fragmentation of collagen and calcium deposition.

Initial surgery mortality for patients with aortic valve replacement who have good left ventricular function should be less than 5%; five-year life expectancy for patients with aortic valve replacement is approximately 75–80%.

Aortic Regurgitation

The etiology of aortic regurgitation can be divided into those diseases that affect the valve leaflets and those diseases that cause aortic regurgitation by dilating the aortic

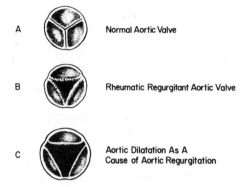

A — Normal Aortic Valve

B — Rheumatic Regurgitant Aortic Valve

C — Aortic Dilatation As A Cause of Aortic Regurgitation

Figure 4 (*a*) Normal aortic valve. (*b*) Rheumatic regurgitant aortic valve. The valve leaflets are fibrotic and shortened. (*c*) Aortic dilatation as a cause of aortic regurgitation. The valve leaflets are bowed and unable to coap during diastole. There may be commissural separation as well.

root (Fig. 4). Diseases that cause aortic regurgitation by affecting the valve leaflet include bacterial endocarditis; rheumatic endocarditis; trauma; ventricular septal defect, in which the aortic leaflet is pulled downward toward the ventricular cavity; bicuspid aortic valve; and discrete subvalvular aortic stenosis. Diseases that cause aortic regurgitation by dilatation of the aortic root include syphilitic aortitis; aortic dissection; prolonged systemic hypertension; Marfan's syndrome; and systemic illnesses including ankylosing spondylitis, rheumatoid arthritis, Ehlers-Danlos syndrome, Reiter's syndrome, and psoriasis. Finally, aortic regurgitation may occur secondary to rupture of a sinus of Valsalva aneurysm; or its cause may be idiopathic. Aortic regurgitation may be acute, such as occurs with acute bacterial endocarditis, dissection of the aorta, or trauma; it may be chronic, such as in rheumatic heart disease; systemic hypertension; syphilitic aortitis; collagen vascular diseases; or in association with congenital abnormalities, such as bicuspid aortic valve or ventricular septal defect.

With acute aortic regurgitation, the left ventricle is suddenly presented with an increase in volume, resulting in severe elevations of left ventricular end-diastolic pressures. In the chronic form of aortic regurgitation, the left ventricle gradually adapts to the increase in volume by dilating and developing hypertrophy. The left ventricle eventually becomes markedly dilated and fails—with elevated end-diastolic pressure and, finally, a decreased stroke volume. In the chronic form, low peripheral diastolic blood pressure secondary to a rapid run-off into the left ventricle leads to the peripheral manifestations discussed below. The low aortic diastolic pressure, which may lead to reduced coronary perfusion pressure plus increased left ventricular work (increase in myocardial oxygen consumption), may precipitate angina.

With acute aortic regurgitation, patients complain of the sudden onset of dyspnea, orthopnea, and paroxysmal nocturnal dyspnea. With the more common chronic aortic regurgitation, patients are often asymptomatic for long periods of time (often up to 20 years in patients with rheumatic carditis). One of the earliest symptoms is increased awareness of the heart beat due to the increased stroke volume. With progression of the disease, patients complain of symptoms due to left ventricular failure: dyspnea, orthopnea, and paroxysmal nocturnal dyspnea. Patients may experience palpitations and complain of unusual symptoms, such as heat intolerance and diaphoresis. When the aortic regurgitation is severe, angina may be present. With long-standing left ventricular failure, the right ventricle may fail as well, with the resultant symptoms of peripheral edema and GI complaints.

The physical examination in chronic aortic regurgitation manifests signs resulting from increased volume ejected in systole and rapid run-off in diastole. The diastolic blood pressure is reduced; the systolic blood pressure increased, with a resultant wide pulse pressure. The peripheral pulses exhibit a "water-hammer" quality, with a rapid upstroke and rapid collapse (also known as Corrigan's pulse). The carotid pulse may be double-peaked in severe aortic regurgitation or when aortic regurgitation is associated with aortic stenosis. Duroziez's sign is the diastolic murmur heard when the stethoscope compresses the femoral artery ("fro" portion of a "to and fro" murmur). Quincke's pulse refers to the visible capillary pulsation in the nailbed in patients with aortic regurgitation. Pistol-shot pulse refers to a loud systolic sound heard with auscultation over the femoral artery. With severe aortic regurgitation, popliteal arterial pressure is higher by 40 mm Hg or more than the brachial arterial pressure (Hill's sign). Musset's sign refers to bobbing of the head during each systole. These peripheral manifestations may be entirely absent if the aortic regurgitation is acute or after severe left ventricular failure develops. With acute aortic regurgitation, sinus tachycardia usually is present.

The left ventricular impulse is forceful and displaced downward and to the left in chronic aortic regurgitation. With acute aortic regurgitation, cardiomegaly usually is not present when the patient is first seen; thus the left ventricular impulse is not displaced laterally. S_1 and A_2 may be soft. A diastolic high-pitched blowing decrescendo murmur begins just after S_2 and continues through part or all of diastole. This murmur is heard best using the diaphragm of the stethoscope, with the patient sitting up and leaning forward. If this diastolic murmur radiates down the left sternal border, the aortic regurgitation is likely to be secondary to damage to the valve leaflets; if the diastolic murmur radiates down the right sternal border, the aortic regurgitation is more likely to be secondary to a dilated aortic root. An S_3 is often audible; an S_4 may be present as well. A concomitant systolic ejection murmur represents increased flow across the aortic valve. The Austin Flint murmur is a low pitched middiastolic rumbling murmur caused by forward flow across a mitral valve that is partially closed due to the regurgitant aortic stream. Differential diagnosis is shown in Table 7.

In chronic aortic regurgitation, the chest x-ray film reveals a markedly enlarged left ventricle, with the apex displaced downward and to the left and dilatation of the aortic root. Syphilitic aortitis is associated with calcification of the ascending aorta. The aortic valve may appear calcified on chest x-ray film (rheumatic, bicuspid). Signs of left ventricular failure, including pulmonary vascular redistribution and interstitial pulmonary edema may be present. With acute aortic regurgitation, the chest x-ray film does not initially show cardiomegaly, but pulmonary vascular redistribution is usually present.

Electrocardiographic features of aortic regurgitation include left atrial enlargement and left ventricular hypertrophy. The left ventricular hypertrophy may show a diastolic overload pattern with an elevated J point and tall T waves. Sinus tachycardia is present in patients with acute aortic regurgitation, while left ventricular hypertrophy is not.

The echocardiogram may be quite helpful in assessing patients with aortic regurgitation. The left ventricular cavity is dilated (chronic aortic regurgitation) with hyperdynamic left ventricular wall motion. High frequency vibrations of the anterior leaflet of the mitral valve and septum occur due to the regurgitant jet of blood. In acute aortic regurgitation, the left ventricular cavity is not dilated. With severe acute

Table 7. Differential Diagnosis of Aortic Regurgitation

Disease Entity	Differentiating Features
Pulmonary regurgitation (diastolic murmur may be confused with aortic regurgitation)	Murmur of pulmonary insufficiency usually occurs in setting of pulmonary hypertension due to mitral stenosis or right-to-left cardiac shunt. Associated right ventricular enlargement. Absence of peripheral manifestations of aortic regurgitation.
Mitral stenosis (murmur may be confused with aortic regurgitation and Austin Flint murmur)	Murmur is low-pitched diastolic rumble with presystolic accentuation. Differentiated from Austin Flint murmur by using amyl nitrite. Austin Flint murmur diminishes with amyl nitrite; murmur of mitral stenosis remains unchanged or increases. Characteristic echocardiographic features of mitral stenosis.
Aortic stenosis (patients with aortic regurgitation may have a prominent aortic systolic murmur due to the increased flow of blood volume across the aortic valve)	With aortic stenosis, there is a delayed carotid upstroke; the murmur tends to peak later in systole; and the echocardiographic features of aortic regurgitation (a hyperdynamic left ventricle and high frequency vibrations of the anterior leaflet to the mitral valve during diastole) are absent.
Patent ductus arteriosus (murmurs may be confused with those of aortic insufficiency)	Murmur is continuous throughout systole and diastole with peak of the murmur at S_2. Systolic ejection murmur accompanying aortic regurgitation usually peaks in midsystole. Left-to-right shunt with radionuclide angiography and cardiac catheterization.

and sometimes severe chronic regurgitation, the mitral valve closes prematurely due to the rapid rise in left ventricular pressure. The echo of vegetations in bacterial endocarditis or a torn cusp may be seen. Aortic regurgitation can be detected by pulsed Doppler ultrasound (in one study, sensitivity was 94%, specificity was 82%, and accuracy was 91%). In a study by Quinones et al., an estimation of the severity of aortic regurgitation was possible from inspection of the Doppler ascending aortic flow velocity curve.

Other noninvasive studies that may be helpful include phonocardiography for confirmation of the auscultatory findings. Phonocardiography can help distinguish an Austin Flint murmur from the murmur of mitral stenosis. Administration of amyl nitrite reduces the Austin Flint murmur but either has no effect or increases the murmur of mitral stenosis. Carotid pulse tracings in aortic regurgitation reveal a rapid upstroke and may have a bisferiens quality. Radionuclide ventriculography at rest and during exercise may aid in determining the extent of left ventricular dysfunction. As discussed under mitral regurgitation, gated radionuclide angiography is a useful technique for estimating the regurgitant fraction.

Cardiac catheterization reveals a decreased diastolic systemic pressure and increased left ventricular end-diastolic pressure. There is a rapid diastolic fall on the aortic pressure tracing. Systolic arterial pressure is normal or increased, and pulmonary capillary wedge pressure may be increased. Aortic root angiography is performed to estimate the degree of aortic regurgitation that is expressed semiquantitatively from $1+$ to $4+$. Morphologic abnormalities of the aorta may be seen, such as dissection, aortic root aneurysm, sinus of Valsalva aneursym, calcification of the ascending aorta and aortic valve. Left ventricular angiography is performed to assess the extent of left ventricular dysfunction that is important for determining prognosis following surgery. If the patient has a history of angina, coronary angiography should be performed as well.

Initial medical therapy for symptomatic aortic insufficiency includes digoxin and diuretics. Recent studies indicate that the afterload reducing agents hydralazine, prazosin, and nifedipine have beneficial effects on cardiac performance in patients with aortic regurgitation. All patients with aortic regurgitation should receive antibiotic prophylaxis for dental and general surgical procedures.

There is controversy as to the exact optimal timing for aortic valve replacement in patients with chronic aortic insufficiency. Some physicians recommend aortic valve replacement even in asymptomatic patients who have cardiomegaly and evidence of left ventricular dysfunction. When patients develop definite symptoms of left ventricular failure due to aortic regurgitation, aortic valve replacement should be considered. Waiting too long for valve replacement may be dangerous, since the chronically volume-overloaded left ventricle develops irreversible dysfunction. Assessing cardiac function noninvasively and at the time of cardiac catheterization is important, since prognosis is poor if left ventricular function is already severely impaired. An echocardiographic study by Henry et al. showed that preoperative echocardiographic measurements of end-systolic left ventricular dimension greater than 55 mm and fractional shortening less than 25% were associated with high mortality due to congestive heart failure; while patients with left ventricular dimensions of less than 55 mm in general did well. A study by Samuels et al. defined the following preoperative variables that discriminated between patients who had a good postoperative result and those who died of heart failure: increased severity and duration of dyspnea, extent of treatment for heart failure, physical findings suggesting left ventricular failure, increased cardiothoracic ratio and resting pulmonary capillary wedge pressure, and cardiac index less than 2.2 L/min/m^2 were all associated with poorer prognosis. These authors concluded that evidence of early left ventricular failure, even of a mild degree is an indicator for operation in patients with significant aortic insufficiency. Other studies have shown that patients with left ventricular end-systolic volumes of less than 30 ml/m^2 do well postoperatively; those with end-systolic volumes of greater than 90 ml/m^2 do poorly.

Most studies have shown some degree of improvement in left ventricular function following aortic valve replacement for aortic regurgitation. However, residual functional impairment appears to be greater in patients with aortic regurgitation than in those with aortic stenosis or combined aortic stenosis plus aortic regurgitation. A radionuclide study by Borer et al. showed that aortic valve replacement can improve but usually does not normalize left ventricular function during exercise in patients operated on for symptomatic aortic insufficiency. Echocardiographic studies have shown a reduction in left ventricular end-diastolic dimensions from 73.8 mm preoperatively to 58.7 mm six months postoperatively, with the greatest reduction in left ventricular size occurring within the first 22 postoperative days. Samuels et al.

showed that 78% of patients became asymptomatic following valve replacement for aortic insufficiency and 58% were alive 5–9 years postoperatively. One study reported a reduction in left ventricular end-diastolic volume following aortic valve replacement but no change in ejection fraction. There is a subgroup of patients who do have regression of hypertrophy following valve surgery. In patients with acute aortic regurgitation, aortic valve replacement is indicated if medical therapy does not control left ventricular failure. The types of prosthetic aortic valves used to treat aortic regurgitation are similar to those used for aortic stenosis.

Right-Sided Valvular Heart Disease

Tricuspid Regurgitation

The etiology of tricuspid regurgitation is often functional, due to dilatation of the right ventricle as occurs in (1) pulmonary stenosis; (2) pulmonary hypertension either primary or secondary to other causes such as mitral stenosis or intracardiac shunt (Eisenmenger's syndrome); or (3) when right ventricular infarction has occurred. Etiologies in which the tricuspid valve itself is altered include rheumatic heart disease (there is usually coexisting mitral and/or aortic valve disease), endocarditis (intravenous heroin users), malignant carcinoid, trauma, Ebstein's anomaly, and prolapse due to myxomatous degeneration.

The symptoms of tricuspid regurgitation are due to the increased systemic venous pressure with reduced right ventricular output and include peripheral edema, hepatic congestion with right upper quadrant tenderness, ascites, GI symptoms due to splanchnic congestion (including nausea, vomiting, anorexia), awareness of pulsations in the neck, symptoms due to concomitant valve or myocardial disease. The decreased right ventricular output may reduce the pulmonary congestion of mitral stenosis. However, severely reduced right ventricular output leads to an overall reduction in forward cardiac output, resulting in the symptoms of fatigue, weight loss, weakness, and hypotension. The symptoms of coexisting mitral valve disease including dyspnea, orthopnea, and paroxysmal nocturnal dyspnea may also be present.

Physical examination reveals distended neck veins with tall regurgitant v waves and rapidly collapsing y descent. A parasternal right ventricular impulse is present. If mitral stenosis is present, the patient may be in atrial fibrillation and have the characteristic murmur of mitral stenosis. If pulmonary hypertension is present, the pulmonic component of the second heart sound typically is accentuated. The murmur of tricuspid regurgitation is holosystolic, high pitched, located along the left lower sternal border and characteristically increases with inspiration. A right-ventricular S_3 may be heard in this region as well; the S_3 also characteristically increases with inspiration. The liver may be enlarged and pulsatile with hepatojugular reflux. Peripheral edema and ascites are often present. Severe, chronic tricuspid regurgitation may be associated with mild jaundice due to hepatic congestion and peripheral cyanosis due to low forward cardiac output.

Chest x-ray film reveals an enlarged right atrium, right ventricle, superior vena cava, and azygous vein. Electrocardiogram shows right atrial enlargement with tall peaked P waves in 2, 3, and aV_F. Right axis deviation and evidence of right ventricular hypertrophy with tall positive R waves in V_1 and V_2 may be present.

Echocardiography reveals a dilated right ventricular chamber with paradoxical septal motion. Echocardiography may provide clues as to the etiology of tricuspid regurgitation. For example, exaggerated motion of the tricuspid valve is typically seen with Ebstein's anomaly; vegetations may be visualized with endocarditis. Tricuspid valve prolapse or rheumatic thickening of the valve may be observed. Echocardiographic contrast agents injected peripherally can be visualized moving back and forth across the tricuspid valve with the aid of two dimensional echocardiography.

The jugular venous pulse wave form shows tall regurgitant systolic v waves and a rapid y descent. Radionuclide angiography reveals a dilated right ventricular cavity, which often has a reduced ejection fraction.

At cardiac catheterization, patients with tricuspid regurgitation demonstrate tall right atrial regurgitant v waves with a rapid y descent and elevated right atrial mean pressure. With right ventricular failure, there is an elevation of right ventricular end-diastolic pressure. Right ventricular angiography reveals a dilated right ventricle and regurgitation of contrast material into the right atrium, which is also dilated in cases of chronic tricuspid regurgitation.

Once patients develop symptoms and signs of right ventricular failure, mild salt restrictions, diuretics, and digitalis should be instituted. If tricuspid regurgitation is not severe and is due to right ventricular dilatation because of mitral valve disease, surgical correction for the mitral disease may be sufficient to correct or reduce the tricuspid regurgitation. Some medical centers perform tricuspid valve anuloplasty for moderate regurgitation secondary to right ventricular dilatation. Patients with severe tricuspid regurgitation that is either organic or functional, may require tricuspid valve replacement with either a porcine heterograft or mechanical prostheses. All patients with tricuspid regurgitation should receive antibiotic prophylaxis for dental or surgical procedures.

Tricuspid Stenosis

The origin of tricuspid stenosis is usually rheumatic disease, in which case there is nearly always concomitant rheumatic mitral valve disease. Less common causes include tricuspid atresia and, occasionally, large vegetations in bacterial endocarditis.

The symptoms are due to increased systemic venous pressure and reduced right ventricular output and, hence, are similar to those of tricuspid regurgitation. Peripheral edema, right upper quadrant discomfort, GI symptoms, and fatigue are the main complaints. With severe venous congestion of the GI tract, protein losing enteropathy may occur. When the tricuspid stenosis is due to rheumatic disease, the symptoms of coexisting mitral stenosis may be present.

Physical examination reveals distended jugular neck veins with a prominent a wave and a slow y descent. The right heart border is displaced to the right. The characteristic murmur of tricuspid stenosis is a diastolic rumbling murmur that increases in intensity with inspiration and is heard best at the left lower sternal border. An opening snap, which also increases in intensity with inspiration, may precede the murmur. If the patient is in sinus rhythm, presystolic accentuation of the murmur may be heard. The murmur can be distinguished from that of mitral stenosis by its increase during inspiration and by its location at the left lower sternal border, while the murmur of mitral stenosis is heard best at the apex. In addition, the murmur of tricuspid stenosis tends to be higher pitched than that of mitral stenosis. Of course, if the tricuspid stenosis is secondary to rheumatic disease, the physical findings of coexisting mitral stenosis and aortic valve disease are usually present. The liver is enlarged and tender, often a presystolic pulsation of the liver and hepatojugular reflux are present. Peripheral edema, ascites, pleural effusions, cyanosis, and icterus may be observed.

Chest x-ray film shows right atrial enlargement with distension of the superior vena cava and azygous veins. Findings of coexisting mitral stenosis may also be seen. The ECG demonstrates tall peaked P waves in the inferior leads, characteristic of right atrial enlargement. Echocardiogram demonstrates thickening and, in some cases, calcification of the valve and a reduced tricuspid valve E-F slope is present. Jugular venous pulse tracings may aid in the diagnosis and show a prominent a wave and a slow y descent.

On cardiac catheterization, there is a diastolic pressure gradient between the right atrium and right ventricle. The gradient may be small (3–5 mm Hg), and is best measured simultaneously with a double-lumen catheter. Right atrial pressure is increased with prominent a waves.

Therapy is largely dependent on associated mitral and aortic valve disease. Severe tricuspid stenosis with signs of low cardiac output usually requires valve surgery— either tricuspid valvuloplasty or valve replacement, most often performed at the same time that mitral valve surgery is undertaken. Symptoms of peripheral venous congestion are initially treated with diuretics; however, overdiuresis should be avoided, as this may result in reduced cardiac output. Digitalis is used for ventricular rate control in patients with atrial fibrillation. Patients with tricuspid stenosis should receive antibiotic prophylaxis against endocarditis for dental and surgical procedures.

Pulmonary Stenosis

Pulmonary stenosis (also see Chapter 18) is usually congenital in etiology, in which case it may be valvular, subvalvular, or supravalvular. Valvular pulmonic stenosis is rarely due to rheumatic heart disease or carcinoid syndrome. Patients with mild valvular stenosis are usually asymptomatic; these patients often first present in adulthood with a systolic murmur. Patients with moderate to severe stenosis as youths may develop increasing stenosis with their physical growth and with gradual fibrosis of the valve. Symptoms include fatigue, dyspnea on exertion, light-headedness, syncope, and, in severe cases, symptoms of right ventricular failure (peripheral edema, ascites, abdominal tenderness, nausea, vomiting).

Physical examination reveals a prominent jugular venous a wave, a right ventricular lift, widely split S_2 with a soft P_2 component, and a right-sided S_4 and S_3. The murmur of pulmonic stenosis is a harsh systolic ejection murmur heard best at the pulmonic area and along the left sternal border. When the murmur is preceeded by an ejection click, this finding suggests that the stenosis is valvular rather than sub- or supravalvular. The more severe the pulmonic valvular stenosis, the later in systole the murmur peaks. Unlike most right-sided cardiac sounds, the ejection click of pulmonic stenosis softens during *inspiration*. It occurs closer to S_1 with increasing severity of the stenosis. Cyanosis may be present if the patient has markedly reduced cardiac output or if there is a right-to-left shunt through an atrial septal defect or patent foramen ovale. With right ventricular failure, peripheral edema, a tender enlarged liver, and ascites are present. Chest x-ray film reveals poststenotic dilatation of the main and left pulmonary arteries, and, with moderate to severe stenosis, the right ventricle and right atrium are enlarged. The pulmonary vasculature may be diminished.

The ECG in patients with mild pulmonic stenosis may be normal. With moderate to severe stenosis, right axis deviation, right ventricular hypertrophy, and right atrial enlargement are seen. Right bundle branch block, complete or incomplete, may be present.

Echocardiography reveals a dilated and hypertrophied right ventricle in cases of severe pulmonic stenosis. The valve itself may demonstrate a prominent a wave. Stenosis of the valve may be visualized by two-dimensional echocardiography. Jugular venous pulse tracing reveals a prominent a wave.

Cardiac catheterization is performed to determine the severity of the stenosis as assessed by the right ventricular-pulmonary artery systolic pressure gradient. If the gradient is less than 50 mm Hg, the stenosis is mild; if the gradient is 50–80 mm Hg, the stenosis is moderate; if the gradient is greater than 80 mm Hg, the stenosis is severe. In moderate to severe stenosis, the right ventricular systolic pressure is elevated. The pulmonary artery pressure typically is normal. Right ventricular or pulmonary artery angiograms help to locate the site of obstruction. Coexistent cardiac abnormalities (atrial septal defect, ventricular septal defect, and tetralogy of Fallot) are ruled out by cardiac catheterization.

Mild to moderate pulmonic stenosis is often asymptomatic and therapy consists of prophylactic antibiotic therapy for dental and surgical procedures. Patients with severe pulmonary stenosis who are symptomatic or have signs of right ventricular failure should be considered for either pulmonary valvulotomy or prosthetic valve replacement. Treatment of asymptomatic patients who have severe pulmonary stenosis is controversial. Some physicians recommend surgery in all patients with severe pulmonary stenosis; others advise waiting for symptoms.

Pulmonary Regurgitation

The most common cause of pulmonary regurgitation is functional regurgitation due to dilatation of the pulmonary valve ring in patients with pulmonary hypertension. The pulmonary hypertension is usually secondary to rheumatic mitral valve disease, cor pulmonale, or primary pulmonary hypertension. Organic abnormalities of the pulmonic valve that result in regurgitation include: isolated congenital pulmonary regurgitation; infective endocarditis (especially among heroin addicts); and, rarely, rheumatic heart disease. Patients who have undergone surgical correction for pulmonary stenosis or tetralogy of Fallot may also have pulmonary regurgitation.

Patients are often asymptomatic as this lesion, in general, is well tolerated. However, with severe pulmonic regurgitation, right ventricular dilatation and failure eventually occur leading to symptoms of peripheral edema, right upper quadrant abdominal discomfort, anorexia, nausea, vomiting, and, with low forward output, the symptoms of fatigue and dyspnea on exertion.

Physical examination reveals a hyperdynamic right ventricular impulse and a wide and physiologically split S_2. The pulmonic component of the S_2 may be accentuated if pulmonary hypertension is present. The murmur of pulmonic regurgitation is a decrescendo diastolic murmur, which increases with inspiration and is heard along the upper left sternal border. When the murmur is high-pitched and blowing in quality (Graham Steell murmur), the etiology of pulmonary regurgitation is more likely to be functional, due to pulmonary hypertension. When the murmur is low-pitched and harsh, the etiology of the regurgitation is more likely to be on an organic basis. The murmur of congenital isolated pulmonary regurgitation may have a diastolic crescendo-decrescendo quality. In addition to a diastolic murmur, a systolic ejection murmur due to increased flow across the pulmonary valve, may be heard. With the development of right ventricular failure, a right-sided S_3 (increases with inspiration) is present. In addition, patients with right ventricular failure demonstrate distended jugular veins, hepatic enlargement and tenderness, hepatojugular reflux, peripheral edema, and ascites.

The chest x-ray film reveals pulmonary artery and right ventricular enlargement. Electrocardiography may show right axis deviation and, in some cases, right ventricular hypertrophy. On echocardiography, the right ventricle may be dilated with paradoxical interventricular septal motion. Cardiac catheterization reveals regurgitation of contrast media from the pulmonary artery to right ventricle during angiography, and the pulmonary artery diastolic pressure is reduced.

Patients with isolated pulmonary regurgitation who do not have pulmonary hypertension usually tolerate the lesion without difficulty. If the pulmonary regurgitation is functional, the prognosis and treatment depends on the underlying disease (mitral stenosis, cor pulmonale). Patients with mild and moderate pulmonary regurgitation usually are asymptomatic and require no specific therapy other than antibiotic prophylaxis for dental or surgical procedures. If the pulmonary regurgitation is more severe and symptoms of right heart failure develop, pulmonary valve replacement is considered.

Bibliography

Aaron BL, Mills M, Lower RR: Congenital tricuspid insufficiency: Definiton and review. *Chest* 69:637, 1976.

Abdulla AM, Frank MJ, Erdin RA Jr, et al: Clinical significance and hemodynamic correlates of the third heart sound gallop in aortic regurgitation: A guide to optimal timing of cardiac catheterization. *Circulation* 64:464, 1981.

Barlow JB, Pocock WA: Mitral valve prolapse, the specific billowing mitral leaflet syndrome, or an insignificant nonejection systolic click. *Am Heart J* 97:277, 1979.

Barnett HJ, Boughner DR, Taylor DW, et al: Further evidence relating mitral valve prolapse to cerebral ischemic events. *N Engl J Med* 302:139, 1980.

Bekheit SG, Ali AA, Deglin SM, et al: Analysis of QT interval in patients with idiopathic mitral valve prolapse. *Chest* 81:620, 1982.

Biddison JH, Dembo DH, Spalt H, et al: Familial occurrence of mitral valve prolapse in X-linked muscular dystrophy. *Circulation* 59:1299, 1979.

Blanchard D, Dieblo B, Peronneau P, et al: Noninvasive diagnosis of mitral regurgitation by Doppler echocardiography. *Br Heart J* 45:589, 1981.

Bland EF, Jones TD: Rheumatic fever and rheumatic heart disease: A 20-year report on 1,000 patients followed since childhood. *Circulation* 4:836, 1951.

Blount SG Jr, Komesu S, McCord MC: Asymptomatic isolated valvular pulmonary stenosis. *N Engl J Med* 248:5, 1953.

Bogart DB, Murphy BL, Wong BY, et al: Progression of aortic stenosis. *Chest* 76:391, 1979.

Bonner AJ Jr, Sacks MN, Tavel ME: Assessing the severity of aortic stenosis by phonocardiography and external carotid pulse recordings. *Circulation* 48:247, 1973.

Borer JS, Rossing DR, Kent KM, et al: Left ventricular function at rest and during exercise after aortic valve replacement in patients with aortic regurgitation. *Am J Cardiol* 44:1297, 1979.

Boudoulas H, Reynolds JC, Mazzaferri E, et al: Metabolic studies in mitral valve prolapse syndrome. A neuroendocrine-cardiovascular process. *Circulation* 61:1200, 1980.

Bough EW, Grandsman EJ, Norin DL, et al: Gated radionuclide angiographic evaluation of valve regurgitation. *Am J Cardiol* 46:423, 1980.

Canepa-Anson R, Emanuel RW: Elective aortic and mitral valve surgery in patients over 70 years of age. *Br Heart J* 41:493, 1979.

Carroll JD, Gaasch WH, Naimi S, et al: Regression of myocardial hypertrophy: electrocardiographic correlations after aortic valve replacement in patients with chronic aortic regurgitation. *Circulation* 65:980, 1982.

Cevese PG, Gallucci V, Monea M, et al: Heart valve replacement with the Hancock bioprosthesis: Analysis of long-term results. *Circulation* 56(Supp II):III, 1977.

Chandraratna PA, Vlahovick G, Kong Y, et al: Incidence of mitral valve prolapse in one hundred clinically stable newborn baby girls: An echocardiographic study. *Am Heart J* 98:312, 1979.

Chen CC, Morganroth J, Mardelli TJ, et al: Tricuspid regurgitation in tricuspid valve prolapse demonstrated with contrast cross-sectional echocardiography. *Am J Cardiol* 46:983, 1980.

Ciobanu M, Abbasi AJ, Allen M, et al: Pulsed Doppler echocardiography in the diagnosis and estimation of severity of aortic insufficiency. *Am J Cardiol* 49:339, 1982.

Coghlan HC, Phares P, Cowley M, et al: Dysautonomia in mitral valve prolapse. *Am J Med* 67:236, 1979.

DeLeon AC Jr: Mitral valve prolapse: etiology, diagnosis, and management. *Postgrad Med* 67:66, 72, 1980.

Devereux RB, Perloff JK, Reichek JV, et al: Mitral Valve Prolapse. *Circulation* 54:3, 1976.

Duran CMU, Pomar JL, Colman T, et al: Is tricuspid valve repair necessary? *J Thorac Cardiovasc Surg* 80:849, 1980.

Engle MA, Ito T, Goldberg HP: The fate of the patient with pulmonic stenosis. *Circulation* 30:554, 1964.

Ferrahs VJ, Boyce SW, Billingham ME, et al: Infection of glutaraldehyde-preserved porcine valve heterografts. *Am J Cardiol* 43:1123, 1979.

Fioretti P, Benossi B, Scardi S, et al: Afterload reduction with nifedipine in aortic insufficiency. *Am J Cardiol* 49:1728, 1982.

Fish RG, Takara T, Crymes T: Prognostic considerations in primary isolated insufficiency of the pulmonic valve. *N Engl J Med* 261:739, 1959.

Fisher ML, Parisi AF, Plotnick GD, et al: Assessment of severity of mitral stenosis by echocardiographic leaflet separation. *Arch Intern Med* 139:402, 1979.

Frank S, Johnson A, Ross J Jr: Natural history of valvular aortic stenosis. *Br Heart J* 35:41, 1973.

Fuchs RM, Heuser RR, Yin FC, et al: Limitation of pulmonary wedge V waves in diagnosing mitral regurgitation. *Am J Cardiol* 49:849, 1982.

Geha AS, Laks H, Stansel HC Jr, et al: Late failure of porcine valve heterografts in children. *J Thorac Cardiovasc Surg* 78:351, 1979.

Giuffrida G, Bonzani G, Betocchi S, et al: Hemodynamic response to exercise after propranolol in patients with mitral stenosis. *Am J Cardiol* 44:1076, 1979.

Gorlin R, Gorlin SG: Hydraulic formula for calculation of the area of stenotic mitral valve, other cardiac valves, and central circulatory shunts. *Am Heart J* 41:1, 1951.

Gottdiener JS, Borer JS, Bacharach SL, et al: Left ventricular function in mitral valve prolapse. Assessment with radionuclide cineangiography. *Am J Cardiol* 47:7, 1981.

Greenberg BH, Demots H, Murphy E, et al: Beneficial effects of hydralazine on rest and exercise hemodynamics in patients with chronic severe aortic insufficiency. *Circulation* 62:49, 1980.

Hakki AH, Iskandrian AS, Bemis CE, et al: A simplified valve formula for the calculation of stenotic cardiac valve areas. *Circulation* 63:1050, 1981.

Hamby RI, Gulotta SJ: Pulmonic valvular insufficiency: Etiology, recognition and management. *Am Heart J* 74:110, 1967.

Hansing CE, Rowe GG: Tricuspid insufficiency: A study of hemodynamics and pathogenesis. *Circulation* 45:793, 1972.

Hanson MR, Conomy JG, Hodgman JR: Brain events associated with mitral valve prolapse. *Stroke* 11:499, 1980.

Harvey WP: Auscultation is obvious—or is it? *Med Times* 3:48, 1971.

Henry WL, Bonow RO, Borer JS, et al: Evaluation of aortic valve replacement in patients with valvular aortic stenosis. *Circulation* 61:814, 1980.

Henry WL, Bonow RO, Borer JS, et al: Observations on the optimum time for operative intervention for aortic regurgitation. I. Evaluation of the results of aortic valve replacement in symptomatic patients. *Circulation* 61:471, 1980.

Hockings BE, Cope GD, Clarke GM, et al: Comparison of vasodilator drug prazosin with digoxin in aortic regurgitation. *Br Heart J* 43:550, 1980.

Holen J, Simonsen S: Determination of pressure gradient in mitral stenosis with Doppler echocardiography. *Br Heart J* 41:529, 1979.

Ibrahim MM: Left ventricular function in rheumatic mitral stenosis. Clinical echocardiographic study. *Br Heart J* 42:514, 1979.

Janowitz WR, Fester A: Quantitation of left ventricular regurgitation fraction by first pass radionuclide angiocardiography. *Am J Cardiol* 49:85, 1982.

Johnson LW, Grossman W, Dalen JE, et al: Pulmonic stenosis in the adult: Long-term follow-up results. *N Engl J Med* 287:115, 1972.

Kavey RE, Sondheimer HM, Blackman MS: Detection of dysrhythmia in pediatric patients with mitral valve prolapse. *Circulation* 62:582, 1980.

Kitchin A, Turner R: Diagnosis and treatment of tricuspid stenosis. *Br Heart J* 26:354, 1964.

Knotsen KM, Bae EA, Sivertssen E, et al: Detection of mitral regurgitation by Doppler ultrasound. A comparison with left ventricular angiography. *Acta Med Scand* 210:349, 1981.

Krayenbeuhl HP, Turina M, Hess OM, et al: Pre and postoperative left ventricular contractile function in patients with aortic valve disease. *Br Heart J* 41:204, 1979.

Lakier JB, Khaja F, Magilligan DJ, et al: Porcine xenograft valves long term (60–89 month) follow up. *Circulation* 62:313, 1980.

Lam W, Pavel D, Byron E, et al: Radionuclide regurgitant index: value and limitations. *Am J Cardiol* 47:292, 1981.

Lieppe W, Behar VS, Scallion R, et al: Detection of tricuspid regurgitation with two-dimensional echocardiography and peripheral vein injection. *Circulation* 57:128, 1978.

Lipson LC, Kent KM, Rossing DR, et al: Long-term hemodynamic assessment of the porcine heterograft in the mitral position: Late development of valvular stenosis. *Circulation* 64:397, 1981.

Malcolm AD, Cankoviac-Darracott S, Chayen J, et al: Biopsy evidence of left ventricular myocardial abnormality in patients with mitral-leaflet prolapse and chest pain. *Lancet* 8125:1052, 1979.

Marcus ML, Dury DB, Hiratzka LF, et al: Decreased coronary reserve: A mechanism for angina pectoris in patients with aortic stenosis and normal coronary arteries. *N Engl J Med* 307:1362, 1982.

Mautner RK, Katz GE, Iteld BJ, et al: Coronary artery spasm: A mechanism of chest pain in selected patients with the mitral valve prolapse syndrome. *Chest* 79:449, 1981.

Mellino M, Salcedo EE, Lever HM, et al: Echocardiographic-quantified severity of mitral anulus calcification: prognostic correlation to related hemodynamic valvular, rhythm, and conduction abnormalities. *Am Heart J* 103:222, 1982.

Miller RA, Lev M, Paul MH: Congenital absence of pulmonary valve. *Circulation* 26:266, 1962.

Mills P, Rose J, Hollingsworth J, et al: Long-term prognosis of mitral valve prolapse. *N Engl J Med* 297:13, 1977.

Morganroth J, Jones RH, Chen CC, et al: Two-dimensional echocardiography in mitral, aortic, and tricuspid valve prolapse: The clinical problem, cardiac nuclear imaging considerations, and a proposed standard for diagnosis. *Am J Cardiol* 46:1164, 1980.

Morrow AG, Goldblatt A, Braunwald E: Congenital aortic stenosis. II. Surgical treatment and the results of operation. *Circulation* 2:426, 1963.

Murphy ES, Lawson RM, Starr A, et al: Severe aortic stenosis in patients 60 years of age or older: Left ventricular function and 10-year survival after valve replacement. *Circulation* 64(2 PT 2):184, 1981.

Nair CK, Sketch MH, Desai R, et al: High prevalence of symptomatic bradyarrhythmias due to atrioventricular node-fascicular and sinus node-atrial disease in patients with mitral anular calcification. *Am Heart J* 103:226, 1982.

Newman GE, Gibbons RJ, Jones RH: Cardiac function during rest and exercise in patients with mitral valve prolapse. Role of nuclear angiocardiography. *Am J Cardiol* 47:14, 1981.

Nolan CM, Kane JJ, Gronow WA: Infective endocarditis and mitral prolapse: A comparison with other types of endocarditis. *Arch Intern Med* 141:447, 1981.

Ogawa S, Hayashi J, Sasaki H, et al: Evaluation of combined valvular prolapse syndrome by two-dimensional echocardiography. *Circulation* 65:174, 1982.

Olsen EG, Al-Rufaie HK: The floppy mitral valve: Study of pathogenesis. *Br Heart J* 44:674, 1980.

Osterberger LE, Goldstein S, Khaja F, et al: Functional mitral stenosis in patients with massive mitral annular calcification. *Circulation* 64:472, 1981.

Perloff JK, Harvey WP: The clinical recognition of Tricuspid Stenosis. *Circulation* 22:346, 1960.

Phillips HR, Levine FH, Carter JE, et al: Mitral valve replacement for isolated mitral regurgitation: Analysis of clinical course and late postoperative left ventricular ejection fraction. *Am J Cardiol* 48:647, 1981.

Pickering NJ, Brody JI, Barrett MJ: Von Willebrand Syndromes and mitral-valve prolapse: Linked mesenchymal dysplasias. *J Thorac Cardiovasc Surg* 82:127, 1981.

Quinones MA, Young JB, Waggoner AD, et al: Assessment of pulsed Doppler echocardiography in detection and quantification of aortic and mitral regurgitation. *Br Heart J* 44:612, 1980.

Raeder EA, Burckhardt D: Noninvasive assessment of myocardial function in young patients with mitral valve prolapse. *Am Heart J* 97:432, 1979.

Rapaport E: Natural history of aortic and mitral valve disease. *Am J Cardiol* 35:221, 1975.

Reeves WC, Leaman DM, Buonocore E, et al: Detection of tricuspid regurgitation and estimation of central venous pressure by two-dimensional contrast echocardiography of the right superior hepatic vein. *Am Heart J* 102(3 Pt. 1):374, 1981.

Reichek N, Shelburne JC, Perloff JK: Clinical aspects of rheumatic valvular disease. *Prog Cardiovasc Dis* 15:491, 1973.

Rigo P, Alderson PO, Robertson RM: Measurement of aortic and mitral regurgitation by gated cardiac blood pool scans. *Circulation* 60:306, 1979.

Rippe J, Fishbein MC, Carabello B, et al: Primary myxomatous degeneration of cardiac valves: Clinical, pathological, haemodynamic, and echocardiographic profile. *Br Heart J* 44:621, 1980.

Rippe JM, Angoff G, Sloss LJ, et al: Multiple floppy valves: an echocardiographic syndrome. *Am J Med* 66:817, 1979.

Roberts WC, Sjoerdsma A: The cardiac disease associated with the carcinoid syndrome (carcinoid heart disease). *Am J Med* 36:5, 1964.

Roberts WC: Anatomically isolated aortic valvular disease. The case against its being a rheumatic etiology. *Am J Med* 49:151, 1970.

Roberts WC: The congenitally bicuspid aortic valve: A study of 85 autopsy cases. *Am J Cardiol* 26:72, 1970.

Roberts WC, Perloff JK, Costantino T: Severe valvular aortic stenosis in patients over 65 years of age. A clinicopathologic study. *Am J Cardiol* 27:497, 1971.

Roberts WC: Valvular, subvalvular and supravalvular aortic stenosis. Morphologic features. *Cardiovasc Clin* 5(Suppl. 1):97, 1973.

Ross J Jr: Left ventricular function and the timing of surgical treatment in valvular heart disease. *Ann Intern Med* 94(4 PT 1):498, 1981.

Salazar E, Levine HD: Rheumatic tricuspid regurgitation: The clinical spectrum. *Am J Med* 33:111, 1962.

Samuels DA, Curfman GD, Friedlich AL, et al: Valve replacement for aortic regurgitation: Long-term follow-up with factors influencing the results. *Circulation* 60:647, 1979.

Santos AD, Mathew PK, Hilal A, et al: Orthostatic hypotension a commonly unrecognized cause of symptoms in mitral valve prolapse. *Am J Med* 71:746, 1981.

Schlant RC, Felner JM, Miklozek CL, et al: Mitral valve prolapse. *DM* 26:1, 1980.

Schutte JE, Gaffney FA, Blend L, et al: Distinctive anthropometric characteristics of women with mitral valve prolapse. *Am J Med* 71:533, 1981.

Selzer A, Cohn KE: Natural history of mitral stenosis: a review. *Circulation* 45:878, 1972.

Shoenfeld Y, Eldar M, Bedazovsky B, et al: Aortic stenosis associated with gastrointestinal bleeding: A survey of 612 patients. *Am Heart J* 100:179, 1980.

Siegel JR, Roberts WC: Electrocardiographic observations in severe aortic valve stenosis: Correlative necropsy study to clinical, hemodynamic, and ECG variables demonstrating relation of 12-lead QRS amplitude to peak systolic transaortic pressure gradient. *Am Heart J* 103:210, 1982.

Smith N, McAnulty JH, Rahimtoola SH: Severe aortic stenosis with impaired left ventricular function and clinical heart failure: Results of valve replacement. *Circulation* 58:255, 1978.

Sorenson SG, O'Rourke RA, Chaudhuri TK: Noninvasive quantitation of valvular regurgitation by gated equilibrium radionuclide angiography. *Circulation* 62:1089, 1980.

St. John Sutton MG, St. John Sutton M, Oldershaw P, et al: Valve replacement without preoperative cardiac catheterization. *N Engl J Med* 305:1233, 1981.

Sung CS, Prices EC, Cooley DA: Discrete subaortic stenosis in adults. *Am J Cardiol* 42:283, 1978.

Tei C, Shah PM, Ormiston JA: Assessment of tricuspid regurgitation by directional analysis of right atrial systolic linear reflux echoes with contrast M-mode echocardiography. *Am Heart J* 103:1025, 1982.

Teply JF, Grunkemeier GL, Starr A: Cardiac valve replacement in patients over 75 years of age. *Thorac Cardiovasc Surg* 29:47, 1981.

Thompson R, Yacoub M, Ahmed M, et al: Influence of preoperative left ventricular function and results of homograft replacement of the aortic valve for aortic stenosis. *Am J Cardiol* 43:929, 1979.

Toussaint C, Cribier A, Cazor JL, et al: Hemodynamic and angiographic evaluation of aortic regurgitation 8 and 27 months after aortic valve replacement. *Circulation* 64:456, 1981.

Udoshi MB, Shah A, Fisher VJ, et al: Incidence of mitral valve prolapse in subjects with thoracic skeletal abnormalities: A prospective study. *Am Heart J* 97:303, 1979.

United Kingdom and United States Joint Report on Rheumatic Heart Disease: The evolution of rheumatic heart disease in children: Five-year report of a cooperative trial of ACTH, cortisone, and aspirin. *Circulation* 22:503, 1960.

United Kingdom and United States Joint Report on Rheumatic Heart Disease: The natural history of rheumatic fever and rheumatic heart disease: Ten-year report of a cooperative clinical trial of ACTH, cortisone, and aspirin. *Circulation* 32:457, 1965.

Venkatesh A, Pauls DL, Crowe R, et al: Mitral valve prolapse in anxiety neurosis (panic disorder). *Am Heart J* 100:302, 1980.

Waller BF, Zoltick JM, Rosen JH, et al: Severe aortic regurgitation from systemic hypertension (without aortic dissection) requiring aortic valve replacement: Analysis of four patients. *Am J Cardiol* 49:473, 1982.

Walsh PN, Kansu TA, Corbett JJ, et al: Platelets, thromboembolism, and mitral valve prolapse. *Circulation* 63:552, 1981.

Wei JY, Fortuin NJ: Diastolic sounds and murmurs associated with mitral valve prolapse. *Circulation* 63:559, 1981.

Weyman AE, Hurwitz RA, Girod DA, et al: Cross-sectional echocardiographic visualization of the stenotic pulmonary valve. *Circulation* 56:769, 1977.

Yacoub M, Halim M, Radley-Smith R, et al: Surgical treatment of mitral regurgitation caused by floppy valves: Repair versus replacement. *Circulation* 64(2 PT 2):210, 1981.

Zone DD, Botti RE: Right ventricular infarction with tricuspid insufficiency and chronic right heart failure. *Am J Cardiol* 37:445, 1976.

CHAPTER 14 | CARDIOMYOPATHY

Robert A. Kloner

Cardiomyopathy is defined as a disorder in which the signs and symptoms are primarily a result of dysfunction of the myocardium itself. The dysfunction may be due to a disease that primarily affects the heart (primary cardiomyopathy) or due to a generalized disease state that affects the heart secondarily (secondary cardiomyopathy). Disease of the myocardium due to hypertension, valvular heart disease, and congenital heart disease are excluded. While some cardiologists exclude disease of the myocardium due to coronary artery disease, Burch et al. (1970) described the condition of ischemic cardiomyopathy in which patients with known coronary disease have clinical manifestations similar to primary myocardial disease. Many types of classifications of cardiomyopathy have appeared in the medical literature. These include classification as primary or secondary; by etiology; or by clinical, pathologic, or as functional features. Perhaps the most helpful classification for the clinician is a functional one in which cardiomyopathies are classified as either dilated (congestive), restrictive, or hypertrophic in type (Fig. 1).

Dilated (Congestive) Cardiomyopathy

Dilated or congestive cardiomyopathy is characterized by a large, dilated heart with reduced systolic pump function, frequently associated with the clinical features of congestive heart failure. There are numerous etiologies of dilated cardiomyopathy (Table 1), but the most common form is called idiopathic cardiomyopathy, a type for which no known cause can be determined. Pathology of the heart reveals dilatation of all four chambers. The degree of hypertrophy of the ventricular walls is disproportionately small in relation to the extent of ventricular dilatation. Various degrees of interstitial and perivascular fibrosis also may be present.

The clinical manifestations are those of congestive heart failure. They include dyspnea on exertion, orthopnea, fatigue, and paroxysmal nocturnal dyspnea. Peripheral edema, ascites, and hepatomegaly occur late, resulting from right-sided cardiac dysfunction. Palpitations and symptoms due to emboli (systemic or pulmonary) may be present.

Physical examination reveals a number of findings depending on the severity of the cardiomyopathy. These may include a narrow pulse pressure; low or normal blood pressure; pulsus alternans; cool skin due to peripheral vasoconstriction; jugular venous distention with prominent a waves; and, if tricuspid regurgitation is present, prominent regurgitant systolic v waves. The cardiac apical impulse typically is displaced leftward with a left ventricular heave, and in some cases, right ventricular heave. A palpable precordial a wave may be present. Auscultation reveals a number

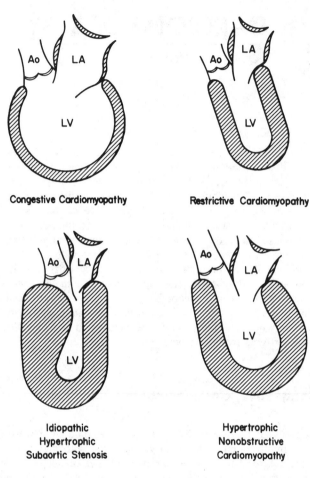

Congestive Cardiomyopathy

Restrictive Cardiomyopathy

Idiopathic
Hypertrophic
Subaortic Stenosis

Hypertrophic
Nonobstructive
Cardiomyopathy

Figure 1   Schematic showing the three general categories of cardiomyopathy: Dilated or congestive, restrictive, and hypertrophic (obstructive [idiopathic hypertrophic subaortic stenosis] and nonobstructive). Key: Ao, aorta; LA, left atrium; LV, left ventricle.

of features, including paradoxical splitting of S_2 when left bundle branch block is present, an S_3 gallop, and, in some cases, an S_4 gallop. The murmurs of mitral and tricuspid regurgitation may be heard. Other signs of left heart failure are common, including pulmonary rales or dullness at the lung bases due to pleural effusion; when right ventricular failure ensues, peripheral edema, ascites, and hepatomegaly are present as well.

The chest x-ray film reveals diffuse cardiac enlargement and when hemodynamic decompensation occurs, signs of congestive heart failure are seen, including pulmonary vascular redistribution, interstitial and alveolar edema, and pleural effusions. When right-sided heart failure is present, the azygous and superior vena cava are dilated; the lung fields may be surprisingly clear. The ECG often shows sinus tachycardia in the presence of congestive heart failure or other arrhythmias, including atrial fibrillation and ventricular ectopy. Conduction disturbances, such as left anterior hemiblock and incomplete or complete left bundle branch block are common. Left atrial enlargement and either left ventricular hypertrophy or low QRS voltage may be present. If there is diffuse myocardial necrosis or fibrosis, even in the absence of a discrete infarction, the ECG may reveal pathologic Q waves. ST-T wave abnormalities are usually nonspecific in nature.

Both M-mode and two-dimensional echocardiography reveal left ventricular dilatation and a poorly contracting left ventricle. When tricuspid regurgitation is present, the septum may show paradoxical motion. The end-diastolic and end-systolic volumes are increased, and the calculated ejection fraction is reduced. Mitral valve closure may be delayed, and aortic valve closure may occur earlier than normal. In later stages of the disease, the right ventricle is dilated as well. The two-dimensional echocardiogram especially is useful for detecting left ventricular thrombus.

Radionuclide ventriculography reveals increased ventricular volumes and reduced ejection fraction. Both two-dimensional echocardiography and radionuclide ventriculography have been shown to be helpful for assessing response to therapy by assessing serial systolic ventricular wall motion and ejection fraction and by helping to rule out large ventricular aneurysms.

Systolic time intervals also may be helpful in following the severity of ventricular dysfunction. The preejection period (PEP) is prolonged and the left ventricular ejection time (LVET) is reduced, resulting in an increased PEP/LVET ratio.

Cardiac catheterization reveals an elevated left ventricular end-diastolic pressure, and left atrial pressure (pulmonary capillary wedge pressure), and modest elevation in the pulmonary arterial pressure. When right ventricular failure occurs, the right ventricular end-diastolic, right atrial, and central venous pressures rise as well. The

Table 1. Etiologies of Dilated (Congestive) Cardiomyopathy

Idiopathic

Peripartum

Postmyocarditis due to infectious agent (viral, parasitic, Rickettsiae, mycobacterial)

Alcoholic

Neuromuscular (muscular dystrophy; myotonic dystrophy)

Connective tissue disorders (systemic lupus erythematosus, rheumatoid disease, polyarteritis).

Beri beri

Glycogen storage diseases

Toxins (cobalt, lead, arsenic)

Doxorubicin hydrochloride, cyclophosphamide, vincristine

Infiltrative: amyloid, hemochromatotic, sarcoid (may have congestive or restrictive features)

Inherited disorders: Fabry's disease, Gaucher's disease

Metabolic: Chronic hypophosphatemia, hypokalemia, hypocalcemia, uremia

left ventricular end-diastolic pressure is usually higher than that in the right ventricle and the cardiac index is reduced. Left ventricular angiography reveals left ventricular dilatation, diffusely hypokinetic wall motion, elevated systolic and diastolic volumes, and a reduced ejection fraction. This procedure also rules out the possibility that the congestive heart failure is due to ventricular aneurysm. Mitral regurgitation can be detected and its severity determined. Mural thrombi appear as intracavitary filling defects. Coronary arteriography can be used to exclude extensive myocardial infarctions (MIs) in patients who have Q waves due to diffuse fibrosis.

Some centers have performed cardiac biopsy at the time of cardiac catheterization. The severity of idiopathic congestive cardiomyopathy or its prognosis, in general, cannot be assessed from histologic changes. There is marked topographic variation in biopsy material and a poor correlation between morphology and function. However, some studies have shown a correlation between hemodynamic and morphologic abnormalities in patients with anthracycline-induced cardiomyopathy.

Therapy for patients with dilated cardiomyopathy includes treatment for the underlying disease (if known), such as alcoholism or systemic lupus erythematosus. Congestive heart failure is treated with salt restriction, diuretics, and the use of digitalis. Some patients with cardiomyopathy may be more prone to digitalis toxicity (especially if the cardiomyopathy is due to amyloidosis). Afterload reduction with vasodilators, such as prazosin and hydralazine, has also been found to improve symptoms and hemodynamics. Patients should curtail those activities that result in symptoms. Some studies have shown that prolonged bed rest may benefit not only the patient's symptoms and heart size but prognosis as well; however, this form of therapy remains controversial. Arrhythmias should be treated with antiarrhythmic agents, but because many of these agents (quinidine, procainamide, disopyramide) have negative inotropic effects, dosages must be carefully titrated and patients assessed frequently as these drugs are begun. If congestive heart failure is severe or the patient has experienced embolic events, long-term systemic anticoagulation is instituted if no contraindications exist. Newer forms of therapy, such as cardiac transplantation, new inotropic agents (amrinone, pirbuterol, prenalterol), and the artificial heart are under study. Recent studies have suggested that there may be prolonged improvement of cardiac function and ultrastructure after a three day infusion of dobutamine.

There have been several studies suggesting that beta blockade may have beneficial effects in patients with dilated cardiomyopathy. Some studies have even described an improvement in ejection fraction and survival with long-term use of these agents. However, in a study by Ikram et al., acebutolol, a cardioselective beta blocking agent, reduced left ventricular contractility, mean aortic pressure, and ejection fraction in patients with dilated cardiomyopathy. The authors concluded that beneficial effects of the beta blockers to reduce myocardial energy requirements, improve ventricular compliance, and lower arterial blood pressure would be advantageous. However, the authors warned that reduced contractility and further cardiac dilatation could lead to hemodynamic deterioration.

A recent study by Fuster et al. evaluated the prognosis of patients with idiopathic congestive cardiomyopathy. Seventy-seven percent of patients in this study had an accelerated course, with the majority of patients dying within the first two years of diagnosis. Twenty-three percent of patients improved or stabilized. Three factors were highly predictive of a poorer prognosis: age (over 50 years old); a cardiothoracic ratio greater than 0.55; and a cardiac index of less than 3 L/min/m^2. In this study, systemic emboli occurred in 18% of the patients who did not receive anticoagulant therapy and in none of those who did, suggesting that anticoagulant therapy probably should be administered if there are no contraindications.

ALCOHOLIC CARDIOMYOPATHY

It has been shown that regular use of moderate alcohol (one or two drinks a day) is associated with a reduced risk of major coronary events, while use of three or more drinks daily is associated with an increased risk of hypertension. Very heavy alcohol ingestion may lead to congestive cardiomyopathy. In one study by Fuster et al., 21% of patients with congestive cardiomyopathy had a history of excessive alcohol consumption. On the other hand, the incidence of severe heart failure in alcoholics is low according to studies by Klatsky et al. and Kino et al. Patients with chronic alcoholism who are asymptomatic may have abnormal systolic and diastolic ventricular function. Echocardiographic findings in such patients include increased left ventricular mass, dimension, septal and left ventricular wall thickness, and left atrial size. Atrial fibrillation is a common arrhythmia in this disorder. The cessation of alcohol may reverse the disease or interrupt its progression in many patients. However, the pathogenic process may continue unabated in some patients who abstain.

CARDIOMYOPATHY INDUCED BY NEOPLASTIC AGENTS

Doxorubicin (Adriamycin), cyclophosphamide, and vincristine may produce both pathological and clinical cardiomyopathy. Doxorubicin induced cardiomyopathy has been studied extensively and its toxic effects are dose-related. In adults, the total dose of doxorubicin should not exceed approximately 500 mg/m^2. Morphologic damage is proportional to cummulative doxorubicin dose, and some studies have shown that cardiac performance correlates with dose and shows a threshold effect. Cofactors which appear to worsen the cardiotoxicity of this agent include concomittant treatment with vincristine, bleomycin, or radiation therapy. Doxorubicin cardiotoxicity may be associated with a sudden fall in QRS voltage.

Peripartum Cardiomyopathy See Chapter 27.

Hypertrophic Cardiomyopathy

Hypertrophic cardiomyopathy is the condition in which the left ventricle develops increased wall thickness of unknown etiology. The hypertrophy may be symmetric, in which the left ventricular septal wall is hypertrophied to the same extent as the left ventricular free wall, or asymmetric (asymmetrical septal hypertrophy, ASH) in which the septal hypertrophy is greater than the free wall hypertrophy. The hypertrophic cardiomyopathy may be obstructive or nonobstructive to outflow of blood from the ventricles. Patients with ASH may have the condition historically termed idiopathic hypertrophic subaortic stenosis (IHSS), in which the septum plus anterior leaflet of the mitral valve encroach on the left ventricular outflow tract during systole, resulting in a significant intraventricular pressure gradient. This obstruction to outflow may be present at rest or only occur when provoked by maneuvers that reduce ventricular volume. This condition has also been termed hypertrophic obstructive cardiomyopathy (HOCM), which may be more appropriate nomenclature. Other patients have ASH in which no outflow obstruction exists either at rest or with provocative maneuvers. Recent studies have suggested that there is an abnormality in diastolic relaxation of the myocardium in patients with hypertrophic cardiomyopathy.

Some patients with hypertrophic cardiomyopathy have hypertrophy involving unusual locations, such as the cardiac apex, posterior ventricular septum, anterior or lateral left ventricular free wall, and even the right ventricle.

Patients with hypertrophic cardiomyopathy may develop transmural myocardial infarction (MI) with insignificant or absent coronary atherosclerosis. Some investigators have postulated coronary spasm as a cause.

Hypertrophic cardiomyopathy recently has been implicated in cases of sudden death of young athletes. Sudden death usually occurred just after severe exertion. Cardiac disease usually was not suspected in these patients.

Hypertrophic cardiomyopathy has also been associated with several unusual conditions, including Friedreich's ataxia, lentiginosis, and untreated hypoparathyroidism. There is debate in the literature as to whether there are differences in frequencies of HLA antigens between patients with hypertrophic cardiomyopathy and control populations.

HYPERTROPHIC OBSTRUCTIVE CARDIOMYOPATHY

Hypertrophic cardiomyopathy with ASH and a left ventricular outflow gradient historically has been referred to as IHSS, although the term hypertrophic obstructive cardiomyopathy (HOCM) is now preferred by many cardiologists. Since the original papers that described the clinical features of this entity used the term IHSS, the description below of clinical features will use the original terminology.

IHSS often exhibits autosomal dominant inheritance with incomplete penetrance. The anterior-superior portion of the interventricular septum is disproportionately thickened and encroaches on the left ventricular outflow tract. Histologic studies reveal myofiber disarray in the region of the hypertrophied septum and, to a lesser degree, in the free wall of the left ventricle. As the left ventricle contracts, the anterior leaflet of the mitral valve is pulled anteriorly toward the thickened left ventricular septum, resulting in an intracavitary obstruction of the outflow tract. In addition, displacement of the anterior papillary muscle and anterior mitral valve leaflet results in mitral regurgitation in some patients. Maneuvers that decrease left ventricular cavity size and increase left ventricular contractility tend to increase the outflow tract gradient; maneuvers that increase cavity size and reduce contractility tend to reduce the gradient.

Symptoms of IHSS include dypsnea on exertion, orthopnea, paroxysmal nocturnal dyspnea, angina, syncope or near-syncope, and palpitations. Syncope typically occurs *after* exertion (when peripheral muscles are no longer pumping increased amounts of blood back to the heart and, hence, there is a relative decrease in left ventricular cavity size in the face of increased ventricular contractility, with an overall increase in obstruction). Instances of sudden death may occur and are presumably related to malignant ventricular arrhythmias. Signs of congestive heart failure may become progressive in the later phases of the disease and are complicated by concomitant mitral regurgitation. Other complications include systemic embolization and bacterial endocarditis (of the aortic or mitral valves). Although the average age of presentations of symptoms is in the middle 20s, this condition is not uncommonly first diagnosed in patients over 60.

It should be pointed out that there is considerable variation from patient to patient in the degree of symptomatology with hypertrophic cardiomyopathy, from totally asymptomatic to severely symptomatic with congestive heart failure. Relatives of patients with documented IHSS may have ASH on echocardiography but often are asymptomatic.

There are several prominent physical findings in patients with intracavitary obstruction. The carotid pulse rises rapidly and typically has a double peak; the jugular venous pulse may reveal a prominent a wave. The apical impulse is displaced leftward, is forceful, and typically consists of a presystolic followed by a double systolic impulse. A systolic thrill may be palpated. Auscultation reveals an S_4 gallop and an S_2 that may be split normally, narrowly, or widely (in patients with severe obstruction). An S_3 may or may not be present. The systolic ejection murmur of IHSS is a harsh crescendo-decrescendo murmur heard best between the lower left sternal border and apex. The murmur radiates toward the base of the heart and clavicle but, unlike that of aortic stenosis, does not radiate into the neck. The murmur *increases* with maneuvers that reduce the size of the left ventricular cavity by reducing preload and/or reducing afterload (Valsalva maneuver, standing, or administration of amyl nitrite or nitroglycerin) and with those maneuvers that increase left ventricular contractility (administration of isoproterenol). The murmur *decreases* with maneuvers that increase left ventricular cavity size by increasing preload (passive leg raising, squatting) and maneuvers that increase afterload (squatting, phenylephrine administration, isometric handgrip). These maneuvers help differentiate the murmur of IHSS from other conditions (see Table 2). The murmur of mitral regurgitation is commonly heard along with the systolic ejection murmur of IHSS. Rarely, the murmur of aortic regurgitation is also present.

Chest x-ray film reveals various degrees of cardiomegaly and, unlike valvular aortic stenosis, post-stenotic aortic dilatation and calcification of the aortic valve are absent but calcification of the mitral anulus may be present. The ECG reveals left

Table 2. Effect of Various Maneuvers on Systolic Murmurs

	Valsalva	Phenylephrine handgrip	Squatting	Amyl nitrite	Leg raising
Aortic stenosis	↓	↓	↑ ↓	↑	↑
IHSS	↑	↓	↓	↑	↓
Ventricular septal defect	↓	↑	→	↓	↑
Mitral regurgitation	↓	↑	→	↓	↑

Key: ↓ decrease; ↑ increase; ↓ slight decrease; → no change; ↑ ↓ increase or decrease

ventricular hypertrophy and ST-T wave abnormalities. Abnormal Q waves give rise to a pseudoinfarction pattern in 20–50% of patients and typically are present in the inferior and/or lateral electrocardiographic leads. Ventricular arrhythmias are common; 5–10% of patients develop atrial fibrillation, and these patients often develop clinical deterioration due to loss of the atrial contribution of left ventricular filling. Left atrial enlargement may also be present on the ECG.

The echocardiogram is extremely useful in establishing the diagnosis of hypertrophic cardiomyopathy with left ventricular outflow gradient but is not always conclusive. The left ventricular walls are hypertrophied, and if the ratio of septal thickness to free wall thickness is greater than 1.3:1, ASH is present (see Chapter 5). Left ventricular outflow obstruction during systole is suggested by finding systolic anterior motion of the anterior leaflet of the mitral valve. The left ventricular internal diameters are small, producing a crowded appearance to the left ventricular cavity. During midsystole, the aortic valve leaflets may appear to close partially or to flutter, due to the Venturi effect produced by the subvalvular stenosis. Provocative maneuvers, such as Valsalva maneuver and administration of amyl nitrite, enhance echocardiographic evidence of left ventricular obstruction.

Phonocardiography may aid in interpretation of the effects of various maneuvers on the intensity of the systolic murmur of IHSS. Carotid pulse tracings are especially helpful, in that they reveal a brisk carotid upstroke in contrast to aortic stenosis; and the wave form often reveals a bisferiens pulse contour. Valsalva maneuver (the strain phase) or amyl nitrite enhances the bisferiens nature of the pulse. Radionuclide ventriculography allows visualization of the thickened septum and obliteration of the left ventricular cavity. Studies using thallium-201 may reveal the asymmetrically thickened septum.

Holter monitoring has been recommended for patients with IHSS, since some studies have shown that patients with high grades of ventricular ectopy and ventricular tachycardia are at risk for sudden death.

Cardiac catheterization studies of patients with IHSS reveal an elevated left ventricular end-diastolic pressure and a systolic pressure gradient between the body of the left ventricular cavity and the area below the aortic valve. This pressure gradient is often quite labile and can be provoked with Valsalva maneuver, amyl nitrite, and isoproterenol. A characteristic feature of IHSS is that the beat following a premature beat has an increased gradient, with a concomitant fall in aortic pulse pressure (Brockenborough's sign, Fig. 2). The systolic arterial wave form may reveal a "spike and dome" configuration. There is usually a prominent a wave in the left atrial and left ventricular wave forms, due to diminished left ventricular compliance. Mild pulmonary hypertension is present in 25% of patients with IHSS, and 15% have a pressure gradient across their right ventricular outflow tract. Left ventricular angiography allows visualization of the obstruction and estimation of the degree of hypertrophy. Anterior motion of the anterior leaflet of the mitral valve and mitral regurgitation may be visualized. The left ventricular cavity is small and often appears to be obliterated at the end of systole. Patients with symptoms of angina may have no evidence of coronary artery disease, but in those who are over 50 years old, concomitant coronary disease is not uncommon.

The main therapy for IHSS is beta blockade with propranolol. The dose that results in symptomatic improvement is usually 40 mg qid. or more. Beta blockade reduces the outflow obstruction caused by isoproteronol and associated with exercise, im-

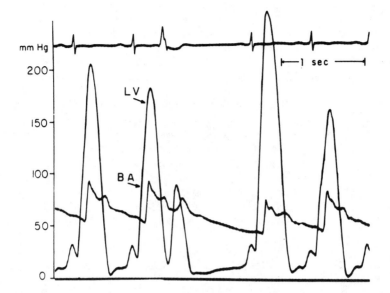

Figure 2 Simultaneous left ventricular (LV) and brachial artery (BA) pressures in a patient with IHSS. The contraction following the premature ventricular beat reveals a reduction in brachial artery pressure and an accentuation of the "spike and dome" configuration of the systemic arterial pressure tracing. (From Braunwald E et al.: Idiopathic hypertrophic subaortic stenosis. *Circulation* 30, Suppl IV, 78, 1964, by permission of the American Heart Association, Inc.)

proves ventricular compliance, and reduces myocardial oxygen demand and, hence, the frequency or severity of angina. It does not appear to provide absolute protection against sudden death.

Recent studies suggest that the calcium blocking agents may be useful in the treatment of IHSS. Verapamil has been shown to reduce the left ventricular outflow gradient, improve exercise capacity, and improve peak left ventricular filling rate. One study showed electrocardiographic evidence of regression of hypertrophy following long-term verapamil therapy. Nifedipine has also been shown to be effective in these patients and, like verapamil, improves the left ventricular diastolic abnormalities of hypertrophic cardiomyopathy.

Patients with IHSS should avoid strenuous exercise, due to the risk of sudden death. In general, digitalis should be avoided, as it increases contractility and, hence, the severity of the outflow obstruction. Vasodilators should also be avoided, as they may increase the obstruction. However, late in the course of the disease, some patients demonstrate clinical signs suggestive of congestive cardiomyopathy and may benefit from digitalis, diuretics, and vasodilators, especially if mitral regurgitation or atrial fibrillation are contributing to their symptoms. Atrial fibrillation should be treated promptly as it may result in hemodynamic deterioration due to loss of the atrial component of left ventricular filling. If the patient is hemodynamically unstable, electrical cardioversion may be required. Surgical myomectomy may be necessary in those patients who do not benefit from medical therapy. A portion of the hypertrophied septum is resected, and this may relieve outflow tract obstruction and symptoms.

Anticoagulation with warfarin should be administered to patients in atrial fibrillation due to the risk of systemic emboli. All patients with IHSS should receive prophylactic antibiotics before dental or surgical procedures, because of the risk of endocarditis.

The prognosis of IHSS is variable. In two-thirds of patients with obstruction, symptoms remain stable or improve. The remaining one-third have a worsening of symptoms. Unfortunately, some patients who have appeared stable develop sudden death. Sudden death in IHSS bears no relationship to the severity of the outflow gradient. It is more common in young people, among certain families, in patients with syncope, and in patients with severe dyspnea on the last follow-up visit. Sudden death does not seem to be prevented by the usual medical or surgical therapy. In patients with severe ventricular arrhythmias despite beta blockade, additional antiarrhythmic agents are indicated.

Nonobstructive Hypertrophic Cardiomyopathy

Nonobstructive hypertrophic cardiomyopathy may represent symmetrical hypertrophy of the left ventricular walls or ASH. There is a wide range of clinical symptomatology, from totally asymtomatic to patients with severe dyspnea on exertion, orthopnea, and paroxysmal nocturnal dyspnea. Angina may be present. Late in the course of this illness, hypertrophic cardiomyopathy may be difficult to differentiate from congestive cardiomyopathy. Physical examination reveals a left ventricular heave and palpable and audible S_4. In patients with ASH, even without obstruction, a systolic ejection murmur may be present due to mitral regurgitation or an increased rate of systolic flow. Chest x-ray film reveals various degrees of left ventricular enlargement; left atrial enlargement may be visualized as well. ECG reveals left ventricular hypertrophy and left atrial enlargement.

Echocardiography is helpful in assessing whether the degree of septal wall thickening is equal to free wall thickening or whether the septum is disproportionately hypertrophied. Evidence of outflow obstruction (abnormal anterior systolic motion of the mitral valve, partial closure of the aortic valve in midsystole) is absent. Radionuclide studies with thallium can be used to demonstrate whether the septal thickening is disproportionate. Cardiac catheterization reveals no evidence of a left ventricular intracavitary gradient either at rest or with provocative maneuvers. Left ventricular end diastolic pressure is usually elevated. Angiography shows a hypercontractile left ventricle with a characteristic "banana-shaped" cavity, which is also seen with IHSS.

In patients with symptomatic symmetic hypertrophic cardiomyopathy, digitalis and diuretics may be instituted. Calcium blockers may be beneficial in reducing the abnormal diastolic properties of hypertrophic cardiomyopathy. Late in the course of nonobstructive asymmetric and symmetric hypertrophic cardiomyopathy, the clinical picture is similar to congestive cardiomyopathy and therapy is similar as well: low salt diet, restriction of activity that results in symptoms, diuretics, digitalis, vasodilators, antiarrhythmic and anticoagulant therapy for atrial fibrillation.

Restrictive Cardiomyopathy

Restrictive cardiomyopathy is characterized by a restriction of ventricular filling during diastole due to reduced ventricular compliance (increased left ventricular stiffness). Systolic contractile function of the ventricles is relatively intact. The clinical picture resembles that of constrictive pericarditis. There are several etiologies of restrictive cardiomyopathy, and these are presented in Table 3.

The clinical symptoms reflect the inability of the ventricles to fill during diastole and to provide an increase in cardiac output with increased demand. Fatigue, weakness, and poor exercise tolerance with dyspnea on exertion are common. Symptoms of reduced filling of the right ventricle include edema, ascites, right upper quadrant discomfort, and anorexia. Chest pain, similar in quality to that caused by myocardial ischemia, may be present in a small percentage of patients. Complications include atrial and ventricular arrhythmias and systemic emboli.

Physical examination reveals signs of systemic venous congestion, including distended neck veins, Kussmaul's sign (jugular venous pressure does not fall normally but rises with inspiration), edema, ascites, an enlarged tender liver, and hepatojugular reflux. The peripheral arterial pulse is typically narrow; the jugular venous pulse reveals a prominent a wave with a rapid x and y descent. The apex is displaced laterally, but in general, cardiomegaly is moderate and not as severe as in patients with congestive cardiomyopathy. Sinus tachycardia is often present. The heart sounds are often soft and an S_3 and S_4 are common. The murmurs of tricuspid and/ or mitral regurgitation may be present.

Table 3. Etiologies of Restrictive Cardiomyopathy

Infiltrative
    Sarcoidosis
    Amyloidosis
    Hemochromatosis
    Neoplasia

Endocardial fibroelastosis: Cardiac dilatation with diffuse endocardial hyperplasia. Thickened aortic and mitral valve; distorted papillary muscle; primary form affects infants.

Endomyocardial fibrosis: Fibrous endocardial lesions of the inflow portion of the ventricles; may involve AV valves and cause regurgitation. Occurs in tropical and subtropical Africa.

Scleroderma

Radiation

Postmyocarditis

Glycogen storage disease

Becker's disease: Cardiac dilatation with fibrosis of the papillary muscles and subendocardium associated with necrosis and mural thrombosis. Occurs in South Africa.

Löffler's endocarditis: dense endocardial fibrosis with overlying thrombosis occurs following an arteritis and eosinophilic infiltrate of the myocardium.

Table 4. Differentiating Features of Restrictive Cardiomyopathy versus Constrictive Pericarditis

	Restrictive Cardiomyopathy	Constrictive Pericarditis
Pulmonary capillary wedge pressure (PCW)	PCW > right atrial pressure	PCW = right atrial pressure
Pulmonary artery systolic pressure	Usually > than 40–50 mm Hg	Usually < 40–50 mm Hg
Right vs left ventricular end-diastolic pressures	Left ventricular > right ventricular end-diastolic pressure	Left ventricular usually = right ventricular end-diastolic pressures
Right ventricular end-diastolic pressure	Usually less than $\frac{1}{3}$ of right ventricular systolic pressure	Usually about $\frac{1}{3}$ of right ventricular systolic pressure
Cardiac output	Depressed	Often normal or only slightly depressed
Square-root sign in ventricular pressure tracings	More prominent in left ventricular tracing. May diminish with therapy	Sign is equally prominent in right and left ventricular pressure tracing
Right atrial pressure	< 15 mm Hg if PCW not markedly elevated	Usually > 15 mm Hg

On chest x-ray film, the heart is normal in size or demonstrates mild cardiomegaly with left ventricular and left atrial enlargement. Signs of pulmonary congestion may be present as well. Calcification within the pericardium suggests constrictive pericarditis rather than restrictive cardiomyopathy. Electrocardiographic features include diffuse low QRS voltage, nonspecific ST-T wave abnormalities, conduction disturbances, including first, second, and third degree heart block, bundle branch blocks, and atrial and ventricular arrhythmias.

Echocardiography often reveals thickening of the left ventricular walls (due to inflitrative processes, such as amyloid) and left atrial enlargement. The diagnosis of cardiac tamponade, sometimes confused with restrictive cardiomyopathy, is aided by the use of echocardiography. The left ventricular cavity may be normal, small, or slightly dilated. Left ventricular wall excursions are often reduced. In patients with amyloid cardiomyopathy, there is an inverse correlation between ECG voltage and muscle cross-sectional area by echocardiography. ^{99m}Tc pyrophosphate scans may show intense diffuse cardiac uptake in patients with amyloid. In patients with metastatic neoplasms or sarcoid granulomas, thallium-201 studies reveal defects in the myocardial walls.

Jugular venous pulse tracings reveal a prominent a wave; the v wave may be prominent as well with rapid x and y descents resulting in a characteristic "M" shaped tracing. Apexcardiography also reveals a prominent a wave.

There are a number of ancillary tests that aid in the diagnosis of the underlying disorder. These include high serum iron levels with hemochromatosis, hypercalcemia, which occurs in approximately 9% of patients with sarcoidosis, and rectal biopsy for diagnosing amyloidosis.

Cardiac catheterization reveals elevated end-diastolic pressures (left ventricular end-diastolic pressure is greater than the right ventricular end-diastolic pressure, in contrast to constrictive pericarditis, in which the left and right ventricular end-diastolic pressures are often equal). The diastolic portion of the ventricular pressure pulse reveals a dip and plateau configuration, resembling a square root sign. This occurs because of the limitation of ventricular filling by the restrictive process. The right atrial pressure curve is "M" shaped and similar to jugular venous pulse tracings described above. Right atrial and left atrial pressures are elevated as well. The systemic arterial pulse pressure is usually reduced. Myocardial biopsy is sometimes performed at the time of cardiac catheterization and can distinguish tumor from other infiltrative processes such as amyloidosis, hemochromatosis, or sarcoidosis. Left ventricular angiography may reveal diffusely reduced wall excursion. Differentiating between constrictive pericarditis and restrictive cardiomyopathy may be difficult and Table 4 lists some of the cardiac catheterization findings which help distinguish the two entities.

Therapy for symptomatic restrictive cardiomyopathy includes low-salt diet, use of diuretics, and vasodilator therapy with long acting nitrates. Digitalis is beneficial in some patients but should be used with caution, since patients with restrictive cardiomyopathy, especially amyloidosis, may be prone to digitalis toxicity. Isolated amyloid fibrils bind digoxin, suggesting that this interaction may play some role in the sensitivity of these patients to digitalis. Specific treatment is available for some forms of restrictive cardiomyopathy, depending upon the underlying etiology of the disease. For example, repeated phlebotomy for hemochromatosis may improve the cardiomyopathy, sarcoidosis may be treated by steroids, and neoplasms by chemotherapy or radiation. Patients with restrictive cardiomyopathy due to an infiltrative process, such as sarcoid, may develop complete heart block, requiring permanent pacemaker therapy. A-V sequential pacing may aid ventricular filling in this setting. Antiarrhythmic agents are sometimes required, and, in some patients with severe myopathy, anticoagulation is indicated to prevent thromboembolic complications.

Bibliography

Ali MR, Soto A, Maroongroge D, et al: Electrocardiographic changes after adriamycin chemotherapy. *Cancer* 43:465, 1979.

Baandrup U, Florio RA, Roters F, et al: Electron microscopic investigation of endomyocardial biopsy samples in hypertrophy and cardiomyopathy: A semiquantitative study in 48 patients. *Circulation* 63:1289, 1981.

Baandrup U, Florio RA, Rehahn M, et al: Critical analysis of endomyocardial biopsies from patients suspected of having cardiomyopathy. II: Comparison of histology and clinical haemodynamic information. *Br Heart J* 45:487, 1981.

Bashour T, Basha HS, Cheng TO: Hypocalcemic cardiomyopathy. *Chest* 78: 663, 1980.

Benjamin TJ, Schuster EH, Bulkley BH: Cardiac hypertrophy in idiopathic dilated congestive cardiomyopathy: A clinicopathologic study. *Circulation* 64:442, 1981.

Benotti JR, Grossman W, Braunwald E: Effects of amrinone on myocardial energy metabolism and hemodynamics in patients with severe congestive heart failure due to coronary artery disease. *Circulation* 62:28, 1980.

Benotti JR, Grossman W, Cohn PF: Clinical profile of restrictive cardiomyopathy. *Circulation* 61:1206, 1980.

Bjarnason I, Jonsson S, Hardarson T: Mode of inheritence of hypertrophic cardiomyopathy in Iceland: Echocardiographic study. *Br Heart J* 47:122, 1982.

Bonow RO, Rosing DR, Bacharach, et al: Effects of verapamil on left ventricular systolic function and diastolic filling in patients with hypertrophic cardiomyopathy. *Circulation* 64:787, 1981.

Bristow MR, Mason JW, Billingham ME, et al: Dose-effect and structure-function relationships in doxorubicin cardiomyopathy. *Am Heart J* 102:709, 1981.

Brigden W: Symposium on cardiomyopathy. *Postgrad Med J* 51:271, 1975.

Bulkley BH, Weisfeldt ML, Hutchins G: Idiopathic hypertrophic subaortic stenosis: Myocardial disarray with isometric contraction. *N Engl J Med* 296:135, 1971.

Burch GE: Cardiomyopathy. In Burch GE (ed). *Cardiovasc Clinics*. Philadelphia, FA Davis, 1972, p 395.

Burch GE, Giles TD, Colcolough HL: Ischemic cardiomyopathy. *Am Heart J* 79:291, 1970.

Carroll JD, Gaasch WH, McAdam KP: Amyloid cardiomyopathy: Characterization by a distinctive voltage/mass relation. *Am J Cardiol* 49:9, 1982.

Casanova M, Gamallo C, Quero-Jimenez M: Familial hypertrophic cardiomyopathy with unusual involvement of the right ventricle. *Eur J Cardiol* 9:145, 1979.

Chew C, Ziady GM, Raphael MJ, et al: The functional defect in amyloid heart diseases: The stiff heart syndrome. *Am J Cardiol* 36:438, 1975.

Cutler DJ, Isner JM, Bracey AW: Hemochromatosis heart disease: An unemphasized cause of potentially reversible restrictive cardiomyopathy. *Am J Med* 69:923, 1980.

Demakis JG and Rahimtoola SH: Peripartum cardiomyopathy. *Circulation* 64:964, 1971.

Epstein SE, Henry WL, Clark CE, et al: Asymmetric septal hypertrophy. *Ann Intern Med* 81:650, 1974.

Frank S, Braunwald E: Idiopathic hypertrophic subaortic stenosis: Clinical analysis of 126 patients with emphasis on the natural history. *Circulation* 37:759, 1968.

Fuster V, Gersh BJ, Giuliani ER, et al: The natural history of idiopathic dilated cardiomyopathy. *Am J Cardiol* 47:525, 1981.

Goldman MR, Boucher CA: Value of radionuclide imaging techniques in assessing cardiomyopathy. *Am J Cardiol* 46:1232, 1980.

Goodwin JF: Treatment of the cardiomyopathies. *Am J Cardiol* 32:341, 1973.

Goodwin JF: Prospects and predictions for the cardiomyopathies. *Circulation* 50:210, 1974.

Grosberg SJ: Hemochromatosis and heart failure: Presentation of a case with survival after three years treatment by repeated venesection. *Ann Intern Med* 54:550, 1961.

Ikram H, Chan H, Bennett SI, et al: Haemodynamic effects of acute beta-adrenergic receptor blockade in congestive cardiomyopathy. *Br Heart J* 42:311, 1979.

Kaltenbach M, Hopf R, Kober G, et al: Treatment of hypertrophic obstructive cardiomyopathy with verapamil. *Br Heart J* 42:35, 1979.

Kino M, Imamitchi H, Morigutchi M, et al: Cardiovascular status in asymptomatic alcoholics, with reference to the level of ethanol consumption. *Br Heart J* 46:545, 1981.

Klatsky AL, Friedman GD, Siegelaub AB: Alcohol use and cardiovascular disease: the Kaiser-Permanente experience. *Circulation* 64(3 Pt 2):III32, 1981.

Klein W, Brandt D, Maurer E: Hemodynamic assessment of prenalterol: a cardioselective beta agonist in patients with impaired left ventricular function. *Clin Cardiol* 4:325, 1981.

Krikler DM, Davies MJ, Rowland E, et al: Sudden death in hypertrophic cardiomyopathy: Associated accessory atrioventricular pathways. *Br Heart J* 43:245, 1980.

Lorell BH, Paulus WJ, Grossman W, et al: Improved diastolic function and systolic performance in hypertrophic cardiomyopathy after nifedipine. *N Engl J Med* 303:801, 1980.

Lorell BH, Paulus WJ, Grossman W, et al: Modification of abnormal left ventricular diastolic properties by nifedipine in patients with hypertrophic cardiomyopathy. *Circulation* 65:499, 1982.

McDonald CD, Burch GE, Walsh JJ: Alcoholic cardiomyopathy managed with prolonged bed rest. *Ann Intern Med* 74:681, 1971.

Maron BJ, Bonow RO, Seshagiri TN, et al: Hypertrophic cardiomyopathy with ventricular septal hypertrophy localized to the apical region of the left ventricle (apical hypertrophic cardiomyopathy). *Am J Cardiol* 49:1838, 1982.

Maron BJ, Gottdiener JS, Bonow RO, et al: Hypertrophic cardiomyopathy with unusual locations of left ventricular hypertrophy undetectable by M-mode echocardiography. Identification wide-angle two-dimensonal echocardiography. *Circulation* 63:409, 1981.

Maron BJ, Roberts WC, Epstein SE: Sudden death in hypertrophic cardiomyopathy: A profile of 78 patients. *Circulation* 65:1388, 1982.

Maron BJ, Roberts WC, McAllister HA, et al: Sudden death in young athletes. *Circulation* 62:218, 1980.

Maron BJ, Savage DD, Wolfson JK, et al: Prognostic significance of 24 hour ambulatory electrocardiographic monitoring in patients with hypertrophic cardiomyopathy: A prospective study. *Am J Cardiol* 48:252, 1981.

Mathews EC, Gardin JM, Henry WL, et al: Echocardiographic abnormalities in chronic alcoholics with and without overt congestive heart failure. *Am J Cardiol* 47:570, 1981.

Matsumori A, Hirose A, Wakabayashi, A, et al: HLA and hypertrophic cardiomyopathy. *Am Heart J* 97:428, 1979.

Mauther RK, Thomas I, Dhurandhar R, et al: Hypertrophic obstructive cardiomyopathy and coronary artery spasm. *Chest* 76:636, 1979.

McKenna W, Deanfield J, Faruqui A, et al: Prognosis in hypertrophic cardiomyopathy: Role of age and clinical electrocardiographic and hemodynamic features. *Am J Cardiol* 47:532, 1981.

McKenna WJ, England D, Doi YL, et al: Arrhythmias in hypertrophic cardiomyopathy. I: Influence on prognosis. *Br Heart J* 46:168, 1981.

Newman PE: Acute myocardial infarction with angiographically demonstrated normal coronary arteries in the presence of hypertrophic cardiomyopathy. *Chest* 78:893, 1980.

Olsen EGJ: Congestive cardiomyopathy. *Postgrad Med J* 54:429, 1978.

Pasternac A, Noble J, Streulens Y, et al: Pathophysiology of chest pain in patients with cardiomyopathies and normal coronary arteries. *Circulation* 65:778, 1982.

Perloff JK: The cardiomyopathies: Current perspective. *Circulation* 44:942, 1971.

Praga C, Beretta G, Vigo PL, et al: Adriamycin cardiotoxicity: A survey of 1,273 patients. *Cancer Treat Rep* 63:827, 1979.

Regan TJ, Haider B: Ethanol abuse and heart disease. *Circulation* 64:(3 PT 2):III-14, 1981.

Roberts WC, Ferrans VJ: Pathologic anatomy of the cardiomyopathies. *Hum Pathol* 6:287, 1975.

Rosing DR, Kent KM, Maron BJ: Verapamil therapy: A new approach to pharmacologic treatment of hypertrophic cardiomyopathy. *Chest* 78(Suppl I):239, 1980.

Rosing DR, Kent KM, Borer JS: Verapamil therapy: A new approach to the pharmacologic treatment of hypertrophic cardiomyopathy. I: Hemodynamic effects. *Circulation* 60:1201, 1979.

Rubin E: Cardiovascular effects of alcohol. *Pharmacol Biochem Behav* 13 Suppl 1:37, 1980.

Rubinow A, Skinner M, Cohen AS: Digoxin sensitivity in amyloid cardiomyopathy. *Circulation* 63:1285, 1981.

Santos AD, Miller RP, Mathew PK, et al: Echocardiographic characterization of the reversible cardiomyopathy of hypothyroidism. *Am J Med* 68:675, 1980.

Savage DD, Seides SF, Maron BJ, et al: Prevalence of arrhythmias during 24-hour electrocardiographic monitoring and exercise testing in patients with obstructive and nonobstructive hypertrophic cardiomyopathy. *Circulation* 59:866, 1979.

Schoolmaster WL, Simpson AG, Sauerbrunn BJ, et al: Radionuclide angiographic assessment of left ventricular function during exercise in patients with severely reduced ejection fraction. *Am J Cardiol* 47:804, 1981.

Short EM, Winkle RA, Billingham ME: Myocardial involvement in idiopathic hemochromatosis. Morphological and clinical improvement following venesection. *Am J Med* 70:1275, 1981.

Silverman KJ, Hutchins G, Bulkley B: Cardiac sarcoid: A clinicopathologic study of 84 unselected patients with systemic sarcoidosis. *Circulation* 58:1204, 1978.

Spodick DH: Effective management of congestive cardiomyopathy: Relation to ventricular structure and function. *Arch Intern Med* 142:689, 1982.

St. John Sutton MG, Iajik AJ, Gioliani ER: Hypertrophic obstructive cardiomyopathy and lentiginosis: A little known neural ectodermal syndrome. *Am J Cardiol* 47:214, 1981.

Swedberg K, Hjalmarson A, Waagstein F, et al: Beneficial effects of long-term beta-blockade in congestive cardiomyopathy. *Br Heart J* 44:117, 1980.

Unverferth DV, Leier CV, Maguriea RD, et al: Improvement of human myocardial mitochondria after dobutamine: A quantitative ultrastructural study. *J Pharmacol Exp Ther* 215:527, 1980.

Unverferth DV, Magorien RD, Lewis RP: Long-term benefit of dobutamine in patients with congestive cardiomyopathy. *Am Heart J* 100:622, 1980.

VonHoff DD, Layard MW, Basa P: Risk factors for doxorubicin-induced congestive heart failure. *Ann Intern Med* 91:710, 1979.

Weber KT, Andrews V, Janicki JS: Cardiotonic agents in the management of chronic cardiac failure. *Am Heart J* 103:(4 PT 2):639, 1982.

Wizenberg TA, Moz J, Sohn YH, et al: Value of positive myocardial technetium-99-m pyrophosphate scintigraphy in the noninvasive diagnosis of cardiac amyloidosis. *Am Heart J* 103(4 PT 1):468, 1982.

Wynne J, Braunwald E: The cardiomyopathies and myocarditis, in Braunwald E (ed): *Heart Disease. A Textbook of Cardiovascular Medicine.* Philadelphia, Saunders, 1980, p. 1437.

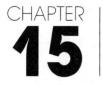

CHAPTER **15** | # MYOCARDITIS
Robert A. Kloner

Myocarditis is an inflammatory process that involves the heart. There is a wide variety of causes, including infectious agents (viruses, bacteria, mycobacteria, rickettsia, protozoa, metazoa), physical agents, chemicals, drugs, and radiation (Table 1). Myocarditis may be an acute process, as in most cases due to virus, or a chronic process, such as the chronic phase of Chagas' disease. Idiopathic congestive cardiomyopathy may, in some patients, be due to a prior unrecognized episode of viral myocarditis. Mild episodes of myocarditis are, in fact, often difficult to diagnose, especially when the symptoms are overshadowed by the presence of a systemic illness and when there is little in the way of cardiac dysfunction. In such cases, nonspecific electrocardiographic abnormalities may be the only clinical manifestation. From 4 to 10% of all routine autopsies show evidence of focal or diffuse myocarditis.

General Clinical Manifestations

There is a wide range of clinical manifestations of myocarditis from the asymptomatic patient with electrocardiographic abnormalities only (usually ST-T wave changes) to the patient with severe congestive heart failure. Symptoms consist of fatigue, dyspnea, palpitations, and chest pain suggesting pericarditis or myocardial ischemia. Tachycardia is out of proportion to the degree of fever. The S_1 is soft; ventricular gallops, a transient apical systolic murmur, and pericardial friction rub may be heard. In severe cases associated with congestive heart failure, pulmonary rales and pulsus alternans may be present. Systemic or pulmonary emboli are complications of myocarditis. The physical findings related to the underlying cause of the myocarditis should be sought; for example, the suppurative pharyngeal membrane of diphtheria or skin rashes associated with Rickettsial infection.

Chest x-ray film is either normal or reveals cardiac dilatation, in severe cases, with or without signs of pulmonary congestion. ECG demonstrates ST-T wave abnormalities and, commonly, ventricular and atrial arrhythmias. Other electrocardiographic features include low QRS voltage, conduction disturbances, and occasionally Q waves.

Echocardiography may demonstrate reduced ventricular contractile function and pericardial effusion. Radionuclide ventriculography also can detect reduced left ventricular function. A recent study by Das et al. showed that asymptomatic patients with prior myocarditis may have left ventricular dysfunction during exercise as assessed by radionuclide ventriculography.

313

Table 1. Etiologies of Myocarditis

Infectious myocarditis
a. Viral: Coxsackie (especially group B), echovirus, poliovirus, influenza, mumps, Ebstein–Barr virus, viral hepatitis, rabies, rubella, rubeola, varicella
b. Bacterial: Diphtheria, tuberculosis, salmonella (typhoid fever), streptococcus (rheumatic fever or direct streptococcal myocarditis), meningococcus, clostridia (gas gangrene or tetanus), myocarditis associated with bacterial endocarditis, brucellosis
c. Spirochetal myocarditis: Syphilis, leptospirosis (Weil's disease), relapsing fever
d. Rickettsial myocarditis: Typhus, Rocky Mountain spotted fever, Q fever
e. Psittacosis
f. Primary atypical pneumonia (mycoplasma)
g. Fungal: candidiasis, aspergilosis, histoplasmosis, actinomycosis, blastomycosis
h. Protozoal myocarditis: Trypanosoma cruzi (Chagas' disease), African trypanosomiasis (sleeping sickness), malaria, toxoplasmosis, amebiasis
i. Metazoal myocarditis: Schistosomiasis, trichinosis, ascarisis, cysticercosis, echinococcus
Myocardial damage due to chemicals, drugs, toxins
a. Antineoplastic agents: Anthracyclines, cyclophosphamide
b. Metal poisoning: Lead, mercury, arsenic
c. Antiparasitic agents: Emetine, chloroquine, antimony compounds
d. Catecholamines (e.g., pheochromocytoma)
e. Psychotropic drugs: Phenothiazines, lithium
f. Animal toxins: Snake bite, wasp, spider, scorpion stings
g. Carbon monoxide
h. Phosphorus
Physical agents: Radiation, hypothermia, heat stroke
Hypersensitivity reactions: Methyldopa, penicillin, sulfonamides, tetracycline, phenylbutazone, serum sickness, rejection of cardiac transplant, collagen vascular diseases

Although most patients recover rapidly from acute myocarditis, a minority develop chronic myocarditis and subsequent dilated cardiomyopathy. A small percentage of patients develop a fulminant illness and die from severe left ventricular failure.

In general, therapy is supportive. Adequate rest and oxygenation are important, as exercise and hypoxemia may increase the damage of myocarditis. Congestive heart failure is treated with salt restriction, diuretics, and digitalis. Patients with myocarditis tend to be sensitive to digitalis; hence, caution is needed with its use. Patients should be monitored for the development of conduction disturbances and arrhythmias. In general, corticosteroids are avoided in patients with viral myocarditis, as viral replication and myocardial necrosis may be hastened by these agents. Although, at present, there are no definite antiviral agents for the therapy of viral myocarditis, experimental animal studies suggest that interferon-stimulating agents may become beneficial. Antibiotics are used for treating specific myocarditides, such as those associated with bacteria (salmonella, meningococcus, diphtheria), psittacosis, mycoplasma, and tuberculosis. Antitoxin is used for diphtheria myocarditis. If the myocarditis is due to chemicals, drugs, or physical agents, the offending substances or agents are withdrawn.

Selected Specific Myocarditides

VIRAL MYOCARDITIS

The clinical manifestations of myocarditis often do not present until several weeks after an initial systemic viral infection. Coxsackie B and echovirus are two of the most common causes of viral myocarditis. In the adult, most Coxsackie infections are probably subclinical or obscured by upper respiratory tract symptoms, arthralgia, myalgia, pleurodynia, and fever. Cardiac manifestations in adults include pericardial chest pain and palpitations, and in severe cases include cardiac dilatation and symptoms and signs of congestive heart failure. The ECG shows ST-T wave abnormalities; arrhythmias and conduction abnormalities are common. Helpful laboratory tests include isolation of virus from blood, throat, or rectal swabs and antibody titer determinations during acute and convalescent phases. Cardiac enzymes may be elevated. Rest is indicated; exercise and corticosteroids may exacerbate viral myocarditis. Most patients recover within weeks, although electrocardiographic abnormalities often persist for months. Coxsackie myocarditis occasionally is fatal in adults; neonates tend to have a more malignant course than adults. Some patients who have viral myocarditis may eventually develop congestive cardiomyopathy.

ACUTE RHEUMATIC FEVER See Chapter 13.

DIPHTHERIA

Myocardial involvement occurs in approximately 25% of cases of diphtheria and may lead to severe cardiac dysfunction and, in some cases, death. The myocarditis is due to a toxin produced by the diphtheria bacillus. Clinical manifestations of myocarditis typically appear at the end of the first week of illness and include congestive heart failure, arrhythmias, conduction defects, and ST-T wave abnormalities on the ECG. Cases of sudden cardiovascular collapse have been reported. Treatment includes administration of antitoxin, respiratory support, antibiotics (penicillin G or erythromycin), and salt restriction and diuretics for congestive heart failure. Digitalis should be administered cautiously because of the complication of increased atrioventricular (AV) block. Transvenous pacemaker therapy is instituted for complete AV block.

CHAGAS' DISEASE (TRYPANOSOMIASIS)

Chagas' disease is the most common form of heart disease in Central and South America and is caused by the protozoan Trypanosoma cruzi. The protozoan is transmitted to humans through the bite of an insect. In the acute phase of the illness, patients are usually asymptomatic or experience constitutional symptoms of fever, sweating, muscle pains, vomiting, and diarrhea along with myocarditis and hepatosplenomegaly. Tachycardia and congestive heart failure may be present. Most patients recover over the course of months. There is a latent phase of approximately 10–30 years, followed by a chronic phase in 30% of infected patients.

Chronic Chagas' disease may be due to an autoimmune mechanism and is characterized by cardiac hypertrophy and fibrosis, mononuclear cell infiltration in the region of the sinoatrial and AV node, bundle of His and subepicardial ganglions, degeneration of myocardial fibers, and, often, mural thrombi. The clinical manifestations include signs of right-sided (fatigue, edema, ascites, hepatic congestion) greater than left-sided (dyspnea, orthopnea) congestive heart failure, cardiomegaly, arrhythmias, and right bundle branch block. Physical examination reveals a widely split S_2 due to right bundle branch block and a loud P_2 due to pulmonary hypertension. The murmur of tricuspid regurgitation is common. Ventricular ectopic activity is a frequent finding, and some patients develop syncope and sudden death due to ventricular fibrillation even before signs of heart failure have developed. Laboratory evidence of Chagas' disease includes a positive complement fixation test (Machado-Guerreiro test) or detection of parasites in the blood of patients with the illness. Electrocardiographic abnormalities include AV and bundle branch block, decreased QRS voltage, prolonged QT interval, T wave abnormalities, and bradycardia.

In general, therapy is supportive; prevention includes control of the insect vector. Patients with high degree of AV block may require pacemaker therapy; antiarrhythmic agents, in combination with pacemaker therapy, are used for treating patients with both arrhythmias and high degrees of AV block. Digitalis may be used with caution. Two agents for treating acute Chagas' disease (nifurtimox and benznidazole) have shown promise in decreasing the length of illness and in reducing parasitemia and early mortality. In general, there is no specific therapy for the chronic form of the illness, although in selected subgroups, the latter two agents may be effective. Congestive heart failure is treated with diuretics, afterload reducing agents, and cautious use of digitalis.

TRICHINOSIS

Trichinosis is an illness due to infestation with the helminth Trichinella spiralis. It is the most common helminthic infestation in humans, and myocarditis is its most serious complication. Although the parasites invade the heart, they do not encyst in the myocardium. Cardiac damage may be due to inflammation or a hypersensitivity reaction produced in response to the parasites. The initial clinical manifestations include muscle tenderness, periorbital edema, and eosinophilia. Cardiac symptoms include dyspnea, palpitations, and chest pain; these typically occur approximately three weeks after the initial onset of the illness. Arrhythmias and congestive heart failure may be present. Electrocardiographic abnormalities are common and include T wave changes, prolongation of the QRS interval, low QRS voltage, and prolonged PR interval. The diagnosis is established by demonstration of larval forms in gastrocnemius muscle biopsies; eosinophilia and a positive skin test provide supportive evidence of the diagnosis. The myocarditis has been successfully treated with corticosteroids. Thiabendazole is also an effective mode of therapy.

Bibliography

Abelmann WH: Viral myocarditis and its sequelae. *Ann Rev Med* 24:145, 1973.
Abelmann WH: Myocarditis. *N Engl J Med* 275:832, 1966.

Cambridge G, MacArthur CGC, Waterson AP, et al: Antibodies to Coxsackie B viruses in congestive cardiomyopathy. *Brit Heart J* 41:692, 1979.

Das SK, Brady TJ, Thrall JH, et al. Cardiac function in patients with prior myocarditis. *J Nucl Med* 21:689, 1980.

Gerzen P, Granath A, Holmgren B, et al: Acute myocarditis: A follow-up study. *Br Heart J* 34:575, 1972.

Grey DF, Morse BS, Phillips WF: Trichinosis with neurologic and cardiac involvement: Review of the literature and report of three cases. *Ann Intern Med* 57:230, 1962.

Helle EP, Koskenvua K, Heikkila J, et al: Myocardial complications of immunizations. *Ann Clin Res* 10:280, 1978.

Levine HD: Virus myocarditis: A critique of the literature from clinical, electrocardiographic, and pathologic standpoints. *Am J Med Sci* 277:132, 1979.

Monif GRG, Lee CW, and Hsiung GD: Isolated myocarditis with recovery of ECHO type 9 virus from the myocardium. *N Engl J Med* 277:1353, 1967.

Morales AR, Vichitbandh P, Chandraung P, et al: Pathologic features of cardiac conduction disturbances in diphtheritic myocarditis. *Arch Pathol Lab Med* 91:1, 1971.

Rosenbaum MB: Chagasic myocardiopathy. *Prog Cardiovasc Dis* 7:199, 1964.

Sainani GS, Dekate MP, Rao CP: Heart disease caused by Coxsackie virus B infection. *Br Heart J* 37:819, 1975.

Solarz SD: An electrocardiographic study of one hundred and fourteen consecutive cases of trichinosis. *Am Heart J* 34:230, 1947.

Steere AC, Batsford WP, Weinberg M, et al: Lyme carditis: Cardiac abnormalities of Lyme disease. *Ann Intern Med* 93:8, 1980.

DIAGNOSIS AND MANAGEMENT OF CARDIAC ARRHYTHMIAS

Thomas B. Graboys
Elliott M. Antman

This chapter will present a unified, concise approach to the cardiac arrhythmias. Management of patients presenting with rhythm disorders requires judgment, experience, and integration of the electrocardiographic abnormality within the context of each patient's clinical status.

Differential Diagnosis of Tachyarrhythmias

The differential diagnosis of cardiac arrhythmias is facilitated by a classification based upon the width of the QRS interval and the regularity or irregularity of the RR cycle. Thus, when one encounters a tachycardia, a logical progression in the differentiation of the rhythm is to determine if the QRS is wide or narrow and the cycling regular or irregular (Table 1). The major differential diagnosis of any wide regular tachycardia would be ventricular tachycardia (VT), supraventricular tachycardia (SVT) with aberration, or preexcitation with antegrade accessory tract conduction.

Wide irregular tachyarrhythmia would probably be atrial fibrillation with either aberrancy, fixed, or rate related bundle branch block. Narrow QRS regular tachycardias fall into the following categories: sinus, supraventricular tachycardia (SVT), junctional tachycardia (JT), or atrial flutter (AFL). Irregular narrow complex tachycardias would then either be atrial fibrillation (AF) or multifocal atrial tachycardia (MAT).

WIDE, REGULAR TACHYCARDIA

Ventricular Tachycardia

By standard definition, three or more consecutive rapid ventricular beats constitute a salvo of ventricular tachycardia. The QRS is wide and, at times, bizarre, particularly if the origin of the tachycardia is sufficiently distant from the normal specialized conduction system. Ventricular activity is independent of that within the atrium, resulting in atrioventricular (AV) dissociation (Fig. 1). The hallmark on the ECG is partial capture if the sinus mechanism coincides with ventricular depolari-

Table 1.   A Classification of Tachycardia

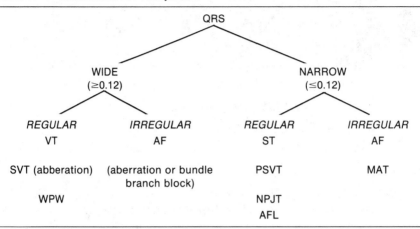

	WIDE (≥0.12)		NARROW (≤0.12)	
	REGULAR	*IRREGULAR*	*REGULAR*	*IRREGULAR*
	VT	AF	ST	AF
	SVT (abberation)	(aberration or bundle branch block)	PSVT	MAT
	WPW		NPJT	
			AFL	

Key: VT, ventricular tachycardia; SVT, supraventricular tachycardia; WPW, Wolff-Parkinson-White; AF, atrial fibrillation; ST, sinus tachycardia; PSVT, paroxysmal supraventricular tachycardia; NPJT, nonparoxysmal junctional tachycardia; AFL, atrial flutter; MAT, multifocal atrial tachycardia.

zation from the VT focus, resulting in a fusion beat. It is important to emphasize that, if possible, a full 12 lead ECG be obtained, so as not to base the diagnosis of a tachyarrhythmia on a single lead, in which the QRS may be spuriously narrow.

The rate of VT is quite variable and dependent on the clinical circumstances. The form of VT occurring within the setting of an acute myocardial infarction (so-called VT of the vulnerable period, VT vp) is typically rapid and accelerating, and it deteriorates to ventricular fibrillation, often within 30–60 seconds. This is in contrast to paroxysmal VT in the nonischemic setting, in which the rate may be a constant 150 beats per minute (bpm). Typically, VT salvos are in the range of 150–200 bpm. Therapy with antiarrhythmic drugs may result in slower nonsustained salvos, with

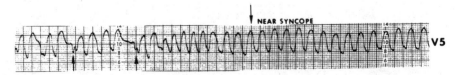

Figure 1   Ventricular tachycardia with AV dissociation (arrows).

rates between 100–150 bpm. The rate of VT may exceed 200; SVT with aberration should be suspected if the rate exceeds 250 bpm and the QRS is between 120–140 ms.

Slow ventricular foci may represent an idioventricular escape mechanism (60–100 bpm), VT with 2:1 exit block from the site of tachycardia, or the electrophysiologic effect of antiarrhythmic drugs producing periods of "slow VT." At times, it may be difficult to differentiate electrocardiographically an accelerated idioventricular focus from VT in which the rate has been slowed.

Supraventricular Tachycardia with Aberrancy

In this condition (see Table 2), the rate of the tachycardia is usually between 160–220 bpm, although frequently exceeds 250 bpm in the presence of concealed bypass tracts or known preexcitation. The QRS is between 0.11 and 0.13 s. More commonly a right bundle branch block pattern is noted, although left ventricular tachycardia may also appear as right-sided intraventricular conduction disturbance. One helpful differentiation is that SVT with aberration usually does not result in QRS durations beyond 0.13 seconds. A vigorous search for P waves preceding each QRS should be undertaken, utilizing special leads if necessary (Lewis, esophageal, or right atrial). Frequently, differentiation from VT is facilitated if the onset of the tachycardia has been recorded. The initial premature beat is noted to be narrow, followed by progressive widening of the QRS as rate-related aberrancy ensues.

Carotid sinus massage (CSM) is one maneuver that often assists in differentiating SVT with aberration from ventricular tachycardia. CSM may interrupt the reentrant mechanism by inducing vagotonia and terminating the tachycardia. If the mechanism

Table 2. Factors in the ECG Diagnosis of VT or SVT with Aberration

	VT	SVT aberration
AV dissociation	+	−
Fusion beats	+	−
QRS width	>140 msec	<140 msec
QRS morphology		
RBBB	Monophasic, LAD	Triphasic, normal axis
LBBB	Wide RV$_1$	−
	RAD	−
Regularity	80%	95%
Onset	VPB	APB with ↑ QRS
CSP	− (<2%)	+ (30%)
Rate (bpm)	150–200	>200

Key: VT, ventricular tachycardia; SVT, supraventricular tachycardia; LAD, left axis deviation; RAD, right axis deviation; VPB, ventricular premature beat; APB, atrial premature beat; CSP, carotid sinus pressure; RBBB, right bundle branch block; LBBB, left bundle branch block.

23 yr. m.

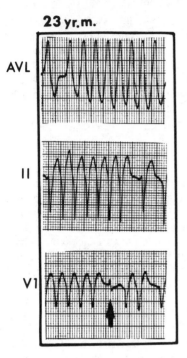

AVL

II

V1

Figure 2 Atrial fibrillation with rapid ventricular response in a patient with WPW indicating anterograde accessory tract conduction.

is atrial flutter, CSM may slow conduction, converting a 2:1 or 1:1 response transiently to 2:1 or 4:1, resulting in normalization of conduction and confirming the presence of aberration. Rarely, CSM may terminate an episode of ventricular tachycardia.

Certain physical findings are helpful in differentiating an aberrated rhythm from ventricular tachycardia. Heart sounds are constant in SVT, as opposed to the variable intensity and splitting of both S_1 and S_2 during ventricular tachycardia. The presence of Cannon a waves observed in the jugular pulse indicates AV dissociation and a ventricular origin of the tachycardia.

Preexcitation Syndromes

These syndromes will be discussed in detail in a separate section. Among those patients with Wolff-Parkinson-White syndrome whose atrial mechanism is fibrillation or flutter, the refractory period of the anomalous pathway may be sufficiently short that rapid conduction with rates in excess of 300 bpm ensues (Fig. 2).

WIDE, IRREGULAR TACHYCARDIA

Torsade de Pointes

Torsade de pointes (Fig. 3) represents chaotic nonsustained ventricular activity that is invariably associated with serious symptoms. The electrocardiographic hallmark is rapid, bizzare QRS complexes, with recurrent alteration of the QRS axis. Etiologic

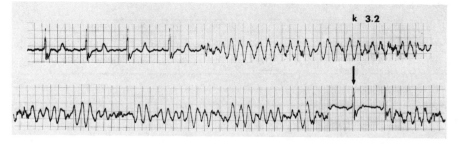

Figure 3 Torsade de pointes (nonsustained ventricular flutter) in a hypokalemic patient receiving quinidine.

factors include antiarrhythmic drugs (the most common being quinidine); phenothiazines; electrolyte disturbances (particularly hypokalemia), hereditary and acquired QT prolongation, AV block, and coronary vasospasm.

Atrial Fibrillation with Aberrancy or Bundle Branch Block

Occasionally, patients with acute onset of atrial fibrillation, particularly in the setting of left ventricular failure, will present with a wide QRS, slightly irregular tachycardia that may be confused with VT. Close scrutiny of the cycle lengths and carotid sinus pressure that slows the ventricular response invariably secure the diagnosis.

NARROW, REGULAR TACHYARRHYTHMIAS

Sinus Tachycardia

Sinus tachycardia is defined as acceleration of the normal sinus mechanism beyond 105 bpm. P waves with the same general morphology as the normal sinus P wave precede each QRS. As the rate increases, the P wave may appear somewhat peaked, and the PR interval may shorten, indicating facilitation of AV conduction. Rates rarely exceed 160 bpm in the adult. However, under unusual circumstances (e.g., thyrotoxicosis), sinus tachycardia may range from 150–200 bpm. The rhythm is typically regular, and the response to carotid sinus massage is gradual slowing, with prompt resumption of the tachycardia. CSM is particularly helpful if there is either rate related or underlying bundle branch block. In this circumstance, particularly if the PR interval is somewhat prolonged, the P wave becomes fused with the preceding T wave at rapid rates; and the rhythm may appear to be ventricular tachycardia. With CSM, slowing unveils the P waves and confirms the presence of a sinus mechanism.

Supraventricular Tachycardia

When there is a rapid atrial mechanism, 150–250 bpm, the diagnosis of paroxysmal supraventricular tachycardia (PSVT) should be entertained (see Figs. 4, 5). Recent

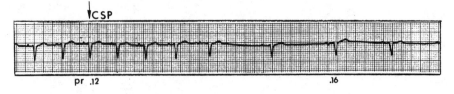

Figure 4 Slow paroxysmal supraventricular tachycardia (PSVT) at 100 bpm reverts to sinus rhythm with carotid sinus pressure (CSP).

development in the techniques of intracardiac recordings have led to a greater understanding of the pathophysiologic mechanisms responsible for PSVT. The two basic mechanisms are reentry and enhanced automaticity. Reentrant rhythms involve a complex mechanism, the substrate of which is electrophysiologic inhomogeneity of adjacent cardiac tissue.

AV nodal reentrant tachycardias account for approximately 60% of cases of PSVT. In approximately ¾ of patients with AV nodal (juntional) reentrant tachycardia, dual AV nodal pathways can be demonstrated in the electrophysiology laboratory. The AV node contains two functionally different pathways, designated alpha and beta. The alpha pathway is slower conducting, but its refractory period is shorter than the faster conducting beta pathway. Atrial premature beats that are sufficiently early block in the beta pathway and conduct slowly in the anterograde direction down the alpha pathway. The beta pathway is then available for retrograde conduction, and the appropriate substrate for reentrant tachycardias is established. As with most forms of reentrant SVT, either an atrial premature beat (APB) or ventricular premature beat (VPB) can initiate AV nodal reentrant tachycardias.

If the genesis of the atrial tachycardia is enhanced automaticity, one will observe a P wave preceding each QRS. The P wave will be morphologically different from the sinus P wave and it will fire at a constant rate of 160–250 bpm.

The response to vagal maneuvers, such as carotid sinus massage, is variable. Thus, if the mechanism is reentry, there may be slowing or abrupt termination of the reentrant tachycardia. If the genesis of the arrhythmia is based on automaticity, such maneuvers may have no effect, or only briefly return to sinus rhythm.

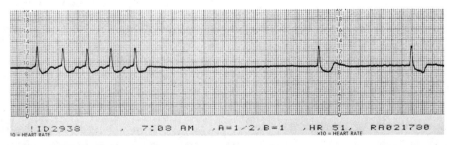

Figure 5 Spontaneous termination of PSVT with asymptomatic offset pause and junctional escape beat.

Atrial Flutter

Atrial flutter is categorized by coarse, regular, "saw tooth" undulations of the baseline referred to as F waves. The rate of appearance of these F waves is approximately 300 bpm (Fig. 6). The majority of episodes of atrial flutter are associated with 2:1 AV block and a resultant ventricular response of 150 bpm. Indeed, any regular narrow tachycardia at 150 bpm should be considered atrial flutter until proven otherwise. CSM, as noted, is most helpful in diagnosis by inducing an increase in AV block, a slowing of the ventricular response, and a disclosure of the flutter waves. The bulk of evidence to date suggests that atrial flutter is due to a reentrant mechanism involving pathways in the atrium. This reentrant mechanism commonly results in a predominantly negative deflection of the flutter waves in the inferior leads. A less common type of atrial flutter involves an oppositely directed reentrant circuit, such that the flutter waves are predominantly positive in the inferior leads.

When the frequency of the atrial rate is as low as 250, it must be differentiated from SVT; at higher frequencies, such as 400, atrial flutter must be differentiated from atrial fibrillation. Pharmacologic interventions may alter the rate of the flutter mechanism. Thus, drugs that prolong the effective refractory period, such as quinidine, procainamide, and disopyramide, will reduce the flutter rate from 300 to 200–250. Drugs that shorten repolarization, such as digitalis, may enhance the flutter rate, as is commonly observed during digitalization; approximately $\frac{1}{3}$ of patients in atrial flutter will convert to atrial fibrillation.

Nonparoxysmal Junctional Tachycardia (NPJT)

NPJT is a manifestation of enhanced automaticity of the AV junction. The average rate is 70–130 bpm. This arrhythmia may be a manifestation of digitalis toxicity, or it may be associated with inferior myocardial infarction (MI) or be seen in the postoperative cardiac surgical patient or observed in patients with severe mitral valvular disease. Patients with acute rheumatic fever and rare individuals who have no other significant heart disease may manifest NPJT.

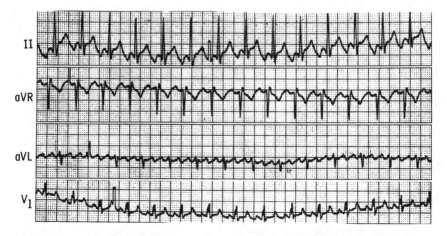

Figure 6   Atrial flutter with atrial rate of 315 and 3:1 atrioventricular response.

NARROW IRREGULAR TACHYCARDIAS

Atrial Fibrillation

It has been suggested that both atrial flutter and fibrillation are part of a spectrum of intraatrial reentry. A shift of atrial flutter to fibrillation can be seen when the flutter waves break down into multiple smaller reentrant wavelets. The creation of such wavelets depends on the circulating impulses encountering areas of inhomogeneous refractoriness, resulting in secondary wavelets in multiple areas of reentry. This produces the chaotic small amplitude fibrillatory waves seen in atrial fibrillation. Borderline cases are seen and may be described as impure flutter or flutter-fibrillation. Because of the extremely high rate of discharge of the fibrillating atrium (500–600 cycles per minute), impulses arriving in the AV junction present a disorganized wave front with insufficient potency to be consistently conducted to the ventricular specialized conduction system (also see Chapter 3).

Although atrial fibrillation at times may be paroxysmal, it is often a chronic stable rhythm. The critical determinant of the clinical response to atrial fibrillation is the rapidity of the ventricular rate. The average ventricular response among patients not receiving beta blockers or digitalis drugs to atrial fibrillation is 160 bpm. More rapid ventricular responses are noted in certain clinical conditions. Thus, patients with thyrotoxicosis, preexcitation, or serious myocardial or valvular disease; patients receiving sympathomimetic agents, such as those utilized in chronic obstructive pulmonary disease; alcoholic cardiomyopathics; and patients with certain electrolyte disorders, such as hypokalemia and hypomagnesemia, may exhibit a ventricular rate over 160 (Fig. 2). Among patients with intrinsic AV junctional conduction abnormality, slower ventricular responses may be observed. Thus, the patient who is not on medication and presents with a ventricular response to atrial fibrillation between 60 and 100 beats per minute should be considered to have an intrinsic AV junctional conduction disorder. Occasionally, athletes with extreme vagotonia may present with atrial fibrillation and a slow ventricular response.

Multifocal Atrial Tachycardia

Multifocal atrial tachycardia is defined as a tachyarrhythmia in which the atrial rate is greater than 100 bpm (Fig. 7). There are well organized discrete P waves of at least three separate morphologies, and there is an irregular variation in the P to P interval. An isoelectric baseline is noted between P waves. MAT is associated with a high mortality rate, primarily due to its association with severe decompensated pulmonary disease. It is important to distinguish this mechanism from other supraventricular rhythm disturbances. Although sinus tachycardia with multifocal APBs usually has a rate greater than 100 bpm, it can be differentiated from MAT by the predominantly uniform P to P intervals and P wave morphology except for isolated APBs. The most important differentiation is atrial fibrillation versus MAT. The indistinct morphology of atrial activity and undulating baseline of atrial fibrillation stand in contrast to the discrete P waves and isoelectric baseline seen in MAT. CSP may transiently decrease the rate of atrial activity in MAT, but this quickly returns to control levels after release of CSP. At times, patients exhibiting MAT will also experience atrial fibrillation, thus making a unified diagnosis of the dysrhythmia difficult.

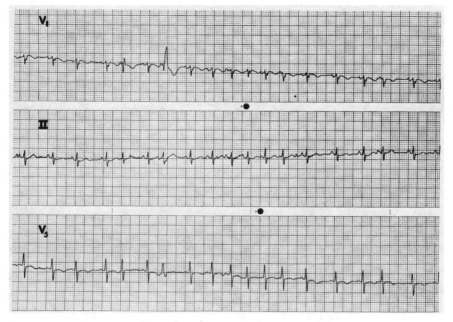

Figure 7 Multifocal atrial tachycardia (MAT). Note variable rate and P wave morphology.

Therapy for Cardiac Arrhythmias See Tables 3 and 4.

Ventricular Tachycardia

Ventricular tachycardia, when it occurs in the acute stage of MI, must be treated immediately. The clinical circumstances dictate acute management. Patients who are hemodynamically unstable during VT and exhibit a change in mental status should be promptly cardioverted. If the patient has lost consciousness, a precordial blow may be successful in reverting VT to sinus rhythm. The small amount of energy delivered by a precordial thump (1 watt second) is frequently sufficient to depolarize enough myocardium and initiate a propagated response by electromechanical transduction. Once ventricular tachycardia has degenerated to ventricular fibrillation, the steep rise in energy requirement for termination of VF then renders chest thumping ineffective. The present recommendation is that chest thump be reserved for monitored patients only, the concern being that a thump delivered during the ventricular vulnerable period may result in VF. However, the possibility that this event will occur is less than 5%. Lidocaine is the drug of choice for complex forms of ventricular premature beats (repetitive, early cycle), ventricular premature beats occurring during acute MI, and would be the initial agent used for paroxysmal VT. Second line agents include intravenous procainamide and bretylium.

Therapy for torsades de pointes requires special mention. Ordinarily, traditional agents are ineffective, although lidocaine or phenytoin are certainly worth an initial trial. Prevention of torsades de pointes requires shortening of the refractory period.

Table 3. Clinical Pharmacology of Antiarrhythmic Drugs

Drug	Indications	Effect on ECG	Dose	Adverse Effects	Therapeutic Plasma Levels
Bretylium	VT–VF		5 mg/kg IV; 5–10 mg/kg q6h	Hypotension; GI (nausea, vomiting) possible aggravation of arrhythmia	
Disopyramide	VEA AEA	QRS, QT, PR prolongation	100–200 mg q6h	Anticholinergic effects; hypotension; heart failure; heart block; tachyarrhythmia	2–8 mcg/ml
Lidocaine	VEA	± QT shortening	Loading: 200–300 mg given as 50–100 mg every 5 min with rebolus after 20–40 min prn. Maintenance: 2–4 mg/min	CNS (drowsiness, agitation, seizures) rarely CHF or heart block	1–5 mcg/ml
Phenytoin	VEA	± QT shortening	100–300 mg IV given as 50 mg every 5 min (ineffective as oral agent)	CNS (ataxia, nystagmus, drowsiness); hypotension and heart block with rapid IV injection	5–20 mcg/ml
Procainamide	VEA AEA	QRS, QT prolongation	500–1000 mg q4–6 hr (po). 1 gm IV load as 100 mg every 3–5 min. Maintenance: 2–6 mg/min	Lupus-like syndrome; GI; Insomnia; rash; hypotension; aggravation of arrhythmia; blood dyscrasias	3–8 mcg/ml
Quinidine	VEA AEA	QRS, QT prolongation	200–600 mg q4–6 hr (po) (average oral dose 300 mg q6h)	Aggravation of arrhythmias ("quinidine syncope"); thrombocytopenia; fever, rash; cinchonism; GI symptoms; digoxin-quinidine interaction (elevation of digoxin levels)	2–7 mcg/ml
Beta-adrenergic blocking agents	AEA VEA	PR prolonged	Propranolol (80–160 mg daily); atenolol (50–100 mg/d); nadolol (40–100 1–2 x/d); metoprolol (50–100 mg 2–3 x/d)	Cardiac (heart block, hypotension, heart failure); asthma; hypoglycemia; lethargy; impotence	
Verapamil	AEA	—	5–15 mg IV; 40–160 mg po q8h	Congestive heart failure, asystole, constipation	

Key: VEA, ventricular ectopic activity; AEA, atrial ectopic activity.

Table 4. New Investigational Antiarrhythmic Agents

Drug	Indications	IV dose	Oral dose	Side effects	Comments
Mexiletine	VEA	Loading: 1200 mg/12 h Maintenance: 250–500 mg/12 h	Loading: 400–600 mg Maintenance: 200–300 mg q 8 h	G.I.; neurologic	Lidocaine-like drug. Local anesthetic; half-life, 8–14 h
Tocainide	VEA	Loading: 0.5–0.75 mg/ kg/min for 15 min	Loading: 400–600 mg Maintenance: 400–800 mg q 8 h	G.I.; neurologic	Lidocaine-like drug. Half-life, 11 h in normals; 14–16 h in patients with high grade VEA
Aprindine	VEA AEA	Loading: 25 mg q 5 min to total of 300 mg	Maintenance: 25–75 mg Loading: 200 mg bid × 2 days	G.I.; neurologic; agranulocytosis; negative inotropic effects; cholestatic jaundice	Local anesthetic properties; Half life, 27 h. Interferes with prothrombin time
Amiodarone	AEA (especially in patients with Wolff-Parkinson-White syndrome) VEA	IV Loading: 300 mg Maintenance: 50 mg/h	Loading: 400–1200 mg per day × 5 d Maintenance: 200–800 mg per day	Constipation; skin rash; may uncover hypo- or hyperthyroidism; nausea; headache; corneal deposits; pulmonary infiltrates	Very long half-life (20–40 days). May increase digoxin level. May worsen existing cardiac conduction disturbances. May prolong coumadin effect.

This can be accomplished either by the use of an isoproterenol infusion or pacing at rates sufficient to overdrive ectopic activity. The inciting agent (i.e., quinidine) or contributing factors (hypokalemia) should be eliminated.

Supraventricular Tachycardia

Management of the acute event is generally directed towards increasing vagal tone with methods such as carotid sinus massage, Valsalva maneuver, or evoking the dive reflex by applying ice water to the forehead. If the basis of the arrhythmia is a reentry circuit involving the AV junction, drugs such as digitalis, beta-adrenergic blocking agents, and verapamil are often effective in restoring normal rhythm. Cardioversion is rarely necessary in PSVT. Stimulants such as caffeine, which can exacerbate PSVT, should be avoided.

Atrial Flutter

This arrhythmia is more difficult to treat pharmacologically. Cardioversion is the treatment of choice. Rapid atrial pacing has also been used to revert flutter. Digitalis glycosides may reduce the ventricular response to atrial flutter, but this is quite variable. At times, high doses of digoxin are necessary, with the risk of development of digitalis toxicity, including paroxysmal atrial tachycardia (PAT) with block. If the patient is receiving quinidine concomitantly, the differentiation of atrial flutter with a slow flutter mechanism and PAT with block is often quite difficult. Diminutive atrial complexes in the inferior leads with an isoelectric baseline favors PAT with block. In approximately $\frac{1}{3}$ of patients, digitalization will convert the patient to atrial fibrillation (AF), and in the remaining $\frac{1}{3}$, sinus rhythm will be restored after a brief period of atrial fibrillation. Once sinus rhythm is restored, maintenance with quinidine, procainamide, or disopyramide may decrease the chance of recurrence.

Atrial Fibrillation

The treatment of atrial fibrillation is dependent upon whether the rhythm disturbance is a paroxysmal event in the absence of congestive heart failure, or whether the arrhythmia is a manifestation of decreased left ventricular function. In the former, membrane stabilizing drugs (quinidine, disopyramide, or procainamide) or cardioversion will be effective in reverting atrial fibrillation to sinus rhythm. In the latter, digitalization with other measures to improve left ventricular function will result in restoration of sinus rhythm.

Management of the paroxysmal (lone) atrial fibrillator may present a complex problem. Typically, these patients have no overt heart disease, normal left atrial size and fine (<2 mm) fibrillatory waves on the ECG. Many such patients are sensitive to changes in vagal tone, and digitalis drugs may then be profibrillatory because of the heterogeneity of cholinergic fibers within the atria. Quinidine and disopyramide are useful agents in this condition.

Verapamil administered either orally or intravenously will slow the response to both atrial fibrillation and flutter. We have not been impressed that this agent is an effective prophylactic drug for the prevention of atrial fibrillation. However, for the patient in whom atrial fibrillation is a fixed rhythm, verapamil may be quite helpful in effecting proper rate control.

The most common cause of atrial fibrillation, particularly in the acute phase of MI, is elevated left ventricular filling pressures. Thus, slowing of the ventricular response is mandatory before sinus rhythm can be established and maintained. Cardioversion offers little advantage in the patient with decompensated cardiac function and atrial fibrillation. Once optimal ventricular function and control of the ventricular response is effected, electrical reversion may then be undertaken if necessary. In our experience, quinidine has been helpful in stabilizing the atrium prior to cardioversion and will result in a 10–15% chance of pharmacologic reversion.

Multifocal Atrial Tachycardia

The treatment of MAT primarily is the treatment of the underlying pulmonary disease.

"Cocktail" Therapy for Paroxysmal Arrhythmias

If the patient's dysrhythmia occurs infrequently, that is, once or twice yearly, and if the patient tolerates the arrhythmia, then the physician might use a therapeutic "cocktail" to revert the arrhythmia. In these situations, it is felt to be unnecessary to have the patient on chronic antiarrhythmic therapy. The use of a single agent or group of drugs only at the time of the cardiac arrhythmia becomes the treatment of choice. Thus, for the patient experiencing PSVT, the use of a digitalis drug, a beta-adrenergic blocking agent, and mild sedatives such as meprobamate may be most effective in controlling infrequent episodes of tachycardia. Paroxysmal atrial fibrillation may be treated with a "cocktail" of quinidine, beta-adrenergic blocking agent, and sedative. Atrial flutter usually does not respond to this approach.

PREEXCITATION SYNDROMES (PES) AND THERAPY

Preexcitation syndromes include those electrocardiographic and clinical entities resulting from accelerated transmission of impulses from atrium to ventricle via accessory tracts which bypass the normal physiologic delay in the AV junction. Electrocardiographic findings reflect the pathoanatomic tracts. Classical syndromes include those described by Wolff-Parkinson-White (WPW) and Lown-Ganong-Levine (LGL), although a number of variations may be encountered. In WPW patients, a short or normal PR interval is inscribed; the "slurring" of the QRS is a result of fusion of early ventricular depolarization via the accessory Kent bundle and that which occurs over the normal His-Purkinje system. In the Lown-Ganong-Levine syndrome, the ECG hallmark is a short PR interval with normal QRS complex. Conceptually, an anomalous connection circumvents a portion of the AV junction. This tract, described by James, is believed to be the explanation for the short PR interval (less than 0.12 s and normal QRS) in the LGL syndrome. A rare form of preexcitation involves the fibers of Mahaim. Accessory pathways from either the lower AV junction or His bundle pass directly to the ventricular myocardium. Thus, the PR interval is normal, as there is no bypass of the AV junction. The QRS complex exhibits a delta wave that is due to premature depolarization of the ventricle as in the WPW syndrome. Preexcitation syndromes are common entities. There is a slight predominance of men, and approximately ⅔ of patients have no associated evidence of organic heart disease. An array of congenital heart defects have been associated with preexcitation syndromes, of which the most common is Ebstein's anomaly of the tricuspid valve.

The majority of patients with symptomatic preexcitation exhibit SVT. The mechanism is a reciprocating, or reentrant, tachycardia. Most commonly, there is antegrade conduction down the AV node with retrograde conduction from ventricle to atrium by the anomalous pathway. The QRS morphology is regular. In a small percent of WPW patients, antegrade conduction down the anomalous pathway with retrograde conduction through the AV node or a second accessory pathway occurs. This results in a regular tachycardia, but with a wide and aberrant QRS complex. This tachyarrhythmia is clinically significant in the acute setting because of its electrocardiographic similarity to ventricular tachycardia.

Atrial fibrillation, which may be seen with increasing age of the WPW patient, can result in rapid depolarization of the ventricle resulting in ventricular fibrillation and sudden death. Atrial flutter can be a significant problem when 1:1 conduction occurs over the accessory tract.

Therapy is guided by the clinical circumstances. These are the patient's symptoms, the rate of the tachyarrhythmia, and the nature of the atrial mechanism (fibrillation, flutter, or reciprocating tachycardia). In an emergency setting, when a patient presents with a bizarre extremely rapid tachycardia (rates in excess of 250 bpm), expedient treatment is mandatory. Intravenous lidocaine will often block the accessory pathway, reducing the ventricular response and allowing for more definitive therapy. Cardioversion is the therapy of choice if the atrial mechanism is flutter or fibrillation. Quinidine, procainamide, and disopyramide will also impede conduction through accessory pathways and are alternate agents to intravenous lidocaine. Digitalis drugs, verapamil, and beta-adrenergic blocking agents are useful if the arrhythmia is a regular reciprocating tachycardia (rates less than 200 bpm) with antegrade conduction through the His-Purkinje system. Digitalis drugs and verapamil are contraindicated in some WPW patients if the tachyarrhythmia is atrial fibrillation. The concern being that digitalis or verapamil will shorten the refractory period of the accessory pathway in a small number of patients, thus promoting enhanced conduction with potential deterioration to ventricular fibrillation. It is not possible to predict which patients are susceptible to this problem by ECG analysis above. It has been suggested that patients with an effective refractory period of the bypass tract of approximately 200 milliseconds (corresponding to a ventricular rate of 300 bpm) are at highest risk.

SICK SINUS SYNDROME (SSS) AND THERAPY

This is a heterogenous entity, both in terms of definition and underlying pathophysiologic mechanisms. Originally coined by Lown in reference to patients after cardioversion who exhibited bradycardia, sinoatrial arrest, and escape junctional mechanisms, it now refers to evidence of sinus node dysfunction producing clinical symptoms; it is also used to describe an asymptomatic individual who has evidence of failure of proper sinoatrial pacemaker function. In effect, SSS represents a generalized disorder of the conduction system of the heart, sinus node dysfunction being only one aspect. Evidence of sinus node dysfunction is observed in diverse populations of patients. The spectrum may range from individuals with extreme vagotonia and minor sclerodegenerative changes in the conduction system to bradycardia-tachycardia syndromes, in which the patient experiences ventricular or atrial tachyarrhythmias and becomes symptomatic during prolonged offset pauses. Therapy must be tailored to each patient, and it is prudent to limit the insertion of pacemakers to those individuals who experience symptomatic bradyarrhythmias. One should not assume a priori that patients who exhibit asymptomatic offset pauses of as long as three seconds following a bout of tachyarrhythmia require permanent pacing. Antiarrhythmic drugs that suppress the tachyarrhythmia may eliminate offset pauses and may not provoke sinoatrial (SA) or AV conduction problems in and of themselves. Patients should undergo careful monitoring to establish their response to antiarrhythmic therapy.

CARDIOVERSION AND DEFIBRILLATION

The use of electrical energy for reverting cardiac tachyarrhythmias has become standard practice in the last 20 years because of its safety and reliability. The term *defibrillation* generally applies to depolarization during ventricular fibrillation (VF) of the entire heart, or a major portion of it, by an unsynchronized electrical discharge. The ensuing cardiac asystole is then terminated by emergence of the cardiac pacemaker with the highest automaticity (usually the SA node).

Cardioversion is the use of electrical energy to revert specific cardiac arrhythmias. It differs from defibrillation in that the electrical discharge is synchronized with the R wave to avoid triggering VF by accidental discharge during the vulnerable period of the ventricle. The vulnerable period is approximately a 30 millisecond span just before inscription of the apex of the T wave on the surface ECG, but may be considerably longer under conditions of ischemia. Discharge of a low intensity shock will produce VF only when delivered during a vulnerable period. For the sake of simplicity, the R wave has been selected for triggering the electrical discharge. The physiologic basis for cardioversion is that an electrical discharge depolarizes a part of the reentrant pathway that is nonrefractory and interrupts the circus movement.

Method of Defibrillation

The vast majority of cardiac arrests are due to VF. Defibrillation constitutes definitive treatment for this condition, and success is assured only if prompt defibrillation is accomplished. Initial defibrillation of adults should be conducted with a setting between 300–400 watt seconds. At present, there is no evidence that energies in excess of 400 watt seconds are needed in humans for defibrillation, provided one strictly adheres to proper technique. Higher energies may result in prolonged periods of asystole or complete heart block, resulting in resumption of VF. Paddle position for defibrillation and cardioversion are the same. Both anteroposterior and anterolateral electrode positions have been employed. The anterior electrode is held *firmly* along the right sternal border at the level of the second and third intercostal spaces while the posterior electrode is placed at the angle of the left scapula. If a lateral paddle is used, it should be placed between the apex and anterior axillary line. The electrodes must be completely covered with conductive gel, particularly along the edges, to reduce the likelihood of skin burns.

Table 5. Average Energy Level Required for Cardioversion

Rhythm	Energy (watt second)
VT	10
Atrial flutter	20
Atrial fibrillation	100
SVT	150

Method of Cardioversion

Cardioversion may be done in both elective and nonelective circumstances. The conscious patient with VT that is hemodynamically compromised should be promptly cardioverted after receiving small amounts of intravenous diazepam. Alternatively, the patient with AF who is to be electively cardioverted should have the procedure fully explained to allay as much anxiety as possible. Digitalis drugs are not necessarily withheld. Serum levels of digoxin and electrolytes should be obtained prior to the procedure; and, if the patient has been anticoagulated, a recent prothrombin time is necessary. Cardioversion may be done at the patient's bedside or in a room equipped for cardiopulmonary resuscitation. There should be a minimum of personnel and activity. A short-acting barbiturate should be administered 1–2 hours before the procedure. This sedation reduces the amount of diazepam given subsequently. At the time of cardioversion, an initial intravenous dose of 5 mg of diazepam is administered followed by 2.5 mg increments every two or three minutes. Both blood pressure and respiratory rates are monitored prior to each dose. The average amount of diazepam required to achieve adequate sedation is usually 15 mg, although the range is quite variable.

The main danger in transthoracic electric discharge is the provocation of VF. The current generation of cardioverters incorporates a display that indicates the portion of the QRS to which the circuit is synchronized. The lead that displays the highest R wave amplitude should be selected for discharge synchronization. Improper synchronization may result when the electrocardiographic signal contains artifactual spikes, when there are extremely prominent T waves, and in bundle branch block when the R′ wave is taller than the R-wave. The energy levels required to terminate specific arrhythmias are detailed in Table 5. It is important to note that during elective cardioversion, energy titration should be employed. Low energies may disclose rhythm disturbances in patients with subclinical digitalis toxicity or electrolyte disturbance, and they also reduce myocardial damage.

INDICATIONS FOR PACEMAKER INSERTION See Chapters 11 and 17.

Table 6 details the indications for both temporary and permanent pacemaker placement. As discussed elsewhere, during acute MI, indications for temporary pacemaker are the occurrence of complete heart block or advanced AV block in the setting of anterior wall MI. Progressive first and second degree AV block in the setting of acute bundle branch block would be another indication for temporary pacing. Controversy

Table 6. Indications for Pacing

Temporary

   The occurrence of the following events during an
acute myocardial infarction:

      Complete heart block

      Mobitz II AV block (anterior wall infarct)

      AV block and acute bifascicular block

      Overdrive suppression of ventricular
arrhythmia

Permanent

   Complete heart block

   Bradycardia tachycardia syndrome

   Symptomatic bradyarrhythmia

   Proven efficacy of overdrive suppression

remains as to the absolute need for pacing in the otherwise stable patient with acute bundle branch block and no evidence of AV conduction disorder.

Placement of a permanent pacemaker should be reserved for patients with symptomatic bradyarrhythmia, brady-tachy syndromes, and evidence of Stokes-Adams syncope. The use of pacemaker technology in the management of patients with recurrent atrial and ventricular tachyarrhythmias is reserved for only a minority of patients with drug-refractory tachycardia.

Because of the rapidly increasing complexity of types of pacemakers, a code for pacemaker identification (Parsonnet, et al.) has been developed for describing essential features of each type. The code consists of five letters. The first letter represents the chamber (or chambers) that is (are) paced (A, atrium; V, ventricle; D, double chamber); the second letter represents the chambers that is (are) sensed (A, V, D, or O [none]); the third letter represents the mode of response (I, inhibited; T, triggered; D, double [atrial triggered and ventricular inhibited]; O, not applicable). The fourth and fifth letter indicate more sophisticated pacing features, such as programmability or special tachyarrhythmia functions. The bulk of current pacemaker therapy involves the standard ventricular demand pacemaker. The first three letters of the code used to describe this type of device are VVI (ventricular paced, ventricular sensed, and inhibited by natural electrical activity in the ventricular chamber).

In some patients, if there is no competing atrial rhythm, synchronized atrial and ventricular contraction may improve cardiac performance. Such devices are capable of sensing and/or pacing the atrium followed by sequential ventricular pacing (VAT, DVI, DDD). If AV conduction is intact, then atrial demand pacing may be used (AAI).

STRATEGIES IN THE APPROACH TO CARDIAC SUDDEN DEATH

Sudden death from heart disease remains the leading cause of mortality in developed countries. In the past two decades, many advances have been made in the man-

Table 7. Indications for the Chronic Treatment of Ventricular Arrhythmias

Primary (noninfarction related) ventricular fibrillation

Sustained symptomatic ventricular tachycardia

Complex ventricular premature beats (defined as repetitive or early cycle, R-on-T) on ECG monitoring or exercise stress testing within 6–12 months following acute MI

Complex VPBs in the patient with unstable, new onset, or active angina or when associated with ST segment depression during exercise testing

Mitral valve prolapse in patient with family history of sudden cardiac death and with paroxysms of symptomatic VT

Long QT syndrome with syncope or family history of sudden death

Obstructive cardiomyopathies, particularly with a family history of sudden death

Symptomatic VPBs

agement of the patient with malignant ventricular arrhythmia, as well as in the use of antiarrhythmic drugs for long-term survival.

While the VPB has been shown to be associated with an enhanced risk for sudden cardiac death, it lacks specificity. The finding of advanced forms of ectopic activity in an asymptomatic otherwise healthy person is cause for neither alarm nor treatment. Table 7 details the current indications for treatment of VPBs. Only a few people exhibiting VPBs require chronic antiarrhythmic therapy. For patients exhibiting so-called malignant ventricular arrhythmia, defined as noninfarction-related ventricular fibrillation or hemodynamically compromising ventricular tachycardia, a systematic approach to antiarrhythmic drug testing and therapy is mandated by the risk of recurrence and high annual mortality of such patients. Most of these patients can be successfully treated with a combination of antiarrhythmic drugs, increasing the chances of long-term survival. A minority of patients with true drug refractory malignant arrhythmia may be candidates for either surgical resection, employing cardiac mapping to define the VT focus, or specialized permanent pacemaker techniques.

Bibliography

Barold SS, Coumel P: Mechanisms of atrioventricular junctional tachycardia: Role of reentry and concealed accessory bypass tracts. *Am J Cardiol* 39:97, 1977.

Cranefield PF, Wit AL, Hoffman BF: Genesis of cardiac arrhythmias. *Circulation* 47:190, 1973.

DeSilva RA, Graboys TB, Podrid PJ, et al: Cardioversion and defibrillation. *Am Heart J* 100:881, 1980.

Doering W: Quinidine-digoxin interaction: Pharmacokinetics, underlying mechanism and clinical implications. *N Engl J Med* 301:400, 1979.

Fisch C: Relation of electrolyte disturbances to cardiac arrhythmias. *Circulation* 47:408, 1973.

Godman MJ, Lassers BW, Julian DG: Complete bundle branch complicating acute myocardial infarction. *N Engl J Med* 282:237, 1970.

Harrison DL, Meffin PJ, Winkle RA: Clinical pharmacokinetics of antiarrhythmic drugs. *Prog Cardiovasc Dis* 20:217, 1978.

Hindman MC, Wagner GS, Jaro M, et al: The clinical significance of bundle branch block complicating acute myocardial infarction: *Circulation* 58:689, 1978.

Josephson ME, Kastor JA: Supraventricular tachycardia: Mechanisms and management. *Ann Intern Med* 87:346, 1977.

Lown B, Graboys TB: Ventricular premature beats and sudden cardiac death, in McIntosh H (ed): *Baylor Cardiology Series*. Vol 3, 1980, p 1.

Lown B, Podrid PJ, DeSilva RA, et al: Sudden cardiac death: Management of the patient at risk. Chicago; *Year Book Medical Publications*, Vol IV, 1980.

Lown B, Graboys TB: Management of patients with malignant ventricular arrhythmias. *Am J Cardiol* 39:910, 1977.

Lown B: Electrical reversion of cardiac arrhythmias. *Br Heart J* 29:469, 1967.

Lown B, Ganong WF, Levine SA: The syndrome of short RR interval, normal QRS complexes and paroxysmal rapid heart action. *Circulation* 5:693, 1952.

Margolis B, DeSilva RA, Lown B: Episodic drug treatment in the management of paroxysmal arrhythmias. *Am J Cardiol* 45:621, 1980.

McAnulty JH, Rahimtoola S, Murphy ES: A prospective study of sudden death in "high risk" bundle branch block. *N Engl J Med* 299:209, 1978.

Moss AJ, Davis RJ: Brady-tachy syndrome. *Prog Cardiovasc Dis* 16:439, 1974.

Parsonnet V, Furman S, Smyth NPD: A revised code for pacemaker identification. *PACE* 4:400, 1981.

Rigby WFC, Graboys TB: Current concepts and management of the preexcitation syndromes. *J Cardiovasc Med* 6:277, 1981.

Shine KI, Kastor JA, Yurchak PM: Multifocal atrial tachycardia: Clinical and electrocardiographic features. *N Engl J Med* 179:344, 1968.

Velebit V, Podrid PJ, Lown B, et al: Aggravation and provocation of ventricular arrhythmias by antiarrhythmic drugs. *Circulation* 65:886, 1982.

Wolff L, Parkinson J, White PD: Bundle branch block with short PR interval in healthy young people prone to paroxysmal tachycardia. *Am Heart J* 5:685, 1930.

Zipes DP, Troup PJ: New antiarrhythmic agents. *Am J Cardiol* 41:1005, 1978.

CHAPTER

17

ATRIOVENTRICULAR CONDUCTION DISORDERS

Peter L. Friedman

Atrioventricular (AV) conduction disturbances represent a frequently encountered problem in contemporary cardiology, often posing both a diagnostic and therapeutic dilemma to the clinician. Whereas the symptomatic patient with complete AV block and a slow idioventricular rhythm clearly requires an artificial pacemaker, the prognostic implications and proper management of lesser degrees of AV block may be less certain or even controversial. This chapter will discuss currently available methods for assessing AV conduction, review the wide array of chronic AV conduction disturbances one is likely to encounter, and, finally, provide a framework for the rational approach to patients with such problems. AV conduction disturbances occurring in the setting of acute myocardial infarction (MI) are considered separately elsewhere (Chapter 11).

Physiology and Pathophysiology of Atrioventricular Conduction

Optimal cardiac performance depends greatly upon an ordered sequence of atrial systole and then, after an appropriate delay, ventricular systole. This ordered sequence of mechanical events, in turn, requires a normally functioning cardiac conduction system, in which pacemaker impulses originating in the sinus node must first depolarize atrial myocardium, then propagate slowly through the AV node, and finally be distributed quickly over the His-Purkinje network to ventricular myocardium. The function of each link in this electrophysiologic chain is best appreciated by examining the time relationships between P waves and QRS complexes of the surface electrocardiogram (ECG) together with simultaneously recorded intracardiac bipolar electrograms from the high right atrium (near the sinus node), left atrium, and His bundle region (Fig. 1). An electrode catheter in the His bundle region, because of its strategic position across the AV ring, is in close proximity to both atrial and ventricular myocardium. Consequently, the electrogram recorded from such a lead consists of three deflections: the first of these represents low right atrial muscle depolarization (A in Fig. 1) near the origin of the AV node; the second is a rapid deflection signifying His bundle depolarization (H in Fig. 1); and the third a large deflection that represents depolarization of the right ventricular septal myocardium (V in Fig. 1). In the surface ECG, the PR interval represents the total time required for transmission of the cardiac impulse from its point of origin in the sinus node to

339

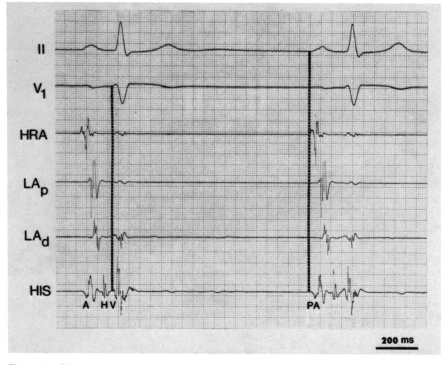

Figure 1 Simultaneous recordings during sinus rhythm of (top to bottom) surface ECG leads II and V_1 as well as intracardiac bipolar electrograms from the high right atrium (HRA), proximal left atrium (LA_p), distal left atrium (LA_d) and His bundle region (HIS). The dark vertical lines denote onset of the QRS complex (left) and P wave (right). See text for discussion.

the ventricular myocardium. This interval is actually a sum of conduction times over each different segment of the AV conducting system; namely, conduction time between the sinus and AV nodes, conduction time through the AV node itself, and conduction time from the His bundle to ventricular myocardium. Although specific information about conduction over each of these segments is not apparent from the surface ECG, it is available from simultaneous recordings of the surface ECG and a His bundle electrogram.

The interval between onset of a normal sinus P wave in the surface ECG and depolarization of the low right atrial myocardium (A in the His bundle electrogram) represents intraatrial conduction time from the sinus node to the AV node. This time is referred to as the PA interval, normally requiring between 10–55 ms, and is determined by conduction velocity over the specialized internodal tracts and through atrial myocardium (Fig. 1). Because intraatrial conduction normally is quite rapid, the PA interval accounts for only a small part of the PR interval. However, conditions that slow intraatrial conduction velocity (atrial infarction, chronic atrial hypertension, and infiltrative diseases, such as amyloidosis or hemochromatosis) all may prolong the PR interval by virtue of prolongation of the PA interval.

Most of the normal delay during AV transmission occurs within the AV node, where cells generate slowly rising low amplitude action potentials, and conduction velocity is accordingly slow. AV nodal conduction time, therefore, accounts for a majority of the PR interval. Since the atrial deflection recorded by a His bundle electrode catheter represents depolarization of atrial muscle near the cranial border of the AV node, the AH interval provides an accurate measure of AV nodal conduction time (Fig. 1). AV nodal conduction times in normal persons span a wide range, usually between 50–140 ms, due largely to variations in sympathetic and parasympathetic tone within the richly innervated AV node. There are many conditions and diseases that can impair AV conduction by interfering with AV nodal conduction. Pharmacologic agents may depress AV nodal conduction via direct electrophysiologic effects on AV nodal cells (verapamil, procainamide) or indirectly, by altering autonomic tone (propanolol, digitalis). Ischemia can also result in AV nodal conduction delay and block. Usually, this is a reflection of compromised flow in the right coronary artery, which is the origin of the AV nodal artery in 90% of patients. Ischemic AV nodal block may be transient, due to hypoxia, parasympathetic reflexes, or various metabolic products liberated by ischemic myocardium. It may also be permanent, usually reflecting actual infarction of all or part of the AV node. Inflammation of any etiology involving the AV node may result in AV nodal delay or block. This is most often seen in acute rheumatic myocarditis, but may also accompany viral myocarditides and occur in association with Lyme arthritis. Other conditions that can result in impaired AV nodal conduction are infiltrative cardiomyopathies (amyloidosis, sarcoidosis, hemochromatosis), open heart surgery (particularly after replacement of heavily calcified aortic or mitral valves), and, on rare occasions, primary or metastatic cardiac tumors. Finally, AV nodal block may be congenital.

The terminal portion of the PR in the surface ECG represents conduction through all segments of the AV conducting system distal to the AV node. This includes conduction over the His bundle, down the right and left bundle branches and through the subendocardial ramifications of the Purkinje network to ventricular myocardium. Total conduction time in this subnodal portion of the AV conduction system is reflected in the HV interval, measured from the H spike in the His bundle electrogram to the earliest point of ventricular depolarization in any intracardiac or surface lead (Fig. 1). In the presence of normal conduction distal to the AV node, the HV interval ranges between 35–55 ms. Unlike AV nodal conduction, conduction velocity in the His-Purkinje system does not change appreciably despite wide fluctuations in autonomic tone. However, subnodal conduction can be severely impaired by a variety of conditions or disease states. Perhaps the most common cause of abnormal His-Purkinje conduction is hypertensive cardiovascular disease, which accelerates aging of the cardiac skeleton and may result in fibrosis of the subnodal conduction system. Ischemic heart disease may also lead to disturbances in intraventricular conduction, either because of fibrosis or actual infarction of the His bundle or bundle branches, as well as underlying myocardium. This is most commonly seen in association with anteroseptal MI, since the left anterior descending coronary artery provides most of the blood supply to the His bundle and bundle branches. However, it may also occur with right coronary artery occlusion with resultant compromise of flow in the posterior descending artery. Infiltrative diseases, such as amyloidosis, hemochromatosis, and sarcoidosis may involve the His-Purkinje system, resulting in impaired subnodal conduction. Other common causes include cardiomyopathy, congenital heart disease, trauma associated with cardiac surgery, and most antiarrhythmic drugs, particularly toxic concentrations of agents with local anesthetic properties. Occasionally one may encounter impaired His-Purkinje conduction due to sclerodegenerative changes in this tissue in the absence of any other cardiac disease (Lev's disease, Lenegre's disease). Infectious causes of impaired His-Purkinje conduction include Chagas' disease and septal abscess formation as a consequence of infective endocarditis. Other uncommon causes of subnodal conduction disturbances are polymyositis, myotonia dystrophica, and Kearns-Sayre syndrome.

Diagnosis and Management of AV Block

First degree AV block is defined as a PR interval of greater than 0.20 second and is probably the most commonly encountered manifestation of altered AV conduction. Of course, the single important exception to this definition is prolonged intraatrial conduction time, which, as pointed out above, may result in a prolonged PR interval in the absence of any true disturbance of AV transmission. Usually, first degree AV block is due to slow conduction through the AV node. Intracardiac recordings in

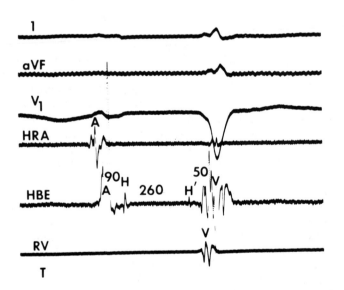

Figure 2   Simultaneous recordings of (top to bottom) surface ECG leads I, aV$_F$, and V$_1$, as well as intracardiac electrograms from the high right atrium (HRA), His bundle region (HBE), and right ventricular apex (RV). First degree AV block is present due to prolonged intra-His conduction time (260 ms). See text for discussion. (From Josephson, ME, Saides, SF: *Clinical Cardiac Electrophysiology.* Philadelphia, Lea & Febiger, 1979).

such cases typically reveal a prolonged AH interval, with normal PA and HV intervals.

First degree AV nodal block may be a manifestation of intrinsic AV node disease or may simply be a reflection of heightened vagal tone or drug effect. In the absence of evidence of higher degrees of block, it requires no therapy. However, prolongation of the PR interval does not always imply slow conduction through the AV node. Figure 2 is an example of a patient with a PR interval of 0.43 second in whom conduction time through the AV node is normal. Note that in this patient the His bundle electrogram is comprised of two separate deflections separated by an interval of 260 ms, rather than a single, discrete spike. This is referred to as a split His potential and represents extremely slow conduction between the proximal and distal portions of the His bundle. In this particular example, conduction time between the distal His bundle and ventricular myocardium is normal; thus, the PR prolongation is due to first degree intra-His block. In some patients with prolonged PR intervals, the site of conduction delay occurs in the more peripheral segments of the conducting system and appears as a prolonged HV interval, with normal PA and AH intervals. This is referred to as first degree infra-His block. Unlike first degree AV nodal block, first degree intra-His or infra-His block is a manifestation of serious disease in the conduction system. Many of these patients eventually develop higher degrees of block. In patients with syncope, the presence of first degree intra-His or infra-His block is an indication for pacemaker therapy. Whether asymptomatic patients with first degree intra or infra-His block should receive prophylactic pacemakers is still a matter of conjecture.

Second degree AV block is defined as intermittent failure of AV conduction and can be recognized as any of several well-known electrocardiographic patterns. Type I second degree AV block is characterized by Wenckebach periodicity of AV conduction, in which the PR interval lengthens and the RR interval shortens during each cycle until a P wave fails to conduct to the ventricles, resulting in a long RR interval (Fig. 3). Occasionally, these long RR intervals may be interrupted by the appearance of junctional escape beats. In its typical form, the PR interval is always shortest following the dropped QRS, and the greatest increment in PR interval occurs in the second cycle following the blocked P wave. However, this typical pattern may not always occur, and, particularly during long Wenckebach cycles, the PR interval may seem to stabilize for several beats; or, alternatively, the greatest increment in PR interval may occur with other than the second beat after the dropped QRS. The most common site of type I second degree AV block is the AV node. His bundle recordings in such cases (Fig. 3) reveal progressive lengthening of the AH interval with a constant HV interval, until conduction through the AV node fails. As with first degree AV nodal block, type I second degree AV nodal block can occur in a wide variety of circumstances, including congenital or acquired disease of the AV node, digitalis intoxication, and inferior MI. Its presence does not always imply intrinsic disease, since it can occur spontaneously in well-trained endurance athletes and can usually be provoked in normal people by incremental atrial pacing. In some instances, type I second degree AV block may occur, not in the AV node, but rather within the His bundle or in the more distal segments of the conducting system. During type I second degree intra-His block, one sees a split His potential with progressive prolongation of conduction time between the proximal and distal portions of the His bundle, culminating in failure of transmission to the distal His bundle and, thus, dropout of

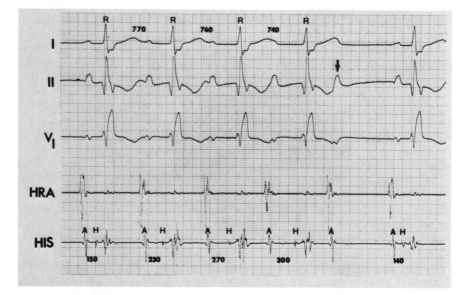

Figure 3 Simultaneous recordings of surface ECG leads I, II, and V₁, as well as intra-cardiac electrograms from the high right atrium (HRA) and His bundle region (HIS). Right bundle branch block is present. The surface ECG demonstrates typical 5:4 type I second-degree AV block, with progressive prolongation of the PR interval until the fifth P wave fails to conduct to the ventricle (arrow). In this example, type I second-degree AV block is due to progressive slowing of AV nodal conduction time (AH interval) until conduction through the AV node fails. See text for discussion.

the QRS. In such cases the AH interval remains constant throughout, even though the ECG reveals Wenckebach periodicity. Type I second degree infra-His block is also characterized by Wenckebach periodicity, but is due to progressive lengthening of conduction time in the *distal* conducting system. This appears as progressive prolongation of the HV interval until complete failure of transmission beyond the His bundle to the ventricles occurs with dropout of the QRS. When evaluating a patient whose ECG reveals Wenckebach periodicity of AV conduction, the occurrence of particularly long Wenckebach cycles with very little increment in PR interval or atypical Wenckebach cycles should raise the suspicion of block within or below the His bundle. In such cases, particularly in patients with a prior history of syncope or presyncope, the diagnosis should be confirmed with a His bundle recording.

Type II second degree AV block differs from type I in that sudden intermittent failure of AV transmission occurs without any detectable prolongation of conduction time prior to the dropped beat. The electrocardiographic appearance of this is the sudden failure of a P wave to conduct to the ventricles in the setting of a constant PR interval prior to and following the blocked beat (Fig. 4a). Unlike type I second degree AV block, which can occur within the AV node, within the His bundle, or below the His bundle, type II second degree AV block occurring within the AV node has never been conclusively demonstrated. Rather, when this type of block occurs, its presence is always a reflection of conduction disease either within or below the bundle of His.

A third type of second degree AV block one may encounter clinically is that in which the ratio of P waves to QRS complexes is 2:1, 3:1, or even higher. Obviously, such cases cannot be labeled either type I or type II and, instead, are simply referred to as high grade second degree AV block. This type of second degree AV block may occur either in the AV node itself or within or below the His bundle. Occasionally, having a patient exercise may be useful in determining the most likely site of block in such cases. The increased sympathetic tone associated with exercise usually improves conduction through the AV node and may, thus, change the conduction ratio from 2:1 to 1:1. In contrast, block within or below the His bundle is usually exacerbated during rapid heart rates and, thus, is made worse during exercise. Nevertheless, it is rarely possible to predict the site of block reliably from the surface ECG. Since these distinctions may have important therapeutic implications, patients with high grade second degree AV block should always undergo electrophysiologic study before pacemaker therapy is advised.

In general, decisions about how best to treat patients with second degree AV block should be based on the clinical circumstances in which the block occurs, as well as knowledge about the precise site in the conducting system that is diseased. As mentioned previously, type I second degree AV nodal block usually occurs in association with some transient active problem such as acute rheumatic fever, digitalis intoxication, or acute inferior MI. Although, in such cases, temporary pacing may be required if higher degrees of block occur, the AV conduction disturbance usually disappears as the underlying active process subsides; and permanent pacing is sel-

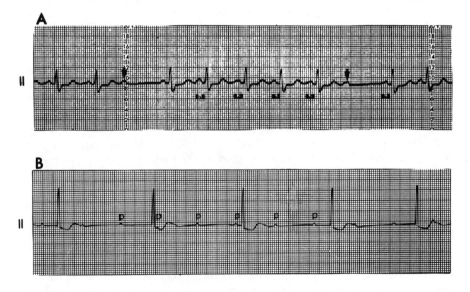

Figure 4   (*a*) Lead II of the surface ECG during type II second degree AV block. The PR interval remains constant preceding and following P waves, which fail to conduct to the ventricles (arrows). (*b*) Lead II of the surface ECG during complete AV block. There is dissociation between P waves and QRS complexes. Atrial rate is typically faster than the ventricular rate. The normal QRS complex suggests block in the AV node with an escape focus high in the His bundle.

dom, if ever, required. Moreover, in this setting, His bundle recording to document the site of block is not essential. On the other hand, patients who develop type I second degree block in the absence of some acute intercurrent process, particularly elderly patients with severe coronary artery disease or calcific aortic or mitral disease, should undergo electrophysiologic testing to determine the site of the block. If type I second degree block in such patients is localized within or below the His bundle, particularly in the setting of prior syncope or presyncope, the likelihood of progression to higher degrees of block is high and permanent pacing should be recommended. Similarly, patients with type II second degree block or high grade second degree block should also undergo His bundle studies to confirm the diagnosis before having a permanent pacemaker implanted.

Third degree, or complete AV block is simply defined as complete failure of conduction between the atria and ventricles. In the presence of sinus rhythm, third degree AV block can readily be distinguished electrocardiographically as dissociation between the P waves and QRS complexes, the ventricles being governed by a subatrial pacemaker that is invariably slower than the sinus node (Fig. 4b). Occasionally, a supraventricular rhythm other than sinus (atrial fibrillation, for example) may be present. Third degree AV block, like the lesser degrees of block, may occur at any site in the AV conducting system, such as in the AV node or within or below the His bundle. In some instances, it may be possible to define precisely the site of block electrocardiographically by examination of the ventricular rate and morphology of the QRS complexes. The rate at which subatrial pacemakers depolarize, in general, decreases as one proceeds distally along the His bundle and bundle branches. Thus, third degree AV block with a ventricular rate greater than 50/min and QRS complexes that are normal in duration is almost certainly due to block in the AV node, with an escape focus high in the His bundle; whereas, ventricular rates of 30–40/min, with wide aberrant QRS complexes, suggest subnodal block with an escape focus in the bundle branches or distal Purkinje system. However, considerable overlap in spontaneous firing rates occurs at different sites in the His-Purkinje system, and bundle branch block patterns may be present even with pacemaker foci located high in the AV junction. Thus, His bundle recording is often necessary to localize the site of block accurately.

The management of patients with third degree AV nodal block is usually straightforward. If such block occurs in association with a transient active problem, such as acute inferoposterior MI, myocarditis, drug intoxication, or recent cardiac surgery, it will usually resolve spontaneously with time. Such patients are best managed expectantly, without resorting to temporary or permanent pacemakers, provided the junctional escape rate is sufficiently rapid to prevent symptoms or hemodynamic compromise. In some patients, most notably those with congenital complete heart block, the third degree AV nodal block is fixed rather than transient. Fortunately, most of these patients are asymptomatic, since the rate of the junctional escape pacemaker is adequate to maintain a normal cardiac output. These patients also do not require permanent pacemakers. However, occasional patients with congenital third degree AV nodal block will have a history of syncope, despite an apparently adequate junctional escape rate. In such cases, observing the patient's response to exercise and electrophysiologic testing are important steps in determining the advisability of pacemaker therapy.

Most instances of third degree AV block are due not to block in the AV node, but rather block within or below the His bundle. In most reported series, third degree intra-His or infra-His block accounts for nearly 80% of patients with complete heart block. His bundle recordings from patients with third degree intra-His block typically reveal split His potentials and complete AV dissociation occurring between the proximal and distal His deflections. Alternatively, in cases of third degree infra-His block, one would instead see a single His spike following each atrial electrogram and dissociated ventricular complexes without a preceding His spike. Functionally, third degree intra and infra-His blocks can be considered together. In these cases, the ventricular rate is always slow and unresponsive to autonomic interventions. Typically, patients with such blocks present with a history of syncope and should always be managed with a permanent pacemaker.

Management of Intraventricular Conduction Defects

Management of the patient with electrocardiographic evidence of an intraventricular conduction defect, who does not yet exhibit overt AV block but who may be at risk for eventual development of complete heart block, has generated an enormous amount of controversy over the past decade and remains a perplexing issue. In order to understand the prognostic implications of the bundle branch blocks and nonspecific intraventricular conduction defects, an understanding of the functional anatomy of the His-Purkinje system is essential. The His bundle in the normal human heart originates near the central fibrous body at a point where fibers from the distal end of the AV node coalesce into large longitudinal Purkinje fibers. Anatomically, it forms a discrete bundle that usually courses down the left side of the membranous interventricular septum to the crest of the muscular septum, where it bifurcates into the right and left bundle branches. The right bundle branch is itself a discrete bundle that continues down the right side of the muscular septum to the right ventricular apex, at which point it arborizes into the septal and right ventricular free wall myocardium. In contrast, the left bundle branch fans out broadly over the left septal surface shortly after its origin. The left bundle branch functions electrophysiologically as though it were composed of two separate divisions, the anterior and posterior fascicles. This is based upon commonly observed electrocardiographic patterns of left ventricular conduction defects. When conduction delay or block occurs in the anterior fascicle, the result is delayed activation of the upper anterior wall of the left ventricle. This pattern of intraventricular conduction is referred to as left anterior hemiblock. The electrocardiographic hallmarks of left anterior hemiblock include a QRS axis in the frontal plane equal to or more negative than $-45°$, small initial R waves in the inferior leads, and then large S waves inferiorly, with dominant R waves in leads I and aV_L. Conduction delay or block in the posterior fascicle of the left bundle branch results in a different electrocardiographic pattern, referred to as left posterior hemiblock. The salient electrocardiographic features of left posterior hemiblock include a QRS axis in the frontal plane greater than or equal to $+110°$, a small initial r wave in lead I, small inferior Q waves, and an initial R wave in lead V_1. This electrocardiographic diagnosis, however, can only be made in the absence of clinical evidence for right ventricular hypertrophy or pulmonary disease. Left posterior hemiblock is less common than left anterior hemiblock, in all likelihood because the posterior fascicle usually has a dual blood supply from both the left anterior descending and posterior descending coronary arteries.

In view of the trifascicular nature of the intraventricular conducting system (right bundle branch, left anterior fascicle, and left posterior fascicle) it is clear that as long as one of these major fascicles is able to conduct normally, the risk of developing complete heart block below the His bundle should be quite small, even in the presence of bundle branch block or hemiblock involving the remaining two fascicles. In such a situation, one would still expect the HV interval, which is a direct measure of conduction below the bundle of His, to be normal or nearly normal. Thus, in approaching patients with intraventricular conduction defects, there are two important questions that must be considered. First, what is the most effective method for assessing the functional integrity of the apparently uninvolved fascicle or fascicles? And second, if conduction disease can be demonstrated in all three fascicles, does this reliably predict subsequent development of complete heart block?

The answer to the first of these two questions is reasonably straightforward. Clinical electrophysiologic studies in patients with various intraventricular conduction defects have demonstrated that, in most circumstances, the QRS morphology and length of the PR interval in the surface ECG are of little value in assessing the functional integrity of the His-Purkinje system. For example, in patients who have right bundle branch block associated with either left anterior or left posterior fascicular block, the ECG shows evidence of conduction disease in two out of the three major fascicles. The same is true for patients who have complete left bundle branch block. Unfortunately, the PR interval in such cases is a notoriously poor indicator of disease in the remaining fascicle. In many cases, PR prolongation in patients with electrocardiographic evidence of bifascicular block is due to first degree AV nodal block, the HV interval being quite normal. In such patients, conduction in the third fascicle clearly is not jeopardized. Conversely, there are some patients who have nonspecific intraventricular conduction defects without complete bundle branch block, hemiblock, or even a prolonged PR interval in whom the HV interval may be markedly prolonged. Thus, trifascicular conduction disease can rarely be documented on the basis of a surface ECG; patients with a history of syncope or presyncope and intraventricular conduction defects, who are suspected of having trifascicular disease, should undergo His bundle recording with measurement of the HV interval. There are, however, two important exceptions to this generalization. Patients who have right bundle branch block associated with alternating left anterior and left posterior hemiblock or patients who demonstrate alternating complete right and complete left bundle branch block clearly have significant trifascicular disease and do not require measurement of the HV interval.

Having accepted the concept that, in most circumstances, measurement of the HV interval is a prerequisite for conclusively demonstrating trifascicular conduction disease, the next issue one must consider is whether HV prolongation in patients with intraventricular conduction defects is a reliable predictor of eventual complete heart block. Obviously, a related question is whether implantation of permanent pacemakers in such patients will have a measurable impact on their prognosis. Unfortunately, there is still considerable controversy about the correct answers to both of these questions. Consequently, it is not possible to list precise recommendations about how best to evaluate and manage patients with bifascicular or trifascicular disease. However, there are broad guidelines regarding the management of such patients that most investigators agree upon. In general, patients who have symptoms of syncope or presyncope in the absence of neurologic disease to explain their symptoms, and who also have evidence of an intraventricular conduction defect, including complete or incomplete bundle branch block with or without associated hemiblock, should undergo electrophysiologic study. This study should include assessment of sinus node function, measurement of baseline HV interval, and also provocative maneuvers such as rapid atrial pacing to unmask inapparent conduction disease in the His-Purkinje system. If HV intervals are prolonged in such patients or if second or third degree intra or infra-His block can be provoked, such patients should probably be treated with a permanent pacemaker. Another category of patients who should probably undergo electrophysiologic testing are those with serious underlying heart disease and intraventricular conduction defect who are scheduled for major cardiac surgery. If HV prolongation or provokable high grade infra-His block is found, then serious consideration should be given to implanting permanent epicardial pacing wires at the time of surgery, although the subsequent use of these pacing wires should depend on the patient's postoperative course. With regard to patients who have intraventricular conduction defects but who are asymptomatic, it is more difficult to recommend electrophysiologic testing with any conviction. It has been suggested that markedly prolonged HV intervals in such patients, for example in excess of 100 ms, may predict subsequent development of complete heart block and, thus, may be a reasonable indiction for prophylactic pacemaker therapy. However, this view has been challenged, and it may be equally prudent simply to follow such patients, relying on the surface ECG and presence or absence of symptoms.

Bibliography

Denes P, Dhingra RC, Wu D, et al: Sudden death in patients with chronic bifascicular block. *Arch Intern Med* 137:1005, 1977.

Denes P, Levy L, Pick A, et al: The incidence of typical and atypical AV Wenckebach periodicity. *Am Heart J* 89:26, 1975.

Dhingra RC, Denes P, Wu D, et al: Prospective observations in patients with chronic bundle branch block and marked HV prolongation. *Circulation* 53:600, 1976.

Josephson ME, Seides SF: *Clinical Cardiac Electrophysiology.* Philadelphia, Lea and Febiger, 1979.

McAnnulty JH, Rahimtoola SH, Murphy ES, et al: A prospective study of sudden death in "high risk" bundle branch block. *N Engl J Med* 299:209, 1978.

Narula OS: *His Bundle Electrocardiography and Clinical Electrophysiology.* Philadelphia, F. A. Davis, 1975.

Narula OS, Narula JT: Junctional pacemakers in man. Response to overdrive suppression with and without parasympathetic blockade. *Circulation* 49:925, 1970.

Rosen KM, Dhingra RC, Loeb HS, et al: Chronic heart block in adults. *Arch Intern Med* 131:663, 1973.

Samet P, El-Sherif N (eds): *Cardiac Pacing.* New York, Grune & Stratton, 1980.

Scheinman MM, Peters RW, Modin G, et al: Prognostic value of infranodal conduction time in patients with chronic bundle branch block. *Circulation* 56:240, 1977.

CONGENITAL HEART DISEASE IN THE ADULT

Richard R. Liberthson

This chapter focuses on the most common congenital heart lesions seen in the adult. Included are atrial septal defect, ventricular septal defect, patent ductus arteriosus, coarctation of the aorta, pulmonic stenosis, and tetralogy of Fallot. Together they comprise more than 80% of the adult congenital heart population. Under each entity, the salient anatomic and physiologic features, natural history, clinical manifestations, noninvasive and invasive evaluation, surgical intervention(s), and postoperative management are discussed. For further details and for discussion of less common entities, readers are referred to more specialized textbooks dealing specifically with congenital heart disease (see Bibliography). Both mitral valve prolapse and bicuspid aortic valve are dealt with elsewhere in this book (Chapter 13).

Atrial Septal Defect (ASD)

ASD accounts for approximately 25% of congenital heart lesions seen in the adult. Patients who have eluded earlier diagnosis as well as those who have had prior correction present to the adult cardiologist. Women outnumber men by three to one.

ANATOMY

ASD size and contour is variable. Defects are subgrouped into secundum (70%), primum or partial atrioventricular (AV) canal (15%), and sinus venosus types (15%); based upon the location of the defect within the septum; whether in the region of the fossa ovalis, the AV junction, or the posterior septum respectively. This subgrouping is useful because each has different associated anomalies. Approximately one-third of secundum defects have associated mitral valve prolapse; two-thirds of primum defects have a cleft anterior mitral valve leaflet; and one-half of sinus venosus defects have anomalous drainage of the right pulmonary veins.

PHYSIOLOGY

Regardless of ASD type, the physiology of uncomplicated defects (those with normal pulmonary arteriolar resistance) is the same. Shunting from the left to the right atrium occurs during diastole and is determined by the relative right and left ventricular compliance (the former being greater in the uncomplicated patient), and by defect size. Pulmonary blood flow is increased. When defect size is small, the shunted volume is small and hemodynamic sequelae are minimal. In those with larger defects,

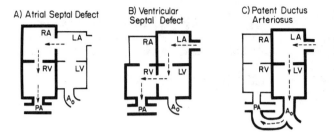

Figure 1 (*a*) Diagramatic illustration of the pathophysiologic consequences in an uncomplicated ASD revealing right atrial (RA), right ventricular (RV), and pulmonary artery (PA) dilation and preservation of normal left atrial (LA), left ventricular (LV), and aortic (Ao) size. (*b*) Uncomplicated VSD showing LA, LV, RV, and PA enlargement, with preservation of normal RA and Ao size. (*c*) Uncomplicated PDA, including LA and LV enlargement, dilation of both the Ao and PA, and preservation of normal RA and RV size.

chronic left-to-right shunting causes right atrial and right ventricular volume overload (Fig. 1*a*). In the uncomplicated patient, the left heart is conspicuously spared; and left atrial, left ventricular, and aortic size are normal.

CLINICAL COURSE

Symptoms and complications, except for an increased incidence of pulmonary infections, are uncommon in the infant and small child, and early findings are subtle even with large defects. Adolescents and young adults also have few symptoms. When present, these include fatigue, palpitations, and mild dyspnea. It is common that ASD is neither suspected nor diagnosed until adult life. Pregnancy is well tolerated. By the fifth decade, however, exercise intolerance, fatigue, and dyspnea are increasingly common and are nearly universal after age 50 years. By this time, the right atrium and ventricle are irreversibly dilated and exhibit decreased contraction. After the sixth decade, atrial fibrillation is present in 50% of the patients and its onset often heralds progressive symptoms and findings of heart failure. Both primum and secundum ASD may have mitral regurgitation. In the former, this manifests early in life and is secondary to the associated cleft mitral valve. With secundum defects, it is rare before age 50 years and is secondary to myxomatous and fibrotic degeneration of the mitral valve. Severe pulmonary vascular obstruction with Eisenmenger's physiology is uncommon, approximately 5%. It is rare before adolescence and is also rare after age 50 years. Severe irreversible pulmonary vascular obstruction causes reversal of shunt flow through the ASD from left-to-right to right-to-left. Progressive right heart failure, systemic desaturation, erythrocytosis, and paradoxical embolus occur; death generally occurs within 10 years of diagnosis. Both pulmonary and paradoxical systemic embolization occur in the older ASD patient, particularly in those with atrial arrhythmia and heart failure. Infective endocarditis is rare, and, when it occurs, it usually involves an associated mitral valve lesion or the pulmonic valve. Although endocarditis is rare, it nevertheless does occur; therefore, we feel that all patients require chemoprophylaxis, regardless of prior surgical repair. Lutembacher's syndrome (associated mitral stenosis) is rare. The average age of death in uncorrected ASD is 50 years.

CLINICAL FINDINGS

Body habitus is generally normal. Patients with the Holt-Oram syndrome (congenital hypoplasia of the thumb and radial bones) often have associated ASD. In the absence of severe pulmonary vascular obstruction, patients are acyanotic. The salient clinical findings include an enlarged hyperdynamic right ventricle and a widely and nearly fixed split second sound (S_2). Even when standing, the S_2 does not become single. A grade II/VI basal systolic ejection murmur secondary to increased blood flow across the pulmonic valve is present, and increases with inspiration. Thrills are exceptional. In older patients, heart failure and atrial fibrillation are common, and an apical holosystolic murmur secondary to mitral incompetence may be present. With severe pulmonary vascular obstruction and shunt reversal, the right ventricle hypertrophies, the pulmonic closure sound becomes loud, and the pulmonic flow murmur becomes soft. A high-pitched diastolic decrescendo murmur of pulmonary in-

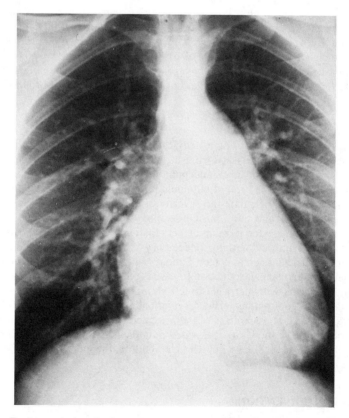

Figure 2 Posteroanterior chest roentgenogram of a 22-year-old woman with a large secundum atrial septal defect. There is a large right atrium and right ventricle, a dilated pulmonic truck, and increased pulmonary blood flow. (From Liberthson RR: Congenital heart disease in the child, adolescent and adult, in Johnson RA, Haber E, Austen WG, eds: *Practice of Cardiology.* Boston: Little, Brown, 1980. Reprinted by permission.)

competence, a pulmonic ejection sound, a right-sided S_4, cyanosis, and clubbing are late findings in these patients.

The *electrocardiogram* reflects the right ventricular volume overload, showing incomplete right bundle branch block in younger patients and often a complete right bundle after middle age. Secundum and sinus venosus defects typically have right axis deviation, although one-quarter have a normal frontal plane QRS axis. Left axis deviation is rare and suggests associated coronary, myocardial, or mitral valve disease. In contrast, in primum type defects, marked left axis deviation is the rule. It is secondary to congenital hypoplasia and attenuation of the anterior radiations of the left bundle branch. Atrial fibrillation is common in the elderly patient.

The *chest x-ray* film reveals right atrial and ventricular enlargement, dilation of the main and proximal pulmonary arteries, and increased pulmonary vascular markings (Fig. 2). The aorta appears to be small, and with uncomplicated ASD, the left heart is conspicuously normal sized (Fig. 1). If left atrial enlargement is present, mitral incompetence should be suspected.

M-mode *echocardiography* shows right ventricular enlargement, paradoxical interventricular septal movement, and tricuspid anular dilation. It also demonstrates associated mitral valve prolapse, if present, or a mitral valve cleft in primum lesions. The two-dimensional echocardiogram also shows the actual ASD.

Intravenous *technetium-99m pertechnetate scanning*, with gamma imaging, identifies both the presence and magnitude, but not the level, of left-to-right shunting.

CARDIAC CATHETERIZATION

Catheterization is indicated prior to surgical repair. Confirmation of the defect is accomplished by catheter passage from the right to the left atrium. Essential data include assessment of right heart and pulmonary artery pressures, pulmonary arteriolar resistance, and the ratio of pulmonic to systemic blood flow. Table 1 shows those formulas used to calculate the severity of the shunt. After the fourth decade, coronary angiography and left ventriculography are advisable to identify acquired heart disease. For suspected primum defects (patients with left axis deviation on the ECG), biplane left ventriculography is necessary to evaluate an associated cleft mitral valve or interventricular septal defect. Patients with pulmonary hypertension should have a trial of pulmonary vasodilation to assess reversibility of pulmonary vascular obstruction. Patients with net right-to-left shunting—Eisenmenger's physiology—are inoperable. In contrast, as a general rule, patients with net left-to-right shunting are surgical candidates, regardless of the presence of pulmonary hypertension, systemic desaturation, or moderately elevated pulmonary vascular resistance. In these latter patients, the larger the net left to right shunt is, the more favorable will be the postoperative result.

SURGICAL INTERVENTION

Surgery consists of either suture closure (usually possible in the young patient) or patch closure in older patients, those with large defects, and in those with primum or sinus venosus defects. For best results, surgery should be performed before school age. Thereafter, ASD closure is indicated when the diagnosis is confirmed. This population is predominantly women. Efforts should be made to repair defects before

Table 1. Calculations of Shunts by Oximetry Analysis[a]

1. Shunts are expressed as:

    Qp/Qs: The ratio of pulmonary blood flow (Qp) to systemic blood flow (Qs)

    and

    Qp−Qs: This value is positive if there is a net left to right (L → R) shunt, and negative if there is a net right to left (R → L) shunt

2. Calculation of pulmonary blood flow (Qp) in l/min

$$Qp = \frac{O_2 \text{ consumption (ml/min)}}{PVO_2 \text{ content} - PAO_2 \text{ content}}$$
$$\text{(ml/l)} \qquad \text{(ml/l)}$$

    Where PV = pulmonary venous blood; PA = pulmonary arterial blood

    If a pulmonary vein has not been entered, systemic arterial O_2 content may be used for PVO_2 if systemic arterial O_2 saturation is 95% or more. If it is <95%, a determination must be made as to whether a R → L shunt is present. If a R → L shunt is present, an assumed value for PVO_2 content is determined as 98% × O_2 capacity. If systemic arterial saturation is <95% and no R → L shunt is present, the observed systemic arterial O_2 content is used.

3. Systemic blood flow (Qs) in l/min

$$Qs = \frac{O_2 \text{ consumption (ml/min)}}{\text{Systemic arterial} - \text{Mixed venous}}$$
$$O_2 \text{ content (ml/l)} \quad O_2 \text{ content (ml/l)}$$

    Where mixed venous O_2 content is average O_2 content of blood in chamber immediately proximal to the shunt. If the shunt is at the level of the right atrium, one commonly used method for estimating mixed venous O_2 content (Flamm, et al), is calculated as:

$$\frac{3 \text{ SVC } O_2 \text{ content} + 1 \text{ IVC } O_2 \text{ content}}{4}$$

    Where SVC = superior vena cava; IVC = inferior vena cava

    Some institutions use the SVC O_2 content as the mixed venous sample, as this sample gives the maximal shunt size.

4. If bidirectional shunting is present, a more complex formula is used.[a]

[a] (See Bibliography: Barry WH and Grossman W)

marriage and childbearing to avoid the tendency for further delay while raising a young family. Repair before the fourth decade usually results in return of normal heart size and function. Thereafter, although both improve, they rarely become normal. Safe repair may be performed even through the seventh decade. Clinical improvement, even in older patients, may be marked, particularly when associated mitral valve incompetence was present and is relieved. In older patients, chronic anticoagulation is advisable, particularly if heart failure, pulmonary hypertension, or atrial fibrillation is present. We do not anticoagulate young patients or those with primary suture closure. Mitral valve clefts may require plasty revision at the time of ASD closure. Older adults with secundum defects should have intraoperative assessment for mitral valve replacement.

The *postoperative course* in patients repaired before the fourth decade is typically benign and lifestyle is normal. No restriction is indicated. The course of pregnancy and delivery is normal. I believe that chemoprophylaxis for bacterial endocarditis should be a lifetime commitment, regardless of surgical repair. This is particularly important because of the frequent association with mitral valve prolapse. With pregnancy, prophylaxis for vaginal organisms should be started with the onset of labor and continued for several days after delivery. In the absence of surgical damage to the sinus node or its vascular supply, young patients retain normal rhythm. For those with supraventricular ectopy or atrial fibrillation, digitalization is indicated. Patients who have new atrial fibrillation following surgery warrant a trial of electrocardioversion after six weeks; anticoagulation and digitalization should precede this, and quinidine is often needed to maintain sinus rhythm. After the sixth decade, postoperative arrhythmia is typical. Routine postoperative clinical evaluation is indicated for all patients, particularly for those having repair past middle age. Longevity in those repaired before that time is normal. Thereafter, residual (but improved) heart failure may be present, and pulmonary or systemic embolization may occur. In the older patient, late progressive mitral insufficiency may occur in spite of ASD closure. In the young patient undergoing repair, the postoperative examination, chest x-ray film, and ECG become normal except for a residual right ventricular conduction defect. Older patients with preoperative heart failure, pulmonary hypertension, and arrhythmia generally have some persisting right heart enlargement.

DIFFERENTIAL DIAGNOSIS

Entities sometimes confused with ASD include persisting patency of the foramen ovale, which occurs in 10–20% of normal autopsies; but this is of no hemodynamic consequence and has no clinical sequelae unless the pulmonary pressure is elevated. Partial anomalous pulmonary venous drainage with intact atrial septum has similar clinical findings, but rarely causes symptoms or requires correction. Mitral valve stenosis, pectus abnormalities, and pulmonic stenosis may all have similar clinical findings; however, both ultrasound and radionuclide scanning are usually sufficient to differentiate them from ASD.

Ventricular Septal Defect

Although ventricular septal defect (VSD) occurs in almost one in 500 normal births, nearly 50% close spontaneously during childhood; thus, in adults it is less common and comprises approximately 12% of patients with congenital heart disease. Adult patients presenting to the physician include those with small inconsequential defects, those who have had prior palliative or corrective surgical procedures, and those with acquired complications. Although there are exceptions, in general, if a patient survives unimpaired to adult age, and does not have Eisenmenger's physiology, the VSD is likely to be small.

ANATOMY

VSD*s* are subgrouped according to location within the interventricular septum. Seventy percent are membranous defects and involve the pars membranacea. They are variably sized and shaped and often close spontaneously. Muscular defects occur within the muscular portion of the septum, toward the apex, mid, and posterior regions. They may be multiple and also often close spontaneously. In both of these circumstances, associated cardiac defects are uncommon. AV canal type defects involving the posterobasal septum are usually large and are associated with mitral and tricuspid valve clefts, as well as a primum type ASD. These are common in patients with Down's syndrome. Supracristal (subaortic) defects are uncommon (5%). They are usually small; however, their strategic location beneath the aortic anulus undermines aortic leaflet support and may cause progressive aortic incompetence.

PHYSIOLOGY

The hemodynamic consequences of VSD vary with defect size. When small, they are minimal. With uncomplicated VSD (those with normal right ventricular pressure and normal pulmonary artery resistance), shunting occurs from the left ventricle to the right ventricle. When defect size is significant, both ventricles enlarge and pulmonary blood flow is increased. Left atrial return is increased; thus left atrial enlargement occurs. When left-to-right shunt flow is very large, heart failure may be present. The right atrium is conspicuously normal sized in uncomplicated VSD (Fig. 1*b*). With large defects, pulmonary hypertension and pulmonary vascular obstruction may develop, which leads to pulmonary artery and right ventricular hypertension, decreased left-to-right shunting, and eventually right-to-left shunting (Eisenmenger's syndrome).

CLINICAL COURSE

The clinical course of patients with VSD is variable because of the variable defect size, the common occurrence of spontaneous defect closure, development of complications in the unoperated patient, and the now common practice of early surgical intervention for those with large defects.

Patients with small defects have a history of a loud murmur present from early infancy, but they are asymptomatic. These patients do not develop complications, with the exception of bacterial endocarditis.

Overt clinical heart failure occurs in the infant with large VSD and may be fatal. Chronic left heart volume overload may cause dyspnea and both symptoms and findings of heart failure may be late sequelae in adult life.

Patients who had large shunts, often with heart failure, during infancy may develop pulmonary vascular obstruction and Eisenmenger's syndrome. In these, the chronic effects of increased pulmonary artery pressure and flow cause pulmonary arteriolar narrowing, pulmonary artery and right ventricular hypertension and reversal of interventricular shunt flow from the previous left-to-right direction to right-to-left. These patients develop systemic desaturation, cyanosis (which is often increased with exertion), and erythrocytosis. Late right heart failure and hemoptysis and systemic embolization may occur. Because of right-to-left shunting, iatrogenic systemic embolization occurs secondary to careless intravenous technique. Bacterial endocarditis occurs regardless of VSD size or earlier repair and usually involves the right ventricular outflow tract. Approximately 5% of patients with VSD develop progressive hypertrophy of the right ventricular infundibulum, which obstructs pulmonary blood flow, causes right ventricular hypertension and hypertrophy, and may cause right-to-left interventricular shunting (see pink tetralogy, under Tetralogy of Fallot, below). Patients with supracristal defects may have aortic insufficiency, which may be severe. Patients with AV canal defects commonly have heart failure during infancy and often develop Eisenmenger's syndrome (also see Chapter 24).

CLINICAL FINDINGS

Body habitus in VSD is normal except with Down's patients, who have characteristic features. The uncomplicated VSD patient has a systolic thrill at the left sternal border, an enlarged hyperdynamic left ventricle, and a loud holosystolic murmur heard best at the left sternal border on expiration and with isometric maneuvers. In general, the louder the murmur, the smaller the defect. This murmur begins with the S_1 and ends with S_2. With muscular defects, the murmur may end before the S_2 if the defect closes with ventricular contraction. Pulmonary vascular obstruction causes this murmur to diminish in intensity. In these patients, right ventricular hypertrophy, a loud pulmonic closure sound, an ejection sound, and late cyanosis develop. With late right ventricular failure, pulmonary and tricuspid incompetence occur. Patients with aortic incompetence have a high-pitched diastolic decrescendo murmur. With canal defects, mitral or tricuspid incompetence murmurs may be present.

The *electrocardiogram* is helpful in diagnosing the type of defect and the presence of complications. With small defects, the ECG is normal. Larger defects have a right ventricular conduction defect and both left atrial and left ventricular enlargement. Uncomplicated defects have a normal frontal plane QRS axis. The QRS axis is an accurate indicator of right ventricular pressure in older children and adults. A normal axis (between -30 and $+90$ degrees) usually rules out right ventricular hypertension, thus making pulmonary vascular obstruction or right ventricular infundibular obstruction unlikely; right axis deviation suggests their presence. As in the primum type ASD, canal type VSD patients have marked left axis deviation (more negative than -30 degrees).

In the uncomplicated patient with a small VSD, the *chest x-ray* film is normal. With larger defects, findings are characteristic (Fig. 3). These include increased pulmonary vascular markings, left atrial and left ventricular enlargement, a small aortic shadow, and sometimes right ventricular enlargement. The right atrium is normal sized (Fig. 1*b*).

Two-dimensional *ultrasound* examination may be diagnostic. It delineates the septal defect and shows left atrial and often biventricular enlargement. When present, associated defects including mitral or tricuspid valve clefts in canal defects, and the prolapsing aortic leaflets in supracristal defects may be seen. Identification of associated great artery abnormalities including transposition, double outlet right ventricle, and truncus arteriosus; and differentiation from single ventricle is readily made by ultrasound study.

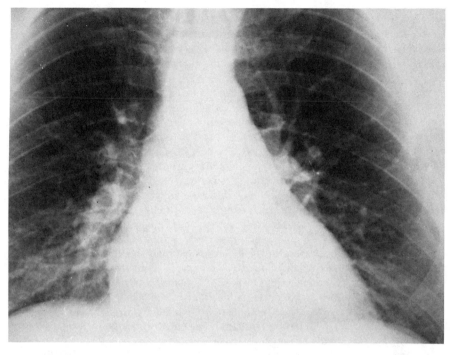

Figure 3 Posteroanterior chest roentgenogram of a 30-year-old man with a large ventricular septal defect. There is biventricular and left atrial enlargement, a dilated pulmonic truck, and increased pulmonary blood flow.

Intravenous *technetium-99m pertechnetate scanning* identifies the presence and approximates the magnitude of left-to-right shunting, but is not specific for the level at which the shunt occurs.

CARDIAC CATHETERIZATION

Not all patients with VSD warrant catheterization. In general, asymptomatic patients with small defects, normal sized hearts, normal ECGs (including a normal axis), and no evidence for associated valvular abnormalities do not require catheterization. Catheterization is necessary prior to surgical intervention. Its objectives include assessment of left-to-right shunt size, pulmonary artery pressure and resistance, and right ventricular pressure. Angiographic delineation of the defect and, when present, associated valvular lesions is necessary. Those with Eisenmenger's syndrome (net right-to-left shunting) must be identified, as these patients are not surgical candidates. Because cateheterization in these latter patients carries increased risk, it should be undertaken only after careful noninvasive assessment and should be performed only by those experienced with this problem. Patients with pulmonary hypertension should have a trial of pulmonary vasodilators during catheterization to identify those in whom there is reversible obstruction.

SURGICAL INTERVENTION

Asymptomatic patients with small defects, normal heart size, normal ECG, and no associated valvular defects do not require surgery. *Palliative banding of the pulmonary artery* is infrequently performed today; however, it was common in early years. Therefore, there are still patients who have had this procedure. It was performed in those with large VSDs to prevent the development of pulmonary vascular obstruction by protecting the pulmonary circulation from increased flow and pressure. However, in so doing, it caused right ventricular hypertension, often with right-to-left shunting through the VSD and its associated complications. The late sequelae of pulmonary banding include cyanosis, erythrocytosis, and systemic embolization. Pulmonary bands sometime distort the pulmonary arteries as well. Patients who have had prior banding require catheterization to delineate the pulmonary artery anatomy and the VSD prior to VSD closure and band removal.

Corrective surgery consists of either suture or prosthetic patch closure of the VSD. It is indicated for patients who have symptoms, cardiomegaly, elevated pulmonary pressure (including elevated pulmonary resistance, provided there is still net left-to-right shunting), and for those with significant left-to-right shunting (greater than two to one). Patients with associated infundibular stenosis should have VSD closure and often also require infundibulectomy. Those with valvular aortic incompetence may warrant repair to buttress the aortic anulus. This sometimes obviates aortic valve replacement. Emergency surgery is indicated for infants with medically refractory heart failure. Patients with severe pulmonary vascular obstruction and net right-to-left shunts are not surgical candidates.

Following successful VSD closure, *postoperative problems* are minimal and a normal lifestyle is usual. Patients may have a residual VSD that was not appreciated at the time of repair or may have incomplete patch closure, but only when left-to-right shunting is large do these require repair. The late course of the buttressed aortic valve in supracristal defects or of the palliated AV valvular incompetence in canal defects is not yet known, and these patients require close follow-up.

Patients with *Eisenmenger's syndrome* have a reduced survival (usually less than 10 years from the time of diagnosis). They are not candidates for VSD closure. They are at increased risk for arrhythmic death when subjected to any form of surgery or to general anesthesia. These patients are also at increased risk with physical exertion or exposure to high altitude. Pregnancy carries an increased risk of death and should be prevented. However, this is often not an easy matter. Birth control pills hasten the progression of the pulmonary vascular obstruction and are contraindicated. Intrauterine devices carry a risk of bacterial endocarditis and should not be used. The procedure of tubal ligation itself is a risk. Bacterial endocarditis chemoprophylaxis is essential. Cautious phlebotomy with replacement of excessive volume loss with volume expanders may be helpful for those with severe erythrocytosis and hematocrit greater than 65%. Digitalization for those with heart failure may improve symptoms.

DIFFERENTIAL DIAGNOSIS

The differential diagnosis of VSD includes single ventricle with small outlet chamber and VSD associated with abnormality of the great artery position including complete transposition, double outlet right ventricle, and truncus arteriosus. Although in some ways similar clinically to patients with large VSD, the above patients also often have cyanosis. Ultrasound examination is useful in differentiating these patients from those with simple VSD.

Patent Ductus Arteriosus

Although patent ductus arteriosus (PDA) is an obligatory component of the normal fetal circulation, persistent patency beyond early infancy is abnormal. PDA is present in 10% of adult congenital heart patients. Both unoperated and previously corrected patients present to the adult physician. It is particularly common in infants whose mothers had rubella infection during their first trimester of pregnancy, in premature infants, in infants with lung disease, and in infants born at high altitude. Girls outnumber boys two to one.

PATHOPHYSIOLOGY

The *anatomic* spectrum includes a wide range of duct caliber, length, and shape. The ligamentum arteriosus is the fibrotic remnant of the obliterated ductus. The *physiologic* consequences vary, depending upon the cross-sectional area of the ductus lumen. In the uncomplicated ductus (those with normal pulmonary arteriolar resistance), flow of blood is from the aorta to the pulmonary circulation (left to right). Large ducts allow large volume pulmonary blood flow, which causes increased pulmonary artery pressure, increased left atrial return, left ventricular enlargement, and enlargement of the aorta proximal to the ductus (Fig. 1*c*). The right atrium and ventricle are normal sized with uncomplicated ductus.

CLINICAL COURSE

The natural history depends on ductus size. Many ducts close spontaneously during early infancy. Thereafter, an annual spontaneous closure rate of 0.6% has been reported. Patients with small ductus are asymptomatic. Heart failure occurs in infants with large ductus and may be fatal. Both symptoms and findings of heart failure occur in adults with large ductus. Patients with large ductus may develop pulmonary vascular obstruction early in life. In these, the late sequelae of Eisenmenger's physiology (right-to-left shunting) include cyanosis and right heart failure. Regardless of ductus size, infective endocarditis may occur. It typically involves the pulmonary side of the ductus. There may be infected pulmonary embolization. Rare elderly patients develop ductal calcification, aneurysmal dilation, and dissection. These may be preceded by hoarseness, secondary to left vocal cord paralysis due to left recurrent laryngeal nerve compression.

CLINICAL FINDINGS

Body habitus is normal except in those with the congenital rubella syndrome, who have cataracts, are deaf, and are retarded. Patients with uncomplicated ducts of

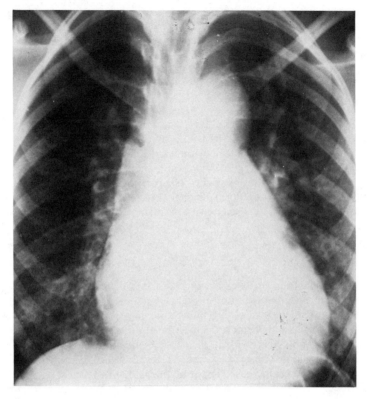

Figure 4 Posteroanterior chest roentgenogram of a 19-year-old woman with a large patent ductus arteriosus and pulmonary artery hypertension. There is cardiomegaly with left atrial and left ventricular enlargement, an enlarged pulmonic truck and aortic knob, and increased pulmonary blood flow. (From Liberthson RR: Congenital heart disease in the child, adolescent and adult, in Johnson RA, Haber E, Austen WG, eds: *Practice of Cardiology*. Boston: Little, Brown, 1980. Reprinted by permission.)

large size have hyperdynamic arterial pulses, wide pulse pressure, and an enlarged hyperdynamic left ventricle. These are absent in those with small ductus. Regardless of ductus size, there is typically a loud continuous machinery-like murmur, heard best in the left infraclavicular area. It obliterates the heart sounds in this region. With severe pulmonary vascular obstruction, the diastolic murmur shortens and becomes softer, and pulmonic closure intensity increases. When reversal of shunt direction occurs in patients with PDA, the lower extremities receive the desaturated pulmonary artery blood flow, and cyanosis and clubbing of the toes develop. In contrast, the upper extremities still receive fully oxygenated blood flow from the ascending aorta; therefore, the fingers are pink and are not clubbed. This differential cyanotic distribution is diagnostic of PDA with Eisenmenger's physiology.

The *electrocardiogram* reveals left ventricular and left atrial enlargement when shunt flow is large. It is normal with a small ductus.

The *chest x-ray* film is normal with small ductus but may be diagnostic in those with large ductus (Fig. 4). Pulmonary plethora, dilation of the proximal pulmonary artery and of the ascending aorta, a prominent aortic knob (in contrast to those with intracardiac shunts, who have a small aortic knob), and left atrial and left ventricular enlargement are present. The right heart is conspicuously normal sized with uncomplicated PDA (Fig. 1c). Calcification of the ductus occurs in older adults.

The *echocardiogram* identifies left atrial and left ventricular enlargement, but delineation of the actual ductus is difficult. Standard gamma imaging following intravenous *technetium-99m pertechnetate* identifies the presence and magnitude of left-to-right shunting, but does not differentiate the level at which shunting occurs.

CARDIAC CATHETERIZATION

Catheterization is indicated in all patients. Its objectives include assessment of shunt size and pulmonary pressure and resistance. The catheter should be passed through the ductus to confirm its existance and to differentiate ductus from other great artery shunts, such as aorticopulmonary window. Angiographic delineation of the ductal anatomy is useful in the older adult to alert the surgeon to aneurysms or atypical anatomy. Patients with elevated pulmonary artery pressure should have a trial of pulmonary vasodilation to identify those with reversible pulmonary vascular obstruction. Patients with net left-to-right shunting should have surgery, while those with net right-to-left shunting are not appropriate candidates.

SURGICAL INTERVENTION

Surgical intervention for PDA consists of double ligation of the ductus with either division or additional ligation to insure obliteration. It does not require heart-lung bypass. It is performed through a left posterior thoracotomy. In children, all ducts should be closed. The optimal age for elective ligation is at one year. Emergency surgery is indicated for infants with medically refractory heart failure. Elective ligation is indicated thereafter at the time of confirmed diagnosis. Older adults with aneurysmal dilation or calcification of the ductus warrant appropriate surgical precautions, including the availability of cardiac bypass, as dissection and rupture may occur.

The *postoperative* patient typically has no further difficulties. Very rarely, recanalization of an improperly ligated and undivided ductus occurs. I believe patients with large ductus and those having repair after early childhood should have postoperative bacterial endocarditis chemoprophylaxis because of the presence of residual endothelial irregularity, which may be a nidus for infection.

It is not yet established whether the *asymptomatic young adult* with small PDA with normal heart size, normal pulmonary artery pressure, and normal pulmonary resistance must have duct closure. In these patients, heart failure, pulmonary vascular obstruction, and symptoms are unlikely ever to develop. Furthermore, some may have spontaneous closure. Aneurysmal dilation and dissection are very rare possibilities; thus, we favor elective ligation. However, close medical follow-up may also be an acceptable alternative. Infective endocarditis precautions are mandatory.

Indomethacin may stimulate ''medical'' closure of PDA in the perinate, but is of no value in older children or adults. It acts by inhibition of prostaglandin activity, which functions to sustain ductal patency.

DIFFERENTIAL DIAGNOSIS

An innocent venous hum is often confused with PDA. Appropriate clinical maneuvers, including auscultation with the patient lying flat or cervical venous occlusion readily differentiate these patients. More critical is identification of patients with aorticopulmonary window at catheterization, because these require heart-lung bypass surgery and median sternotomy. Patients with VSD and aortic incompetence have some similar clinical findings, but can usually be differentiated both clinically and noninvasively. Sinus of Valsalva's fistulae and coronary arteriovenous fistulae may resemble PDA clinically; but in both, the murmur is typically louder over the heart than beneath the left clavicle. Angiography is the confirmatory procedure in both. Angiography is also required to differentiate patients with pulmonary or systemic arteriovenous fistulae in whom the physical examination may closely resemble that in PDA.

Coarctation of the Aorta

Coarctation comprises 15% of adults with congenital heart disease. Hypertensive screening programs and closer scrutiny of hypertensive patients identify increasing numbers with coarctation. The diagnosis is frequently not made until adult life. Both undiagnosed patients and those who have had prior repair are seen by adult physicians. Men outnumber women by two to one. This discussion will concern adult type, or periductal, coarctation.

PATHOPHYSIOLOGY

Coarctation is a fibrotic narrowing of the aortic lumen in the region of the insertion of the ductus or ligamentum arteriosus. The caliber, configuration, and extent of narrowing varies, as does its relationship to the origin of the left subclavian artery and the insertion of the ductus. In some patients, the left subclavian artery arises distally to the coarctation. At least one-third of patients have an associated bicuspid aortic valve. Infants who have early symptoms usually have significant associated VSD, PDA, or aortic stenosis.

The *physiology* of coarctation is that of obstruction to left ventricular outflow. The left ventricle, the proximal aorta, and its proximally arising branches (the carotids and the subclavian arteries) have elevated blood pressure and strong pulse relative to the distal aorta and lower limbs, which have lower blood pressure and delayed arterial pulse. Concentric left ventricular hypertrophy occurs, although in late adult life, there may be heart failure and left ventricular dilation. With significant coarctation narrowing, blood flow to the lower body comes in part from collateral arterial circulation, which arises from the subclavian arteries. The internal mammary and posterior intercostal arteries carry most of this flow and are enlarged. The more severe the coarctation, the more extensive the collateral development.

CLINICAL COURSE

Symptoms are minimal or absent in the young patient and, when present, are secondary to hypertension, which occurs in nearly all patients regardless of age. Headache, epistaxis, forceful carotid pulsations, and lower extremity claudication with exertion occur. Infants who have signficant associated defects can have heart failure, which may be fatal, but, with isolated coarctation, this is not common. Heart failure is rare after infancy and before the fourth decade, but thereafter occurs in two-thirds of patients. Cerebral vascular accident occurs in approximately 8% of patients. It is rare in infants, uncommon in children, but occurs in 20% of older adults. It is attributed to both chronic hypertension and to the increased incidence of congenital berry aneurysm of the circle of Willis associated with coarctation. Cerebral vascular accident is less common after correction but may still occur. Infective endocarditis occurs in 5% of patients, including some who have had repair. It may involve the coarctation or the surgical resection site, or associated lesions, notably a congenitally bicuspid aortic valve, which is present in approximately 25% of patients. Significant stenosis of the bicuspid aortic valve is uncommon until late in life, when calcification and fibrosis develop. Significant obstruction may develop regardless of prior coarctation repair, and late aortic valve replacement may be necessary. Aortic dissection at or near the site of the coarctation is rare. Rarely, coarctation may complicate pregnancy. Both severe hypertension and toxemia are more common in these pregnant women, and aortic dissection is a risk. In the absence of earlier repair, survival beyond age 50 years is unusual.

CLINICAL FINDINGS

Body habitus is usually normal, although some have underdeveloped lower extremities and hypertrophy of their arms and upper body. With Turner's syndrome, coarctation is common and these patients have a typical appearance. The clinical findings in patients with coarctation are diagnostic. Upper extremity hypertension is nearly always present. The upper extremity pulses are forceful relative to the lower extremity pulses, which are typically weak and delayed or absent. All pulses should be checked, as aberrant subclavian artery origin distal to the coarctation occurs. In those patients with extensive collaterals, femoral pulses may be surprisingly strong, but careful comparison with the carotid or brachial pulses reveals a relative difference. Extensive collaterals are evident by both palpation and auscultation over the chest wall. It is worthy of note that unlike the normal person, whose blood pressures in the lower extremities are slightly higher than in their upper extremities, in the patient with coarctation, the legs are always relatively hypotensive. Left ventricular hypertrophy is present. There is often an ejection sound that derives from an associated bicuspid aortic valve or from the dilated ascending aorta. A soft systolic ejection murmur, secondary to a bicuspid valve, may be present; and a systolic murmur over the left upper back, originating from the coarctation, is typical. Findings of heart failure are common in older patients.

The *electrocardiogram* is not specific. The left ventricle is the dominant chamber; however, frank left ventricular hypertrophy and strain are often absent until the third or fourth decade. In younger patients, a right ventricular conduction abnormality is common.

The *chest x-ray* film is often diagnostic (Fig. 5). The coarctation itself is demarcated by an indentation bordered proximally by the dilated left subclavian artery and distally by poststenotic aortic dilation "figure 3 sign." The ascending aorta is dilated. Notching of the posterior inferior ribs develops by adolescence, and increases with

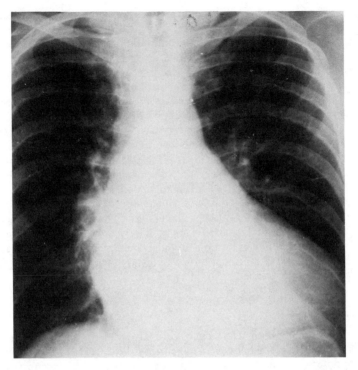

Figure 5 A posteroanterior chest roentgenogram of a 64-year-old woman with coarctation of the aorta. The heart is enlarged owing to left ventricular hypertrophy. The aortic knob shadow is small. The left subclavian artery is enlarged, and there is postcoarctation dilation; thus, a figure-3 sign. There is prominent rib notching. (From Liberthson RR: Congenital heart disease in the child, adolescent and adult, in Johnson RA, Haber E, Austen WG, eds: *Practice of Cardiology*. Boston: Little, Brown, 1980. Reprinted by permission.)

age. Notching may resolve after correction. Heart size is normal, except in those with heart failure who have left ventricular and left atrial enlargement. Calcification of an associated bicuspid aortic valve may be a late finding.

CARDIAC CATHETERIZATION

Catheterization is indicated prior to repair. Its objectives include delineation of the specific coarctation anatomy; assessment of the presence of adequate collateral circulation to permit safe aortic cross-clamping, without risk of spinal cord ischemia; and identification of associated cardiac lesions, particularly aortic stenosis, VSD, and patent ductus arteriosus. In older patients, evaluation to rule out acquired coronary and myocardial disease is advisable. Determination of the pressure gradient across the coarctation is not essential and has limited value, because the severity of the coarctation varies directly with the degree of collateral development that will tend to decrease the transcoarctation gradient.

SURGICAL INTERVENTION

Surgery consists of coarctectomy and either primary aortic reanastomosis (sometimes using a proximal left subclavian flap and distal subclavian ligation), or insertion of a tubular prosthetic graft. Emergency surgery is lifesaving in infants with medically refractory heart failure. Elective repair, optimally, should be performed before school age to avoid the problem of residual hypertension. Thereafter, surgery is still indicated at the time of diagnosis regardless of age. Even older adults who have longstanding hypertension should have correction, as 50% still become normotensive postoperatively and the remainder have more manageable pressures. Older patients with heart failure are also improved by correction.

Postoperative problems include residual coarctation, which is limited to those having correction during infancy and occurs in 25%. Residual hypertension with a blood pressure gradient greater than 20 mm Hg systolic between the arms and legs is an indication for recatheterization and reoperation, after angiographic delineation of the obstruction. Children who had repair before school age rarely have postoperative hypertension, and have a normal lifestyle free of any restriction. However, 30 to 50% of those repaired thereafter have hypertension. Although hypertension is usually mild in these patients, some require treatment with antihypertensive medication. In those with an associated bicuspid aortic valve, late stenosis must be watched for. Chemoprophylaxis for infective endocarditis should be a lifetime commitment, regardless of prior repair.

DIFFERENTIAL DIAGNOSIS

The clinical findings in acquired aortic obstruction secondary to arteritis, notably Takayasu's disease, may closely resemble those of coarctation, although the two are readily differentiated by angiography. Aortic dissection and traumatic paraaortic hematoma or tumor also may have similar findings. Preoperative differentiation of the above greatly alters management. Pseudocoarctation has radiologic features similar to coarctation, but does not have its clinical sequelae, since there is neither aortic obstruction nor hypertension. It does not warrant correction. So-called fetal coarctation is sometimes confused semantically with adult type coarctation. The difference is great, however, in that the former is a variant of the hypoplastic left heart syndrome and has associated hypoplastic left ventricle and ascending aorta, and often aortic and mitral stenosis or atresia. The right heart perfuses the systemic circulation via a large patent ductus. These infants are inoperable and generally die within weeks of birth.

Pulmonic Stenosis

Pulmonic stenosis is present in approximately 10% of adults with congenital heart disease. Both unoperated and postoperative patients present to adult physicians. Men outnumber women by two to one.

PATHOPHYSIOLOGY

Most pulmonic stenosis is valvular and secondary to a partially fused, bicuspid or tricuspid valve. These valves have a domed "fish mouth" appearance. Because of the chronic pressure load imposed on the right ventricle, that chamber hypertrophies. Sometimes there is selective hypertrophy of the infundibulum beneath the pulmonic valve, which contributes to the overall right ventricular outflow tract obstruction.

The *physiologic* consequences of pulmonic stenosis vary with its severity. When severe, there is right ventricular hypertension with decreased right ventricular compliance and elevation of end-diastolic pressure. The severity of pulmonic stenosis is commonly divided into mild, moderate, and severe, according to the pressure gradient between the right ventricle and the pulmonary artery. These gradients approximate less than 40 mm Hg in mild stenosis, between 40 and 70 mm Hg in moderate, and greater than 70 mm Hg in severe.

CLINICAL COURSE

Patients with mild and moderate pulmonic stenosis have few or no symptoms, and lifestyle is normal. They may go undetected until adult life, but often have a long standing history of a loud asymptomatic murmur. Complications, even late in life, are few. Some patients with moderate stenosis have progressive fatigue and dyspnea late in life. Severe stenosis may cause heart failure and cyanosis (owing to right-to-left shunting through a patent foramen ovale) during infancy. Fatigue and dyspnea occur in children and adults with severe cyanosis, but overt clinical failure and atrial arrhythmia are not common. With severe stenosis, chest pain can mimic angina pectoris. It is attributed to the excessive demand placed on coronary flow by the hypertrophied right ventricle. Right ventricular ischemia and infarction occur, but are rare. Infective endocarditis is also rare. With severe stenosis and chronic heart failure, some patients develop cardiac cirrhosis secondary to passive congestion. Paroxysmal dyspnea is uncommon but ominous, and sometimes heralds sudden death with severe stenosis.

CLINICAL FINDINGS

Body habitus is normal and patients are acyanotic, unless there is an associated patent foramen ovale or ASD, which permits right-to-left shunting and, therefore, systemic desaturation. With valvular stenosis, there is an ejection sound. Its position relative to the S_1 correlates inversely with the severity of stenosis. When very close or merged with the S_1, stenosis is severe. Of note, the ejection sound is louder during expiration than inspiration, unlike other right heart auscultatory phenomena. Patients have a systolic ejection murmur heard best at the upper left sternum and loudest with inspiration. Its intensity and duration correlate directly with the stenosis. Very loud and long murmurs that reach to the S_2 indicate severe stenosis. The later the peaking of the murmur, the more severe the stenosis. Pulmonic valve closure intensity correlates inversely with the severity of stenosis. The more severe the stenosis, the softer the pulmonic closure intensity. In addition, the more stenotic the valve, the more delayed the pulmonic closure sound from aortic closure. Patients with moderate or severe stenosis have palpable right ventricular hypertrophy and,

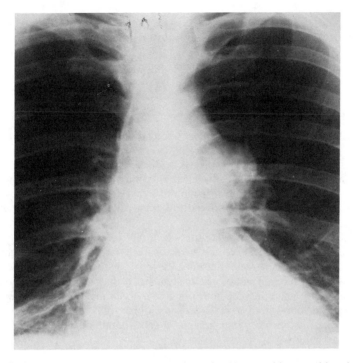

Figure 6 Posteroanterior chest roentgenogram of a 48-year-old man with valvular pulmonic stenosis. There is prominent poststenotic dilation of the main and left pulmonary artery. (From Liberthson RR: Congenital heart disease in the child, adolescent and adult, in Johnson RA, Haber E, Austen WG, eds: *Practice of Cardiology*. Boston: Little, Brown, 1980. Reprinted by permission.)

typically, a systolic thrill at the upper left sternal border. A prominent jugular venous a wave and a right ventricular S_4 are present with severe stenosis.

The *electrocardiogram* shows right atrial and right ventricular hypertrophy and right axis deviation with moderate and severe stenosis, and is normal with mild gradients.

The *chest x-ray* film is often diagnostic. Those patients with moderate or severe stenosis have right ventricular and right atrial enlargement. Patients with valvular stenosis have characteristic poststenotic dilation of the main and left pulmonary arteries (Fig. 6). Poststenotic dilation does not correlate with the severity of stenosis. Pulmonary blood flow is normal.

Cardiac *ultrasound* examination delineates the pulmonic valvular and infundibular anatomy as well as the hypertrophied right ventricle in those patients with significant stenosis. It may be normal with mild stenosis.

CARDIAC CATHETERIZATION

Patients with mild stenosis and no symptoms do not require catheterization. Those with cardiomegaly or symptoms or clinical findings suggesting moderate or severe stenosis should be studied. Catheterization is always indicated prior to surgical intervention. Its objectives include assessment of right ventricular pressure, both absolute and relative to systemic pressure, and determination of the right ventricular outflow tract gradient. Detailed angiographic delineation of the right ventricular outflow tract is essential.

SURGICAL INTERVENTION

Patients with mild stenosis do not require surgery. Those with cardiomegaly, symptoms, and severe stenosis should have surgical revision.

For most patients, pulmonic valve surgery consists of plasty revision to open the valvular commissures and relieve obstruction. Pulmonic valve replacement is rarely necessary. Some patients require resection of hypertrophied and obstructing infundibular muscle, and some require an outflow tract patch if the pulmonary anulus is hypoplastic.

The *postoperative course* following successful relief of obstruction is excellent and patients are asymptomatic. There may be a soft residual systolic murmur and sometimes also a pulmonic diastolic murmur. Residual stenosis occurs, but usually is limited to those with unicuspid or anular stenosis. It may necessitate reoperation if severe. Pulmonary valve incompetence is common but generally well tolerated. In the older adult who has fibrosis secondary to chronic right ventricular hypertrophy, right ventricular dysfunction with fatigue, dyspnea, and sometimes ventricular arrhythmia may persist.

DIFFERENTIAL DIAGNOSIS

Patients with the "straight back syndrome," pectus deformity of the sternum, small ASD, and idiopathic dilation of the pulmonic artery have some findings on physical examination that resemble mild pulmonic stenosis. These conditions are rarely confused with more significant stenosis, however. They can usually be differentiated noninvasively.

Tetralogy of Fallot

Ten percent of adults with congenital heart disease have tetralogy of Fallot. It is the most common cyanotic cardiac lesion encountered after infancy and accounts for more than 50% of adults with cyanotic heart disease. Internists now see the unoperated patient infrequently, but see increasing numbers who have had either prior palliative surgery or definitive corrective procedures.

ANATOMY

By definition, tetralogy has four anatomic components: (1) Right ventricular obstruction is secondary to both infundibular and pulmonic valvular stenosis. Both are of variable severity. Some patients have complete atresia of the right ventricular outflow tract. The pulmonary arteries themselves may also be small and sometimes hypoplastic, which may obviate surgical correction. (2) The VSD is membranous and large and approximates the size of the aortic anulus. (3) Aortic overriding across the ventricular defect is of variable degree and may approach 50% in those with severe pulmonic stenosis. (4) The right ventricle is hypertrophied, secondary to its chronic pressure load; and patchy fibrosis occurs in older adults.

PHYSIOLOGY

There are two essential physiologic components in tetralogy. (1) The right ventricular outflow tract obstruction causes decreased pulmonary blood flow; and (2) the large VSD allows blood to flow from the right ventricle to the systemic circulation (right-to-left shunting). Systemic desaturation is variable, depending on the severity of right ventricular obstruction. When severe, desaturation is marked. In the absence of surgical intervention, patients with severe pulmonic stenosis or atresia must develop collateral blood flow from the systemic to the pulmonary circulation in order to survive. In older patients, these natural collateral channels are extensive. When right ventricular obstruction is mild, right-to-left shunting is minimal and patients may be acyanotic (pink tetralogy).

CLINICAL COURSE

Cyanosis is typically present from early infancy and is progressive and worsened by exertion. A history of "tet spells" during the first years of life is sometimes given. Spells typically occur in hot weather, follow exertion or feeding, and are characterized by irritability, dyspnea, hyperventilation, cyanosis, and sometimes syncope and seizure. Some patients have late residua of these spells, including seizure disorders and cerebral vascular accident. Spells are rare after the age of two years. Squatting is learned from infancy and is often incorporated into a child's activities, allowing him or her periods of comfort during play. More socially acceptable postures, such as crossing the legs when sitting, are sometimes adopted by adults. Squatting increases systemic resistance and, therefore, decreases right-to-left blood flow across the ventricular defect and forces more blood to the lungs. Patients with chronic right-to-left shunting and systemic desaturation compensate by increased erythropoietin secretion and develop erythrocytosis. When the erythrocytosis becomes excessive, however, (hematocrit greater than 65%), dyspnea, fatigue, and in situ thrombosis may occur. Some patients who have not had surgical intervention give a history of repeated phlebotomy. With longstanding erythrocytosis, there may be uric acid elevation and symptomatic gout. Chronic right-to-left shunting subjects both uncorrected patients and those who have had only palliative surgical procedures to the risk of systemic embolization. These may occur with careless intravenous technique. Cerebral abscess is another sequelae of chronic right-to-left shunting, and must be suspected in patients with neurologic symptoms or findings. Bacterial endocarditis occurs in uncorrected patients and in those with palliated and corrected tetralogy. It usually involves the right ventricular outflow tract or the overriding aortic valve, but it may occur at the site of palliative shunt insertion. Chemoprophylaxis is, therefore, a lifetime obligation. In the adult, ventricular tachyarrhythmia is an ominous finding and may herald sudden death. Maternal mortality is increased in pregnant women with uncorrected tetralogy, and the incidence of fetal death is also greatly increased.

CLINICAL FINDINGS

The salient findings in unoperated patients include generalized cyanosis and digital clubbing. Body habitus is normal, although kyphoscoliosis occurs in 20%. Those who have had a prior palliative procedure have a thoracotomy incision. Corrective procedures are performed via a median sternotomy. In the adult who has not had prior surgery, there are continuous collateral bruits throughout the chest. Those with a functioning palliative shunt will have a similar sounding continuous bruit beneath their thoracotomy scar.

The actual cardiac examination in patients with palliative shunts and those who have not had prior surgery is the same because both still have the anatomic components of tetralogy. Successfully palliated patients differ only in having less cyanosis, because their pulmonary blood flow has been augmented; often they have no digital clubbing. However, previously palliated patients may outgrow or close their shunts and develop progressive cyanosis. In both uncorrected and palliated patients, there is palpable right ventricular hypertrophy, and a palpable systolic thrill secondary to pulmonic stenosis. The S_1 is normal; the S_2 is single and often loud. Patients with very mild tetralogy (pink tet) may have an audible pulmonic closure sound, which is otherwise atypical in tetralogy. An ejection sound is common and arises from the overriding aortic valve and is best heard on expiration. A systolic ejection murmur secondary to right ventricular outflow tract obstruction is typical. The length, intensity, and contour of this murmur help the clinician assess the severity of pulmonic stenosis. Long, loud, late-peaking murmurs indicate less severe right ventricular obstruction than do short, soft, early-peaking murmurs. With pulmonary atresia, there is no outflow tract murmur.

The *electrocardiogram* is not specific for tetralogy of Fallot, but reveals right ventricular hypertrophy and right axis deviation in both uncorrected and palliated patients.

The *chest x-ray* film is often diagnostic. In the young patient, pulmonary vascular markings are diminished. However, with age and proliferation of collateral circulation, pulmonary vascular markings may actually be increased (Fig. 7). Functioning palliative shunts also cause increased pulmonary markings and enlargement of the pulmonary branch into which they enter. In unoperated patients and in those with palliative shunts, the cardiac silhouette is typical. There is an upturned apex, secondary to right ventricular enlargement, and a concave left basal region caused by the small main pulmonary artery. This combination gives the heart a boot shape. Approximately 25% of patients with tetralogy have a right-sided aortic arch.

Ultrasound examination delineates the morphology of the right ventricular obstruction, the VSD, the overriding aorta, and the hypertrophied right ventricle. It also differentiates tetralogy from more complex entities, including single ventricle and variants of transposition of the great arteries.

CARDIAC CATHETERIZATION

Catheterization is always necessary prior to surgical intervention. Its objectives include detailed angiographic study of the right ventricular obstruction, including assessment of the caliber of the pulmonary arteries; assessment of the VSD and exclusion of multiple or atypical septal defects; and evaluation of the coronary arteries

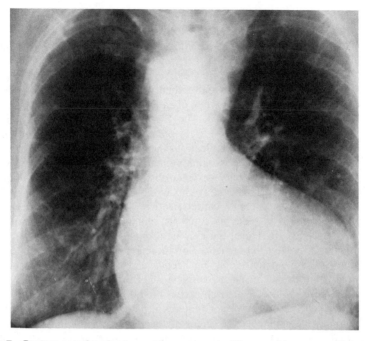

Figure 7 Posteroanterior chest roentgenogram of a 59-year-old woman with tetralogy of Fallot and extensive systemic to pulmonary collateral vasculature with secondary rib notching. The cardiac silhouette has a distinctive "boot" shape secondary to the upturned apex, secondary to right ventricular hypertrophy and the concave pulmonary artery segment. There is a right aortic arch. (From Liberthson RR: Congenital heart disease in the child, adolescent and adult, in Johnson RA, Haber E, Austen WG, eds: *Practice of Cardiology.* Boston: Little, Brown, 1980. Reprinted by permission.)

to identify the approximately 5% of patients who have anomalous origin of major left coronary branches from the right coronary. These branches cross the anterior right ventricle and can be damaged at the time of right ventriculotomy if not identified. In patients who have had prior palliative shunts, it is important to assess pulmonary artery pressure and resistance, as longstanding shunts may cause severe pulmonary vascular obstruction. Angiographic study of these surgical shunts is also important prior to surgical revision. Catheterization must also exclude more complex entities.

SURGICAL INTERVENTION

Surgery for tetralogy of Fallot began with the *palliative* procedures involving creation of a shunt between the systemic and pulmonary circulations to increase pulmonary blood flow and to alleviate systemic desaturation. The *Blalock-Taussig* shunt involves ligation of the distal subclavian artery and insertion of its proximal end into the ipsilateral pulmonary artery. Complications with this procedure are rare, and excellent long-term alleviation of desaturation is typical. Both pulse and blood pressure in the ipsilateral arm are sacrificed, but arm function and development are usually normal. The *Potts* shunt involves creation of a surgical window between the left pulmonary artery and the descending aorta. It also achieves excellent long-term palliation of desaturation. However, about one-quarter of patients develop either early heart failure because of excessive pulmonary flow or late pulmonary vascular obstruction. Patients with these shunts require assessment of pulmonary artery pressure and resistance at the time of catheterization. When the latter is high, corrective surgery may be precluded. The *Waterston* shunt is a surgical window between the ascending aorta and the right pulmonary artery. It also provides excellent palliation. However, its complications include hypoplasia and stenosis of the right pulmonary artery secondary to kinking; early heart failure if the shunt is too large; and, occasionally, pulmonary vascular obstruction. Regardless of shunt type, patients may outgrow them, or they may kink or close, and recurrent and progressive cyanosis occurs. In these patients, catheterization and further surgery is indicated. In spite of their success in relieving cyanosis, shunts do not alter the intracardiac pathology of tetralogy; therefore, the chronic sequelae of right-to-left shunting and right ventricular hypertension remain. For these reasons, patients with palliative shunts should still have definitive surgical repair and shunt closure.

Correction of tetralogy consists of surgical relief of right ventricular obstruction (which may require the use of a patch across the outflow tract), and patch closure of the VSD. When the outflow tract requires a patch to enlarge it, patients have residual pulmonic incompetence. Most centers perform elective total correction during early childhood. Infants who have spells require either emergency palliation or definitive repair. Thereafter, surgery should be performed when the diagnosis is confirmed. After the fifth decade, risks of total correction increase because of right ventricular dysfunction, secondary to chronic hypertrophy and fibrosis.

Following successful tetralogy repair, patients become acyanotic, clubbing resolves over a period of years, exercise tolerance markedly improves, and lifestyle becomes normal. Some patients still have residual problems and all require continued surveillance. Problems include residual right ventricular obstruction which, when severe (gradient greater than 50 mm Hg), requires reoperation, and incompletely closed VSD. In the latter, when shunt size exceeds two to one, repeat operation is appropriate. Patients with right ventricular outflow tract patches have pulmonic incompetence, but this is usually well tolerated. If an anomalous coronary artery was damaged at the time of repair, patients may have anterior wall myocardial infarction. Ventricular ectopy usually arises from the right ventricle and may be secondary to fibrosis or to aneurysm or infarction in those patients with a damaged anomalous coronary artery. It is an ominous finding and requires intensive antiarrhythmic treatment. When ventricular ectopy is associated with significant residual right ventricular obstruction, VSD, or severe pulmonic incompetence, patients may require reoperation. Right bundle branch block and left anterior hemiblock occur in 10% of patients following repair, but rarely leads to more advanced degrees of heart block. Syncope in these patients is uncommon.

DIFFERENTIAL DIAGNOSIS

Patients with pulmonic stenosis and VSD who also have variants of transposition of the great arteries, as well as those who have single ventricle rather than just a

VSD, may be impossible to differentiate from tetralogy of Fallot clinically. Both ultrasound and angiography are important in identifying these patients. The latter is essential, because in some reparative surgery is precluded and in others its risk may be great.

Bibliography

Barry WH, Grossman W: Cardiac Catheterization, Braunwald E (ed): in *Heart Disease*. Philadelphia, Saunders, 1980, p 278.

Flamm MD, Cohn KE, Hancock EW: Measurement of sytemic cardiac output at rest and exercise in patients with atrial septal defect. *Am J Cardiol* 23:258, 1969.

Liberthson RR: Congenital heart disease in the child, adolescent, and adult patient, in Johnson RA, Haber E, Austen WG (eds): *The Practice of Cardiology*. Boston, Little, Brown, 1980, p 755.

Perloff J: *The Clinical Recognition of Congenital Heart Disease*. Philadelphia, Saunders 1980.

Roberts WC: *Congenital Heart Disease in Adults*. Philadelphia, Davis, 1979.

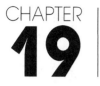

CHAPTER 19 | HEART FAILURE

Victor J. Dzau
Robert A. Kloner

Definition and Mechanisms of Heart Failure

Heart failure may be defined as that condition in which the heart cannot pump blood at a volume adequate to meet the metabolic needs of the tissues of the body, due to an abnormality of cardiac function. The abnormality in cardiac function may be due to an abnormality in the myocardial cells themselves (*myocardial failure*) or due to some other abnormality within the structure of the heart, such as valvular stenosis or regurgitation.

Myocardial failure may be due to a quantitative loss of functioning myofibers, such as heart failure associated with a large myocardial infarction (MI), or to a generalized qualitative abnormality in myocyte function, as occurs with congestive cardiomyopathy. The exact mechanism of the abnormal myocyte function in myocardial failure remains controversial, but there are several likely causes. One possible mechanism is the reduction in myofibrillar ATPase, which has been observed in the hearts of patients and experimental animals with congestive heart failure. Another possible mechanism comes from animal studies that suggest that sarcoplasmic reticulum is defective in its ability to pump calcium. Normally, the sarcoplasmic reticulum takes up intracellular calcium during the relaxation phase of the cardiac cycle. During electrical depolarization, extracellular calcium enters the cell and intracellular calcium is released from the sarcoplasmic reticulum. The calcium interacts with the contractile apparatus, resulting in a contraction. Experimental studies suggest that, in myocardial failure, the sarcoplasmic reticulum is defective in its ability to take up calcium during relaxation. As a result, there is little calcium available for release to the contractile apparatus during systole. In myocardial failure, the mitochondria may become the main site of uptake of calcium and source of calcium for contraction. Release of calcium from the mitrochondria is a slow process, however, and this could lead to reduced amounts of calcium available to activate the contractile mechanism.

Other possible explanations for myocardial failure include reduced coronary blood flow and myocardial oxygen consumption per unit of tissue. Depletion of norepinephrine from myocardial stores has been observed in myocardial failure. Although regional norepinephrine stores do not play a role in the intrinsic contractile state of the myocardium, the adrenergic nervous system is an important compensatory mechanism for the failing heart. The depleted norepinephrine levels may impede this compensatory mechanism.

Compensatory Mechanisms in Heart Failure

There are several compensatory mechanisms that the heart relies upon for maintenance of its pumping ability in the setting of either myocardial failure or an excessive hemodynamic burden (such as systemic hypertension, aortic regurgitation, or stenosis). The first is the Frank-Starling mechanism, in which the force of contraction or extent of shortening is dependent upon the initial muscle length. When the muscle and, therefore, sarcomere length is increased by an increase in preload to provide optimal overlap between the actin (thin) and myosin (thick) filaments, cardiac performance is enhanced. The optimal overlap of the thick and thin filaments occurs when sarcomere length is between 2.0–2.2 µm. At this length, the number of force-generating cross links between the actin and myosin filaments is maximal. When sarcomere length is less than 2.0 µm, developed tension is reduced; when sarcomere length is greater than 2.2 µm, there is a fall in developed tension.

Figure 1 shows a typical example of Frank-Starling curves. Ventricular end-diastolic volume (preload) is plotted on the horizontal axis, while ventricular performance (this could be expressed as stroke volume) is plotted on the verticle axis. As ventricular end-diastolic volume or preload increases, so does ventricular performance. Braunwald et al. have described those factors resulting in changes along a given curve (changes in preload resulting in different degrees of stretching of the myocardium) and those changes shifting the curve (alterations of the contractile state of the myocardium). Factors that alter ventricular end-diastolic volume and, hence, result in movement along a given Frank-Starling curve include total blood volume; body position; intrathoracic and intrapericardial pressure; venous tone; the pumping action of skeletal muscle that returns blood to the heart; and the atrial contribution to ventricular filling. Factors that shift the Frank-Starling curve upward and to the left (increase in the contractile state of the myocardium as shown in curve B) include sympathetic nerve stimulation; circulating catecholamines; positive inotropic agents, such as digitalis; and the force-frequency relationship (an increase in heart rate resulting in an increase in contractility). Factors that shift the Frank-Starling curve down and to the right (depressed contractile state of the myocardium; curve C)

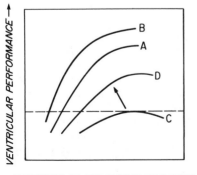

Figure 1 Starling curves showing ventricular end-diastolic volume plotted on the horizontal axis and ventricular performance on the vertical axis. The horizontal axis could also be ventricular end-diastolic pressure, and the vertical axis could be stroke volume or stroke work. Curve A represents the normal curve; curve B represents a curve of increased contractile state; curve C represents that of reduced contractile state; curve D represents the curve of a failing heart following digitalis treatment.

include anoxia, hypercapnia, acidosis, pharmacologic depressants (such as quinidine and local anesthetic agents), loss of myocardium, and intrinsic myocardial depression.

Patients with myocardial failure function along this depressed (curve C) Frank-Starling curve. In order to maintain the same ventricular performance as in a normal heart, they must have a higher ventricular end-diastolic volume. If the metabolic demands of the body increase, requiring increased cardiac performance, this occurs in such patients at the expense of a higher ventricular end-diastolic volume, which may in turn result in the symptoms of dyspnea or even pulmonary edema.

The second compensatory mechanism of heart failure is an increase in release of catecholamines by sympathetic cardiac nerves and an increase in circulating catecholamines by release from the adrenal medulla, which enhance myocardial contractility.

Other neurohumoral systems are activated, including the renin angiotensin-aldosterone system and vasopressin. These factors plus increased sympathetic tone result in increased systemic vascular resistance, and promote salt and water retention. The former restores systemic blood pressure, but results in increased afterload. The latter increases ventricular filling (preload).

Long term compensatory mechanisms of the heart to valvular or myocardial abnormalities include myocardial hypertrophy and dilatation. In the initial stages of heart failure, the compensatory mechanisms may sustain the circulatory needs of the body. Eventually, however, as myocardial failure progresses, the compensatory mechanisms can no longer maintain the pump function of the heart and the clinical syndrome of heart failure emerges.

The Clinical Syndrome of Heart Failure

THE CONCEPT OF FORWARD VERSUS BACKWARD HEART FAILURE

The clinical syndrome of heart failure has been hypothesized to arise from either backward or forward cardiac failure, or both. Backward failure refers to blood damming up behind one or both ventricles, due to the inability of the ventricle to discharge its contents. Symptoms result from an increase in systemic venous pressure with right ventricular failure resulting in transudation of fluid into the interstitium of the liver, mesentery, and subcutaneous tissue; or from an increase in pulmonary venous pressure with left ventricular failure, resulting in transudation of fluid into the interstitium of the lung. The forward failure hypothesis refers to the inability of the heart to pump an adequate amount of blood into the arterial tree, resulting in symptoms of underperfusion of the vital organs. Reduced perfusion to the kidneys results in increased sodium and water retention, leading to an increase in extracellular fluid and tissue congestion. The renal mechanisms for increased water retention are complex; they include reduced renal water excretion due to decreased renal blood flow with reduced glomerular filtration rate, enhancement of the renin angiotensin-aldosterone system, and enhanced antidiuretic hormone release. Reduced forward output to the brain results in mental confusion; to the skeletal muscles, in weakness.

In the majority of patients with chronic heart failure, both backward and forward failure result in symptoms.

THE CONCEPT OF RIGHT- VERSUS LEFT-SIDED HEART FAILURE

Right ventricular failure, associated with blood "damming up" in the systemic vasculature, includes symptoms and signs of edema, congestive hepatomegaly, ascites, and eventually signs of low forward output including weakness and mental confusion. Symptoms and signs of left ventricular failure are due to blood "damming up" behind the left ventricle and to pulmonary congestion. Long-standing left ventricular failure may eventually result in signs of right ventricular failure, with generalized accumulation of fluid. Experimental studies have shown that failure of one ventricle induced by a hemodynamic stress eventually results in biochemical changes (depletion of norepinephrine and abnormalities in the activity of actinomyosin ATPase) of the other ventricle. This may be secondary to the fact that muscle bundles composing one ventricle are in continuity with those of the other ventricle.

LOW VERSUS HIGH OUTPUT CARDIAC FAILURE

Heart failure causing low cardiac output is the most common form of heart failure and is usually due to an ischemic, valvular, hypertensive, congenital, or cardiomyopathic process. Heart failure also may result from several high output states such as beriberi, Paget's disease, thyrotoxicosis, arteriovenous fistula, and anemia. While low output failure is characterized by reduced stroke volume, peripheral vasoconstriction with cold and pale extremities, reduced pulse pressure, and widened arteriovenous oxygen difference, high output failure is characterized by a widened pulse pressure and peripheral vasodilatation, with warm and flushed extremities. High output states are associated with reduced arteriovenous oxygen difference. There is not as much of a decrease in arteriovenous oxygen difference in patients with high output states once congestive heart failure develops.

Causes of Heart Failure

The general underlying causes of heart failure are outlined in Table 1. It is important to realize that 50% of episodes of clinical heart failure are secondary to a precipitating cause. Thus, in treating heart failure, it is important to recognize both the underlying and precipitating causes.

The Clinical Symptoms of Left-Sided Heart Failure

The major clinical symptoms of left ventricular heart failure include exertional dyspnea, orthopnea, paroxysmal nocturnal dyspnea, dyspnea at rest, pulmonary edema, weakness, fatigue, nocturia, and mental confusion.

Table 1. Causes of Heart Failure

Primary abnormality of myocardial cells
  Cardiomyopathy and myocarditis
Secondary abnormality of myocardial cells
  Due to prolonged exposure to a hemodynamic burden (i.e., aortic regurgitation, hypertensive heart disease, primary or secondary pulmonary hypertension)
  Due to reduced O_2 delivery (ischemia)
Structural abnormalities
  Valvular heart disease
  Congenital heart disease
  Pericardial disease
  Coronary artery disease (ischemia, myocardial infarction, LV aneurysm)
  Intracavity outflow obstruction
High output states
Precipitating causes
  Increased salt intake
  Inappropriate reduction of a drug regimen
  Excess exertion or emotion
  Arrhythmias
  Systemic infection
  Onset of high output states: anemia, hyperthyroidism, pregnancy
  Pulmonary embolism
  Increased fluid load
  Renal failure
  Myocardial ischemia
  Cardiac depressants (e.g., disopyramide)

Dyspnea is the sensation of breathlessness, difficulty in breathing, or increased awareness of breathing, which occurs with elevation in left atrial pressure resulting in pulmonary capillary hypertension. It is associated with a restrictive ventilatory defect due to the replacement of air with fluid or blood in the lungs. The work of breathing is increased in order to distend the stiffened lungs. In the early phases of left ventricular heart failure, the dyspnea occurs only with exertion; with increasing heart failure, the level of exertion resulting in dyspnea diminishes until, in severe heart failure, dyspnea occurs at rest. Orthopnea is dyspnea that occurs while the patient is recumbent and is relieved by standing or sitting. It is caused by redistribution of fluid from the dependent parts of the circulation to the thorax, where the depressed left ventricle cannot pump the additional volume of delivered blood. Orthopnea results from pulmonary venous and capillary congestion. The severity of the orthopnea can often be determined by asking the patient how many pillows he sleeps on.

Paroxysmal nocturnal dyspnea (PND, an extreme form of orthopnea) occurs when a patient wakes from sleep with a sense of severe breathlessness and suffocation. It is often associated with bronchospasm and, hence, has been referred to as "cardiac

Table 2. Noncardiac Causes of Pulmonary Edema

Decreased plasma oncotic pressure: hypoalbumenemia due to renal, hepatic disease, nutritional cause, or protein-losing enteropathy

Altered alveolar-capillary membrane permeability (often referred to as Adult Respiratory Distress Syndrome, ARDS

    Pneumonia: viral, bacterial, parasite, aspiration

    Inhaled toxins: smoke, nitrogen dioxide, phosgene

    Circulating toxins: bacterial endotoxins, snake venom

    Radiation pneumonitis

    Endogenous vasoactive substances: kinins, histamines

    Disseminated intravascular coagulation

    Uremia

    Immunologic reactions: hypersensitivity pneumonitis

    Associated with drowning

Lymphatic insufficiency: carcinomatosis, fibrosing lymphangitis

Unknown or not well understood

    Narcotic overdose: heroin

    High altitude pulmonary edema

    Neurogenic: subarachnoid hemorrhage, central nervous system trauma

    Eclampsia

    Postcardiopulmonary bypass

    Postcardioversion

    Postanesthesia

---

asthma.'' PND occurs at night, usually, and is frequently not relieved by sitting upright. The pathophysiology of this condition includes interstitial edema.

Pulmonary edema occurs when there is marked elevation of the left atrial pressure and transudation of fluid into the alveoli. It is the severest form of breathlessness associated with heart failure. In acute pulmonary edema, patients are severely short of breath at rest, with associated agitation or dizziness. Pulmonary edema, which is considered a medical emergency, can be caused by any entity causing heart failure (Table 1). In addition, there are several noncardiac causes of pulmonary edema (increased capillary "leakage" without elevation of atrial pressures), which should be kept in mind (Table 2).

Differentiating between dyspnea due to cardiac disease and dyspnea due to pulmonary disease may be difficult, especially when both disease processes coexist. Table 3 presents some useful differentiating features.

Other symptoms of left-sided heart failure reflecting reduced forward output include fatigue; weakness; and, in severe cases, mental confusion.

The New York Heart Association (NYHA) has devised a functional classification of heart disease that grades the severity of heart failure according to the amount of exertion required to cause symptoms. While the classification is based on subjective findings, it has proved useful in following the course of patients during their disease, assessing results of therapy, and comparing groups of patients.

Table 3. Differentiation of Cardiac versus Pulmonary Dyspnea

Cardiac dyspnea	Pulmonary dyspnea
Onset of dyspnea more sudden	Dyspnea tends to occur more gradually (except with infectious bronchitis, pneumonitis, pneumothorax, asthma)
Dyspnea usually not associated with sputum production	Dyspnea at night often associated with sputum production and relieved by coughing up sputum
No history of pulmonary disease	History of chronic obstructive lung disease; smoking history; noxious inhalants
No history of smoking	
No evidence of lung disease on chest x-ray film	Chest x-ray evidence of lung disease
Restrictive ventilatory defect by pulmonary function tests	Obstructive or restrictive ventilatory defect by pulmonary function tests
Arm to tongue circulation time usually increased (>16 sec)[a]	Arm to tongue circulation time more likely to be normal

[a] The circulation time may be a useful test to perform when trying to distinguish pulmonary from cardiac dyspnea and low output from high output heart failure. Three to five ml of Decholin is injected rapidly intravenously and the time until the patient senses a bitter taste is measured. Normal values are 9–16 seconds. In patients with low-output heart failure, values are >16; in patients with high-output failure, circulation time is normal or reduced; in patients without heart failure, values are normal.

Class I. No limitation of physical activity. No dyspnea, fatigue, palpitations with ordinary physical activity.

Class II. Slight limitation of physical activity. These patients have fatigue, palpitation, dyspnea with ordinary physical activity but are comfortable at rest.

Class III. Marked limitation of activity. Less than ordinary physical activity results in symptoms but patients are comfortable at rest.

Table 4. Specific Etiologies of Right-Sided Heart Failure

Mitral stenosis with pulmonary hypertension
Cor pulmonale due to chronic obstructive lung disease
Pulmonary valve stenosis
Pulmonary hypertension due to other causes
    Congenital heart disease
    Primary pulmonary hypertension
    Collagen vascular disease
Tricuspid valve regurgitation (causes right ventricular [RV] failure)
Tricuspid valve stenosis; obstruction of flow into RV without RV myocardial failure
Right ventricular myocardial infarction
Cardiomyopathy
Chronic left-sided congestive heart failure due to valvular, ischemic disease

Class IV. Symptoms are present at rest and any physical exertion exacerbates the symptoms.

The Symptoms of Right-Sided Heart Failure

The common specific etiologies of right-sided heart failure are listed in Table 4. Symptoms of predominantly right-sided heart failure are those of systemic venous congestion, including dependent edema; right upper quadrant pain due to stretching of the hepatic capsule from liver engorgement; anorexia, nausea, and bloating due to congestion of the mesentery and liver; and fatigue as forward output diminishes. It is unusual to have pulmonary symptoms unless there is concomitant left-sided heart failure.

Signs of Heart Failure

The general appearance of patients in left-sided heart failure is affected by the severity of the heart failure. With mild failure, patients may appear entirely comfortable sitting at rest and do not appear breathless or in any distress until they undertake physical activity or lie flat. With severe failure, patients at rest may appear to be in severe distress, tachypneic, pale, with cool extremities. They may be cyanotic.

Examination of the lungs in patients with mild heart failure reveals moist rales at the bases; with severe failure, and pulmonary edema rales may be heard over the entire lung fields and may be associated with blood-tinged sputum. Dullness on percussion at the lung bases may reflect a pleural effusion.

If heart failure is secondary to left ventricular failure, evidence of dilatation and/ or hypertrophy of that chamber may be present, including displacement of the apical impulse downward and towards the axilla (dilatation) and a left ventricular heave, which is a localized sustained outward motion of the ventricle during systole (left ventricular hypertrophy). With right ventricular enlargement, the right heart border may be percussed to the right of the sternum and a right ventricular heave may be felt as a diffuse lift over the lower portion of the sternum.

The S_1 is often normal; P_2 may be accentuated with the development of left ventricular failure and pulmonary hypertension. A protodiastolic or S_3 gallop, heard 0.13 to 0.16 seconds after the S_2, is a common sign of congestive heart failure. This sound occurs in association with increased ventricular volumes and is caused by a rapid deceleration of ventricular inflow occurring just after the early filling phase of the ventricle. Reduced ventricular distensibility may contribute to the gallop sound.

Fourth heart sounds (presystolic gallop) may be heard when congestive heart failure is associated with conditions in which the atrium contracts forcibly into a noncompliant left ventricle and occur with left ventricular hypertrophy. Gallops emanating from the left ventricle are best heard at the apex with the patient in the left lateral decubitus position; gallops emanating from the right ventricle are best heard at the lower left sternal border and, typically, increase with inspiration. Murmurs due to mitral regurgitation or tricuspid regurgitation secondary to ventricular dilatation are not uncommon in heart failure.

Tachycardia is another common manifestation of heart failure and is a compensatory mechanism whereby the heart attempts to maintain cardiac output in the setting of reduced stroke volume.

Pulsus alternans is characterized by a regular rhythm in which there is an alternation of strong and weak contractions as detected by palpation of the pulse or by sphygmomanometry. This phenomenon occurs secondary to alternating stroke volume due to incomplete recovery of contractile cells on every other beat.

Cheyne-Stokes respiration occurs in advanced cardiac failure and is characterized by alternating periods of apnea and hyperpnea. This condition is due to a reduced sensitivity of the respiratory center to CO_2 and prolonged circulation time from lung to brain associated with left ventricular failure. When congestive failure is severe and long standing, cardiac cachexia occurs with anorexia and weight loss.

Signs of right ventricular failure include jugular venous distension, hepatojugular reflux, hepatomegaly, right upper quadrant tenderness, edema, and ascites. When severe congestion of the viscera occurs, a protein-losing enteropathy may exacerbate the development of ascites by a reduction in plasma oncotic pressure. With the development of tricuspid regurgitation, a systolic regurgitant v wave may be seen and palpitated in the jugular veins.

Laboratory Examination in Congestive Heart Failure

A typical chest x-ray feature of congestive heart failure includes cardiomegaly with a cardiothoracic ratio of more than 0.5 to 0.6. The appearance of the lung fields serves as an estimate of the pulmonary capillary pressure. Normally the apices of the lung are less well perfused than the bases. With pulmonary capillary pressures of 15–20 mm Hg, there is equalization of apical and basal perfusion; with pulmonary capillary pressures of 20–25 mm Hg, upper lobe pulmonary veins become more prominent than those in the lower lobe. With pulmonary capillary pressures of greater than 25 mm Hg interstitial pulmonary edema and Kerley B Lines (interlobular edema) occurs and with pressures exceeding 25–30 mm Hg alveolar edema, and pleural effusions may be seen.

Further details of the chest x-ray film of heart failure appear in Chapter 4.

The electrocardiogram (ECG) may help define the underlying etiology of the heart failure and confirm the presence of ventricular hypertrophy (See Chapter 3).

Echocardiography is useful in assessing the severity and etiology of heart failure and may aid in serial evaluation of the effect of therapy. Radionuclide ventriculography is another useful noninvasive technique for assessing ventricular function. Serial ejection fractions can be followed, and areas of abnormal ventricular wall motion due to infarction detected. Serial exercise testing and exercise radionuclide ventriculography can be used to follow the response of patients with chronic heart failure to treatment regimens. Cardiac catheterization is undertaken for defining the underlying abnormality of heart failure, but is usually not needed for establishing the diagnosis of congestive heart failure. Catheterization may be helpful in assessing the effect of various pharmacologic interventions, such as vasodilators or experimental inotropic agents, on patients whose heart failure is refractory to other forms of medical therapy.

Several blood chemistries may be abnormal in congestive heart failure, including elevated liver enzymes (SGOT, SGPT) and bilirubin secondary to hepatic congestion. Urinalysis may reveal proteinuria and high urine specific gravity. With reduced renal flow, the BUN becomes elevated. With chronic cor pulmonale, polycythemia may occur. Serum electrolytes are usually normal in most cases of mild to moderate congestive heart failure prior to treatment. With severe heart failure, diuretic therapy, salt restriction, and reduced ability to excrete free water result in dilutional hyponatremia.

Hypokalemia may result from thiazide or loop diuretics. Hyperkalemia may also result from spironolactone administration or it may occur in severe heart failure with markedly reduced renal blood flow.

Therapy of Congestive Heart Failure

MANAGEMENT OF ACUTE CARDIOGENIC PULMONARY EDEMA

The major aim of the management of acute cardiogenic pulmonary edema is to improve oxygenation and reduce pulmonary capillary pressure. Oxygen should be administered by nasal prongs or face mask at high flow rate (except with chronic obstructive lung disease and CO_2 retention). At least one large (number 18 or larger) bore intravenous catheter should be placed for access to the circulation. The patient should be sitting upright, which increases venous pooling, reduces central venous pressure, and improves pulmonary perfusion-ventilation matching. Arterial blood gas prior to oxygen administration and a twelve lead ECG should be immediately obtained. Other nonpharmacologic interventions include applying tourniquets in rotation or in three of four extremities and phlebotomy. The value of the former has not been clearly established and the latter is usually reserved for dire emergencies.

The first pharmacologic agent immediately administered in acute pulmonary edema is intravenous morphine. Morphine reduces both preload and afterload. In addition, it reduces the sympathetic overdrive and anxiety, which can worsen pulmonary edema in these patients. Morphine is administered slowly (3–10 mg). Signs of respiratory depression must be closely watched for. Naloxone or nalorphine hydrochloride (morphine antagonists), should be available. Relative contraindications to morphine include severe pulmonary disease, severe kyphoscoliosis, liver failure, and myxedema. Aminophylline given parenterally (250–500 mg IV over 15 to 20 minutes) improves ventilation. More important is the use of intravenous furosemide for diuresis. Furosemide (10–40 mg) induces veno and arteriolar dilatation and also causes diuresis in 10–30 minutes after intravenous administration. The peak effect is in 60 minutes. Digitalization is useful, especially if there is atrial tachyarrhythmia with rapid ventricular response. If the patient has a systolic blood pressure greater than 95 mm Hg, sublingual or intravenous nitroglycerin may be administered in order to reduce ventricular preload.

The acid–base disturbances in acute pulmonary edema include acute respiratory alkalosis, acute respiratory alkalosis with metabolic acidosis, or acute respiratory acidosis with primary metabolic acidosis. In the latter situation, hypoperfusion of tissue produces a lactic acidosis. Furthermore, severe alveolar-arteriolar oxygen gradient and ventilation/perfusion mismatching can lead to respiratory acidosis. Combined acidosis carries a poor prognosis and is frequently a harbinger of cardiopulmonary arrest. In patients with $pCO_2 > 60$ mm Hg and pH <7.2, immediate intubation with assisted ventilation is indicated.

Factors that may have precipitated the pulmonary edema should be identified and treated. For example, atrial fibrillation and ventricular tachycardia must be recognized and rapidly treated. If pulmonary edema occurs due to a severe bradycardia that is unresponsive to medical therapy, a pacemaker should be inserted. Other precipitating causes of pulmonary edema include hypertensive crisis, acute myocardial infarction (MI) or ischemia, anemia, iatrogenic fluid overload, and infection.

MANAGEMENT OF CHRONIC CONGESTIVE HEART FAILURE

Management Strategy

General measures for the treatment of chronic heart failure include restrictions in dietary sodium intake and physical activity; weight reduction for the obese patient; avoidance of precipitating factors; and control of related diseases such as arrhythmias, hypertension, and myocardial ischemia. Dietary restrictions range from eliminating salt at the table to a strict low sodium diet. Elimination of the salt shaker at the table and excessively salty food (such as potato chips, pretzels, salted nuts, salt cured meat) will reduce the average American daily sodium intake from 2.5–6.0 g to 1.6–2.8 g. Salt substitutes such as KCl may be used. Strict adherence to a rigid dietary program is essential for patients with class III–IV symptoms. In these patients, sodium intake may be reduced to 1.2–1.6 g per day by eliminating salt from cooking. In patients with severe class IV symptoms, it may become necessary to reduce daily sodium intake to 0.2–0.5 g daily. This will require avoidance of bread, cereal, milk, canned vegetables, soup, and cheese. There are a large number of specially prepared low salt or salt free foods, which may be useful.

Excessive physical exertion places an extra demand on the heart and should be avoided by heart failure patients. Regular periods of rest are encouraged in all patients. As with dietary restrictions, reduction of physical activity ranges from avoiding heavy labor to total bed rest, depending on the severity of heart failure. The reduction in physical activity should be tailored to the individual patient, depending upon symptoms and degree of cardiac dysfunction. A common sense approach should be used. Thus, if patients develop severe dyspnea when they walk up more than two flights of stairs, they should avoid that particular activity.

In addition, reducing weight, discontinuing smoking, avoiding excess alcohol, and avoiding emotional stress are also important general measures to be initiated early in the treatment of heart failure. Finally, associated clinical conditions, such as recurrent tachy or bradyarrhythmias, uncontrolled hypertension or diabetes, chronic obstructive lung disease, anemia, and thyrotoxicosis can worsen heart failure. Control of these conditions are important for the proper management of heart failure.

Pharmacologic therapy in heart failure includes the systematic use of several classes of drugs: diuretics, digitalis glycosides, vasodilators, and nondigitalis ino-

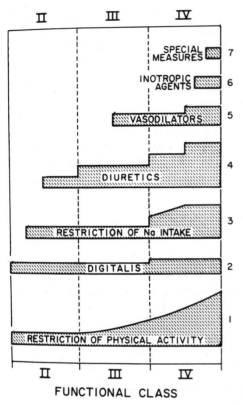

FUNCTIONAL CLASS

Figure 2 Step-care strategy of treatment of congestive heart failure in the adult. Therapy begins with restriction of activities that exacerbate symptoms. Other general measures include decreasing obesity with diet and stopping cigarette smoking. Digitalis, restriction of sodium intake, diuretics, vasodilators, and other inotropic agents follow. In severe cases, special measures include dialysis, paracentesis, heart transplant, and left ventricular assist devices in very severe cases. (Reprinted with permission from "The Management of Heart Failure," by Dr. Thomas Smith and Eugene Braunwald in *Heart Disease*, (ed) Eugene Braunwald. W.B. Saunders Company, Philadelphia, 1980, p. 51.)

tropic agents. Analogous to the treatment of hypertension, the management strategy of chronic heart failure may be approached in a step-care fashion. This has been outlined by Smith and Braunwald (Fig. 2).

Pharmacologic therapy begins with digitalis or diuretics. Most physicians initiate drug therapy with digitalis. If digitalis alone is insufficient in controlling class II symptoms, a thiazide diuretic is usually added. More potent loop diuretics, (e.g., furosemide and ethacrynic acid) are substituted for thiazides in patients with late class II or early class III symptoms or in those patients with reduced glomerular filtration rate. Late class III patients are begun on vasodilators (such as hydralazine, prazosin, or nitrates). Class IV patients are further restricted in sodium intake and may require higher doses of digitalis and more diuretics, such as the potassium-sparing agents spironolactone or triamterene. In refractory patients, metolazone (Zaroxolyn) can be used in place of loop diuretics. If class IV patients show deterioration, they may need hospitalization, in which case intravenous therapy with diuretics as well as more potent inotropic agents as the sympathomimetic amines (dopamine, dobutamine) and more potent vasodilators (nitroprusside, captopril) are added. Experimental inotropic agents, such as amrinone, are options in decompensated patients. Special measures such as phlebotomy, dialysis, and thoracentesis are used under special circumstances. Other special measures include the use of AV sequential pacing in restrictive cardiomyopathy and the use of calcium channel blockers to control rate in atrial fibrillation. Left ventricular assist devices, heart transplants, and the artificial heart are used in specialized centers for severe refractory heart failure.

Response to therapy is gauged by symptomatology; physical exam; chest x-ray; and special tests including echocardiography, rest and exercise radionuclide ventriculography, treadmill exercise tests, and in some cases acute drug testing during the time of cardiac catheterization.

DRUG THERAPY

Digitalis

Digitalis is a class of steroid or steroid glycosides that has a positive inotropic effect on the heart. Its exact mechanism of action is still not completely understood. Evidence suggests that digitalis exerts its inotropic effect by inhibiting Na-K ATPase, increasing intracellular sodium concentration which leads to increases in calcium influx via the Na-Ca exchange mechanism. Increases in cytosolic calcium results in

Table 5. Electrophysiologic Properties of Digitalis

Property	Effect
Pacemaker automaticity	
SA node	→ ↓ (↑ after atropine or toxic doses)
Purkinje fibers	↑
Excitability	
Atrium	→[a]
Ventricle	Variable[a]
Purkinje fibers	↑[a]
Membrane responsiveness	
Atrium	Variable[a] (↓ after atropine)
Ventricle	↓ (toxic doses)
Purkinje fibers	↓ (toxic doses)
Conduction velocity	
Atrium, ventricle	↑ (slight)[a]
AV node	↓
Purkinje fibers	↓
Effective refractory period	
Atrium	↓ (↑ after atropine)
Ventricle	↓
AV node	↑
Purkinje fibers	↑[a]

SOURCE: From Moe, G. K., and Farah, A. E.: Digitalis and allied cardiac glycosides, in Goodman, L. S., and Gilman, A. (eds): *The Pharmacological Basis of Therapeutics,* 5th ed. New York, Macmillan, 1975, p. 661.

Key: The arrows indicate the direction, not the magnitude, of the changes indicated: ↑ = increased; ↓ = decreased; → = no significant change.

[a] Decreased with high toxic doses of digitalis.

the activation of contractile elements. Digitalis also affects the electrophysiologic properties of the heart as shown in Table 5. It exerts both direct and neurally mediated effects resulting in slowing of conduction velocity and increase in effective refractory period of the AV node whereas it increases the excitability and automaticity of Purkinje fibers. In addition, the conduction velocities of the atrium and ventricle are increased, and their effective refractory periods are decreased by digitalis.

Although there are many digitalis compounds, the one that is most widely used in the United States and will be discussed in detail in this chapter is digoxin. Eighty percent of oral digoxin is absorbed. It is excreted predominantly by the kidney. The renal excretion is proportional to the glomerular filtration rate, although recent data suggest that digoxin is also secreted by the tubule. Enterohepatic recycling of digoxin is relatively insignificant. In subjects with normal renal function, one third of body stores are lost daily and the average half-life of the drug is 36 hours. The loading dose of digoxin in a patient depends on the lean body weight (0.0075 mg/lb lean body weight). Thus, an average oral loading dose is 1.25 to 1.5 mg and can be given as 3–4 divided doses in 6–8 hour intervals over 24 hours. The intravenous loading dose is usually 0.75 mg in 3–4 divided doses over 24 hours. Therapeutic digoxin levels can be achieved in 5–7 days of "maintenance" dose without a loading dose since steady state can be reached in 4–5 half-lives. Maintenance dose in a patient with normal renal function is usually 0.25 mg daily, in order to replace the 37% loss to maintain steady state blood levels. In patients with renal impairment, the maintenance dosage has to be adjusted. The loading dose is unchanged but the maintenance dose can be estimated as follows:

$$\text{maintenance dose (mg)} = \% \text{ daily loss} \times \text{loading dose (mg)}$$

$$\% \text{ daily loss in men} = 11.6 + \frac{20}{\text{serum creatinine}}$$

$$\% \text{ daily loss in women} = 12.6 + \frac{16}{\text{serum creatinine}}$$

The Use of Digitalis in Congestive Heart Failure

Digitalis increases contractility and reduces elevated ventricular end diastolic pressure of the dysfunctioning heart. As shown in Figure 1, digitalis shifts the ventricular function curve of the failing heart upwards and to the left (curve D), indicating that the drug increases the force of systolic ejection and thus contractility. The end systolic volume is reduced and end diastolic pressure declines. Thus, the same stroke work can be delivered from a markedly reduced filling pressure. Digitalis also increases the contractile state of the normal ventricle. However, this is not translated into increased cardiac output, since digitalis induces peripheral vasoconstriction in the normal circulation, resulting in increased impedance to ventricular ejection. In contrast, digitalis results in an overall reduction of sytemic vascular resistance in patients with heart failure, due to improved cardiac output and a secondary decrease in peripheral resistance.

The positive inotropic effect of digitalis increases myocardial oxygen consumption in the normal ventricle. In contrast, digitalis results in an overall decrease in myocardial oxygen consumption due to a reduction in heart size and wall tension in heart failure. Thus, digitalis can be beneficial in chronic ischemic heart disease with ventricular dysfunction.

In acute myocardial infarction (MI) without congestive failure, digitalis is contraindicated since it increases myocardial oxygen consumption and may potentially increase myocardial ischemia. However, digitalis may be of great value in acute MI complicated by atrial tachyarrhythmia, especially atrial fibrillation. In mild heart failure due to MI diuretics alone or with vasodilators is the preferred treatment. On the other hand, digitalis may be helpful in patients with cardiomegaly and frank heart failure in the setting of acute MI.

Cor Pulmonale and Digitalis

Digitalis is of no value to patients with chronic obstructive pulmonary disease without heart failure. In patients with right ventricular failure due to cor pulmonale, measures that improve hypoxemia and reduce pulmonary vascular resistance constitute the primary mode of therapy. Digitalis can be used as an adjunct, since it may decrease right ventricular end-diastolic pressure and increase stroke volume. However, in the setting of hypoxemia, sensitivity to digitalis toxicity is increased, probably due to increased cardiac and plasma catecholamine levels.

Mitral Stenosis and Digitalis

Digitalis is of no benefit to patients with mitral stenosis in normal sinus rhythm, except those with right ventricular failure. However, digitalis is useful to patients in atrial fibrillation, since control of ventricular response improves diastolic filling and cardiac output. In patients with mitral stenosis and right ventricular failure, digitalis can be helpful in improving right ventricular contractility and thus improving overall cardiac function.

Hypertrophic Obstructive Cardiomyopathy and Digitalis

Digitalis is of little value and may even be detrimental in hypertrophic obstructive cardiomyopathy. Increased contractility may result in increased obstruction to ventricular outflow. The only setting in which digitalis may be helpful in hypertrophic obstructive cardiomyopathy is end-stage disease, when cardiac dilatation and frank congestive heart failure has developed.

Pericardial Disease and Digitalis

Digitalis is of no help in constrictive pericarditis or pericardial tamponade, except for control of atrial arrhythmias.

Wolff-Parkinson-White (WPW) Syndrome and Digitalis

In the presence of WPW syndrome, atrial fibrillation may develop, with conduction down the accessory pathways at very fast rates. Digitalis can be hazardous in this setting, since it can shorten the refractory period of the accessory pathway, resulting in rapid increases in ventricular responses and increased sensitivity to ventricular fibrillation.

DIGITALIS LEVELS

Serum digoxin levels can be measured by radioimmunoassay. The therapeutic level of serum digoxin in the adult ranges from 0.5 to 2 ng/ml. In this range, most of the patients have evidence of clinical response without toxicity. The mean serum digoxin level in patients receiving 0.25 mg digoxin daily is 1.25 ± 0.4 ng/ml. The serum digoxin level of patients with clinical evidence of toxicity is usually greater than 2 ng/ml. However, 10% of patients without toxicity have serum digoxin concentrations of 2–4 ng/ml. On the other hand, 10% of patients with toxicity have serum digoxin levels of less than 2 ng/ml. In this group of patients, electrolyte abnormalities, hypoxemia, or increased autonomic activity is usually present.

Serum digoxin levels are indicated in patients in whom the status of digitalization is uncertain, particularly in patients with severe congestive heart failure; in patients with GI disease or after surgery, in whom absorption may be a problem; in patients with clinical suspicion of digitalis toxicity without overt ECG manifestations; in those who may be noncompliant; and for follow-up of therapy of digitalis toxicity.

DIGITALIS TOXICITY

It is estimated that 8–25% of hospitalized patients receiving digitalis have drug toxicity. Conditions that predispose to digitalis toxicity are shown in Table 6. The manifestations of toxicity can be divided into noncardiac and cardiac. The former include anorexia; nausea and vomiting; fatigue; restlessness, agitation or drowsiness; psy-

Table 6. Conditions Predisposing to Digitalis Toxicity

Renal insufficiency
Electrolyte disturbances (hypokalemia, hypercalcemia, hypomagnesemia)
Severe heart disease (NYHA class III or IV)
Acute MI
High-output state
Advanced age
Thyroid disease, especially hypothyroidism
Hypoxic states, acute or chronic pulmonary disease
Multiple drug therapy (especially institution of quinidine)
Hypertrophic obstructive cardiomyopathy, WPW syndromes, and amyloid heart disease
Sinoatrial and AV block.

chosis; and visual complaints including hazy vision, yellow halos, and scotomata. The toxic effects of digitalis on cardiac rhythm are listed below:

1. Depression of conduction: second degree AV block of Wenckebach type, third degree AV block with junctional or ventricular escape, sinoatrial or AV junctional exist block.
2. Increased automaticity of subsidiary or ectopic pacemakers: ventricular ectopic beats, ventricular bigeminy or tachycardia, non paroxysmal AV junctional tachycardia.
3. Combination of above: Paroxysmal atrial tachycardia with AV block, AV dissociation with simultaneous atrial and AV junctional tachycardia (bidirectional tachycardia), atrial fibrillation with regularization of ventricular response due to accelerated AV junctional or ventricular pacemaker focus.

Atrial fibrillation or flutter, supraventricular premature beats, sinus tachy or bradycardia, and multifocal atrial tachycardia are usually not manifestations of digitalis toxicity.

TREATMENT OF DIGITALIS TOXICITY

1. Digitalis induced ectopic arryhthmias (ectopic atrial, junctional, or ventricular) can be effectively treated with phenytoin or lidocaine. Phenytoin, if first giv `n as a loading dose (100 mg slowly infused intravenously every 5 minutes until control of arrhythmia or onset of phenytoin toxicity) followed by a maintenance dose of 400–600 mg daily. Phenytoin may also improve sinoatrial block and AV conduction, making it an ideal drug for treatment of digitalis intoxication. Lidocaine is administered as usual (100 mg loading dose and 1–3 mg/min continuously as maintenance dose). Quinidine and procainamide are also useful. However, both drugs carry the risk of cardiac toxicity, especially in eliciting ventricular arryhthmia. Propranolol, although effective in suppressing ectopic arryhthmia, can depress sinoatrial and AV pacemakers, as well as AV conduction, and could result in severe bradycardia or asystole.
2. Depression of conduction: Atropine can be effective in treating sinus bradycardia, AV block, or sinoatrial exist block. However, temporary transvenous pacing is occasionally required in patients with sinoatrial block, sinus arrest, or second or third degree block with extremely slow ventricular rate.
3. In advanced life threatening digitalis toxicity, digoxin-specific antibody Fab fragments have been successfully administered in investigative studies.

In general, potassium replacement is indicated for patients with hypokalemia and ectopic arryhthmias. However, it is contraindicated in the presence of hyperkalemia or conduction abnormalities since elevated serum potassium levels can further depress atrioventricular conduction. DC cardioversion should be avoided if possible since digitalis toxicity increases the likelihood of ventricular fibrillation following electrial cardioversion. Cardioversion should not be withheld if all measures have failed.

DRUG INTERACTIONS

Drugs can alter the serum digoxin concentration by interfering with absorption, excretion, and volume of distribution. Certain drugs can also increase the activity of the myocardium to digitalis effect and toxicity (Table 7).

Quinidine-Digoxin Interaction

Several studies have demonstrated that serum digoxin concentrations increase by 0.5 ng/ml or more in approximately 90% of patients, when standard doses of quinidine are added to a stable chronic regimen of digoxin. The serum digoxin level on the average doubles (range from zero to six-fold), when a new steady state is reached with quinidine treatment. The increase in serum digoxin level can be seen on the first day and reaches a plateau after approximately five days when quinidine is added without a loading dose. With a loading dose, serum digoxin level reaches a steady state within three days.

The exact mechanism of interaction is unclear. Evidence suggests that quinidine reduces the renal clearance of digoxin by up to 40–50%. This may be due to quinidine effect on tubular secretion of digoxin. A decrease in nonrenal rate of excretion has also been noted. Some investigators demonstrated that quinidine reduces the volume of distribution of digoxin by displacing digoxin from tissue compartments to plasma, while others have suggested that some of the increase in cardiac effect of digoxin occurring during quinidine treatment is mediated in the central nervous system.

Whether the occurrence of frank digitalis toxicity increases as a result of this interaction is subject to debate. Retrospective data analysis indicated a 17–41% incidence. However, no prospective study involving a large number of patients has been performed. Our recommendation is to reduce the digoxin maintanence dose to half when quinidine is to be added. Serum digoxin levels should be followed and the digoxin dose readjusted to achieve therapeutic nontoxic levels. Other investigators have advocated careful follow-up without adjustment of digoxin doses. Alternatively, antiarrhythmic agents other than quinidine or other digitalis preparations can be used. Indeed, Bigger pointed out that several type I antiarrhythmic agents do not cause changes in serum digoxin concentrations.

Table 7.   Drug Interaction with Digitalis

Cholestyramine, neomycin, nonabsorbable antacids, and kayopectate	Decrease oral absorption
Diuretic	Decreases glomerular filtration rate Hypokalemia Hypomagnesia Hypercalcemia (Thiazide)
Anesthesia	Increases sympathetic activity Arrhythmogenic
Quinidine	Decreases tubular secretion of digoxin Displaces digoxin from tissue
Verapamil, amiloride, spironolactone, triamterene	Decrease tubular secretion of digoxin

DIURETICS

60–75% of the filtered sodium load is reabsorbed in the proximal tubule of the nephron, 20% in the ascending limb of the loop of Henle, and the rest in the distal tubule and collecting duct. In congestive heart failure, the filtered sodium load is decreased. Furthermore, the proximal tubular sodium reabsorption is increased due to a decrease in peritubular hydrostatic pressure.

Diuretics increase urine flow and sodium excretion by acting at various sites along the nephron to interrupt sodium and water reabsorption. Reduction of sodium and water retention results in reduced ventricular preload and improves congestive symptoms. Furthermore, a reduction in ventricular volume may also decrease afterload and improve ventricular function. Thiazides and furosemide may also have direct vasodilating effects. Diuretics can be classified by their site of action. Table 8 is a list of diuretics, site of action, common oral dosage and side effects.

Special Considerations in the Use of Diuretics

1. Carbonic anhydrase inhibitors, e.g., acetazolamide, act primarily at the proximal tubule. Acetazolamide increases sodium bicarbonate excretion and thus can lead to the development of metabolic acidosis. It reduces glomerular filtration rate. Tolerance to the drug can develop in a few days and, when given to patients with liver impairment, drowsiness and confusion may occur.

2. Thiazide diuretics act in the distal tubule and tend to reduce glomerular filtration rate. They are ineffective in patients with glomerular filtration rates below 30 ml/min. Metabolic alkalosis may occur as a result of hypokalemia or volume contraction. The activity of these agents is not affected by alkalosis or acidosis.

3. Like chlorothiazide, metolazone exerts its action on the distal tubule. However, it does not reduce glomerular filtration rate or renal blood flow. Thus, it may be effective in patients with impaired renal function.

4. Spironolactone, triamterene, and amiloride act on the distal tubule. These agents reduce potassium excretion and may lead to metabolic acidosis and hyperkalemia due to reduced potassium-hydrogen exchange.

5. The effectiveness of loop diuretics are not affected by reduced glomerular filtration rates. These agents inhibit chloride transport in the ascending limb. Metabolic alkalosis may be a complication of these drugs. Their effectiveness is not inhibited by metabolic alkalosis or acidosis.

6. Hyponatremia can occur as a complication of diuretic therapy. Furosemide, ethacrynic acid, and thiazides reduce free water excretion. Furthermore, antidiuretic hormone and thirst may be increased in congestive heart failure. The combination of these factors can result in hyponatremia. Treatment consists of withholding diuretics if tolerated, restricting fluid intake, and improving cardiac function.

7. Patients with severe heart failure may be refractory to oral thiazides or furosemide due to poor gastrointestinal absorption secondary to bowel edema. These patients often respond well to a course of intravenous furosemide or ethacrynic acid. Combination of oral diuretics can also be used. The combined use of a loop diuretic (furosemide) with a distal tubular agent (thiazide, spironolactone,

Table 8. Commonly Used Diuretics in Heart Failure

Drug	Site of Action	Total Daily Dose in CHF	Frequency	Complications
Acetazolamide (Diamox)	Proximal tubule	250–375 mg	qod or qd × 2 days, skip day 3	Metabolic acidosis
Thiazides	Distal tubule			
Hydrochlorothiazide (Hydrodiuril, Esidrix)		50–200 mg	qd to bid	Hyponatremia, hypokalemia, metabolic alkalosis, hyperuricemia, glucose intolerance, lipid abnormalities, hypercalcemia, reduced GFR, allergy
Chlorothiazide (Diuril)		500–1500 mg	qd to bid	
Phthalimidine derivatives	Distal tubule			
Chlorthalidone (Hygroton)		50–200 mg	qd	Similar to thiazides, but hypokalemia may be profound
Metolazone (Zaroxolyn)		2.5–10 mg	qd	
Loop diuretics	Loop of Henle			
Furosemide (Lasix)		40–320 mg	qd to bid	Hyponatremia, hypokalemia, metabolic alkalosis, hyperuricemia, glucose intolerance, interstitial nephritis, ototoxicity
Ethacrynic acid (Edecrin)		50–400 mg	qd to bid	
Potassium-sparing diuretics:	Distal tubule			
Spironolactone (Aldactone)		25–200 mg	qd to tid	Hyperkalemia, mental confusion, nausea, and gynecomastia (spironolactone only)
Triamterene (Dyrenium)		100–300 mg	qd to bid	
Amiloride (Midamor)		5–10 mg	qd	

etc.) may be highly effective in patients refractory to a single diuretic regimen. We have found the regimen of furosemide and hydrochlorothiazide or metolazone particularly effective. However, hypokalemia and hyponatremia frequently complicate this regimen.

VASODILATION THERAPY

As stated earlier, the therapy of heart failure is directed at reducing the workload of the heart and manipulating the various factors that control cardiac performance. Major determinants of cardiac performance are heart rate, wall tension (including preload and afterload), and contractility. These factors determine to a great degree how the heart will be able to meet the metabolic demands of the body as well as the metabolic cost of this cardiac work. In patients with advanced congestive heart failure, special attention has to be paid to the state of preload and afterload. Preload refers to left ventricular fiber length at the end of diastole and, in essense, is left ventricular end-diastolic pressure (LVEDP), which is governed by venous return. In patients with advanced congestive heart failure, LVEDP is elevated. This results in an increase in hydrostatic pressure and transudation of fluid in the pulmonary capillaries, with symptoms of pulmonary congestion. Afterload refers to the tension that has to be generated in the left ventricular wall to open the aortic valve and discharge the stroke volume into the systemic circulation. Afterload is determined by arterial pressure, ventricular radius (according to Laplace's law), systemic vascular resistance, and aortic impedance. In advanced congestive heart failure, systemic vascular resistance is elevated as a compensatory mechanism to maintain systemic blood pressure. The increase in arteriolar tone is maintained by increased neurohumoral activities, such as sympathetic and renin angiotensin system. The increase in systemic vascular resistance results in increased impedance to left ventricular ejection. The vicious cycle leads to a new steady state when cardiac output will be lower and systemic vascular resistance (SVR) higher than is optimal for the patient.

Effects of a venodilator on cardiac performance are dependant on the initial level of left ventricular filling pressure (LVFP). Thus, in heart failure patients who are maximally diuresed to near normal LVFP, the addition of a venodilator can result in decreases in stroke volume and cardiac output. On the other hand, if one starts at a high LVFP, a reduction in filling pressure will occur along the flat portion of the ventricular function curve and will not produce a marked reduction in ventricular performance, but will relieve pulmonary venous congestion (Fig. 3).

The predominant mechanism whereby an arteriolar dilator increases cardiac output is by reducing SVR. This reduction in impedance and instantaneous wall stress results in augmentation of myocardial fiber shortening and increased stroke volume in the failing heart. The reduction of SVR will be offset by the increase in cardiac output and, hence, blood pressure may fall slightly or not at all.

Thus, there are two principal mechanisms by which vasodilators can diminish left ventricular wall tension during systole (ventricular afterload). First, these agents may reduce SVR, decrease aortic impedance to left ventricular ejection, allowing a greater stroke volume and cardiac output. Since the low cardiac output usually increases to the same extent the elevated SVR decreases, there is little or no decline in systemic blood pressure. Second, peripheral vasodilator drugs may also cause venodilatation,

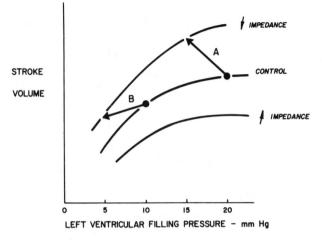

STROKE

VOLUME

IMPEDANCE

A

CONTROL

B

IMPEDANCE

0   5   10   15   20

LEFT VENTRICULAR FILLING PRESSURE – mm Hg

Figure 3 Left ventricular function curves plotting stroke volume as a function of left ventricular filling pressure. The control curve is in the middle. With a vasodilator drug such as nitroprusside, there would be a decrease in impedance, which would shift the curve up and to the left. Note that if a patient on the control curve were given a vasodilator with an initial filling pressure of 20 mm Hg, the reduction of filling pressure would be accompanied by an increase in stroke volume (line A). However, if the same patient began at a filling pressure of 10 mm Hg, with a decrease of filling pressure to 5 mm Hg, there would be a decrease in stroke volume (line B). Thus, the effects of a vasodilator (such as nitroprusside) are dependent on the left ventricular filling pressure. (Reproduced by permission from Grune & Stratton. From K. Chatterjee and W.W. Parmley: The role of vasodilator therapy in heart failure. *Prog Cardiovasc Dis* 19:301, 1977.)

resulting in peripheral pooling of blood and reduced venous return. Consequently, LVFP and LVEDP (preload) are reduced and pulmonary congestion is relieved. In addition, myocardial oxygen requirement (MVO_2) is reduced by the decrease in ventricular wall tension during contraction due to peripheral vasodilator-induced decrease in ventricular volume and aortic impedance.

Choice of Vasodilators

Arteriolar dilators (e.g., hydralazine) are of particular value to patients with a dilated ventricular chamber, low cardiac output and evidence of low forward output, and declining performance in vital organs as a result of intense vasocontriction. In patients with volume overload, such as mitral and aortic regurgitation, afterload reduction decreases the magnitude of regurgitation and improves left ventricular forward stroke volume.

Venodilators (e.g., nitrates) decrease preload and pulmonary venous pressure. They are desirable for those patients in whom the primary manifestation of the heart failure is pulmonary congestion due to increased LVFP. They should be used with caution in patients who have received excessive diuresis, since this may precipitate hypotension.

Balanced vasodilators (e.g., prazosin and captopril) act on both arterial and venous sides and are capable of reducing LVFP and pulmonary congestion as well as SVR, and increasing cardiac output.

Vasodilators are usually added to the treatment regimen when digitalis and adequate doses of furosemide are insufficient in controlling late NYHA class II or early class III symptomatology. When symptoms are primarily those of pulmonary congestion, a pure venodilator (e.g., nitrates: oral, sublingual, ointment, or nitrate patches) should be used. On the other hand, if the patient's symptoms are predominantly those of low forward output, a pure arteriolar dilator (e.g., hydralazine) can be used. Most heart failure patients have symptoms of both low output and pulmonary congestion. They respond well to both veno and arteriolar dilation. Agents with veno and arteriolar dilating properties (i.e., "mixed" vasodilators such as prazosin and captopril) are preferred in these patients. Alternatively, the combination of pure venodilator and arteriolar dilator such as isosorbide dinitrate and hydralazine can be employed. Table 9 is a list of commonly used vasodilators in heart failure, their doses, site of action, and complications.

Special Considerations in the Choice of Vasodilators

Chamber Size
Packer and colleagues observed that the magnitude of changes in stroke volume, LV filling pressure, and stroke work index during hydralazine therapy correlated with pretreatment left ventricular end-diastolic dimensions (LVEDD) as determined by M-mode echocardiography. Over 60% of patients with LVEDD≥60 mm were improved clinically after 2–3 weeks of hydralazine therapy. This was associated with decreases in blood urea nitrogen. In contrast, 60% of patients with LVEDD< 60 mm deteriorated, associated with increases in blood urea nitrogen after hydralazine treatment. The differences in responses of the two groups may be due to a more effective reduction in systolic wall stress and, hence, afterload in the former group. Furthermore, the magnitude of underlying mitral regurgitation secondary to ventricular dilatation may be greater in the former groups, thus rendering these patients more responsive to vasodilator therapy.

Degree of Valvular Regurgitation
Vasodilator therapy has been shown to be effective in patients with mitral or aortic regurgitation and congestive heart failure. In general, the degree of hemodynamic and clinical responses correlates to some extent with the magnitude of reguritant flow.

Blood Pressure
Acute or chronic elevation of systemic blood pressure further increases aortic impedance and can aggravate heart failure in an already compromised heart. The presence of hypertension is a clear indication for aggressive vasodilator therapy (See Chapter 23). In heart failure patients with histories of long standing hypertension, but in whom blood pressures are normal or slightly elevated, further reduction in blood pressure by vasodilators can lead to improvement of cardiac hemodynamics.

Patients with hypertension may have heart failure symptoms without frank ventricular dilation. These patients usually have concentric hypertrophy with a small

Table 9. Commonly Used Vasodilators in Heart Failure

Drug	Site of Action	Route of Administration	Usual Initial Dose	Maximal Dose	Complications
Nitroprusside (Nipride)	Arteriolar and venous	IV	10–25 µg/min IV	Up to 300 µg/min IV	Thiocyanate toxicity, methemoglobinemia
Phentolamine (Regitine)	Arteriolar	IV	0.1 to 1.0 mg/min q 5–10 min		Nausea, vomiting, abdominal pain, tachycardia
Trimethaphan (Arfonad)	Arteriolar and venous	IV	1–15 mg/min IV		Postural hypotension, bowel and bladder atony, respiratory depression
Nitrates nitroglycerin	Venous	Sublingual	0.4 mg SL	–	Headache, postural hypotension, methemoglobinemia
		IV	5–10 µg/min IV	500 µg/min IV	
		Cutaneous ointment	½–1″ q 6 hr	2–3″ q 3–6 hr	
		Patches	5–10 mg/24 hr	–	
isosorbide dinitrate (Isordil)		Oral or sublingual	2.5–10 mg q 2 hr (SL) 10–40 mg qid (oral)	–	Headache, postural hypotension
Hydralazine (Apresoline)	Arteriolar	Oral	10 mg tid to qid	400 mg/day	Headache, positive ANA, SLE-like syndrome (10–20% if dose >400 mg/day), drug fever, skin rash
Prazosin (Minipres)	Arteriolar and venous	Oral	1 mg tid	24 mg/day	Postural hypotension, fluid retention, polyarthralgia
Captopril (Capoten)	Arteriolar and venous	Oral	12.5–25 mg tid	450 mg/day	Skin rash, proteinuria, renal failure, agranulocytosis
Minoxidil (Loniten)	Arteriolar	Oral	2.5 mg qd to bid	40 mg/day	Hirsuitism, sodium retention, pericardial effusion, question of pulmonary hypertension

or normal ventricular cavity size and reduced ventricular compliance during diastole. This subset of patients may be particularly responsive to calcium entry blockers, such as nifedipine, which can effectively improve diastolic relaxation as well as reduce systemic vascular resistance.

Special attention should be paid to the effects of acute vasodilation on the renal function of patients with long standing hypertension. Many of these patients have varying degrees of nephrosclerosis: a precipitous drop in perfusion pressure may worsen renal function.

End Organ Perfusion

Vasoconstriction in congestive heart failure results in reduction and redistribution of blood flow to various organs. Renal, splanchnic, and cutaneous blood flow are particularly reduced, since these organs are greatly influenced by serum angiotensin and the sympathetic nervous system. Vasodilators can affect the distribution of cardiac output. Hydralazine and captopril increase renal blood flow with or without increasing glomerular filtration rate. These agents may improve renal function and potentiate renal response to furosemide. Prazosin has no effect on renal flow, but increases hepatic blood flow and may be particularly effective in patients with hepatic and splanchnic hypoperfusion. All these agents improve exercise tolerance.

Etiology of Congestive Heart Failure

Vasodilator therapy should be initiated cautiously in patients with ischemic cardiomyopathy. Reflex tachycardia with vasodilator treatment is generally not a problem in patients with chronic heart failure, since the myocardial norepinephrine stores are depleted and the baroreceptor reflex blunted in these patients. However, in patients with acute heart failure, vasodilators can induce tachycardia and increase myocardial oxygen consumption. Excessive hypotension may precipitate angina and worsen cardiac function in both acute and chronic heart failure.

Transient decreases in systemic blood pressure to 75 mm Hg systolic and 50 mm Hg diastolic are generally well tolerated in patients whose heart failure is not on the basis of coronary artery disease.

In our experience, vasodilator therapy may be particularly effective in patients with nonischemic viral, idiopathic, alcoholic, or nutritional cardiomyopathy. These patients usually have normal coronary arteries and significant secondary mitral regurgitation. Clinical and hemodynamic improvement may be sustained, particularly after removal of the offending agent.

Drug Tolerance

Attenuation of response to vasodilators, reported with almost all vasodilators, presents a significant problem in the therapy of heart failure. Attenuation of drug effect may reflect progression of the primary myocardial disease; it may also be due to primary or secondary activation of neurohumoral mechanisms, alterations of receptor density and responsiveness, and/or changes in drug metabolism. Indeed, vasodilators can cause reflex increase in neurosympathetic or renin-angiotensin activities by lowering systemic vascular resistance and blood pressure. A recent study showed that within minutes after the withdrawal of nitroprusside, some patients with heart failure developed a transient rebound increase in systemic vascular resistance, arterial blood pressure, and left ventricular filling response associated with an increase in heart rate. This phenomenon can be explained on the basis of carotid baroreceptor reflex activation.

The attenuation of prazosin vasodilator effect in heart failure has been well documented. Prazosin tolerance is associated with increases in plasma norepinephrine concentration and plasma renin activity.

Beta-adrenergic receptor agonists including dobutamine, pirbuterol, and salbutamol, are quite effective in reducing systemic vascular resistance and increasing cardiac output. However, a significant degree of hemodynamic and clinical attenuation occurs during long term treatment. The clinical attenuation seen with these agents may be related to "down regulation" of beta-adrenergic receptors in the myocardium and blood vessels. Similarly, tolerance to hydralazine may be a result of receptor adaptation or alterations in drug metabolism. In contrast, there appears to be little evidence of tolerance to captopril in the therapy of heart failure, although the experience with this drug has been limited. Captopril appears to blunt the baroreceptor reflex and prevent secondary rises in plasma catecholamines in patients with heart failure. Indeed, tachycardia is not observed with this drug, despite the fall in arterial blood pressure. Furthermore, plasma norepinephrine and epinephrine levels remain unchanged after captopril therapy in patients with advanced heart failure. Thus, the sustained effectiveness of captopril may be related to its blockade of both neurohumoral mechanisms.

An important observation made by Packer et al., is that patients who are refractory to one vasodilator may respond to another vasodilator that acts by a different mechanism. Thus, alternating the use of several vasodilators and the combined use of two vasodilators may reduce the incidence of clinical tolerance.

Drug Interaction
Nonsteroidal antiiflammatory agents (NSAI) inhibit prostaglandin synthetase activity. Since vasodilator prostaglandins E_2 and I_2 probably modulate systemic vascular resistance and renal perfusion, those NSAI agents may reduce renal blood flow and glomerular filtration rate. These agents may also attenuate the effects of diuretics and vasodilators. Indomethacin has been shown to attenuate the effect of furosemide, while aspirin blocks the effect of spironolactone. In hypertensive patients, indomethacin reduces the vasodilating effect of captopril. This mechanism is probably also applicable to heart failure patients. Finally, in patients with prerenal azotemia, NSAI may precipitate renal failure.

NONDIGITALIS INOTROPIC AGENTS

Dopamine and Dobutamine

Dopamine is an endogenous catecholamine capable of stimulating dopaminergic, alpha-adrenergic, and beta-adrenergic receptors. A systemic infusion of dopamine at 2–5 μg/kg body weight per minute induces peripheral vasodilatation, increase in renal blood flow, coronary flow, and myocardial contractility with little change in heart rate. The vasodilatory effect of dopamine is mediated by vascular dopaminergic receptors. Dopamine also acts directly on β_1-adrenergic receptors and releases norepinephrine from nerve terminals, resulting in increased cardiac contractility. In doses of >5–10 μg/kg/min, systemic vasoconstriction occurs, leading to increased blood pressure and decreased renal blood flow. This is due to the activation of α-adrenergic receptors by dopamine. In this dose range, increased β_1 stimulation also increases heart rate, myocardial oxygen consumption, and coronary resistance.

Dobutamine is a synthetic sympathomimetic amine capable of stimulating β_1, β_2, and α adrenoreceptors. Its effect on β_1 is greater than on β_2, and its effect on α_1 is greater than on α_2. In low doses (2–5 μg/kg/min), it causes slight vasoconstriction and stimulates increased myocardial contractility. Higher doses of dobutamine (5–10 μg/kg/min) induce a biphasic vasoconstriction-vasodilator response, mediated by α_1 and β_1 receptors respectively. Dobutamine does not directly affect renal blood flow, but causes a redistribution of cardiac output in favor of coronary and skeletal muscle circulation.

Dopamine and dobutamine may be used in patients with advanced acute and chronic decompensated heart failure. The addition of a parenteral vasodilator, such as nitroprusside, to dopamine or dobutamine can further augment cardiac output by reducing afterload. In combination, these agents enhance diuretic activity of furosemide, and have been used successfully in treating patients with heart failure.

Recently, two new drugs under investigation have shown promise as inotropic agents. Amrinone induces significant increase in cardiac contractility, with secondary reductions in ventricular filling pressures and systemic resistance. This agent may induce thrombocytopenia. Pirbuterol is a beta agonist whose primary effect appears to be vasodilation, although a positive inotropic effect has also been demonstrated.

INPATIENT VERSUS OUTPATIENT MANAGEMENT

Cases of mild to moderate congestive heart failure can be successfully treated with outpatient management once etiology and precipitating factors have been worked up. Diet, restriction of salt intake, modification of physical activity, and treatment with digitalis and diuretics are instituted; and patients should be seen at least two weeks after therapy has been started. Follow-up examination should include complete cardiovascular exam, including weight; and electrolytes, BUN, and Cr should be checked if the patient has been started on diuretics. Initial management of severe heart failure, acute or chronic, should be instituted in the hospital.

In summary, the genre "congestive heart failure," is complex and includes different etiologies, pathophysiologies, hemodynamic impairments, and clinical states. A careful evaluation of these factors is necessary in all patients. Although a step-care approach can be used in the treatment of heart failure, treatment should also be tailored to each patient in view of the heterogeneity of patient characteristics.

BIBLIOGRAPHY

Bigger TJ: The quindine-digoxin interaction. *Mod Concepts Cardiovasc Dis.* 51:73, 1982.

Beller GA, Smith TW, Abelman WH, et al: Digitalis intoxication: Prospective clinical study with serum level correlations. *N Engl J Med* 284:989, 1971.

Braunwald E: Clinical manifestations of heart failure, in Braunwald E (ed): *Heart Disease: A Textbook of Cardiovascular Medicine.* Philadelphia, Saunders, 1980, p 493.

Braunwald E: Determinants and assessment of cardiac function. *N Engl J Med* 296:86, 1977.

Braunwald E: *The Myocardium: Failure and Infarction*. New York, H. P. Publishing Co., 1974.

Braunwald E, Mock MB, Watson J: Current research and clinical heart failure, in Braunwald, Mock et al (eds): *Congestive Heart Failure*. New York, Grune and Stratton, 1982.

Braunwald E, Ross J Jr, Sonnenblick EH: Mechanism of Contraction of the Normal and Failing Heart (ed 2). Boston, Little, Brown, 1976.

Colucci WS, Wynn J, Holman BL, et al: Chronic therapy of heart failure with prazosin: A randomized double-blind trial. *Am J Cardiol* 45:337, 1980.

Doherty JE: How and when to use the digitalis serum levels. *JAMA* 239:2594, 1978.

Dzau VJ, Colucci WS, Williams GH, et al: Sustained effectiveness of converting enzyme inhibition in patients with severe congestive heart failure. *N Engl J Med* 302:1373, 1980.

Dzau VJ: Angiotensin converting enzyme inhibition in the treatment of hypertension and congestive heart failure. Update IV. in Isselbacher, et al, *Harrison's Principles of Internal Medicine*. New York, McGraw-Hill 1983, p 137.

Dzau VJ, Hollenberg NK, Williams GH: Neurohumoral mechanisms in congestive heart failure: Role in pathogenesis, therapy and drug tolerance. Fed Proceedings (in press).

Forrester JS, Waters DD: Hospital treatment of congestive heart failure: Management according to hemodynamic profile. *Am J Med* 65:173, 1978.

Franciosa JA, Colin JN: Immediate effects of hydralazine-isosorbide dinitrate combination on exercise capacity and exercise hemodynamics in patients with left ventricular failure. *Circulation* 59:1085, 1979.

Frazier HS, Yager H: The clinical use of diuretics. *N Engl J Med* 288:246, 1973.

Gleason WL, Braunwald E: Studies on Starling's law of the heart. VI. Relationship between left ventricular end-diastolic volume and stroke volume in man with observations on the mechanism of pulsus alternans. *Circulation* 25:841, 1962.

Goldberg LI: Dopamine: Clinical uses of an endogeneous catecholamine. *N Engl J Med* 291:707, 1974.

Jelliffe RW: Factors to consider in planning digoxin therapy. *J Chron Dis* 24:407, 1971.

Lee DCS, Johnson A, Bingham JB, et al: Heart failure in outpatients: A randomized trial of digoxin versus placebo. *N Engl J Med* 306:699, 1982.

Leier CV, Heban PT, Huss P, et al: Comparative systemic and regional hemodynamic effects of dopamine and dobutamine in patients with cardiomyopathic cardiac failure. *Circulation* 56:918, 1977.

Magorien RD, Triffon DW, Desch CE, et al: Prazosin and hydralazine in congestive heart failure: Regional hemodynamic effects in relation to dose. *Ann Intern Med* 95:5, 1981.

Massie B, Ports T, Chatterjee K, et al: Long-term vasodilator therapy for heart failure. *Circulation* 63:269, 1981.

Mckee PA, Castelli WP, McNamara PM, et al: The natural history of congestive heart failure: The Framingham study. *N Engl J Med* 285:1441, 1971.

Miller RR, Awan NA, Joye JA, et al: Combined dopamine and nitroprusside therapy in congestive heart failure. *Circulation* 55:881, 1977.

Moore TJ, Crantz FR, Hollenberg NK, et al: Contribution of prostaglandins to the antihypertensive action of captopril in essential hypertension. *Hypertension* 3:168, 1981.

Packer M, Meller J, Medina M, et al: Importance of left ventricular chamber size in determining the response to hydralazine in severe chronic heart failure. *N Engl J Med* 303:250, 1980.

Parmley WW, Chatterjee K: Vasodilator therapy. *Curr Probl Cardiol* 2:1, 1978.

Patak RV, Mookerjee BK, Bentzel CJ, et al: Antagonism of effects of furosemide by indomethacin in normal and hypertensive man. *Prostaglandins* 10:649, 1975.

Reinock HJ, Stein JH: Mechanisms of action and clinical use of diuretics, in Brenner BM, Rector FC (eds): *The Kidney* (ed 2). Philadelphia, Saunders. 1981, p 1097.

Ross J Jr, Braunwald E: Studies on Starling's law of the heart. IX. The effects of impeding venous return on performance of the normal and failing human left ventricle. *Circulation* 30:719, 1964.

Shah PM, Gramiak R, Kramer DH, et al: Determinants of atrial (S_4) and ventricular (S_3) gallop sounds in primary myocardial disease. *N Engl J Med* 278:753, 1968.

Smith TW, Braunwald E: The management of heart failure, in Braunwald E (ed): *Heart Disease: A Textbook of Cardiovascular Medicine*, (ed 1). Philadelphia, Saunders, 1980, p 509.

Smith TW, Butler VP, Haber E, et al: Treatment of life-threatening digitalis intoxication and digoxin-specific Fab antibody fragments: Experience in 26 cases. *N Engl J Med* 307:1357, 1982.

Sonnenblick EH, Frishman WH, LeJemtel TH: Dobutamine: A new synthetic cardioactive sympathetic amine. *N Engl J Med* 300:17, 1979.

Wellens HJJ: The electrocardiogram in digitalis intoxication, in Yu N, Goodwin JF (eds): *Progress in Cardiology*. Philadelphia, Lea and Febiger, Vol 5, 1976, p 271.

Zelis R, Flaim SF: The circulation in congestive heart failure. *Mod Concepts Cardiovasc Dis* 51:79, 1982.

CHAPTER 20 | PERICARDIAL DISEASES

Haim Hammerman
Robert A. Kloner

The mode of presentation of pericardial disease depends on both the etiology and the type or stage of pericardial inflammatory reaction. Thus, pericardial diseases can be classified in two ways, by etiology and according to stage. The etiologies of pericardial disease can be classified into major categories: infectious, neoplastic, metabolic, autoimmune-related, traumatic and idiopathic (Table 1). The stages of inflammatory reactions include acute, subacute, chronic, with or without effusion or constriction.

Clinically, pericardial involvement may manifest as an acute disease, with or without evidence of pericardial effusion or tamponade. Sometimes it presents as a subacute constrictive disease, or effusive constrictive process. Chronic pericarditis can manifest as (1) relapses of acute attack, (2) chronic pericardial effusion, or (3) chronic constrictive pericarditis (Table 2).

Acute Pericarditis

Common etiologies of acute pericarditis include viral, post myocardial infarction (MI) uremic, idiopathic, and autoimmune related diseases. Acute pericarditis is a clinical entity characterized by three major features: chest pain, friction rub, and fever. The pain of pericarditis characteristically is sharp or stabbing in quality, variable in intensity, persistent, aggravated by respiration, coughing, and movement. Usually the pain is precordial, sometimes substernal, and occasionally it radiates to the neck, arms, and back. It may be relieved by leaning forward or sitting, or exacerbated by lying down. Some patients have acute pericarditis without pain; in others, the pain mimics ischemic disease.

The most characteristic physical sign is a precordial friction rub. This is a scratchy noise, caused by friction between the pericardial layers and may have three components (presystolic, systolic, and protodiastolic). All three components are not always heard in any one patient. The quality of the rub typically changes with patient position and often is transitory in nature. It is best heard during expiration, with the patient leaning forward. Although a pericardial friction rub is pathognominic for pericarditis, it is found in only 60–70% of patients with acute pericarditis. It may be difficult to distinguish the rub from a murmur when only one component of the rub is heard. Therefore, every attempt must be made to repeat the auscultatory examination in order to detect other components or a change in the friction rub. Absence of a friction rub does not rule out pericardial effusion. Other common signs of acute

Table 1.   Etiologic Classification of Pericardial Disease

Infectious
  Viral (Coxsackie B, A; echo; influenza; infectious mononucleosis)
  Bacterial (pneumococci, staphylococci, meningococci, gonococci)
  Tuberculous
  Fungal (histoplasmosis, aspergillosis)
  Parasitic
Pericarditis associated with acute MI (See Chapter II)
Neoplastic
  Primary (mesothelioma)
  Secondary (lung, breast, melanoma, lymphoma, leukemia)
Metabolic
  Uremia
  Myxedema
  Cholesterol
Autoimmune related
  Connective Tissue Diseases (systemic lupus erythematosus, rheumatoid arthritis, scleroderma, polyarteritis nodosa, Takayasu's disease, Wegener's granulomatosis)
  Post Cardiac Injury (late postmyocardial infarction syndrome–Dressler's syndrome, postcardiotomy syndrome; posttrauma syndrome)
  Drug Induced (procainamide; hydralazine; penicillin; isonicotinic acid hydrazide; phenylbutazone; minoxidil; high dose cyclophosphamide in children)
Trauma
  Penetrating chest injury
  Closed chest injury
  After thoracic surgical procedures
  After cardiac catheterization and pacemaker insertion
  Rupture of heart or great vessels
Aortic dissection and rupture of heart
Radiation
Miscellaneous
  Sarcoidosis
  Amyloidosis
  Acute pancreatitis
  Chylopericardium
  Familial mediterranean fever
  Familial pericarditis
Idiopathic

pericarditis are fever and tachycardia. Associated symptoms and signs of systemic disease should be sought. Patients should be evaluated for clinical signs of cardiac compression (e.g., tamponade).

Laboratory findings depend on the etiology of the disease. In cases of viral, immune-related, infectious, or idiopathic pericarditis, there may be an increase in sedimentation rate and leukocyte count. The electrocardiogram (ECG) shows sinus tachycardia and diffuse ST segment elevation in multiple leads in the early stages (see Chapter 3). This diffuse ST elevation is in contrast to acute MI, in which ST elevation is localized and accompanied by Q wave formation. Sometimes only T

Table 2. Stages of
Inflammatory Reaction in
Pericarditis

Acute Pericarditis
  Noneffusive (fibrinous)
  Effusive

Subacute pericarditis
  Effusive constrictive
  Constrictive

Chronic pericarditis
  Effusive
  Constrictive
  Adhesive

wave changes are detected. A decrease in the QRS amplitude is seen in cases with pericardial effusion, and atrial arrhythmias occasionally are detected. Chest x-ray film may be normal; or, with pericardial effusion, the heart shadow may be enlarged.

Management of acute pericarditis includes: (1) observation for development of pericardial effusion and signs of tamponade (monitor heart rate, arterial and venous pressure); (2) determining and treating the underlying etiology; and (3) analgesics and antiinflammatory agents for viral or idiopathic pericarditis. Most patients with viral or idiopathic pericarditis recover rapidly with the help of symptomatic therapy, such as aspirin, for a few days. Indomethacin is often used, but probably has little advantage over aspirin. Glucocorticosteroids are more potent, but should be used only in severe cases that do not respond to nonsteroidal antiinflammatory agents. Chronic recurrent or relapsing pericarditis may follow acute pericarditis. This syndrome often develops in patients who have been treated with glucocorticosteroids and later had the dose reduced. Management of this relapsing syndrome includes very slow reduction of the glucocorticosteroid dose. Pericardiectomy should be considered in relapsing cases that require long periods (more than a year) of steroid therapy.

ACUTE PERICARDITIS WITH PERICARDIAL EFFUSION

Pericardial effusion (accumulation of fluid in the pericardial space) can occur in the acute phase of pericarditis and develop either rapidly or insidiously. Pericardial effusion may or may not be associated with compression of the heart. If fluid has accumulated to a point of causing increased intrapericardial pressure, compression of the heart can develop. The rate at which the fluid accumulates is important, since slow accumulation allows the pericardium to stretch over time, whereas with rapid accumulation this compensatory mechanism does not have time to develop. The primary effect of accumulation of fluid in the pericardial space is eventual restriction of diastolic filling, whereas the influence on systolic contraction is negligible. Systemic arteriolar contraction, salt and water retention and increased venous tone act initially as compensatory mechanisms to preserve cardiac output (see below, under Cardiac Tamponade). Thus, the clinical picture of compensated pericardial effusion with compression is increased systemic venous pressure. In cases of cardiac tamponade, there is failure of the compensatory mechanisms with a drop in cardiac output. It should be stressed that pericardial effusion can present as a wide range of clinical syndromes, from an asymptomatic undetected pericardial effusion without hemodynamic compromise to dramatic life threatening tamponade. The two main factors governing the presentation are the *amount* of fluid and *rate of* accumulation. Extent of prior inflammation or thickening of the pericardium affects its capability to stretch and hence the amount of fluid required for tamponade.

Clinical findings of pericardial effusion include the pain of associated pericarditis (sometimes the pain may become less sharp in quality once fluid accummulates), shortness of breath, orthopnea, cough, tachycardia, elevated central venous pressure, hepatic enlargement, a weak apical cardiac impulse, and faint heart sounds. The friction rub of pericarditis may disappear. In large effusions there may be an area of dullness to percussion and bronchial breathing at the angle of the left scapula, probably caused by lung compression (Ewart's sign).

Electrocardiographic findings are similar to those noted above. In large effusions, typically, there is a decrease in the QRS amplitude.

The chest x-ray film reveals an enlarged cardiac silhouette (Chapter 4) with clear lungs. Epicardial fat lines may be seen within the cardiac shadow. Fluoroscopy shows diminished cardiac pulsations. Echocardiography is an accurate and convenient noninvasive tool for making the diagnosis of pericardial effusion. Both M-mode

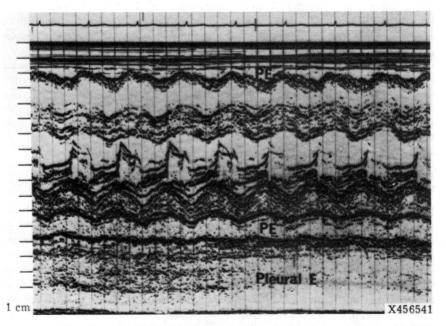

Figure 1   M-mode echocardiogram of a patient with pericardial and pleural effusions (E). In this patient, the pericardial effusion (PE) can be seen both anteriorly and posteriorly. (Reproduced with permission from Feigenbaum H: Pericardial disease, in Feigenbaum H, ed: *Echocardiography*, 3rd ed. Philadelphia, Lea & Febiger, 1981, p. 488.)

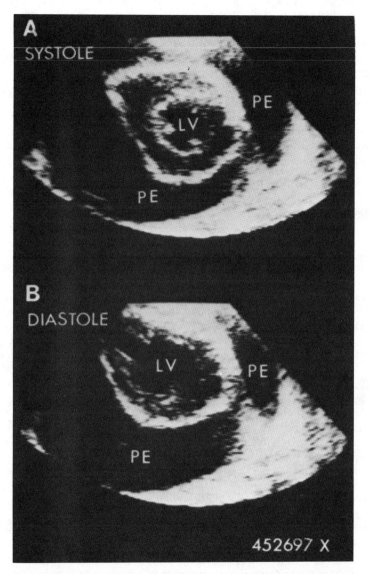

Figure 2 Short-axis two-dimensional echocardiogram of a patient with a large pericardial effusion, demonstrating the shift in cardiac position from systole to diastole. PE, pericardial effusion; LV, left ventricle. (Reproduced with permission from Feigenbaum H: Pericardial disease, in Feigenbaum H, ed: *Echocardiography*, 2nd ed. Philadelphia, Lea & Febiger, 1981, p. 444.)

and two dimensional echocardiograms show fluid accumulation and pericardial thickening. In general, it is possible to semiquantitate the amount of fluid by M-mode echocardiography. In small to moderately sized effusions, fluid appears as an echo-free space posterior to the left ventricle. In the absence of adhesions, fluid also appears anteriorly in moderate to large effusions. Very large effusions often extend behind the lower left atrium. Exaggerated heart movements ("swinging heart") are seen with large effusions, and are often associated with the echocardiographic appearance simulating mitral and tricuspid prolapse (so called "pseudoprolapse"). Two-dimensional echocardiography provides a better idea as to the quantitation of fluid, especially if a large volume has accumulated or if the fluid is loculated (Figs. 1, 2). Serial echocardiography is valuable in following the course of pericardial effusions. Radionuclide scans and intravenous injection of CO_2 with contrast angiocardiography have been used to detect effusion, in cases where echocardiography is unsatisfactory.

Cardiac Tamponade

Cardiac tamponade is an accumulation of fluid in the pericardium in an amount sufficient to cause serious restriction of diastolic filling, with failure of compensatory mechanisms. The development of tamponade is related to the distensibility of the pericardium and the speed of fluid accumulation. It is not proportional to the amount of fluid present, since massive effusions may be present without tamponade, and relatively small amounts of fluid collecting quickly may produce severe compression and tamponade. Circulation cannot be sustained for long, once pericardial pressure exceeds venous pressure. Any cause of pericardial effusion can induce cardiac tamponade. Frequent causes are neoplasms, radiation, trauma, bleeding after cardiac surgery, pyogenic infections, tuberculosis, and uremia (Table 3). Tamponade occasionally occurs during acute viral or idiopathic pericarditis and in patients treated with anticoagulants during the course of acute pericarditis.

The clinical findings are due to a fall in cardiac output and elevated venous pressure. Patients complain of light headedness and dizziness as forward output decreases, as well as other symptoms of pericardial effusion discussed above. Physical examination reveals jugular venous distension, tachycardia, systemic hypotension, narrow pulse pressure, paradoxical pulse and in some cases tender and enlarged liver. When tamponade is severe, there is evidence of shock state with signs of organ hypoperfusion.

Paradoxical pulse is a valuable sign of cardiac tamponade. It is defined as an abnormally large drop in arterial systolic pressure with inspiration; a drop of greater than 10 mm Hg is considered abnormal. This physical sign can be detected by palpation of the pulse. During inspiration there is a pronounced decrease in the amplitude of the pulse. An estimate of the degree of paradoxical pulse can be obtained by measuring blood pressure during the respiratory cycle. Measurements should be made during normal respiration, since deep breathing as well as artificial respiration exaggerate paradoxical pulse. In severe cases with hypotension, this sign is difficult to appreciate. Paradoxical pulse can be accurately determined by means of direct arterial pressure measurements. In chronic constrictive pericarditis, paradoxical

Table 3. Common Causes of Tamponade

Neoplastic disease
Idiopathic pericarditis
Uremia
Trauma
Infection (tuberculous, pyogenic)
Rupture of heart or great vessels
Anticoagulant therapy (during pericardial disease)
Iatrogenic (after thoracic surgery, catheterization, pacemaker)

pulse is often minimal or absent. Although this finding is consistently found in tamponade it is not pathognomonic of it, since it can be observed in acute and chronic obstructive lung diseases, severe myocardial failure, hemorrhagic shock, and in some forms of restrictive cardiomyopathies. Kussmaul's sign (rise in central venous pressure with inspiration) occasionally occurs in cardiac tamponade, but it is more common in patients with constrictive pericarditis; it also occurs in some patients with tricuspid valve disease. Typically, the x and y descents of the jugular venous pulse are approximately equal, or the x descent is predominant. Auscultation typically reveals tachycardia; the heart sounds may be faint with or without a pericardial friction rub.

The ECG shows features similar to those described under effusion. Electrical alternans (alternation of the QRS amplitude on every other beat) appears in severe cases of tamponade.

The chest x-ray film may show either a normal or large heart shadow, with clear lung fields. Symmetrical enlargement of the heart shadow occurs when more than 200–300 ml of fluid accumulates. Fluoroscopy reveals diminished cardiac pulsations.

Echocardiography establishes the presence of pericardial fluid and allows a reasonable estimate of size of effusion. (Figs. 1, 2). Detection of abnormal diastolic right ventricular wall motion may be a sensitive indicator of a hemodynamically significant pericardial effusion. There is posterior motion of the anterior right ventricular wall that represents true collapse of the right ventricle in early diastole. However, it is important to stress that the diagnosis of tamponade depends primarily on the clinical findings and characteristic hemodynamic features, rather than echocardiography. In cases of life-threatening tamponade, performance of echocardiography should not delay the decision to perform pericardiocentesis. The clinical features of right ventricular infarction sometimes mimic tamponade. Detection of fluid by echocardiography with no evidence of right ventricular enlargement or abnormal right ventricular contractility favors the latter diagnosis.

Cardiac catheterization is not required when the diagnosis is certain, but it is of importance in questionable cases or when an element of pericardial constriction is suspected. Characteristically, venous pressure is elevated with normal inspiratory decline (Kussmaul's sign usually absent). Prominent y descent, which is characteristic of constrictive pericarditis (described later), is absent in tamponade. Paradoxical pulse can be recorded from a systemic artery or from left ventricular pressures, and, in extreme cases, pulsus alternans (alteration of systolic pressure amplitude every other beat) can be recorded. Typically, both right and left ventricular diastolic pressures equal intrapericardial pressure. Right atrial pressure is elevated above normal, and right atrial pressure, right ventricular end-diastolic pressure, pulmonary artery diastolic pressure, and pulmonary capillary wedge pressure are within 5 mm Hg of each other. Following pericardial aspiration, pericardial and right atrial pressures fall, right ventricular diastolic pressure comes down to a normal level and cardiac output increases.

Patients with acute pericarditis should be observed carefully for the possibility of developing pericardial effusion with tamponade. In the presence of pericardial effusion, heart rate, arterial and central venous pressure should be monitored continuously, and serial echocardiograms obtained to detect any change in the amount of pericardial fluid. In case of cardiac tamponade, the definitive emergency treatment is removal of pericardial fluid by pericardiocentesis or surgical drainage. Medical support is often necessary to stabilize the patient's condition while preparations are made for the definitive procedures. Intravenous fluids are administered in order to help restore left ventricular filling volumes. Despite venous congestion, significant volumes should be administered (up to 300–500 ml/15 min). Inotropic support may be beneficial in improving cardiac output. Isoproterenol is infused initially at the rate of 2–4 μg/min and increased up to 20 μg/min until improvement or appearance of arrhythmias. Dobutamine may be infused starting at 1–2 μg/kg/min and increased to 15 μg/kg/min. Expansion of blood volume combined with nitroprusside has been shown to increase cardiac output and improve blood pressure in numerous studies of animals with tamponade. However, in humans, the hemodynamic benefits of volume expansion alone or combined with nitroprusside are very limited. Medical support is not an alternative mode of treatment and should not cause a delay in performing pericardiocentesis or surgical drainage.

PERICARDIOCENTESIS

Pericardiocentesis, needle aspiration of the pericardial sac, has been used successfully in the management of pericardial effusion and tamponade. Pericardiocentesis may be performed for two major reasons: (1) therapeutically, for relief of tamponade as an emergency procedure or, in cases of large effusion, for relief of symptoms; and (2) for obtaining fluid for diagnostic purposes. Pericardiocentesis is associated with potentially dangerous complications (e.g., ventricular laceration or puncture, coronary artery laceration, ventricular arrhythmias, MI, and even cardiac arrest), and should be performed by those experienced in this procedure. Some believe that pericardiocentesis should be performed only for emergency relief of cardiac tamponade, and recommend surgical drainage in elective cases.

Optimally, pericardiocentesis should be performed in the cardiac catheterization laboratory under electrocardiographic and fluoroscopic control. However, it can be performed at the bedside with proper monitoring. In general, a needle is inserted 2–4 cm below the junction of the subxyphoid process and the left costal margin at an angle of 20–30°, so that it passes underneath the sternum into the pericardial sac. A chest lead of the ECG is connected to the needle and monitored throughout the insertion. When the needle touches the myocardium, ST elevation is detected. The location of the needle can also be determined, by fluoroscopy (sometimes with the aid of a contrast agent injection), by echocardiography, by measuring pressure contour from the needle, or by the type of fluid aspirated. Aspirated bloody fluid should be compared to venous blood for its hemoglobin content, to determine whether a cardiac chamber was punctured. Bloody pericardial fluid tends not to clot, in contrast to blood aspirated accidentally from a cardiac chamber. The pericardiocentesis tends to be low risk when there is a large anterior pericardial effusion, determined by echocardiography. Intrapericardial pressures should be measured before and after aspiration of fluid. In tamponade, this pressure exceeds or equals central venous pressure, and in some cases it may exceed 20 mm Hg. Intrapericardial pressure drops after removal of fluid. Some pericardial needles have a plastic cannula over them; after successful entry into the pericardial space, the needle is removed, leaving the cannula for drainage. Some cardiologists prefer to exchange the needle for a catheter, and this may be accomplished by passing a guide wire through the needle, and then passing a small multihole catheter over the guide wire into the pericardial sac. This catheter can be left for continuous drainage for a short period of time, or for intrapericardial drug administration.

Open surgical drainage is an alternative mode of treatment for cardiac tamponade. Subxyphoid pericardiotomy under local anesthesia can be performed in acutely ill patients for relief of tamponade. Surgical drainage is indicated in cases with repeated accumulation of pericardial effusion.

The pericardial fluid should be analyzed for color, turbidity, cell counts, cultures, chemistries, and cytology. However, in a number of diseases (viral pericarditis, collagen-vascular diseases, uremia) the pericardial fluid has no pathognomonic features. The quality of fluid inspected visually may be of some diagnostic yield. Serosanguineous or sanguineous effusion is found after cardiac surgery, trauma, pericarditis following acute MI treated with anticoagulants, neoplastic pericarditis, and rupture of the heart and great vessels. Serous effusion commonly is found in viral pericarditis, radiation pericarditis, heart failure, tuberculous pericarditis, collagen diseases, and hypoalbuminemia. Chylous effusion may follow cardiac surgery with injury to lymph vessels, or when neoplasm interferes with lymph drainage. Cholesterol effusion is found in cases of myxedema.

The fluid should be characterized as a transudate (protein < 3 g/100 ml) or an exudate (protein > 3 g/100 ml). Transudates occur in heart failure, hypoalbuminemia, Dressler's syndrome, postpericardiotomy syndrome, drug induced pericarditis, some cases of collagen diseases, and radiation pericarditis. Exudates are more likely to occur in infection, neoplasms, uremia, chylous pericarditis, and collagen diseases. Cholesterol content is elevated in cases of myxedema. Glucose content of the fluid is low in bacterial pericarditis.

Other tests that should be performed include blood cell count and differential; gram stain; Ziehl-Neelsen stain; cultures for aerobic and anaerobic bacteria; cultures for tuberculosis; and, when suspected, fungal cultures. Positive cytologic findings have been reported in 50–75% of patients with neoplastic involvement of the pericardium, depending on the number of samples examined. Pericardiocentesis can provide positive culture diagnosis in 15% of cases of tuberculosis and in almost all cases of pyogenic pericarditis.

As mentioned previously, pericardiocentesis is not without hazards, therefore it, as well as surgical exploration, should be performed only when they are indicated; namely tamponade or high pressure pericardial effusion, suspicion of pyogenic pericarditis, and the need to obtain fluid for diagnosis.

Chronic Pericarditis

Chronic pericarditis may be associated with relapses of acute pericarditis, chronic pericardial effusion or constriction, or adhesion to surrounding structures. Chronic pericardial effusion can follow any cause of pericarditis, presenting as a wide variety of clinical pictures depending on the degree of compression of the heart and the manifestations of the underlying disease. Occasional patients develop chronic asymptomatic pericardial effusion, without progressing to compression or cardiac constriction.

CHRONIC CONSTRICTIVE PERICARDITIS

This condition occurs when the healing of acute pericarditis is followed by formation of scar tissue surrounding the heart, compressing its chambers and restricting diastolic filling. Constrictive pericarditis may follow idiopathic pericarditis, tuberculosis, pyogenic infection, radiation, uremia, neoplasm, trauma, and viral and connective tissue diseases. The etiology of pericarditis often is indeterminable in late stages of constrictive pericarditis. The fundamental pathophysiology in constrictive pericarditis is restriction of diastolic filling, due to limitation imposed by the fibrous scarred pericardium. Stroke volume is diminished, and the end-diastolic pressure in the ventricles, as well as the mean atrial pressures, systemic, and pulmonary vein pressures are equally elevated. Sometimes pericardial fibrosis is associated with myocardial fibrosis, which leads to ventricular contraction abnormality.

Clinical manifestations include shortness of breath, orthopnea, and fatigue due to limited cardiac output reserve, and elevated systemic jugular venous pressure. Kussmaul's sign may be present. The jugular venous pulse has a characteristic wave form. The peak of the v wave is early, and there is a deep y descent. This is followed by an early diastolic rise, terminating in an early h wave and a plateau (Fig. 3). Paradoxical pulse is observed in some cases. Signs of congestive hepatomegaly, splenomegaly, and ascites may be found; dependent edema is less common than ascites. Constrictive pericarditis is a commonly missed diagnosis. Patients with chronic constrictive pericarditis may be erroneously diagnosed as having cirrhosis of the liver; others are suspected of having gastrointestinal malignancy and undergo a lengthy clinical work up. These diagnostic errors can be avoided simply by careful examination of the venous pressure, which is elevated in constrictive pericarditis. The precordial pulse is either imperceptible or appears to retract during systole. Heart sounds typically are faint. A diastolic pericardial knock, which is an early high pitched sound (0.06–0.12 sec following aortic closure), may be heard and is related to the phase of early diastolic filling of the heart. It coincides with the y trough described in the venous pulse. Studies have related this sound to the sudden halt of ventricular filling observed in constrictive pericarditis. This sound, like Kussmaul's sign, occurs with some frequency in constrictive pericarditis but rarely in cardiac tamponade.

Hancock suggested that there are two forms of constriction, one elastic and the other more rigid. These two forms are believed to cause different patterns of diagnostic signs. The elastic form is similar to cardiac tamponade and is associated with prominent paradoxical pulse and systolic descent in venous tracings. The rigid type has a less prominent paradoxical pulse and a more conspicuous diastolic descent in the venous pressure tracing, often associated with a pericardial knock.

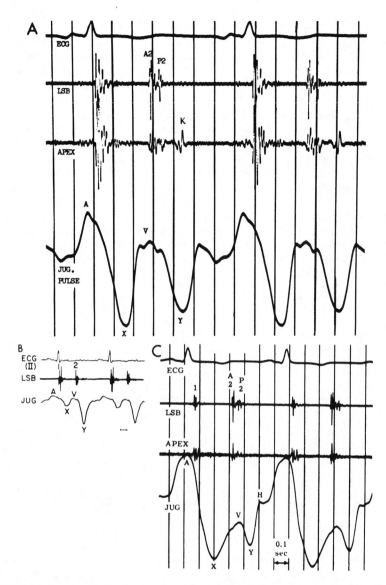

Figure 3 Jugular pulses in three examples of pericardial constriction. In example A, both X and Y descents are deep. A pericardial "knock" (K) coincides with the Y trough. Example B shows a deep Y descent but a shallow X descent. A few sound vibrations are located in early diastole at the expected time of the "knock." Example C displays a deep X descent with a relatively short Y descent. All three examples display early v wave peaking (around the time of S₂), an early Y trough (less than 0.2 second after A₂), and an early, prominent H wave. These features are characteristic of pericardial constriction. (Reproduced with permission from Tavel ME: The jugular pulse tracing: Its clinical application, in Tavel ME, ed: *Clinical Phonocardiography and External Pulse Recording*, 3rd ed. Chicago, Year Book Medical Publishers, 1979, p. 250.)

Electrocardiographic abnormalities include low QRS amplitude, T wave changes, notched P waves, and atrial fibrillation in about 25% of patients. Chest x-ray film shows a normal or slightly enlarged cardiac shadow, with clear lung fields. Pericardial calcification may be seen (see Chapter 4). Pericardial thickening on echocardiography, in the absence of effusion, is a nonspecific finding and cannot be relied upon for diagnosis of constriction. Left ventricular filling, as reflected by a sharp posterior motion of the posterior wall in early diastole followed by a flat segment, can be seen in constrictive pericarditis; and there is prominent early diastolic anterior motion of the ventricular septum. Two-dimensional echocardiography may show small ventricles with enlarged atria, dilatation of the inferior vena cava, and bulging of the interventricular and interatrial septa into the left side of the heart in inspiration.

Cardiac catheterization reveals that ventricular end-diastolic pressures are elevated. Right ventricular pressure shows a consistent steep early-diastolic dip, followed by a plateau ("square-root sign"). The end-diastolic pressure of the right ventricle is higher or equal to one-third of its systolic pressure. The wave form and amplitude of left ventricular diastolic pressure is identical to that of the right ventricle. Pulmonary arterial diastolic pressure is equal to the end-diastolic pressure in

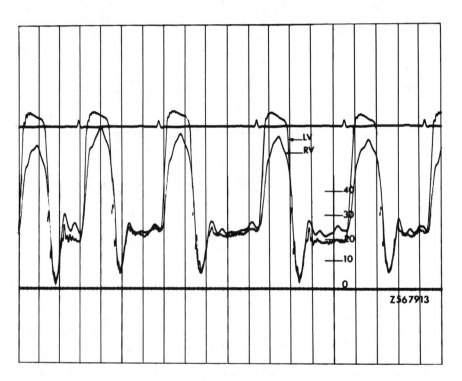

Figure 4 Simultaneous left ventricular and right ventricular pressure recordings in a patient with constrictive pericarditis. The classical "square root" sign of the ventricular pressures during diastole can be noted. (Reproduced with permission from Feigenbaum H: Pericardial disease, in Feigenbaum H, ed: *Echocardiography*, 3rd ed. Philadelphia, Lea & Febiger, 1981, p. 494.)

the ventricles. Severe constriction is associated with filling pressures of 20–25 mm Hg (Fig. 4). The right atrial pressure pulse has an M-shaped pattern. The typical venous M-shaped pattern and ventricular "square root sign" are characteristic of constriction and differentiate it from tamponade. Cardiac catheterization helps differentiate constrictive pericarditis from restrictive cardiomyopathy (see Chapter 14). Transvenous endomyocardial biopsy may be of value when differential diagnosis between restrictive myocardial or constrictive pericardial disease is necessary.

Pericardial resection is the treatment of choice in symptomatic cases. Operative mortality approximates 5%. Long term results are satisfactory, especially in radical resection of the pericardium; however, the hemodynamic improvement may be gradual. In cases with no improvement, one should look for either myocardial involvement or inadequate pericardial resection. Recurrence of constriction is rare.

SUBACUTE EFFUSIVE-CONSTRICTIVE PERICARDITIS

In this condition, constrictive pericarditis coexists with pericardial effusion and tamponade. The constriction in this situation is by the visceral pericardium, rather than by the parietal pericardium. Causes of effusive-constrictive pericarditis include tuberculosis, recurrent relapses of idiopathic pericarditis, trauma, postradiation effects, uremia, and connective tissue diseases. Physcial findings include paradoxical pulse and elevated venous pressure with prominent x descent. An, S_3 or diastolic knock may be present. The ECG demonstrates low or borderline QRS amplitude with T wave changes. Chest x-ray film reveals a large heart, and echocardiography often reveals effusion and pericardial thickening. Following removal of fluid by pericardiocentesis, venous pressure typically remains elevated due to remaining constriction. The intracavitary pressure tracings shift from those typical of tamponade (x = y descent or x > y descent, no square root sign) prior to pericardiocentesis to those typical of constriction (y > x descent, square root sign) after pericardiocentesis. This condition may progress to chronic constrictive pericarditis. Surgical excision of the pericardium is indicated in severe cases.

ADHESIVE PERICARDITIS

This is a condition in which there are adhesions between pericardium and structures in the mediastinum. This condition usually does not interfere with cardiac function.

Features of Specific Forms of Pericardial Disease

VIRAL OR ACUTE BENIGN FORM OF PERICARDITIS

This is a frequent entity and can be caused by a wide range of viruses (Coxsackie B, A, influenza, echo, herpes simplex, mumps, chicken pox, and adenovirus). Viral pericarditis can cause a variety of inflammatory reactions (serous, fibrinous, hemorrhagic, or suppurative), probably depending on the virus. Sometimes acute pericarditis is related or associated to a viral infection by history. Viral cultures are not always helpful; fourfold or greater increases in convalescent serum titer are usual, but because of the benignity of most infections, are not tested. When viral etiology cannot be established but is presumed (by default), the illness is referred to by some physicians as acute benign pericarditis. This disease is more frequent in young adults. Pain is usually accompanied by fever; pneumonitis and pleuritis are frequently present. There is evidence of pericardial effusion but tamponade is unusual. The acute disease lasts for 10–14 days and relapses of the acute disease occur in 20% of cases. No specific therapy is available. Analgesic antiinflammatory drugs may be used (aspirin or indomethacin) and corticosteroids are needed only in severe cases.

NEOPLASTIC PERICARDIAL DISEASE

Metastatic tumors (also see Chapter 22) are of importance, since they are responsible for serious pericardial effusion and tamponade. Common malignancies affecting the pericardium are carcinoma of the lung and breast, melanoma, lymphoma, and leukemia. Neoplasms characteristically produce large pericardial effusions and, sometimes, tamponade.

Pericardial metastases can be detected in some cases by echocardiography. Pericardiocentesis is indicated to relieve tamponade, symptomatic pericardial effusion, and for obtaining cytologic specimens. Positive cytologic findings have been reported in 50–75% of patients with neoplastic pericardial effusion. Open pericardial biopsy taken from suspected foci in the pericardium can be of diagnostic value in up to 90% of the cases with neoplastic involvement. In recurrent pericardial effusion or tamponade intrapericardial chemotherapy administration or surgical procedure should be considered.

RADIATION PERICARDITIS

This condition may occur early after radiation therapy, or even many years after exposure. It is of importance to diagnose this entity in patients with neoplastic diseases and to differentiate it from metastatic involvement of the pericardium, since radiation pericarditis has a better prognosis. Differentiation sometimes can be made by cytologic or histologic examination of the fluid and pericardium. Although acute pericarditis and effusion may follow in radiation of the heart, effusive constrictive pericarditis is the common entity in these patients.

TUBERCULOUS PERICARDITIS

The incidence of tuberculous pericarditis is decreasing in developed countries. It is important to make the diagnosis in the acute stage, since antituberculous drugs are effective. This condition tends to be associated with large pericardial effusions and, if not treated, progresses to an effusive-constrictive phase and eventually to chronic constrictive pericarditis. Pericardiocentesis can provide positive diagnosis in only 15% of the cases.

PYOGENIC PERICARDITIS

Pyogenic pericarditis is a rare condition associated with pneumococcal, staphylococcal, streptococcal, and gram negative infections. Purulent pericarditis may complicate cases of systemic fungal infections. Patients with pyogenic pericarditis are very ill, febrile, and toxic. In suspected cases, pericardiocentesis should be performed immediately, in order to diagnose this etiology and obtain cultures. Surgical drainage should be promptly performed to evacuate the purulent fluid, in addition to specific antibiotic therapy. Pyogenic pericarditis tends to progress to constrictive pericarditis despite antibiotic therapy.

UREMIC PERICARDITIS

This type of pericardial involvement is associated with advanced chronic renal failure and is a serious complication, since it may be associated with tamponade. Intense hemodialysis is indicated for treatment of uncomplicated uremic pericarditis and results in resolution of pericarditis in 40–60% of patients. Serial physical examination, chest x-rays, and echocardiograms are useful for follow-up of chronic dialysis therapy in renal patients and for identifying those patients with fluid accumulation. Resolution of uremic pericarditis complicated by tamponade is accomplished, in most cases, by intense hemodialysis in association with pericardiocentesis. Surgical pericardial excision is recommended in cases with recurrent episodes of pericarditis. Treatment of intractable uremic pericardial effusion by local steroid (triamcinolone hexacetonide) administration into the pericardial sac has been described in a few patients (Popli et al.). Frequently, mild degrees of pericardial effusion are associated with fluid overload, congestive heart failure, and left ventricular dysfunction, which often occurs in chronic renal patients. Cardiac catheterization may be needed to establish whether tamponade is a dominant component in these cases.

TRAUMATIC HEMOPERICARDIUM

Traumatic hemopericardium can result either from penetrating wounds of the heart or as a result of closed chest trauma caused by the steering wheel in automobile accidents. Hemopericardium due to closed chest trauma is sometimes difficult to recognize, since it may develop slowly. Cardiac tamponade may develop following cardiac operations early or late in the patient's course and rarely following cardiac catheterization and pacemaker insertion.

POSTCARDIAC INJURY SYNDROME

This condition occurs as an inflammatory reaction following either pericardial injury induced in the course of a cardiac operation or trauma to the heart or after the first 14 days of an MI (Dressler's syndrome: see Chapter 11). Prominent clinical features include fever, pericarditis, and sometimes pneunonitis and pleuritis. The postcardiac injury syndrome may occur from several days to months after the injury or the infarction. Pericarditis may be accompanied by pericardial effusion. The clinical picture mimics acute viral pericarditis, but it is believed to be a hypersensitivity immune reaction following myocardial injury. Patients are generally managed by analagesic antiinflammatory drugs; in severe disabling or recurring cases, corticosteroids may be effective.

PERICARDIAL EFFUSION ASSOCIATED WITH CONGESTIVE HEART FAILURE

Effusion may accompany cases with heart failure, without evidence of pericarditis. In general, pericardial effusion due to heart failure does not lead to tamponade. In one study, cardiac disease associated with congestive heart failure was found to be the most common cause of pericardial effusion in patients referred for echocardiography. Parameters of left heart function are markedly abnormal in these patients with congestive heart failure and pericardial effusion.

Bibliography

Alcan KE, Zabetakis PM, Mariho ND, et al: Management of acute cardiac tamponade by subxyphoid pericardiotomy. *JAMA* 247(8):1143, 1982.

Applefeld MM, Slawson RG, Hall-Craigs M, et al: Delayed pericardial disease after radiotherapy. *Am J Cardiol* 47:210, 1981.

Armstrong WF, Schilt BF, Helper DJ, et al: Diastolic collapse of the right ventricle with cardiac tamponade: An echocardiographic study. *Circulation* 65:1491, 1982.

Chandraratna PA, Aronow WS: Detection of pericardial metastates by crosssection echocardiography. *Circulation* 63:197, 1981.

Culliford AT, Lipton M, Spencer FC: Operation for chronic constrictive pericarditis: Do the surgical approach and degree of pericardial resection influence the outcome significantly? *Ann Thorac Surg* 29:146, 1980.

Felner JM: Pericardial disease, in Hurst JW (ed): *The Heart*. New York, McGraw-Hill, 1978, p 473.

Feigenbaum H: Pericardial disease, in Feigenbaum H (ed): *Echocardiography*. Philadelphia, Lea and Febiger, 1981, p 478.

Fowler ND: The recognition and management of pericardial disease, in Hurst JW (ed): *The Heart*. New York, McGraw-Hill, 1978, p 1640.

Fowler ND: Pericardial diseases, in Fowler NO (ed): *Cardiac Diagnosis and Treatment*. New York, Harper & Row, 1980, p 976.

Hancock EW: Cardiac Tamponade. *Med Clin North Am* 63:223, 1979.

Hancock EW: Subacute effusive-constrictive pericarditis. *Circulation* 43:183, 1971.

Hancock EW: On the elastic and rigid forms of constrictive pericarditis. *Am Heart J* 100:917, 1980.

Kamar S, Lesch M: Pericarditis in renal disease. *Prog Cardiovasc Dis* 22:357, 1980.

Kerber RE, Gascho JA, Litchfield R, et al: Hemodynamic effects of volume expansion and nitroprusside compared with pericardiocentesis in patients with acute cardiac tamponade. *N Engl J Med* 307:929, 1982.

Kessler KM, Rodriguez D, Rahim A, et al: Echocardiographic observations regarding pericardial effusions associated with cardiac disease. *Chest* 78:736, 1980.

Krikorian JG, Hancock EW: Pericardiocentesis. *Am J Med* 65:808, 1978.

Lewis BS: Real time two-dimensional echocardiography in constrictive pericarditis. *Am J Cardiol* 49:1789, 1982.

Lorell B, Leinbach RC, Pohost GM, et al: Right ventricular infarction: Clinical diagnosis and differentiation from cardiac tamponade and pericardial constriction. *Am J Cardiol* 43(3):465, 1979.

Martins JB, Manuel WJ, Marcus ML: Comparative effects of catecholamines in cardiac tamponade; experimental and clinical studies. *Am J Cardiol* 46:59, 1980.

Popli S, Ing TS, Daugirdas JT, et al: Treatment of uremic pericardial effusion by local steroid instillation via subxyphoid pericardiotomy. J Dial 4:83, 1980.

Posner MR, Cohen GI, Skarin AT: Pericardial disease in patients with cancer: The differentiation of malignant from idiopathic and radiation-induced pericarditis. *Am J Med* 71:407, 1981.

Shabetai R: The pericardium: An essay on some recent developments. *Am J Cardiol* 42:1036, 1978.

Spodick DH: The normal and diseased pericardium: Current concepts of pericardial physiology, diagnosis and treatment. *J Am Coll Cardiol* 1:240, 1983.

Tavel ME: The jugular pulse tracing: Its clinical application, in Tavel ME (ed): *Clinical Phonocardiography and External Pulse Recording*, 3rd ed. Chicago, Year Book Medical Publishers, 1979, p 250.

Tyberg TI, Goodyear AV, Langon RA: Genesis of pericardial knock in constrictive pericarditis. *Am J Cardiol* 46:570, 1980.

Walsh TJ, Baughman KL, Gardner TJ, et al: Constrictive epicarditis as a cause of delayed or absent response to pericardiectomy: A clinicopathological study. *J Thorac Cardiovasc Surg* 83:126, 1982.

Wong B, Murphy J, Chaug CJ, et al: The risk of pericardiocentesis. *Am J Cardiol* 44:1110, 1979.

CHAPTER 21 | INFECTIVE ENDOCARDITIS

Leonard S. Lilly
Robert A. Kloner

Infections of the heart valves and mural endocardium are due to a wide spectrum of microorganisms and may cause a variety of clinical presentations. Such infections may develop in otherwise healthy people, but are more likely to occur when previous cardiac damage is present. Based on an individual patient's clinical course, endocarditis can be divided into an indolent "subacute" form and a fulminant "acute" variety. This division will serve as the skeleton of our discussion after a brief look at the causative organisms and pathogenesis of this disease.

Etiology

Bacteria are responsible for most episodes of infective endocarditis. Although almost all bacterial species have been implicated at one time or another, certain organisms cause most cases, as shown in Table 1. Streptococci are most commonly involved, but staphylococcal infections are increasing in frequency, as a result of the surge in intravenous drug abuse and other factors discussed below. Ten to 15% of the time no organism can be isolated; this syndrome will be discussed later.

The organisms that cause the subacute form of endocarditis tend to be of low invasiveness; and although they are capable of establishing infection on a previously damaged cardiac valve or site of congenital heart abnormality, they are not usually able to infect an otherwise healthy heart. These organisms are most often streptococcal species and are usually found in the body's normal flora in the oral cavity and GI tract. In order to incite intracardiac infection, the bacteria must first enter the bloodstream and be carried to the heart. Table 2 lists the major portals of entry through which streptococci and other organisms may enter the circulation.

The more invasive organisms are responsible for the fulminant acute variety of infective endocarditis; they can localize and establish infection in previously undamaged sites. These agents are usually not part of the normal flora and include *Staphylococcus aureus, Streptococcus pneumoniae, Neisseria gonorrhoeae,* certain gram-negative rods, and fungal species. Possible routes of their entry into the bloodstream are listed in Table 2, but often no apparent source can be localized.

Underlying cardiac structural abnormalities can be found in 70% of patients who develop infective endocarditis. The most commonly associated lesions are listed in Table 3. Implanted hardware, such as prosthetic valves, pacemaker wires, and corrective shunts (e.g., Blalock, Waterston, ventriculoatrial) are also targets of infection.

Table 1. Major Organisms Responsible for Infective Endocarditis

Streptococci	55%
Streptococcus veridans	
Enterococci	
Streptococcus bovis	
Anaerobic streptococci	
Other streptococci	
Staphylococci	20–25%
Staphylococcus aureus	
Staphylococcus epidermidis	
Gram-negative rods	7%
"Culture negative"	10–15%
Fungi, rickettsia, chlamydia, uncommon bacteria	5%

Subacute endocarditis predominently affects the left side of the heart, whereas more pyogenic organisms, as seen in IV drug abusers, also infect the right-sided valves.

Pathogenesis

Development of the subacute form of endocarditis requires certain conditions. First, a previously damaged heart valve or site of congenital abnormality is usually present, which forces a jet of blood to flow from a high pressure area to a low pressure area.

Table 2. Bacterial Portals of Entry Leading to Infective Endocarditis

Portal of Entry	Organisms Involved
Oral cavity (dental manipulation including tooth brushing, dental extractions)	*Streptococcus veridans* Anaerobic streptococci *Staphylococcus epidermidis*
Upper airway (rigid bronchoscopy, orotracheal intubation, tonsillectomy)	*Streptococci* species *Staphylococcus epidermidis* *Streptococcus pneumoniae*
Genitourinary tract (cystoscopy, prostatectomy, pyelonephritis)	Gram-negative rods *Enterococci*
Gastrointestinal tract (rigid sigmoidoscopy, barium enema, percutaneous liver biopsy)	Gram-negative rods *Streptococcus bovis* *Enterococci*
Indwelling IV catheters, hemodialysis access sites, hyperalimentation catheters	*Staphylococcus* species *Candida* species
Skin infections, burns	*Staphylococcus* species
Pneumonia	*Streptococcus pneumoniae* *Hemophilus influenzae*

Table 3. Cardiac Lesions Associated with Development of Infective Endocarditis

Rheumatic valvular disease

Congenital heart disease (especially ventricular septal defect, patent ductus arteriosus, tetralogy of Fallot, coarctation of the aorta, congenitally abnormal aortic valve)

Acquired mitral regurgitation, calcific aortic stenosis, aortic regurgitation

Idiopathic hypertrophic subaortic stenosis

Mitral valve prolapse (if mitral regurgitation is present)

Implanted hardware (prosthetic valves, pacemaker wires, intravascular corrective shunts: e.g., Blalock, Waterston, ventriculoatrial)

For example, mitral regurgitation creates such a jet between the left ventricle and the left atrium. Abnormalities that do not create a forceful jet of blood, such as an ostium secundum atrial septal defect, are not usually associated with endocardial infection. Second, a sterile platelet-fibrin thrombus may form at the site of impact of this jet of blood (in the left atrium in the case of mitral regurgitation). Third, a transient bacteremia allows delivery of organisms to this sterile thrombus, where they can adhere, multiply, and form a vegetation. Although transient bacteremias are quite common (after tooth brushing, for example), endocardial infection occurs rarely, because the organisms associated with these common bacteremias tend to be small in number and of low invasiveness. Why certain bacteremias do adhere and multiply on damaged heart valves is not known, but the role of agglutinating antibody, forming larger clumps of bacteria, may be important.

The pathogenesis of acute endocarditis is quite different from that of the subacute variety. The organisms involved are highly invasive and are required only in small numbers to incite infection. Underlying cardiac structural abnormalities are not necessary, and over 50% of acute endocarditis develops on previously normal valves.

Clinical Features

Subacute infective endocarditis typically begins with nonspecific symptoms including low grade fever, malaise, anorexia with weight loss, and generalized weakness. Headache, low back pain, arthralgias, and chills are common. Often, a diagnosis of upper respiratory tract infection is erroneously made, and oral antibiotics are prescribed. These may temporarily obscure the symptoms. If the diagnosis of endocarditis is suspected, a detailed history may disclose a portal of bacterial entry, such as recent dental work. Although these generalized symptoms may last for months, the diagnosis is usually suspected sufficiently early, so that classic features of subacute bacterial endocarditis, such as Janeway lesions and Osler's nodes (discussed below), are rarely seen today.

The onset of acute endocarditis is more explosive than the subacute variety. The patient rapidly becomes ill with rigors and high fever. Sometimes, preexisting pneumococcal pneumonia, staphylococcal skin infection, or evidence of IV drug abuse may be found.

Table 4.   Cutaneous and Occular Manifestations of Endocarditis

Petechiae	Conjunctiva, oral cavity, skin
Subungual hemorrhages	Linear splinter hemorrhages that do not reach the distal nail bed
Osler's nodes	Small red painful nodules in pulp spaces of terminal phalanges, thenar, and hypothenar eminences
Janeway lesions	Small erythematous nontender macules on the palms and soles
Roth's spots	Small white retinal dots surrounded by hemorrhage

Several physical findings may be associated with infective endocarditis. Heart murmurs are found in 90% of patients with subacute endocarditis, but often this simply reflects a preexisting valvular lesion or "flow" murmur of an accompanying anemia. Changing murmurs are quite uncommon, but are significant, as new regurgitant murmurs may herald severe ventricular compromise.

Petechiae may be present in the conjunctivae, oral cavity, or the skin. Other cutaneous manifestations, which occur rarely, are listed in Table 4. Retinal hemorrhages, exudates, or Roth's spots (Table 4) may be found. Splenomegaly is often present in subacute endocarditis, but not in the acute form, unless a splenic abscess has developed. Renal manifestations are common and reflect both embolic and immune-mediated phenomena. Over 50% of patients demonstrate hematuria (microscopic or gross), which may be associated with immune-complex diffuse or focal glomerulonephritis, or with renal infarction due to arteriolar embolization.

Fragments of infected valvular vegetation may break off, leave the cardiac chambers, and travel to distant sites. Most commonly, the brain, kidneys, spleen, bowel, and coronary arteries are the targets for such embolization, leading to infarction of the involved organ. In acute endocarditis, thromboembolism of infected material may cause abscess formation at these sites. Large emboli, which usually form in the setting of fungal endocarditis, may lodge in large peripheral arteries, resulting in the sudden loss of a major pulse. Septic pulmonary emboli may result from endocarditis involving the right side of the heart.

One third of patients with infective endocarditis manifest neurologic complications. Major cerebral emboli may lead to hemiplegia and hemi-sensory loss. Multiple smaller emboli may cause seizures, confusion, or multiple focal neurologic abnormalities. Brain abscess and purulent meningitis are not seen in the setting of subacute endocarditis, but do occur, rarely, in the acute variety, where more pyogenic organisms are involved. Peripheral ("mycotic") aneurysms may develop as a result of either immune complex deposition in the arterial wall, or from embolic occlusion of the vasa vasorum. Although these usually remain asymptomatic, they may expand, resulting in headache, cranial nerve palsies, and should rupture occur, intracerebral or subarachnoid bleeding.

Many serious cardiac complications may develop, especially during the course of acute endocarditis. Extension of infection may lead to disruption of valve leaflets, chordae tendineae, or supporting structures, resulting in progressive valvular dysfunction and congestive heart failure. Acute pulmonary edema may result from sudden mitral or aortic regurgitation. Myocardial abscess formation (seen with pyogenic organisms) may extend into the conduction tissues, with resultant conduction blocks and arrhythmias. Such an abscess may rupture through the intraventricular septum, forming a ventricular septal defect, or into the pericardial sac with resultant cardiac tamponade. A sinus of Valsalva mycotic aneurysm may also rupture into the right ventricle or right atrium, forming a left-to-right shunt.

Infective Endocarditis in IV Drug Abusers

The rise in parenteral drug abuse in recent decades has been accompanied by an increase in associated bacterial endocarditis. In these patients, bacteremia may arise from cellulitis at an injection site or from microbial contamination of injected material. *Staphylococcus aureus* is responsible for over 50% of these cases; other commonly involved species include *Candida* species and gram-negative rods, especially *Pseudomonas*. Unlike infective endocarditis in the general population, in these infections, streptococcal organisms account for less than 20%. The majority of intravenous narcotic abusers who present with endocarditis have no underlying heart disease, and the clinical presentation is that of an acute fulminant infection. The frequency of valvular involvement is unusual in that the tricuspid valve is most commonly affected. *Staphylococcus aureus* and gram-negative rods are particularly likely to infect the tricuspid valve and may result in septic pulmonary emboli, as an initial finding.

Because of the high frequency of *Staphylococcus aureus* and fungal infections in drug abusers, metastatic abscesses and large peripheral emboli are common. In a patient thought to be an IV drug abuser, in whom a fever and pulmonary infiltrates are found, endocarditis of the tricuspid valve should be strongly suspected.

Prosthetic Valve Endocarditis

Four to 10% of patients with prosthetic heart valves develop endocarditis. This occurs with the same frequency on mechanical and biologic (porcine xenograft) prostheses, and occurs most commonly on prostheses in the aortic position. Two specific syndromes can occur: "early" endocarditis develops within two months of valve replacement; "late" endocarditis occurs after that time. The early variety arises from either intraoperative contamination or from a perioperative complication: pneumonia, urinary tract infection, or sternotomy infection; therefore, the agents responsible include staphylococci, gram-negative rods, diphtheroids, and *Candida* species. The late form, on the other hand, arises from the same sources as endocarditis in the general polpulation. The organisms are, therefore, similar to those in subacute endocarditis, except that *Staphylococcus epidermidis* is more frequently involved, accounting for over 20% of prosthetic valvular infections. Repeated isolation of *Staphylococcus epidermidis* from the blood of a patient with a prosthetic valve must not be dismissed as a mere contaminant.

Complications of prosthetic valve endocarditis can arise from detachment of the sewing ring due to infiltrating infection, perforation of a xenograft cusp, or sticking of the mobile disc or ball due to thrombus formation, any of which can lead to rapid hemodynamic compromise. Embolization of thrombotic material may occur. Clinical clues to the development of endocarditis on a prosthetic valve include fever of unclear origin, muffling of the prosthetic heart sounds, a new murmer, and evidence of peripheral embolization.

Laboratory Findings

The hallmark of infective endocarditis is demonstration of the responsible organism by blood culture. Although the optimum number of blood cultures to obtain prior to initiating therapy has not been determined, five sets is generally accepted. However, as the bacteremia of endocarditis tends to be constant, if one blood culture is positive, all are likely to be positive. In the case of subacute endocarditis, in which immediate therapy is not as crucial as in the acute form, these can be obtained over a period of 12 to 24 hours. In suspected acute endocarditis, therapy must not be delayed, and all cultures should be drawn as rapidly as possible (within one hour). Aerobic and anaerobic cultures should be obtained under sterile conditions, and specimens should be kept for two to three weeks to insure identification of even slowly growing organisms. Special culture requirements may be needed when certain uncommon organisms (Weinstein and Schlesinger, 1974) are suspected.

Ten to 15% of patients with infective endocarditis do not have positive blood cultures. Possible explanations for this include: recent antibiotic therapy (within 10 days); fastidious growth requirements (especially *Brucella, Hemophilus, Histoplasma, Aspergillus*, chlamydial, rickettsial, and certain anaerobic organisms); right-sided endocarditis due to organisms of low invasiveness; and technical difficulties, such as inadequate quantities of blood or inappropriate incubation. Serological tests may help identify endocarditis caused by *Coxiellia burnetti* (Q fever), *Chlamydia psittaci*, and *Brucella* species.

Other laboratory findings are frequently present. A normochromic, normocytic anemia is common, especially in subacute endocarditis. The white cell count may be normal in the subacute form, but is usually elevated in the acute variety, with a shift toward less mature forms. Immunoglobulin abnormalities are seen: rheumatoid factor is detected in one-half of patients who have had the disease for more than six weeks and disappears with appropriate therapy. Circulating immune complexes can be found in over 90% of cases. These complexes are likely to be responsible for the glomerulonephritis seen with endocarditis, and may play a role in the development of the cutaneous manifestations (Table 4). Other common laboratory findings include hematuria, proteinuria, and elevated serum creatinine, if glomerulonephritis has led to acute renal failure. Detection of serum antibodies to teichoic acid, a component of the bacterial cell wall, may be helpful in documenting endocarditis due to *Staphylococcus aureus*, as they are found in the presence of valvular infection, but usually not in other staphylococcal infections.

Echocardiography may be useful in identifying valvular vegetations, but the current limits of resolution of this technique will not detect lesions smaller than 2 mm in size. M-mode examination may demonstrate suggestive findings in one-third to one-half of patients and is more likely to identify fungal vegetations, as these tend to be quite large. Two-dimensional imaging has complimented the M-mode study by increasing the yield of detection further, especially in identifying right-sided valvular lesions. The complications of endocarditis are often more readily visualized than the vegetations themselves. For example, flail valvular leaflets, ruptured chordae tendineae, features of acute aortic regurgitation (see Chapter 13), and evidence of valvular ring abscess may be identified by these methods. Pulsed Doppler recordings in association with two-dimensional echocardiography is under investigation as a means of accurately identifying aortic, mitral, and tricuspid regurgitant lesions.

Prosthetic valve dysfunction may be demonstrated at echocardiography by a rocking motion of the suture ring, disrupted xenograft leaflets, visible vegetations, or thrombus formation manifest by abnormal valvular opening or closing with muffled prosthetic sounds by phonocardiography.

Therapy

Prior to the antibiotic era, infective endocarditis was almost always a fatal condition. Today, antibiotic and surgical therapies have greatly reduced its mortality, but to achieve a cure, appropriate intravenous therapy must be administered for prolonged periods, usually four to six weeks. This is necessary because microorganisms in vegetations are protected from normal host defenses, and every single organism must be irradicated to prevent a recurrence. Bacteriocidal antibiotics must be used, often in combination for resistent organisms, and although dosages have not been standardized, those listed in Table 5 are recommended.

Although initiation of therapy need not be immediate in the subacute form of endocarditis and can await blood culture results, this is not the case with the acute variety. In this, early therapy is crucial to prevent rapid valvular destruction, hemodynamic compromise, myocardial abscess formation, and peripheral embolization of infected material. In the setting of suspected acute endocarditis, a Gram's stain of the peripheral blood buffy coat smear may help to identify the responsible organism, so that appropriate therapy may begin immediately after blood cultures are obtained. If the patient is an IV drug abuser, or if there is a strong suspicion of staphylococcal sepsis, a penicillinase-resistent penicillin or cephalosporin should be used. If urinary or GI sepsis is suspected, initial antibiotics should cover gram negative rods (Table 5). When there is no clue to the identity of the infecting organism, therapy should be directed toward the enterococci, as this provides broad coverage in vivo. Once positive blood cultures have identified the responsible organism, treatment should be adjusted to provide appropriate antibiotic coverage as determined by sensitivity testing in the laboratory. As a rule, the antibiotic dosage should be adjusted such that a 1:8 dilution of the patient's serum, drawn just prior to a dose of antibiotic, is bacteriocidal for the infecting organism in culture.

Recommended antibiotic regimens are listed in Table 5. With the exception of the enterococci, most streptococcal species are highly sensitive to penicillin. In penicillin-allergic patients, vancomycin or erythromycin are the prefered substitutes. In addition, as the risk of cross-reactivity between penicillin and the cephalosporins is low, the latter may also be cautiously considered in penicillin-sensitive patients. As *Steptococcus bovis* infections are often associated with malignancies of the lower

Table 5. Antibiotic Therapy of Common Organisms Responsible for Infective Endocarditis

Organism	Drug of Choice	Dose	Penicillin Allergy
Strepococcus veridans	Penicillin G	2.5 million U IV q6h	Cephalothin 2 g IV q4h or vancomycin 500 mg IV q6h or erythromycin 1 g IV q6h
Enterococcus sp.	Nafcillin (or ampicillin)	2 g IV q4h	Erythromycin 1 g IV q6h or vancomycin 500 mg IV q6h
	plus gentamicin (or tobramycin)	3–5 mg/kg/day in 3 divided doses	*plus* gentamicin (or tobramycin)
Streptococcus bovis	Penicillin G	2.5 million U IV q6h	Cephalothin 2 g IV q4h or vancomycin 500 mg IV q6h or erythromycin 1 g IV q6h
Anaerobic streptococci	Penicillin G	15–20 million U IV q6h	
Staphylococcus aureus	Nafcillin or oxacillin or cephalothin	2 g IV q4h	Vancomycin 500 mg IV q6h
Staphylococcus epidermidis	Vancomycin or cephalothin	500 mg IV q6h 2 g IV q4h	
"Culture negative"	Nafcillin	2 g IV q4h	Erythromycin 1 g IV q6h or vancomycin 500 mg IV q6h
	plus gentamicin (or tobramycin)	3–5 mg/kg/day in 3 divided doses	*plus* Gentamicin (or tobramycin)
Streptococcus pneumoniae	Penicillin G	5 million U IV q6h	Erythromycin 1 g IV q6h
Neisseria gonorrhoeae and meningitidis	Penicillin G	5 million U IV q6h	Erythromycin 1 g IV q6h
Pseudomonas sp.	Gentamicin (or tobramycin)	3–5 mg/kg/day in 3 divided doses	
	plus carbenicillin (or ticarcillin)	500 mg/kg/day in 6 divided doses 250 mg/kg/day in 6 divided doses	
Escherichia coli	Ampicillin	2 g IV q4h	
	plus gentamicin (or tobramycin)	3–5 mg/kg/day in 3 divided doses	

GI tract, a search for such a lesion should be undertaken when treatment for this organism is underway.

Enterococcal endocarditis is relatively resistent to penicillin therapy, which must be administered in high doses in addition to an aminoglycoside. Nafcillin plus tobramycin (or gentamicin) has been shown to act synergistically in vivo against this organism. For those enterococci that prove to be exquisitely sensitive to ampicillin, this drug may be substituted for nafcillin.

Staphylococcus aureus infections are usually resistent to penicillin G, and the antibiotics of choice are nafcillin, oxacillin, or a cephalosporin, for a period of four to six weeks. In penicillin-allergic patients, vancomycin is recommended. Despite the lower invasiveness of *Staphylococcus epidermidis*, this is an extremely difficult organism to irradicate, especially on prosthetic valves; vancomycin or a cephalosporin is the preferred treatment.

Antimicrobial therapy of fungal endocarditis has been disappointing, especially when prosthetic valves are involved. Amphotericin B is currently the only available fungicidal agent and has quite toxic side-effects. An oral fungistatic drug, 5-fluorocytosine, may be added to amphotericin B when an organism has shown sensitivity to both drugs; and this combination can increase the fungicidal activity of the latter. In spite of this, bulky vegetations often form with local myocardial invasion and peripheral embolization, most often requiring surgical removal of the involved valve.

When infection of a prosthetic valve is suspected, antibiotic therapy should begin as early as possible and be continued for six to eight weeks. In general, these infections respond poorly to antibiotic therapy; the overall mortality is 50 to 60% and is least favorable in the group with early involvement. Anticoagulation therapy should be continued in patients with mechanical valvular prostheses, although a risk of bleeding exists if cerebral embolization or mycotic aneurysm rupture should ensue (see Wilson, 1975). Surgical replacement of the prosthesis should be undertaken on an emergent basis if progressive deterioration develops in the form of increasing congestive heart failure due to valvular dysfunction, systemic embolization despite appropriate antibiotic therapy, or continued bacteremia after seven to 10 days of therapy. Because of the high mortality associated with prosthetic endocarditis in general, early valvular replacement should be considered in all cases, except those in which an organism is highly sensitive to antibiotic therapy (e.g., *Streptococcus veridans*). Ideally, surgical replacement should follow several days of antibiotics, which should then be continued for at least two weeks after the operation.

Fever usually resolves within one week of initiating appropriate antibiotic therapy, although petechiae and other embolic phenomena may continue beyond this time. A persistent fever suggests inappropriate antibiotic therapy, localized abscess formation, or antibiotic related fever.

Prophylaxis

In patients with structural heart abnormalities (Table 3), transient bacteremias can initiate infective endocarditis. The common procedures listed in Table 6 have been been responsible for such infection, and antibiotic prophylaxis should be administered prior to their performance in patients with predisposing cardiac lesions. The

Table 6. Procedures that Require Antibiotic Prophylaxis in Patients with Cardiac Lesions Predisposing to Infective Endocarditis

1. Dental manipulations (including hygienic cleaning, extractions, and other procedures in which gingival bleeding is likely to occur)
2. Rigid bronchoscopy, tonsillectomy
3. Urinary tract manipulation (catheter insertion, cystoscopy, prostatectomy)
4. Septic abortion or peripartum infection
5. Percutaneous liver biopsy
6. Gastrointestinal surgery, including cholecystectomy

Committee on Prevention of Bacterial Endocarditis of the American Heart Association recommends the antibiotic prophylaxis listed in Table 7. These regimens are particularly aimed at *Streptococcus veridans* (oral cavity and upper airway) and enterococci (GI and GU tracts). This preventative therapy is especially important in the presence of a prosthetic valve, in which treatment of established infection is quite difficult, as discussed above.

The following procedures do not require antibiotic prophylaxis, unless a prosthetic valve is present: normal vaginal delivery, dilatation and curettage of the uterus,

Table 7. Prophylactic Antibiotic Regimens for the Prevention of Bacterial Endocarditis[a]

Procedure	30 Minutes to 1 Hour before Procedure	Then
Dental and upper respiratory tract procedures	Aqueous penicillin G 1–2 million U IM or IV *plus* Procaine penicillin G 600,000 U IM	Penicillin V 500 mg po q6h for 4–8 doses
Parenteral	In patients with prosthetic valves or who are on chronic rheumatic fever prophylaxis: *add* Streptomycin 1 g IM	
Penicillin allergy:	Vancomycin 1 g IV	Erythromycin 500 mg po q6h for 4–8 doses
Oral	Penicillin V 2 g po	Penicillin V 500 mg po q6h for 4–8 doses
Penicillin allergy:	Erythromycin 500 mg po	Erythromycin 500 mg po q6h for 4–8 doses

Table 7. (Continued)

Procedure	30 Minutes to 1 Hour before Procedure	Then
GI and GU procedures	Aqueous penicillin G 2 million U IM or IV (*or* Ampicillin 1–2 g IM or IV) *plus* Gentamicin 1.5 mg/kg IM	Repeat regimen q8h for two more doses
Penicillin allergy:	Vancomycin 1 g IV *plus* Gentamicin 1.5 mg/kg IM	Repeat regimen q8h for two more doses

[a] (in patients with lesions listed in Table 3)

barium enema, sigmoidoscopy, and fiberoptic gastroscopy without biopsy. In addition, prior to elective valve replacement for congenital or acquired heart disease, poor dentition should be corrected to reduce the incidence of subsequent prosthetic valve endocarditis. During open heart surgery for valvular replacement, prophylaxis against *Staphylococcus aureus* is recommended.

Bibliography

Arnett EN, Roberts WC: Valve ring abscess in active infective endocarditis. Frequency, location and clues to clinical diagnosis from the study of 95 necropsy patients. *Circulation* 54:140, 1976.

Banks T, Fletcher R, Ali N: Infective endocarditis in heroin addicts. *Am J Med* 55:444, 1973.

Bayer AS, Theofilopoulos AN, Tillman DB, et al: Use of circulating immune complex levels in the serodifferentiation of endocarditic and nonendocarditic septicemias. *Am J Med* 66:58, 1979.

Block PC, DeSanctis RW, Weinberg AN: Prosthetic valve endocarditis. *J Thorac Cardiovasc Surg* 60:540, 1970.

Cabane J, Godeau P, Herreman G, et al: Fate of circulating immune complexes in infective endocarditis. *Am J Med* 66:277, 1979.

Cohen PS, Maguire JH, and Weinstein L: Infective endocarditis caused by gram negative bacteria. *Prog Cardiovasc Dis* 22:205, 1979.

Davis RS, Strom JA, Frishman W, et al: The demonstration of vegetations by echocardiography in bacterial endocarditis: An indication for early surgical intervention. *Am J Med* 69:57, 1980.

Dismukes WE, Karchmer AW, Buckley MJ, et al: Prosthetic valve endocarditis: Analysis of 38 cases. *Circulation* 48:365, 1973.

Everett ED, Hirschman JV: Transient bacteremia and endocarditis prophylaxis: A review. *Medicine* (Baltimore) 56:61, 1977.

Gardner P, Saffle JR, Schoenbaum SC: Management of prosthetic valve endocarditis, in Duma RJ (ed): *Infections of Prosthetic Heart Valves and Vascular Grafts*, Baltimore, University Park Press, 1977, p. 123.

Hill DG, Yates AK: Prophylactic antibiotics in open heart surgery. *NZ Med J* 81:414, 1975.

Horowitz MS, Smith LG: Vegetative bacterial endocarditis on the prolapsing mitral valve: Echocardiographic evaluation. *Arch Intern Med* 137:788, 1977.

Hutter AM, Moellering RC: Assessment of the patient with suspected endocarditis. *JAMA* 235:1603, 1976.

Kaplan EL: Committee on Prevention of Rheumatic Fever and Bacterial Endocarditis of the American Heart Association. Prevention of bacterial endocarditis. *Circulation* 56(Suppl 1):139A, 1977.

Karchmer AW, Swartz MN: Infective endocarditis in patients with prosthetic heart valves, in Kaplan EL, Taranta AV, (eds): *Infective Endocarditis*. American Heart Association Monograph 52, 1977, p. 58.

Karchmer AW, Dismukes WE, Buckley MJ, et al: Late prosthetic valve endocarditis: Clinical features influencing therapy. *Am J Med* 64:199, 1978.

Klein RS, Recco RA, Catalano MT, et al: Association of *Streptococcus bovis* with carcinoma of the colon. *N Engl J Med* 297:800, 1977.

Lerner PI, Weinstein L: Infective endocarditis in the antibiotic era. *N Engl J Med* 274:199, 259, 388, 1966.

Melvin E, Berger M, Lutzker LG, et al: Noninvasive methods for detection of valve vegetations in infective endocarditis. *Am J Cardiol* 47:271, 1981.

Manzies CJG: Coronary embolism with infarction in bacterial endocarditis. *Br Heart J* 23:464, 1961.

Mills J, Utley J, Abbott J: Heart failure in infective endocarditis: Predisposing factors, course, and treatment. *Chest* 66:151, 1974.

Mintz GS, Kotler MN, Segal BL, et al: Comparison of two-dimensional and M-mode echocardiography in the evaluation of patients with infective endocarditis. *Am J Cardiol* 43:738, 1979.

Mintz GS, et al: Clinical value and limitations of echocardiography: Its use in the study of patients with infectious endocarditis. *Arch Intern Med* 140:1022, 1980.

Nagel JG, Tuazon CU, CArdella TA, et al: Teichoic acid serologic diagnosis of staphylococcal endocarditis: Use of gel diffusion and counterimmunoelectrophoretic methods. *Ann Intern Med* 82:13, 1975.

Pelletier LL, Petersdorf RG: Infective endocarditis: A review of 125 cases from the University of Washington Hospitals 1963–1972, *Medicine* 56:287, 1977.

Perez GO, Rothfield N, Williams RC: Immune-complex nephritis in bacterial endocarditis. *Arch Intern Med* 136:334, 1976.

Pesanti EL, Smith IM: Infective endocarditis with negative blood cultures: An analysis of 52 cases. *Am J Med* 66:43, 1979.

Pruitt AA, Rubin RH, Karchmer AW, et al: Neurologic complications of bacterial endocarditis. *Medicine* 57:329, 1978.

Reisberg BE: Infective endocarditis in the narcotic addict. *Prog Cardiovasc Dis* 22:193, 1979.

Richardson JV, Karp RB, Kirklin JW, et al: Treatment of infective endocarditis: A 10 year comparative analysis. *Circulation* 58:589, 1978.

Roberts WC, Buchbinder NA: Right-sided valvular infective endocarditis. *Am J Med* 53:7, 1972.

Rubenson DS: The use of echocardiography in diagnosing culture-negative endocarditis. *Circulation* 64:641, 1981.

Rubinstein E, Noriega ER, Simberkoff MS, et al: Fungal endocarditis: Analysis of 24 cases and review of the literature. *Medicine* 54:331, 1975.

Sande M and Scheld WM, et al: Combination antibiotic therapy of bacterial endocarditis. *Ann Intern Med* 92:390, 1980.

Stinson EB, Giepp RB, Vosti K, et al: Operation treatment of active endocarditis. *J Thorac Cardiovasc Surg* 71:659, 1976.

Wang K, Gobel FL, Gleason DF: Bacterial endocarditis in idiopathic hypertrophic subacute stenosis. *Am Heart J* 89:359, 1975.

Weinstein L, Schlesinger JJ: Pathoanatomic, pathophysiologic, and clinical correlations in endocarditis. *N Engl J Med* 291:832, 1974.

Weinstein L, Rubin RH: Infective endocarditis-1973. *Prog Cardiovasc Dis* 16:239, 1973.

Welton DE, Young JB, Raizner AE, et al: Value and safety of cardiac catheterization during active infective endocarditis. *Am J Cardiol* 44:1306, 1979.

Wilson WR, Jaumin PM, Danielson GK, et al: Prosthetic valve endocarditis. *Ann Intern Med* 82:751, 1975.

Wilson WR, Geraci JE, Danielson GK, et al: Anticoagulant therapy and central nervous system complications in patients with prosthetic valve endocarditis. *Circulation* 57:1004, 1978.

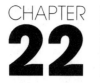

CHAPTER | # CARDIAC TUMORS
22 | Robert A. Kloner

Primary Cardiac Tumors

The incidence of primary cardiac tumors is quite low (less than 0.002 to 0.28 of the general population). Approximately 75% of all primary cardiac tumors are histologically benign; the most common are myxomas, followed by lipomas, papillary fibroelastomas, rhabdomyomas, and fibromas. Twenty five percent of primary cardiac tumors are malignant, the most common being rhabdomyosarcomas and angiosarcomas.

Benign Cardiac Tumors

LEFT ATRIAL MYXOMAS

Myxomas are the most common primary tumor of the heart and account for 30–50% of all cardiac tumors. Although there has been some debate in the past as to whether these tumors actually represent neoplasms or just well-organized thrombi, studies in which tissue from myxomas were grown in culture showed that their cells demonstrated neoplastic properties. Myxomas tend to arise in the atria; in the left atrium three to four times more commonly than in the right atrium. There have been several cases reported of familial occurrences of myxoma. These tumors typically are pedunculated and mobile and prolapse through the mitral valve orifice, resulting in obstruction to flow through the valve, or mitral regurgitation. The symptoms, due to obstruction and regurgitation, may mimic those of rheumatic mitral valve disease and include dyspnea, orthopnea, paroxysmal nocturnal dyspnea, fatigue, cough, and chest pain. Paroxysmal episodes of dizziness, seizures, and syncope are also described. If the tumor becomes lodged in the mitral orifice, acute circulatory failure may occur. Unlike mitral stenosis, the onset of these symptoms is often sudden and may vary with the position of the patient. Tumor emboli are common with atrial myxomas, due to their friability and intracavitary location. Left atrial myxomas result in systemic emboli, while right atrial myxomas cause pulmonary emboli and pulmonary hypertension. If the emboli affect a peripheral vessel, a histologic diagnosis of myxoma can be made by recovering the systemic embolic material. Systemic symptoms may occur in patients with myxoma; these include fever, weight loss, general malaise, arthralgia, and pallor. It has been postulated that these symptoms result from an immunologic mechanism, from products secreted by the tumor, or tumor necrosis. These systemic symptoms plus those of embolization may mimic endocarditis.

439

The physical examination of patients with left atrial myxoma reveals a loud S_1, S_4, and an early diastolic sound called a "tumor plop," which occurs when the tumor strikes the endocardial wall or when its motion is suddenly halted. This tumor plop usually occurs later and is lower in frequency than an opening snap; it occurs earlier and is higher in frequency than an S_3. A low-pitched diastolic rumble due to obstruction of flow through the mitral orifice may mimic the murmur of rheumatic mitral stenosis; a holosystolic murmur at the apex due to mitral regurgitation has also been described. These murmurs typically vary in intensity with the patient's position. Friction rubs due to contact of the tumor with the atrial and ventricular endocardium are occasionally present.

Examination of the lungs may reveal rales due to pulmonary congestion, and examination of the extremities may show clubbing. Laboratory studies usually demonstrate anemia, elevated sedimentation rate, hypergammaglobulinemia, leukocytosis, thrombocytosis, or thrombocytopenia. Chest x-ray findings in patients with left atrial myxoma include an enlarged left atrium, pulmonary congestion, and, in 10% of cases, calcification within the intracardiac tumor. The ECG may show atrial arrhythmias (atrial fibrillation or flutter), right ventricular hypertrophy, and abnormal P waves. M-mode and two-dimensional echocardiography have been extremely useful for assessing the presence of cardiac tumors. Left atrial myxomas can be visualized as a mass of echoes in the left atrium during systole. Since myxomas are commonly pedunculated, they prolapse into the left ventricle during diastole, resulting in a mass of echoes behind the anterior leaflet of the mitral valve (Chapter 5).

Some investigators have suggested that two-dimensional echocardiography may eliminate the need for preoperative angiography. Radionuclide imaging of the tumors by gated blood pool scanning (resulting in a filling defect) or computer assisted tomography are helpful noninvasive tests, if the echocardiogram is nondiagnostic. Angiography (performed by filming the levo-phase of a pulmonary arteriogram in order to avoid dislodging tumor fragments) reveals a mobile left atrial filling defect which may prolapse into the left ventricle during diastole. An atrial ball thrombus may appear similar to a myxoma on angiography, but is usually associated with thrombus in the atrial appendage.

RIGHT ATRIAL MYXOMAS

Right atrial myxomas produce symptoms of right-sided heart failure including peripheral edema, fatigue, ascites, and abdominal discomfort due to obstruction of tricuspid valve flow or tricuspid regurgitation. Tricuspid regurgitation is due to actual valve trauma by the tumor or interference with normal tricuspid closure. Cyanosis, dizziness, and syncope may be related to body position. Tumor emboli to the pulmonary arteries may result in pulmonary hypertension. Physical examination reveals jugular venous distension with a prominent a wave in the jugular venous pulse, hepatomegaly, ascites, peripheral edema, and the murmurs of tricuspid stenosis and/or tricuspid regurgitation. Friction rubs, clubbing, cyanosis, and signs of superior vena caval obstruction may be present. These findings often mimic those of constrictive pericarditis, rheumatic tricuspid disease, Ebstein's anamoly, and right-sided endocarditis. Typical laboratory abnormalities include elevated sedimentation rate, leukocytosis, and hypergammaglobulinemia. If a right-to-left shunt has developed through a patent foramen ovale due to elevated right atrial pressure, polycythemia may occur. ECG abnormalities include large P waves, low voltage, and right bundle branch block; chest x-ray film may show right atrial enlargement and intracardiac tumor calcification. The right atrial tumor may be visualized by echocardiography and angiography; superior vena caval injection is suggested for angiography in order to avoid tumor dislodgement.

The treatment of both left and right atrial myxomas is surgical excision. Many surgeons prefer wide resection of the atrial septum surrounding the attachment of the tumor because recurrence is possible if resection is incomplete. This may necessitate repair of an atrial defect with a Dacron patch.

RHABDOMYOMAS

These tumors are found mainly in infants and children. They involve the ventricular walls, affecting right and left sides equally. Many investigators believe that rhabdomyomas are not true neoplasms but represent hamartomas. Children with rhabdomyomas may have symptoms related to obstruction of a cardiac chamber or valve orifice, may present as stillborn infants or die shortly after birth with severe intracavitary obstruction, or be asymptomatic. Rhabdomyomas commonly occur in association with tuberous sclerosis. Clinical features include symptoms and signs of left- and/or right-sided congestive heart failure, systolic and diastolic murmurs, syncope, cyanosis, and occasionally sudden death. Left axis deviation, left ventricular hypertrophy, and left bundle branch block may be present on electrocardiography. Treatment is surgical excision.

FIBROMAS

Fibromas are another benign tumor that most commonly affects infants and children and occurs within the ventricular myocardium. Fibromas may be asymptomatic or result in obstruction to intracardiac flow, abnormalities in ventricular contraction, or conduction disturbances. A whorled pattern of intracardiac calcification may be present on chest x-ray film.

LIPOMAS

Lipomas may be located within the subendocardium, subepicardium, or intramural myocardium. They may be asymptomatic or produce atrioventricular (AV) or intraventricular conduction abnormalities and arrhythmias or impair ventricular contraction.

MESOTHELIOMAS

Mesotheliomas occur predominantly in women and tend to be located in the area of the AV node. These slow-growing cystic tumors may result in complete heart block, syncope, and sudden death.

There are a number of benign pericardial tumors, including teratomas and leiomyomas, most of which are asymptomatic.

Malignant Primary Tumors of the Heart

Malignant tumors comprise approximately 25% of all primary tumors of the heart and in most cases are sarcomas. The most common of these include angiosarcoma, rhabdomyosarcoma, and fibrosarcoma. The development of these tumors is more common in adults and can involve either atrium or ventricle, but is more common on the right side of the heart. Clinical features include those of progressive right-sided and/or left-sided heart failure, arrhythmias, pericardial effusion, chest pain, and cardiac tamponade. These tumors may be rapidly growing, invading the myocardium, intracardiac chambers and pericardial space; and often they metastasize. They may obstruct either the superior vena cava, resulting in edema of the face and upper extremities, or the inferior vena cava, causing mesenteric, hepatic, and lower extremity edema. Most patients have a progressively downhill course and die within weeks to a few years once symptoms are present.

   In general, various forms of radiation therapy, chemotherapy, and surgery have failed to alter the poor prognosis of cardiac sarcomas.

Metastatic Tumors to the Heart

Metastatic tumors to the heart are more common than primary cardiac tumors. Cardiac metastases occur with many types of tumors (carcinomas more commonly than sarcomas). Malignant melanoma involves the heart in over 50% of cases and cardiac metastases occur in about 33% of cases of bronchogenic carcinoma and carcinoma of the breast. Microscopic cardiac infiltration is present in about half the cases of leukemia and about one-sixth the cases of lymphoma, especially reticulum cell sarcoma. Cardiac metastases occur most frequently in patients over the age of 50 with an equal sex incidence. Metastatic tumors to the heart have been described in up to 6% of unselected autopsies and 2–21% of patients dying with malignancy. Cardiac metastases, in general, are encountered with widespread systemic tumor dissemination—only rarely are metastases limited to the heart or pericardium. Metastatic tumors are thought to reach the heart by hematogenous or lymphatic spread or by direct invasion. Lymphatic spread is particularly frequent with carcinoma of the bronchus and breast. Intracavitary metastatic tumors are disseminated via the great veins. Thus, metastases from carcinoma of the kidney, testis, and thyroid invade the right atrium via the vena cava and may mimic myxoma; metastases from bronchogenic carcinoma may enter the left atrium via the pulmonary veins. Metastases to valvular tissue or the endocardium are unusual, since these structures are avascular. When they do occur, it is probably by direct extension. Endocardial and valve metastases may be polypoid and form emboli mimicking myxomas and endocarditis. They can result in valvular stenosis or regurgitation. Pericardial metastases occur more frequently than myocardial metastases and are common in patients with carcinoma of the breast or lung (by lymphatic spread) or mediastinal lymphoma (by direct extension). Pericardial effusions and tamponade or a constrictive pericarditis may occur. Finally, intramural metastases may be present in either left or right ventricles. Intramural metastases usually do not affect cardiac function in most cases.

Myocardial infarction has resulted from metastatic tumor encircling or compressing the epicardial coronary arteries.

Cardiac symptoms occur in less than 10% of patients with cardiac metastases proven by autopsy. The metastases usually are not a major factor contributing to the death of the patient. Symptoms depend more on the location than the size of the tumor; for example, metastases from a hypernephroma may infiltrate the AV node, resulting in complete heart block. Metastatic tumor to the heart should be suspected when a patient with metastatic disease develops cardiac dysfunction without apparent cause. Common signs and symptoms include those of pericarditis with chest pain, fever, a persistent pericardial rub, evidence of cardiac tamponade or pericardial constriction, rapid increase of heart size, development of heart block, arrhythmias, changing cardiac murmurs, evidence of obstruction to the great vein orifices, and intractable and unexplained cardiac failure. This latter feature may be due to lymphatic obstruction by the tumor, with severe myocardial interstitial edema and secondary pressure on the myofibers resulting in cardiac decompensation.

Electrocardiographic abnormalities are common and include ST-T wave changes, which sometimes mimic myocardial infarction (especially when the cardiac metastases produce necrosis), arrhythmias including supraventricular tachyarrhythmias (especially when the metastases involve the atria), AV block and bundle branch block (due to tumor infiltration of the conducting system), abnormal P waves, and reduced QRS amplitude in cases both with and without pericardial effusion. The arrhythmias often do not respond to digitalis or any other standard therapy. Two-dimensional echocardiography has been shown to be useful for assessing the presence of cardiac tumors. Rarely, malignant or metastatic cardiac tumors may be amenable to surgery. Paliative radiation therapy and systemic chemotherapy may afford symptomatic relief, but radiation to the chest may produce myocardial fibrosis and damage to the conduction system. Radiation has caused regression of pericardial effusion, but pericardiocentesis is required in cases of tamponade. The pericardial fluid may then be examined for cytology. Recurrent effusions resulting in tamponade or the presence of pericardial constriction may require pericardiectomy.

Bibliography

Berge T, Sievers J: Myocardial metastases: A pathological and electrocardiographic study. *Br Heart J* 30:383, 1968.

Bulkley BH, Hutchins GM: Atrial myxomas: A fifty year review. *Am Heart J* 97:639, 1979.

Castaneda AR, Vanco RL: Tumors of the heart: Surgical considerations. *Am J Cardiol* 21:357, 1968.

Cohen GU, Perry TM, Evans JM: Neoplastic invasion of the heart and pericardium. *Ann Intern Med* 42:1238, 1955.

Cohn RE, Stewart JR, Fajardo LF, et al: Heart disease following radiation. *Medicine* 46:281, 1967.

Colucci WS, Braunwald E: Primary tumors of the heart, in Braunwald E (ed): *Heart Disease: A Textbook of Cardiovascular Medicine*. Philadelphia, Saunders, 1980, p 1501.

Come PC, Kurland GS, Vine HS: Two dimensional echocardiography in differentiating right atrial and tricuspid valve mass lesions. *Am J Cardiol* 44:1207, 1979.

Come PC, Riley MF, Markis JE, et al: Limitations of echocardiographic techniques in evaluation of left atrial masses. *Am J Cardiol* 48:947, 1981.

Donaldson RM, Emanuel RW, Earl CJ: The role of two-dimensional echocardiography in the detection of potentially embolic intracardiac masses in patients with cerebral ischemia. *J Neurol Neurosurg Psychiatry* 44:803, 1981.

Farah MG: Familial atrial myxoma. *Ann Intern Med* 83:358, 1975.

Freiman AH: Cardiovascular disturbances associated with cancer. *Med Clin North Am* 50:733, 1966.

Glancy DL, Roberts WC: The heart in malignant melanoma: A study of 70 autopsy cases. *Am J Cardiol* 21:555, 1968.

Godwin JD, Axel L, Adams JR, et al: Computed tomography: A new method for diagnosing tumor of the heart. *Circulation* 63:448, 1981.

Goodwin JF: Symposium on cardiac tumors. Introduction: The spectrum of cardiac tumors. *Am J Cardiol* 21:328, 1968.

Greenwood WF: Profile of atrial myxoma. *Am J Cardiol* 21:367, 1968.

Hanfling SM: Metastatic cancer to the heart: Review of the literature and report of 127 cases. Circulation 22:474, 1960.

Harris TR, Copeland GD, Brody DA: Progressive injury current with metastatic tumor of the heart: Case report and review of the literature. *Am Heart J* 65:392, 1965.

Harvey WP: Clinical aspects of cardiac tumors. *Am J Cardiol* 21:328, 1968.

Heath D, MacKinnon J: Pulmonary hypertension due to myxoma of the right atrium. With special reference to the behavior of emboli of myoxoma in the lung. *Am Heart J* 68:227, 1964.

Huggins TJ, Huggins MJ, Schnapf DJ, et al: Left atrial myxoma: Computed tomography as a diagnostic modality. *J Comput Assist Tomogr* 4:253, 1980.

James TN: Metastasis in hypernephroma to atrioventricular node: Report of a case. *N Eng J Med* 266:705, 1962.

Lappe DL, Bulkley BH, Weiss JL: Two dimensional echocardiographic diagnosis of left atrial myxoma. *Chest* 74:55, 1978.

Larrieu AJ, Jamieson WR, Tyers GF: Primary cardiac tumors: Experience with 25 cases. *J. Thorac Cardiovasc Surg* 83:339, 1982.

Lubell DL, Goldfarb CR: Metastatic cardiac tumor demonstrated by 201 thallium scan. *Chest* 78:98, 1980.

MacGregor GA, Cullen RA: The syndrome of fever, anaemia, and high sedimentation rate with an atrial myxoma. *Brit Med J* 5:158, 1959.

McAllister HA Jr: Primary tumors and cysts of the heart and pericardium, in Harvey WP (ed): *Current Problems in Cardiology*. 1979, vol 4, p 1.

Peterson CD, Robinson WA, Kurnick JE: Involvement of the heart and pericardium in the malignant lymphomas. *Am J Med Sci* 272:161, 1976.

Pohost GM, Pastore JO, McKusick KA, et al: Detection of left atrial myxoma by gated radionuclide cardiac imaging. *Circulation* 55:88, 1977.

Quaife MA, Boschult P, Baltaxe HA, et al: Myocardial accumulation of labeled phosphate in malignant pericardial effusion. *J Nucl Med* 20:392, 1979.

Roberts WC, Glancy DL, DeVita VT Jr: Heart in malignant lymphoma (Hodgkin's disease, lymphosarcoma, reticulum cell sarcoma, and mycosis fungoides): A study of 196 autopsy cases. *Am J Cardiol* 22:85, 1968.

Roberts WC, Bodey GP, Wentlake PT: The heart in acute leukemia: A study of 420 autopsy cases. *Am J Cardiol* 21:388, 1968.

Seibert KA, Rettenmier CW, Waller BF, et al: Osteogenic sarcoma metastatic to the heart. *Am J Med* 73:136, 1982.

Selzer A, Sakai FJ, Popper RW: Protean clinical manifestations of primary tumors of the heart. *Am J Med* 59:9, 1972.

St. John Sutton MG, Mercier LA, Giuliani ER, et al: Atrial myxomas: A review of clinical experience in 40 patients. *Mayo Clin Proc* 55:371, 1980.

Tway KP, Shah AA, Rahimtoola SH: Multiple bilateral myxomas demonstrated by two-dimensional echocardiography. *Am J Med* 71:896, 1981.

Wolfe SB, Popp R, Feigenbaum H: Diagnosis of atrial tumors by ultrasound. *Circulation* 39:615, 1969.

Wolverson MK, Grider RD, Sundaram M, et al: Demonstration of unsuspected malignant disease of the pericardium by computed tomography. CT 4:330, 1980.

Zaret BL, Hurley PJ, Pitt B: Noninvasive scintiphotographic diagnosis of left atrial myxoma. *J Nucl Med* 13:81, 1972.

CHAPTER **23** | EVALUATION AND MANAGEMENT OF HYPERTENSION

Victor J. Dzau

Definition of Hypertension

Systemic arterial pressure fluctuates throughout the day in response to stimuli of stress and physical activity. Blood pressure also tends to increase with age. There is no evidence for a threshold level beyond which cardiovascular risks increase precipitously. Hence, the definition of hypertension is, at best, arbitrary and is based on population distribution analysis. The World Health Organization has recommended the following criteria for epidemiologic studies:

1. Normotension: systolic <140 and diastolic <90 mm Hg
2. Hypertension: systolic >160 and/or diastolic >95 mm Hg
3. Borderline: any reading between the groups above

There is now a general consensus that these criteria may be set too high. The recent studies of the Veterans Administration Hospital and Hypertension Detection and Follow-up Program suggest that vigorous treatment of even the intermediate group (diastolic 90–105 mm Hg) will also reduce mortality.

Physiology

The major determinants of blood pressure are cardiac output and systemic vascular resistance. These factors are controlled by various neurohormonal systems and the kidney. The autonomic nervous system and the renin-angiotensin system are involved with short-term regulation of blood pressure in normal human. The kidney exerts a long-term control on blood pressure by the regulation of sodium and extracellular fluid volume.

The renin-angiotensin system will be discussed in more detail, since recent concepts of blood pressure analysis using plasma renin activity and the development of specific pharmacologic inhibitors are important advances in the area of hypertension.

Renin is a proteolytic enzyme released by the juxtaglomerular cells in the afferent arterioles of the kidney. Renin cleaves its substrate in plasma, angiotensinogen, an α_2-globulin synthesized by the liver. Angiotensin I, a decapeptide, a product of renin and angiotensinogen reaction, is physiologically inactive. Angiotensin I is cleaved by pulmonary and plasma-converting enzymes to the octapeptide, angiotensin II

447

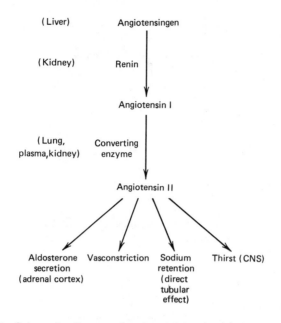

Figure 1 Schematic diagram of renin-angiotensin-aldosterone system.

(AII), which is a potent vasoconstrictor and primary stimulus for aldosterone secretion from the adrenal cortex (Fig. 1).

The release of renin from the kidney into the plasma is determined by (1) renal perfusion pressure; (2) sodium content in the distal tubule; (3) autonomic nervous system; and (4) humoral factors. Thus, systemic and renal hypotension, hypokalemia, hyponatremia, increased sympathetic nervous activity, and circulating catecholamines stimulate renin secretion.

Renin release is the rate-limiting step in angiotensin II production and is subjected to feedback control. An increase in plasma angiotensin II concentration results in decreased renin secretion by (1) increased sodium retention and extracellular fluid (ECF) volume expansion, secondary to aldosterone and direct tubular effect of AII; (2) a direct negative feedback of AII on the juxtaglomerular cells; (3) increased blood pressure; and (4) changes in sodium concentration on the macula densa.

Evaluation of the Hypertensive Patient

Evaluation of the hypertensive patient should include a careful history and physical examination, as well as screening laboratory tests (Table 1) with the following goals:

1. Proper documentation of hypertension
2. Assessment of cardiovascular risk factors
3. Search for evidence of end-organ damage
4. Decision regarding when to perform a work-up for secondary hypertension

Table 1.   Clinical Evaluation of the Hypertensive Patient

History

    Age, sex, duration of hypertension, response to therapy

    Symptoms of headaches, TIA, CVA, CHF, angina, PVD

    Symptoms of episodic headaches, palpitations, perspiration (pheochromocytoma), muscular weakness, cramps and polyuria (primary aldosteronism), headache and lower extremity claudication (coarctation of aorta)

    Family history of hypertension. History of smoking, diet, exercise and other risk factors (diabetes, gout, etc.)

    Medication: birth control pill, amphetamines (diet and cold capsules, nasal sprays) cocaine abuse, large quantities of licorice, adrenal steroid, thyroid hormones.

Physical

    Vital signs including postural BP; arm and leg BP; weight
    Fundi exam for retinopathy

    Cardiac and chest exam for heart size, sounds

    Abdominal exam for masses, bruit

    Peripheral vascular exam

    Neurologic exam

    Check for evidence of gout, hyperlipidemia, thyroid, Cushing's syndrome; signs of neurofibromatosis, cafe au lait spots, etc.

Laboratory (initial)

    Serum K+, creatinine or BUN, FBS, cholesterol, EKG, urinalysis

    Additional: CBC, uric acid, Na+

Key: TIA, transient ischemic attack; CVA, cerebrovascular accident; CHF, congestive heart disease; PVD, peripheral vascular disease; FBS, fasting blood sugar.

The following guidelines should be followed in blood pressure documentation:

1. Appropriate techniques for the measurement of blood pressure is important. It is properly measured in both arms with the patient seated comfortably. An appropriate sized cuff should be placed at the level of the heart. To avoid falsely elevated readings, the cuff width should be greater than $\frac{2}{3}$ of the arm width. Diastolic pressure is measured at Korotkoff's fifth sound (the point at which the sound disappears rather than when it muffles). The patient should sit quietly for five minutes before the blood pressure is taken.

2. Multiple readings should be taken during the visit. The mean of two or three readings taken at one sitting should be used. For patients with borderline readings, three readings separated by one to two minutes on three different days should be used for clear documentation.

3. In addition, during each visit the blood pressures should also be measured with the patient supine, sitting, and standing at least once.

CARDIOVASCULAR RISK FACTORS

Assessment of cardiovascular risk profile is an important aspect of the evaluation of hypertensive patients. The presence or absence of these factors is taken into account in deciding when and how aggressively hypertension should be treated. Furthermore, control of these risk factors can substantially reduce cardiovascular mortality and morbidity. According to the Framingham study (1975), the factors that significantly influence prognosis are:

1. Blood pressure
2. Smoking
3. Serum cholesterol level
4. Glucose intolerance
5. Left ventricular hypertrophy

The incidence of cardiovascular complications increases in the presence of each of these risk factors. The risk of hypertension is related to the height of both systolic and diastolic pressures. Furthermore, hypertension acts in concert with other risk factors, increasing mortality and morbidity in a synergistic fashion, rather than as a simple additive effect.

END-ORGAN DAMAGE: THE COMPLICATIONS OF HYPERTENSION

Patients with prolonged hypertension develop complications of the disease manifested by evidence of anatomic changes within organs (end-organ disease). Evidence of end-organ disease should be sought by both physical examination and certain screening laboratory tests. The fundoscopic examination may reveal signs of arteriolar damage (see below).

A palpable left ventricular heave suggests left ventricular hypertropy. With severe hypertensive cardiovascular disease, signs of frank congestive heart failure may be present. Since hypertension accelerates atherosclerosis, signs of cerebrovascular thrombosis and/or hemorrhage, ischemic heart disease, and impaired renal function due to sclerosis of the arterioles should be sought.

The major purpose of therapy (discussed in a separate section) is to reduce the incidence of end-organ damage. Natural history studies have shown that of patients who do not receive treatment nearly 50% die of heart disease, 33% of stroke, and 10–15% of renal disease.

HYPERTENSIVE RETINOPATHY

The fundoscopic examination provides useful information regarding the severity of vascular damage in hypertensive patients. Keith and Wagner (1939) demonstrated that different grades of hypertensive retinopathy carried different prognosis. Grade I: tortuosity, minimal constriction; grade II: increased arteriole light reflex (copper wiring), AV knicking; grade III: cotton wool exudates and hemorrhages; grade IV: papilledema. The hypertensive patient with severe arterial changes but no hemorrhages or exudates has a life expectancy of about five years without therapy. Patients with untreated malignant hypertension and papilledema live, on the average, only six months. These prognostic statements should be tempered by reports that (1) isolated crossing changes are insignificant; (2) focal narrowings are predictive of mortality from all causes; and (3) arteriolar narrowing and focal narrowing correlate best with blood pressure levels.

SCREENING LABORATORY TESTS

Screening laboratory tests should be performed with the costs of the tests and the yield of useful information in mind. Laboratory evaluation should be directed for the following aims:

1. For cardiovascular risk profiling
2. To assess end-organ function
3. To screen for secondary hypertension

Table 2 summarizes a list of essential laboratory tests and their respective costs. Fasting blood sugar, serum cholesterol, and serum uric acid identify patients with diabetes, hypercholesterolemia, and hyperuricemic risk factors. Serum creatinine, urinalysis, and ECG assess the renal and cardiac status of these patients (end-organ function). Serum potassium concentration, particularly without concomitant diuretic ingestion, is a useful screening test for the existence of hyperaldosteronism (etiology). Complete blood count and chest x-ray are optional tests in the initial evaluation of these patients. The above laboratory tests coupled with a thorough history and physical examination should provide sufficient information for the care and workup of a hypertensive patient.

Table 2. Baseline Laboratory Tests for Evaluation of Hypertension

Tests	Information
Complete blood count	Baseline (stress erythrocytosis)
Serum potassium concentration	Pretreatment baseline (diuretic therapy) Screening for primary or secondary aldosteronism (etiology)
Serum creatinine	End-organ function (complication) Renal hypertension (etiology)
Fasting blood sugar	Risk factor
Serum cholesterol	Risk factor
Serum uric acid	Baseline (diuretic therapy) Indicator of nephrosclerosis (complication)
Electrocardiogram	Risk factor
Urinalysis	Renal hypertension (etiology) End-organ function (complications)

SOURCE: Modified from Slater EE & Haber E. Hypertension, in *The Practice of Cardiology.* Ed. R.A. Johnson, E. Haber and W.G. Austen. 1980. Little, Brown and Co., Boston, MA.

Table 3. Causes of Hypertension

Primary (essential) Hypertension
Secondary Hypertension
  Renovascular hypertension
    Fibromuscular disease
    Atherosclerotic disease
  Primary aldosteronism
    Bilateral adrenal cortical hyperplasia
    Adrenal cortical adenoma
    Adrenal cortical carcinoma
  Cushing's syndrome
    Hypothalamic-pituitary dysfunction
    ACTH producing tumor
    Adrenal neoplasia
  Pheochromocytoma
    Benign vs malignant
    Single vs multiple
    Adrenal vs extra-adrenal
  Other endocrine hypertension
    Mineralocorticoid excess
    Hyperthyroidism
    Hyperparathyroidism
    Growth hormone excess
  Oral contraceptive
  Renal disease
    Acute glomerulonephritis
    Chronic renal failure
    Chronic pyelonephritis
    Hydronephrosis
    Nephrectomy
  Coarctation of aorta

Etiology

Approximately 90% of patients with hypertension have primary or essential hypertension in unselected populations. The remaining have secondary forms of hypertension. These are listed in Table 3.

Secondary Forms of Hypertension

Routine screening of secondary forms of hypertension is not recommended. Factors that should influence the decision to evaluate for secondary hypertension are:

1. Onset of hypertension at a young age (<35).
2. In patients with evidence of diffuse arteriosclerotic disease, multiple high risk factors, and severe disease.

3. Clinical suspicion of secondary disease based on history or physical findings, such as rapid onset with negative family history, symptoms suggestive of pheochromocytoma or hyperaldosteronism, physical stigmata of Cushing's disease, arm and leg pressure discrepancy, presence of abdominal bruit, or hypokalemia on laboratory screening.
4. Those with poor response to vigorous therapy.

The screening tests for specific forms of hypertension are outlined in Table 4. Further work-up of these forms will be discussed below.

Renovascular Hypertension

Renovascular hypertension accounts for about 2% of adults with hypertension. Renal artery stenosis occurs, usually, as a result of atherosclerosis or fibromuscular disease. The former is seen in older patients, usually with evidence of diffuse arteriosclerotic disease. The latter occurs in young patients, predominantly women. The hypertension is usually of recent onset. The family history is often negative; the presence of an abdominal bruit occurs in 50–60% of patients with renovascular hypertension. Hypokalemia is seen in 20% of patients reflecting secondary hyperaldosteronism.

Random plasma renin activity is of little value. Only 50–60% of patients with renovascular hypertension have elevated peripheral plasma activity. There is substantial overlap in basal plasma renin activity (PRA) levels between patients with essential hypertension and those with renal artery stenosis. The stimulated PRA has been used as a screening test by several investigators. This is performed by sodium restriction (10 mEq sodium diet for three days) plus 2–4 hours of upright posture, or the simpler intravenous furosemide test (40 mg IV followed by $\frac{1}{2}$ hour upright posture on an unrestricted diet). PRA of greater than 10 ng/ml/h is suggestive of surgically correctable renovascular hypertension. Unfortunately, a high incidence of false positive results is seen with this test.

The best screening procedure for renovascular hypertension is the hypertensive IVP. Using three major criteria for features suggestive of renal ischemia (i.e., >1.5 cm difference in renal size, delayed appearance of dye, late hyperconcentration),

Table 4. Screening Tests for Specific Forms of Hypertension

Diagnosis	Screening Test
Renovascular hypertension	Hypertensive IVP
Primary aldosteronism	Stimulated PRA 24 hour urine potassium excretion
Cushing's syndrome	Overnight dexamethasone suppression
Pheochromocytoma	24 hour urine metanephrine, VMA, and catecholamines
Renal hypertension	Urinalysis, BUN, creatinine, IVP, ultrasound, urine culture
Coarctation of aorta	Chest x-ray
Hyperparathyroidism	Serum calcium and phosphorus levels
Hyperthyroidism	Serum T4 and thyroglobulin levels

this procedure provides about 10–15% false positive and false negative results. Thus, a negative IVP offers a high degree of assurance that renovascular hypertension is not present. The risk of the procedure is low except in elderly diabetics, patients with impaired renal function, and patients with multiple myeloma.

The blood pressure response to the inhibitors of the renin-angiotensin system such as saralasin (angiotensin antagonist) and the teprotide (converting enzyme inhibitor) have also been used as screening tests for the diagnosis of renovascular hypertension. A mild state of volume contraction is first achieved with a 10 mEq sodium diet for three days or with a single intravenous dose of furosemide (40 mg). Saralasin or teprotide is then given to the patient. A hypotensive response (supine diastolic pressure decrease of greater than 10–20 mm of mercury) accurately identifies patients with proven renovascular hypertension in greater than 90% of cases. At present, however, these tests, which show great promise, are not easy to perform in an uncontrolled office setting.

Isotopic renography is sometimes used in substitution for IVP. The test appears to be slightly less accurate and less sensitive than an IVP. However, the renal scan is a safe procedure and is the preferred screening test for elderly patients with diabetes and/or renal insufficiency, or for patients with history of a dye reaction.

Recently, digital subtraction angiography (DSA) has been introduced for screening patients with suspected renovascular hypertension. DSA provides an image of specified renal vasculature and abdominal aorta. This can be performed in a relatively noninvasive manner in the outpatient setting. In preliminary experience, satisfactory diagnostic information can be obtained in over 75% of patients referred for suspected renovascular hypertension. This is a particularly useful technique in screening young patients with suspected fibromuscular disease. The risks of DSA are similar to those of IVP.

Since renovascular hypertension accounts for a small percentage of total population of hypertension, a negative result from any one of the screening tests generally indicates that no further work-up is necessary, unless clinical findings strongly suggest the presence of renovascular hypertension. The best diagnostic test is renal arteriography.

Renal Vein Renin Ratio
Renal vein renin is a safe procedure, involving simultaneous sampling of venous blood from each renal vein and its major branches. In addition, inferior vena caval blood above and below the renal veins and a peripheral PRA are also measured. Survey of all published data to date reveals that 93% of patients with a lateralizing renal vein renin ratio that is greater than 1.5–2.1 between the abnormal and the contralateral side are cured or improved by operation. On the other hand, only 60% of patients with renovascular hypertension, but nonlateralizing renal vein renin, are cured or improved with surgery. The causes of nonlateralizing renal vein renin include bilateral renal artery stenosis, volume expansion, nonsimultaneous sampling of renal vein blood, assay error, or nonsignificant renal artery lesion. To further increase the sensitivity of the procedure, drugs that inhibit the secretion of renin (such as beta-adrenergic antagonist, reserpine, clonidine, methyldopa) should be stopped three to five days prior to the study. Renin secretion can be further stimulated by a low-salt diet, the administration of intravenous furosemide, hydralazine,

or converting enzyme inhibitor, which can accentuate the differences between the two sides.

Renal Arteriography

Renal arteriography is performed to prove the diagnosis and characterize the anatomy for consideration of surgery or other therapeutic procedures. The information that one looks for in renal arteriography includes:

1. The presence of unilateral, bilateral, or multiple stenotic lesions.
2. Location of these lesions (e.g., close to the origin of the renal artery versus just before the bifurcation of the branches versus in segmental branches).
3. Etiology of the renovascular hypertension, such as atherosclerotic; renal fibromuscular dysplasia; intimal fibroplasia or periarterial fibroplasia; or extrinsic lesions resulting in compression of the renal vasculature.
4. Size of the affected kidney and the contralateral kidney.
5. Presence of collateral vascularity in the affected kidney.
6. Extent of arteriosclerosis in the abdominal aorta.

The information above provides data for the physician in deciding the type of surgical procedure, if indicated, and prognosticating the outcome of the intervention.

Management of renovascular hypertension can involve surgery, medical therapy, or the use of percutaneous transluminal angioplasty. The choice of therapy should be tailored to each patient and will be discussed later (Fig. 2). Surgical procedures

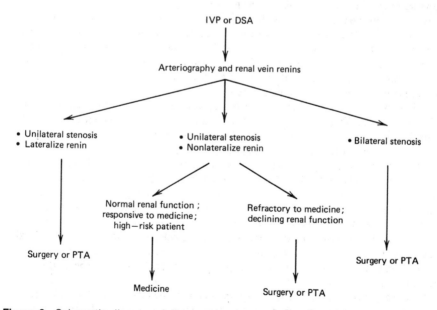

Figure 2 Schematic diagram of diagnosis and management for patients with renovascular hypertension. IVP, hypertensive intravenous pyelography; DSA, digital subtraction angiography; PTA, percutaneous transluminal angioplasty.

include end-arterectomy, aortorenal anastamosis or bypass, splenorenal or mesenterorenal anastamosis, or nephectomy. The choice depends on the location and extent of renal artery disease, state of the abdominal aorta and the function of the ischemic kidney. The outcome of surgical intervention depends on the underlying pathologic process and the pathophysiologic state of the patient. Revascularization produces very good results in patients with fibromuscular disease (85% cured or improved) but less good for those with arteriosclerotic disease (67% cured or improved). In general, the presence of a proximal unilateral lesion in an unshrunken kidney to which the renal vein renin is lateralized carries a very good prognosis for revascularization.

Propranolol (inhibits renin secretion) and captopril (blocks angiotensin II production) are effective medical agents for the control of hypertension in these patients.

Since some patients with renovascular hypertension are exquisitely sensitive to captopril, the author routinely begins with a dose of 12.5 or 25 mg tid and carefully increases the dose by titrating it to the blood pressure response. It is important to note that the acute depressor response in these patients is directly related to the pretreatment plasma renin activity, but the long-term response to captopril is not. Patients with volume-dependent hypertension may not respond to captopril monotherapy. In general, most patients are well managed by the combination of captopril and diuretic. In more severe cases, the addition of propranolol has proven to be effective in controlling blood pressure.

The administration of captopril should be done with care in patients with renovascular hypertension. Several investigators have reported secondary elevations in plasma creatinine after captopril therapy. In fact, a few cases of acute renal failure have been observed. Patients with marked sodium depletion, bilateral renal artery stenosis, or unilateral stenosis with contralateral dysfunction (due to nephrosclerosis) are particularly at risk. Therefore, patients undergoing captopril therapy should be monitored for sudden declines in renal function. In addition, the development of other drug toxicity manifestations such as rash, loss of taste, proteinuria, or leukopenia should be rountinely monitored.

It is important to remember that medical management does not treat the primary disease process. Thus, progression of the renal artery disease should be monitored closely by periodic determinations of blood pressure; renal function, by serum creatinine; size, by ultrasound; and vascular anatomy, by DSA.

Recently, the use of percutaneous transluminal angioplasty (PTA) of stenotic lesions of the renal arteries has shown great promise in the treatment of renovascular hypertension, particularly fibromuscular disease. The results of PTA are similar to those of surgery, insofar as cure rates are dependent on patient selection. The cure rate results of PTA are better in patients with fibromuscular disease compared to atherosclerotic disease and in those with lateralizing renal vein renin. It has also been noted that cure rates are improved if the diseased segment is confined to the renal artery beyond its ostium as compared to lesions involving the aorta and/or renal ostium.

Early reports encourage cautious optimism about the future use of PTA in treating renovascular hypertension. In cases of fibromuscular disease, early reports of high initial cure rates and low recurrence rates suggest that PTA may become the procedure of first choice in this disease. Despite the discouraging results of the study of Grim et al., PTA may still emerge as the treatment of first choice in high risk patients. PTA may also prove to be useful in treating patients with bilateral or multiple lesions to minimize the amount of surgical repair. It should be pointed out that a therapeutic trial of PTA does not preclude other options and can be followed by repeated dilatations or definitive surgery.

PTA should probably not be viewed as a competitive treatment modality to medicine or surgery, but rather as an adjunct whose intermediate role is as yet undefined.

Figure 2 summarizes the author's present approach to the evaluation and management of renovascular hypertension.

Fibromuscular Disease

In the past, surgery has generally been recommended for patients with this disease. If available, a trial of PTA is warranted with close follow-up monitoring of: blood pressure, renal function, status of the lesion by DSA; and renal size by ultrasound. In our opinion, PTA is the procedure of choice for the very young patient with multiple lesions, since the probability of recurrence elsewhere after surgery is high.

Atherosclerotic Disease

Patients with unilateral atherosclerotic stenosis with no associated surgical risks can be treated by either drugs, PTA, or surgery. In view of the associated problems of drug therapy (cost, compliance, inconvenience, side effects, and progression of disease), the author favors surgery or a single trial of PTA prior to surgery. In patients with diffuse atherosclerosis (particularly involving the abdominal aorta) and with associated coronary, cerebrovascular, or pulmonary disease, the author prefers a trial of PTA. Revascularization by PTA may be particularly beneficial in high surgical risk patients with compromised renal function. If necessary, PTA can be repeated once or twice in these patients.

Alternatively, high risk patients with normal renal function can be managed with drugs. However, they should be monitored closely for progression of disease, evidence of renal failure or its sequelae. In general, surgery is usually reserved as a later option in these patients.

Primary Aldosteronism

Primary aldosteronism arises from an autonomous hypersecretion of the mineralocorticoid, aldosterone, from an adrenal adenoma (Conn's syndrome), or from bilateral adrenal hyperplasia. Adrenal adenoma is the more frequent cause of this syndrome. An excess circulating aldosterone level results in increased renal sodium retention and, usually, potassium excretion. Thus, the syndrome is characterized by hypertension, marked expansion of extracellular fluid volume, and hypokalemia. The symptoms of primary aldosteronism are primarily the manifestations of hypertension and hypokalemia. Muscle cramps, weakness, glucose intolerance, cardiac arrhythmias, and loss of urinary concentrating ability, with polyuria, are some of the manifestations associated with this syndrome.

Patients with diastolic hypertension and hypokalemia (serum potassium <3.5 mEq/ L) without a history of diuretic, excess licorice intake, diarrhea, or vomiting should be evaluated for the diagnosis of primary aldosteronism. In addition, the diagnosis should be entertained in any hypertensive patient on diuretic therapy who continues to have persistent and severe hypokalemia despite large doses of potassium supple-

Table 5. Evaluation of the Patient Suspected of Primary Aldosteronism

Tests	Positive Results
1. Hypertension and hypokalemia	K < 3.5[a]
2. Stop diuretic therapy and give K supplement 1–2 weeks	↓ K persists
3. 24 hour urine potassium excretion	>30 mEq/24 hr
4. Stimulated plasma renin activity	Suppressed
5. Plasma aldosterone concentration	Elevated
6. Saline infusion	Plasma aldosterone not suppressed
7. Abdominal CT scan	Bilateral adrenal hyperplasia or cortical adenoma

[a] up to 10% may have K+ 3.5–3.9 mEq/L

mentation. In these patients, diuretic therapy should be stopped and KCl supplement continued for one to two weeks and serum potassium remeasured. Persistent hypokalemia should be a clue for further evaluation. It should be noted that about 10% of patients with primary aldosteronism have a serum potassium of 3.5–3.9 mEq/L. The work-up for the diagnosis of primary aldosteronism is outlined in Table 5. The screening tests include a 24 hour urine potassium excretion and a determination of the stimulated plasma renin activity (PRA). A 24 hour urinary excretion of potassium of greater than 30 mEq documents potassium loss via the renal route. PRA is suppressed in patients with primary aldosteronism due to the markedly expanded extracellular fluid (ECF) volume. Furthermore, PRA remains suppressed despite dietary sodium restriction or furosemide administration and upright posture. In contrast, patients with secondary aldosteronism have elevated PRA, whereas patients with low renin essential hypertension have low plasma aldosterone and usually do not have hypokalemia. Plasma aldosterone concentration is almost invariably elevated in patients with primary aldosteronism. However, aldosterone secretion is also affected by ACTH and serum potassium. Thus, a random plasma aldosterone level is of little diagnostic value. The diagnosis of autonomous hypersecretion of aldosterone is made by the saline loading test. The standard procedure is to obtain a supine basal level of plasma aldosterone followed by an infusion of two liters of normal saline over a four hour interval. Inability to suppress aldosterone excess by volume expansion is diagnostic of this syndrome. Distinction between adenoma and hyperplasia can be made by the abdominal computerized tomography (CT) scan if the tumor is greater than 1 cm in diameter. However, most adrenal tumors are smaller than 1 cm in diameter and are frequently missed by CT scan. Hence, adrenal venography and venous sampling are necessary for accurate localization, in most cases. Furthermore, work-up and management should be performed in consultation with an endocrinologist.

Cushing's Syndrome

Cushing's syndrome is produced by an excess of glucocorticoid secretion by adrenal adenoma, carcinoma, or bilateral hyperplasia. The latter is often the result of an

ACTH secreting pituitary adenoma or extra-pituitary neoplasm (e.g., lung carcinoma). Hypertension is seen in patients with Cushing's syndrome. The pathogenesis of this hypertension is unclear. Glucocorticoid increases hepatic angiotensinogen production and may, in part, increase plasma angiotensin production. Furthermore, there is also evidence of increased vascular sensitivity to vasoconstrictor hormones in these patients. The salt-retaining effect of high glucocorticoid levels may also contribute to the development of hypertension. Only patients who have clinical stigmata of Cushing's syndrome, such as truncal obesity, buffalo hump, moon facies, and violaceous striae should be evaluated for this form of hypertension. A 24 hour urine cortisol excretion is a useful screening test. The dexamethasone suppression test is a more simple alternative. This is performed by the administration of 1 mg of dexamethasone at midnight and plasma cortisol is measured at 8 AM the next morning. Failure of suppression of cortisol level (greater than 5 μg/dl) warrants further investigation (Table 6). The next step is the more prolonged dexamethasone suppression test, which involves the administration of dexamethasone 0.5 mg every six hours for two days, followed by 2 mg every six hours for two additional days. Urinary 17-hydroxycorticoids excretion should be measured on the second day of each dose. Patients with Cushing's syndrome will fail to suppress urinary 17-hydroxycorticoids to below 3 mg per day on the 0.5 mg every six hours regimen. If Cushing's syndrome is caused by an excess pituitary ACTH drive with bilateral adrenal hyperplasia, the urinary 17-hydroxycorticoids will be suppressed to below 50% of the control value on the second day of the 2 mg every six hours regimen. In those patients whose urinary corticoid excretion is not suppressed, ACTH level

Table 6. Evaluation of the Patient Suspected of Cushing's Syndome

Test	Results	Conditions
1. Overnight dexamethasone suppression: 1 mg midnight, 8 AM plasma cortisol	>5 μg/dl	(Suspect Cushing's syndrome)
2. Standard dexamethasone test		
(a) 0.5 mg q6h × 2 days (day 1–2)	≤3mg	(Normal response)
24 hr urine 170H coritcoid day 2	≥3 mg	(Cushing's syndrome)
(b) 2 mg q6h × 2 days (day 3–4)	<50% control	(pituitary ACTH excess)
24 hr urine 170H coritcoid day 4	>50% control	(adrenal neoplasia, or nonendocrine ACTH tumor)
3. Metyrapone (750 mg q4h × 14 doses) 24 hr urine 170H corticoid	>2 × increase	(pituitary-hypothalamic dysfunction)
4. Plasma ACTH	<50 pg/ml	(adrenal neoplasia)
	>80 pg/ml	(non-endocrine ACTH tumor or pituitary ACTH excess)
5. 24 hr urine 17-ketosteroid	>30 mg	(adrenal carcinoma)
6. Miscellaneous Skull x-ray, chest x-ray, abdominal or brain CT scan		

should be measured to differentiate between adrenal neoplasm and adrenal hyperplasia secondary to ACTH producing tumor. Patients with adrenal neoplasm have normal to low ACTH levels that are less than 50 pg/ml. The distinction between adrenal adenoma or carcinoma can be made on the basis of 24 hour urinary 17-ketosteroid production. Adrenal carcinoma is associated with high urinary 17-ketosteroid excretion (greater than 30 mg per 24 hours). Metyrapone testing is also useful in differentiating adrenal tumors from adrenal hyperplasia. Patients with adrenal tumors fail to respond to metyrapone challenge with a rise in urinary 17-hydroxycorticoids. Evaluation of the pituitary by the appropriate roentgenographic and computerized tomographic scanning procedures as well as a search for nonendocrine ACTH producing tumors are sometimes indicated. In summary, in the presence of clinical stigmata of Cushing's syndrome, the overnight dexamethasone suppression test should reliably detect and confirm the diagnosis of Cushing's syndrome. Further work-up and management should probably be performed in consultation with an endocrinologist.

Pheochromocytoma

Ninety percent of pheochromocytoma arise in the adrenal medulla; 10% of these are bilateral and 10% are malignant. Excess catecholamine secretion by chromaffin cell tumors produces hypertension, headache, sweatiness, palpitations, nausea, and vomiting. The symptoms of pheochromocytoma can be sustained or intermittent. Laboratory evaluation may reveal elevated blood sugar, an increase in hematocrit, an elevated white blood cell count with a shift to the left, and cardiac arrhythmias. The most reliable screening test is a timed (e.g., 24 hour) urinary metanephrine. The urinary excretions for total metanephrines, vanillylmandelic acid (VMA), and free catecholamines in normal adults are <1.2, <6.5 and <0.1 mg per day, and in patients with pheochromocytoma are $1.0–100$, $5.0–600$ and $0.1–10$, respectively. In a study performed at the Mayo Clinic, urinary total metanephrines gave the lowest number of false negatives (4%) when compared with VMA (30%) and urinary catecholamines (20%). Basal plasma catecholamines yield a large number of false positives and negatives. Kaplan et al. suggested that a single void urine specimen can be useful for the determination of urinary excretion of metanephrine if a simultaneous urinary creatinine level is determined. Thus, the urinary concentration of metanephrine, when related to that of creatinine, appears to have a close correlation with the 24 hour secretion. Timed urine collection during a symptomatic episode is particularly useful in patients with the episodic secreting type of pheochromocytoma. Many substances and drugs—for example, sympathomimetic and sympatholytic agents—interfere with the assay for catecholamine and its metabolites, but few interfere with the determination of metanephrines (Table 7). A very high plasma catecholamine level in the setting of high 24 hour urine catecholamines confirms the diagnosis of pheochromocytoma. The clonidine suppression test is useful in distinguishing patients with pheochromocytoma from those with essential hypertension and high plasma catecholamines. This is performed by a single oral dose of 0.3 mg clonidine accompanied by sampling of peripheral venous plasma norepinephrine levels before and 180 minutes after clonidine. Plasma norepinephrine is suppressed by clonidine in patients with essential hypertension, but is unaffected in patients with pheochromocytoma. The glucagon stimulation test is not routinely recommended, and it is only

Table 7. Substances Interfering with Assays for Catecholamines/Metabolites

Free catecholamines
Increase: methyldopa, L-dopa, tetracyclines, quinidine, isoproterenol, theophylline
Metanephrines
Increase: chlorpromazine, MAO inhibitors
Decrease: x-ray contrast media containing methylglucamine (e.g., Renografin, Renovist, Hypaque)
Vanillylmandelic acid (VMA)
Increase: nalidixic acid, anileridine, nitroglycerin (slight)
Decrease: monoamine oxidase inhibitors, clofibrate

SOURCE: Reproduced with permission from Ram, C.V.S., and Engelman, K.: Pheochromocytoma: Recognition and Management, in Harvey, W.P., et al. (eds): *CURRENT PROBLEMS IN CARDIOLOGY.* Copyright 1979 by Year Book Medical Publishers, Inc., Chicago.

reserved for diagnosing selected patients suspected of pheochromocytoma but having mildly elevated plasma or urinary catecholamines. This test must be performed with extreme caution.

Localization of tumor can be performed by x-ray of the chest and abdomen, intravenous pyelography, nephrotomography, and abdominal ultrasound. Recently improved techniques of computerized axial tomography of the abdomen have essentially replaced the procedures above. Since 80% of pheochromocytoma are localized in the adrenal medulla and 10% are bilateral, angiography may be necessary for definitive localization of tumor and providing information on the anatomy necessary for surgery. Multiple adrenal tumors are seen in patients with familial pheochromocytoma or multiple endocrine adenomatosis. Workup of patients with pheochromocytoma should include tests that screen for the presence of other endocrine abnormalities, particularly those associated with multiple endocrine adenomatosis (MEA) type II, such as hyperparathyroidism and medullary carcinoma of the thyroid. Further evaluation and therapy should be done with endocrinological and surgical consultations.

Other Endocrine Causes of Hypertension

Congenital adrenal hyperplasia associated with 11-hydroxylase deficiency or 17-hydroxylase deficiency is associated with hypertension. Systemic hypertension can also be seen with hyperthyroidism, hyperparathyroidism and acromegaly.

Hypertension Associated with Oral Contraceptives

Although the blood pressure increases in most women ingesting oral contraceptives, only a small percentage develops frank hypertension (5% in five years). The incidence is 3–5 times higher than among nonpill-users. The largest increase occurs within the first year, but blood pressure continues to rise over five years. The mechanism of oral-contraceptive-related hypertension is unknown. Data indicate that plasma volume and cardiac output are increased in normal women after several months of oral contraceptive ingestion. This may be related to the sodium retentive effects of estrogen and synthetic progesterone. Hepatic synthesis of angiotensinogen is also stimulated by estrogen. Thus, the rate of angiotensin production increases in the plasma. Furthermore, there may be an increase in sympathetic nervous activity as reflected in high levels of plasma dopamine-β-hydroxylase.

The hypertension is usually mild and reversible. If the blood pressure remains elevated three months after discontinuation of the pill, further work-up and therapy should be initiated.

Hypertension Related to Renal Disease

Hypertension can develop with chronic renal failure, renal parenchymal disease without renal insufficiency, acute glomerulonephritis, chronic pyelonephritis, hydronephrosis, or after bilateral nephrectomy. The mechanism of hypertension may be divided simplistically into volume-dependent or renin-dependent hypertension. The former is usually responsive to removal of sodium and fluid excess by diuretics or dialysis. The latter type of hypertension is usually aggravated by volume depletion and may be responsive to propranolol or alpha-methyldopa. In some cases, hypertension may be refractory to standard triple therapy. Captopril and minoxidil are effective agents for the treatment of refractory hypertension associated with renal insufficiency.

Coarctation of Aorta

Congenital narrowing of the aorta usually occurs beyond the origin of the left subclavian artery or distal to the ligamentum arteriosum. Takayasu's arteritis is an acquired form of coarctation that can also lead to hypertension. Clues from history and physical examination usually lead to further evaluation for coarctation. Symptoms include headache, epistaxis, and bounding carotid pulsations. Claudication, stroke, and heart failure may occur. Cardiac findings include a suprasternal notch thrill, left ventricular hypertrophy, loud A_2, S_4 gallop, and systolic flow murmur loudest over the left posterior thorax. Arm and leg blood pressure discrepancy, with a delayed or absent lower extremity pulse, are classical findings. A chest x-ray film can confirm the diagnosis by the characteristic rib notching (due to large intercostal collaterals) as well as the "figure three" sign of the descending aorta. The diagnosis is confirmed by aortography. Patients with coarctation of the aorta have other associated cardiac lesions. In particular, bicuspid aortic valve can be seen in up to one-third of the adolescent and adult population with coarctation. The management of coarctation of the aorta is discussed in details in Chapter 18.

Management of Hypertension

This section deals primarily with the management of patients with essential hypertension. The specific management of secondary forms of hypertension has already been discussed.

DECISIONS IN THERAPY

The Joint Committee on Hypertension recommends that patients with diastolic blood pressure of 120 mm Hg or higher should receive immediate evaluation and treatment. This is particularly important if hypertensive retinopathy is present. In patients with diastolic pressures of 105–119 mm of mercury, treatment is clearly indicated and evaluation should be initiated. Patients with diastolic pressure of less than 90 should be followed at yearly intervals. Individualized treatment is recommended in patients with a diastolic pressure of 90–104 mm of mercury. In this group, the presence of risk factors, evidence of target organ damage, male sex, and a family history of complications of hypertension should push toward treatment of these patients.

THERAPY OF HYPERTENSION

General measures such as weight reduction, exercise, and no-added-salt diet are generally recommended to all patients with essential hypertension. Relaxation response or behavioral modification is also gaining popularity as another nonpharmacologic approach to hypertension management. Although these measures are frequently insufficient in themselves to normalize blood pressure, they constitute an important adjunct to pharmacologic therapy.

The principle of pharmacologic therapy is to inhibit one or several of the factors that can elevate blood pressure. As previously discussed, these determinants include sodium and volume status, vascular tone, the renin-angiotensin system, and the sympathetic nervous system. Thus, the drugs can be broadly divided into the following categories:

1. Diuretics
2. Vasodilators
3. Sympatholytic agents
4. Renin-angiotensin-converting enzyme inhibitors

A list of commonly used antihypertensive drugs and doses is provided in Table 8.

The traditional approach to drug therapy of essential hypertension is the step-care approach. This is outlined as follows:

Start with:

Step 1. Diuretic; if blood pressure (BP) uncontolled, add

Step 2. Sympatholytic agent (beta-adrenergic blocker, alpha-methyldopa, clonidine, reserpine, or prazosin); if BP uncontrolled, add

Step 3. Vasodilator (hydralazine or minoxidil); if BP uncontrolled, add

Step 4. Addition of guanethidine or another sympatholytic agent not used in step 2.

The combination of a diuretic, a sympatholytic agent (usually beta-adrenergic blocker), and a vasodilator is commonly known as triple therapy. This combination is effective in over 90% of patients with moderate or severe hypertension. The rationale for this combination is summarized in Figure 3.

Table 8. Commonly Used Antihypertensive Drugs and Doses

I. Oral Agents Agent	Usual Initiating Dose	Maximal Daily Dose
Diuretics (agents are compiled in equivalent dosage forms)		
Chlorothiazide	500 mg qd	1000 mg
Hydrochlorothiazide	50 mg qd	100 mg
Furosemide	40 mg qd	600 mg
Spironolactone	25 mg tid	100 mg
Adrenergic inhibitors		
Rauwolfia derivatives:		
Reserpine (typical of this group)	0.25 mg qd (oral)	0.25 mg
Methyldopa	250 mg bid or tid	3 g
Guanethidine	10 mg qd	150–250 mg
Clonidine	0.1 mg bid	2.4 mg
Alpha-adrenergic receptor antagonist:		
Prazosin	1 mg tid	24 mg
Phenoxybenzamine	5 mg bid	As necessary
Beta-adrenergic receptor antagonist:		
Propranolol	10 to 40 mg bid	640 mg
Metoprolol	50 mg bid	450 mg/day
Nadolol	40 mg qd	320 mg/day
Atenolol	50 mg qd	100 mg/day
Pindolol	10 mg bid	60 mg/day
Timolol	10 mg bid	60 mg/day
Vasodilators		
Hydralazine	10 mg bid to qid	400 mg
Minoxidil	5 mg qd	100 mg
Converting-enzyme inhibitor:		
Captopril	25 mg tid	450 mg

II. Parenteral Agents Agent	Dose	Onset	Duration
Vasodilators			
Diazoxide	100–300 mg IV	1–3 min	4–18 hr
Nitroprusside	25–300 µg/min IV	<1 min	minutes
Hydralazine	5–20 mg IV or IM	15 min	2–6 hr
Adrenergic inhibitors			
Reserpine	1–5 mg IM (after 0.5 mg test dose)	2–3 hr	4–8 hr
Methyldopa	250–1000 mg IV	1–3 hr	4–8 hr
Trimethaphan	1–15 mg/min IV	<1 min	minutes
Alpha-adrenergic receptor antagonist:			
Phentolamine	5–15 mg IV	<1 min	$\frac{1}{4}$–2 hr
Beta-adrenergic receptor antagonist:			
Propranolol	1–5 mg IV	<1 min	1–2 hr

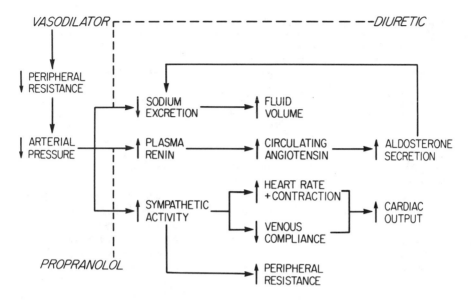

Figure 3 The primary and secondary effects of vasodilator therapy in hypertension. The protective effects of diuretic and beta blocker therapy are shown by the dotted lines. (Adapted from Koch-Weser, J: Vasodilator drugs in the treatment of hypertension. *Arch Intern Med.* 133:1017, 1974.)

With the availability of captopril, the angiotensin-converting enzyme inhibitor, and the increasing popularity of using a beta-blocker as a step 1 drug in young hypertensive patients, the step-care program may be revised as follows:

Start with:

Step 1. Diuretic or beta blocker

Add

Step 2. Addition of diuretic if beta blocker used in 1 or sympatholytic if diuretic used in 1.

Add

Step 3. Vasodilators including captopril, minoxidil

Add

Step 4. Sympatholytic agent not used in 2 or captopril

Laragh and colleagues recently proposed a "volume-vasoconstrictor" analysis of blood pressure control. They pointed out that the two major determinants of blood pressure are the status of circulatory volume (or cardiac output) and the vascular tone. In vasocontricted states, plasma volume is decreased, whereas in volume expanded states, the vascular tone is reduced. Thus, in the former condition, PRA should be elevated; and in the latter states, PRA is suppressed. They proposed that in any patient, a measurement of PRA (in relationship to urinary sodium excretion) provides an index of the dominant component of blood pressure control. Hence, if

Table 9. Common Drug Interactions in Hypertension Therapy

Drug	Antihypertensive	Effect
Tricyclic antidepressant	Clonidine	Attenuate antihypertensive effect
	Alpha-methyldopa	as above
	Reserpine	as above
	Guanethidine	as above
	Bethanidine	as above
Sympathomimetics	Clonidine	Attentuate antihypertensive effect
	Alpha-methyldopa	as above
	Guanethidine	as above
Phenothiazines	Alpha-methyldopa	Paradoxical hypertension
	Guanethidine	Attenuate antihypertensive effect
Monoamine oxidase inhibitors	Guanethidine	Attenuate antihypertensive effect
	Alpha-methyldopa	Paradoxical hypertension
	Reserpine	Paradoxical hypertension
CNS depressants	Clonidine	Increase CNS depression
	Alpha-methyldopa	Increase CNS depression
		Barbiturates reduce alpha-methyldopa effect
	Reserpine	Increase CNS depression
Miscellaneous:		
Digitalis	Diuretics	Hypokalemia, digitalis toxicity
Warfarin	Thiazides	Increase Prothrombin time
Pyridoxine	Hydralazine	Blocks pyridoxine effects
L-dopa	Alpha-methyldopa	Interfere with L-dopa in treatment of Parkinson's disease
	Reserpine	as above
Anesthesia	Central Sympatholytics	Hypotension
Digitalis, quinidine	Reserpine	Arrhythmias

the PRA is low, the patient should be treated vigorously with and respond to diuretics. In contrast, patients with elevated PRA should be responsive to beta-adrenergic blocker, since these drugs reduce renin secretion and sympathetic activity. This simplified concept may sometimes be helpful in the management of some subsets of patients, especially in those who are unresponsive to usual doses of standard therapy.

Table 10. Effects of Antihypertensive Drugs on Cardiovascular and Renal Compensatory Mechanisms

Class of Drugs	Renin-angiotensin Activity	Sympathetic Activity	Sodium Retention
Diuretics	↑	↑	↓
Sympatholytic agents	↓	↓	↔ or ↑
Vasodilator	↑	↑	↑
Captopril	↓	↔ or ↓	↓

Treatment of Refractory Hypertension

In evaluating patients with treatment-resistant hypertension, one must consider several important factors:

1. *Compliance.* The commonest cause of uncontrolled hypertension is patient non-compliance. This is frequently difficult to document. A careful and thorough history is important, paying particular attention to patient's comprehension of his drug regimen and history of drug side-effects. Measurements of plasma or 24 hour urine drug concentrations or the use of pill counts have been useful in documenting patient noncompliance.

2. *Secondary forms of hypertension.* The possibility of secondary forms of hypertension should be evaluated in all patients who require step 4 drugs.

3. *Drug interactions.* Drug interactions that can result in the attenuation of the effect of certain antihypertensives (e.g., tricyclic antidepressants with adrenergic blocking agents) should be excluded. A list of such drug interactions is shown in Table 9.

4. *Inappropriate drug combinations.* In evaluating drug combinations, it is helpful to consider that all antihypertensive agents belong to one of the three broad classes of drugs: diuretics, sympatholytics, or vasodilators. Ordinarily it is not desirable or logical to add a second drug from the same class, since it may have little or no additional effect. For example, a patient refractory to hydrochlorothiazide, propranolol, and alpha-methyldopa should be switched to hydrochlorothiazide, propranolol, and hydralazine. The best combinations are among the three classes of antihypertensive drugs.

5. *Activation of cardiovascular compensatory mechanisms.* Finally, certain drugs can activate cardiovascular compensatory mechanisms which can result in the attenuation of the primary antihypertensive action of the drug. For example, hydralazine stimulates sympathetic nervous system (reflex tachycardia) and activates the renin-angiotensin system. Furthermore, it promotes sodium retention. For these reasons, long-term hydralazine monotherapy is ineffective for blood pressure control.

The effects of different drugs on the sympathetic nervous system, renin-angiotensin system, and sodium excretion are summarized in Table 10. An understanding of drug effects on these cardiovascular compensatory mechanisms allows a more rational choice of combinations of antihypertensive agents.

Hypertensive Crisis

When approaching a patient with severe hypertension, it is important to distinguish between conditions that are hypertensive emergencies requiring immediate control of blood pressure and those that are urgencies, in which hypertension should be controlled over hours to days. The former conditions are associated with immediate grave prognosis if blood pressure remains uncontrolled. Rapid-acting parenteral antihypertensive agents are the treatment of choice in these patients. Table 11, part I, summarizes the conditions that are classified as hypertensive emergencies. The di-

Table 11. Conditions Associated with Hypertensive Crisis

I. Hypertensive Emergencies

    Malignant hypertension: eyegrounds reveal hemorrhages or exudates or papilledema

    Hypertension with acute pulmonary edema

    Hypertensive encephalopathy

    CVA, including hemorrhage and infarction

    Aortic dissection

    Pheochromocytoma with severe hypertension

    Hypertension following tyramine ingestion in patients on monoamine oxidase inhibitors

    Severe toxemia or eclampsia

II. Urgent Conditions Associated with Hypertension

    Accelerated hypertension—eyegrounds reveal hemorrhage and exudates

    Severe hypertension in a patient with myocardial infarction or severe angina

    Occlusive stroke or transient ischemic attack in a hypertensive patient

    Renal failure or significant renal impairment in a hypertensive patient

    Marked hypertension associated with burns, acute glomerulonephritis or preeclampsia

    Severe hypertension in patients with bleeding postoperatively

    The patient with hypertension, new cardiovascular or neurologic symptoms

    New patient with DBP >130

---

agnosis is based on a clinical composite, rather than merely the absolute level of blood pressure.

Table 11, part II, lists the urgent conditions associated with hypertension. Prompt treatment in these patients is mandatory. However, control of blood pressure can be accomplished over several hours to days. In these patients, a rigorous regimen of oral drugs can be used. A list of drugs, their action and indications for use in hypertensive crisis are shown in Table 8, part II, and Table 12. Certain specific conditions are discussed in detail below.

MALIGNANT HYPERTENSION

Malignant hypertension is defined by most clinicians as severe accelerated hypertension with papilledema. It is frequently associated with evidence of severe end-organ damage, such as acute renal failure, microscopic hematuria and proteinuria, congestive heart failure, myocardial necrosis, and microangiopathic hemolysis. Hypertensive encephalopathy and cerebrovascular accidents are also seen in these patients. The underlying pathologic lesion is diffuse fibrinoid necrosis of arterioles with microthrombi and end-organ ischemia.

HYPERTENSIVE ENCEPHALOPATHY

This is an acute but reversible syndrome usually precipitated by an abrupt and sustained increase in blood pressure, which exceeds the limits of cerebral autoregula-

Table 12. Selection of Drugs to Be Given in Various Types of Hypertensive Crises

Type of Hypertensive Crisis	Drug of Choice (parenterally)	Drugs to Avoid or use Cautiously
Acute hypertensive encephalopathy	diazoxide nitroprusside trimethaphan	rauwolfia methyldopa clonidine guanethidine propranolol
Intracerebral or subarachnoid hemorrhage	nitroprusside trimethaphan	sympatholytics
Acute pulmonary edema with hypertension	nitroprusside trimethaphan reserpine methyldopa furosemide hydralazine	diazoxide
Pheochromocytoma *or* Monamine oxidase inhibitor with tyramines *or* sympathomimetics	phentolamine *or* phenoxybenzamine *or* nitroprusside, plus propranolol	sympatholytics
Acute glomerulonephritis or lupus nephritis crisis	nitroprusside diazoxide hydralazine methyldopa furosemide	trimethaphan
Dissecting aortic aneurysm	trimethaphan reserpine nitroprusside methyldopa furosemide	hydralazine diazoxide
Acute myocardial infarction	propranolol nitroglycerin	hydralazine diazoxide

SOURCE: Modified from Onesti, G., and Lowenthal, D.V. (Eds.): *The Spectrum of Antihypertensive Drug Therapy,* Hahnemann Medical Proceeding, Seminar in Therapeutics, Hahnemann College, Nov., 1976, p. 106, with permission.

tion. Symptoms include severe headache, diuresis, lethargy or confusion, and vomiting. Generalized seizures, nonfocal neurologic signs, myoclonus, and coma can develop. The syndrome occurs in the setting of increased intracranial pressure, although papilledema is occasionally absent. Hypertensive encephalopathy must be distinguished from intracerebral hemorrhage, embolic or thrombotic stroke, metabolic encephalopathy, or primary seizure disorders. The cerebrospinal fluid is usually clear but under increased pressure. The protein content may be normal or increased.

The electroencephalogram shows various nonspecific abnormalities. Brain CT scan and isotopic brain scans are usually normal.

Hypertensive encephalopathy is a true emergency; since, if untreated, coma progresses and death ensues within hours. Blood pressure should be promptly reduced with rapid acting agents, such as diazoxide or sodium nitroprusside. The immediate goal is a blood pressure of 150–160/90–100, avoiding more profound decreases that may result in ischemic damage. Central acting antihypertensive drugs such as alpha-methyldopa, or reserpine should be avoided, since these drugs depress central nervous system activity and obscure monitoring.

DISSECTING AORTIC ANEURYSM

Hypertension is seen in a high percent of patients with dissecting aortic aneurysm. Medical management is the main stay of current therapy for this condition. Vigorous control of blood pressure can prevent further progression of dissection. Surgical therapy is frequently necessary, particularly in dissection involving the ascending aorta (type A). The proper selection of antihypertensive drug is of paramount importance. Agents that stimulate reflex increase in heart rate, cardiac output, ventricular ejection rate, myocardial contractility, and shear rate to aortic blood flow must be avoided. The recommended regimen includes a beta-adrenergic blocker such as propranolol, given intravenously in combination with nitroprusside. Alternately, trimethaphan can be used as the primary agent. If beta-adrenergic blockers cannot be used, reserpine can be given parenterally instead. Vasodilators, such as hydralazine and diazoxide, are contraindicated in this condition. Further therapy of dissecting aneurysm is discussed in details in Chapter 28.

HYPERTENSIVE CRISIS ASSOCIATED WITH EXCESS CATECHOLAMINES

These include pheochromocytoma crisis, tyramine ingestion in patients receiving MAO inhibitors, guanethidine plus tricyclic acid antidepressant administration, and hypertensive crisis after cessation of clonidine. In all these conditions, the use of the adrenergic antagonist, phentolamine, intravenously, is the treatment of choice. Beta-adrenergic blockers are usually needed as adjunctive therapy for control of tachyarrhythmias. Beta-adrenergic blockers should never be used alone without the administration of phentolamine first.

SEVERE HYPERTENSION ASSOCIATED WITH MYOCARDIAL INFARCTION

Control of hypertension can reduce myocardial oxygen demand and is thus important during acute myocardial infarction. Agents that induce reflex tachycardia or increase cardiac output must be avoided. Parenteral nitroglycerin or propranolol alone, or in combination, can be effective agents. Calcium channel antagonists, nifedipine or verapamil can also be used. Data suggest that nitroprusside may increase infarct size and should not be used for blood pressure therapy during acute myocardial infarction.

Drug Side Effects

Virtually all antihypertensive medicines have known side effects; the magnitude of side effects varies from minimal to occasionally severe, requiring that the drug be discontinued. Complications of diuretics are reviewed in Table 8, Chapter 19, and of vasodilators in Table 9, Chapter 19. Adverse effects of beta blockers are shown in Table 6, Chapter 9.

Other sympatholytic agents have well-known adverse effects. Methyldopa can cause drowsiness, depression, orthostatic hypotension, impotence, hemolytic anemia (Coombs positive), and hepatitis. Guanethidine can cause orthostatic hypotension, weakness, bradycardia, nasal congestion, diarrhea, and retrograde ejaculation. Reserpine may result in serious depression as well as drowsiness, nasal congestion and bradycardia. Clonidine's side effects include dry mouth, sedation, and rebound hypertension. It is important for the physician to be alert to these untoward effects and, if necessary, to alter the drug regimen.

Summary

In summary, evaluation of the hypertensive patient should include a careful history and physical examination to look for associated risk factors, evidence of end-organ damage, and clues for secondary hypertension. The laboratory evaluation should include those with low cost/high benefit ratio. Unless there is a strong clinical suspicion of secondary forms of hypertension, serum potassium concentration is the only routinely performed screening test.

Secondary forms of hypertension can usually be screened by one or two laboratory tests: for example (1) hyperaldosteronism: serum potassium concentration, stimulated plasma renin activity (PRA); (2) renovascular hypertension: stimulated PRA or IVP; (3) pheochromocytoma: 24 urinary metanephrines; (4) Cushing's syndrome: overnight dexamethasone suppression; (5) coarctation of aorta: chest x-ray.

Finally, decision with respect to therapy involves the utility of all the information gathered from this evaluation.

ACKNOWLEDGMENTS

The author would like to thank Dr. T.J. Moore for helpful suggestions on the section of Endocrine-Hypertension, and Ms. Nancy Orgill, Ms. Laura J. Ducey, Ms. Diane Rioux, and Ms. Carmen Francisco for their secretarial assistance in the preparation of this manuscript.

Bibliography

AMA Committee on Hypertension. 1974. The treatment of malignant hypertension and hypertensive emergencies. *JAMA* 228:1673.

Bravo EL, Tarazi RC, Fouad FM, et al: Clonidine suppression test: A useful aid in the diagnosis of pheochromocytoma. *N Engl J Med* 305:623, 1981.

Brunner HR, Kirshman D, Sealey JE, et al: Hypertension of renal origin: Evidence for two different mechanisms. *Science* 174:1344, 1971.

Brunner HR, Laragh JH, Baer L, et al: Essential hypertension: Renin and aldosterone, heart attack and stroke. *N Engl J Med* 286:441, 1972.

Case DB, Atlas SA, Marion RM, et al: Long-term efficacy of captopril in renovascular and essential hypertension. *Am J Cardiol* 49:1440, 1982.

Dzau VJ: Angiotensin converting enzyme inhibition in the treatment of congestive heart failure and hypertension, in Isselbacher E, et al (eds): *Harrison's Principles of Internal Medicine*, Update IV. New York, McGraw-Hill, 1983, pp 137–146.

Dzau VJ, Gibbons G, Levin D: Renovascular hypertension: An update on pathophysiology, diagnosis, and treatment. *Am J Nephrol* (in press).

Fisch IR, Frank J: Oral contraceptives and blood pressure. JAMA 237:2499, 1977.

Gavras H, Brunner HR, Turini, GA, et al: Antihypertensive effect of the oral angiotensin converting enzyme inhibitor SQ 14225 in man. *N Engl J Med* 298:991, 1978.

Gold EM: The Cushing syndromes: Changing views of diagnosis and treatment. *Ann Intern Med* 90:829, 1979.

Grim CE, Luft FC, Weinberger MH, et al: Sensitivity and specificity of screening tests for renal vascular hypertension. *Ann Intern Med* 91:617, 1979.

Grim CE, Luft HY, Yune EC, et al: Percutaneous transluminal dilation in the treatment of renal vascular hypertension. *Ann Intern Med* 95:439, 1981.

Hunt JC, Sheps SG, Harrison EG Jr, et al: Renal and renovascular hypertension: A reasoned approach to diagnosis and management. *Arch Intern Med* 133:988, 1974.

Hricik DE, Browning PJ, Kopelman R, et al: Captopril-induced functional renal insufficiency in patients with bilateral renal-artery stenosis or renal-artery stenosis in a solitary kidney. *N Engl J Med* (in press).

Hypertension Detection and Follow-up Program Cooperative Group: Five-year findings of the Hypertension Detection and Follow-up Program. I. Reduction in mortality of persons with high blood pressure, including mild hypertension. JAMA 242:2562, 1979.

Hypertension Detection and Follow-up Program Cooperative Group: Patient participation in a hypertension control program. JAMA 239:1507, 1978.

Kannel WB, Sorlie P: Hypertension in Framingham, in Paul O (ed): *Epidemiology and Control of Hypertension*. Miami, Symposia Specialist, 1975, p 553.

Kaplan NM: *Clinical Hypertension*. 2nd ed. Baltimore, Williams and Wilkins Co., 1978.

Kaplan NM, Kramer NJ, Holland OB, et al: Single-voided urine metanephrine assays in screening for pheochromocytoma. *Arch Intern Med* 137:190, 1977.

Kaplan NM, Kem DC, Holland OB, et al: The intravenous furosemide test: A simple way to evaluate renin responsiveness. *Ann Intern Med* 84:639, 1976.

Kaplan NM: Renin profiles: The unfilfilled promises. JAMA 238:611, 1977.

Keith NM, Wagner HP: Some different types of essential hypertension. Their cause and prognosis. *Am J Med Sci* 197:332, 1939.

Kem DC, Weinberger MH, Mayes DM, et al: Saline suppression of plasma aldosterone in hypertension. *Arch Intern Med* 128:380, 1971.

Laragh JH: Modern system for treating high blood pressure based on renin profiling and vasoconstriction-volume analysis: A primary role for beta blocking drugs such as propranolol. *Am J Med* 61:797, 1976.

Lawrence AM: Glucagon provocative test for pheochromocytoma. *Ann Intern Med* 66:1091, 1967.

Marks LS, Maxwell MH, Varady PD, et al: Renovascular hypertension: Does the renal vein renin ratio predict operative results? *J Urol* 115:365, 1976.

Maron BJ, Humphries JO, Rowe RD, et al: Prognosis of surgically corrected coarctation of the aorta: A 20-year post-operative appraisal. *Circulation* 47:119, 1973.

Martin EC, Mattern RF, Baer C, et al: Renal angioplasty for hypertension: Predictive factors for long-term success. *Am J Radiol* 137:921, 1981.

Maxwell RA, Wastila WB: Adrenergic neuron blocking drugs, in Gross F (ed): *Antihypertensive Agents*. New York, Springer-Verlag, 1977, p 161.

McMahon FG: Management of Essential Hypertension. New York, Futura Publishing Company, 1978.

Oparil S, Haber E: The renin-angiotensin system. *N Engl J Med* 291:389–401, 446, 1974.

Ram CVS, Englemen K: Pheochromocytoma, in Current Problems in Cardiology Volume 4, Year Book Medical Publishers, Inc., 1979, p 1–38.

Ram CVS, Kaplan MN: Individual titration of diazoxide dosage in the treatment of severe hypertension. *Am J Cardiol* 43:627, 1979.

Re R, Novelline R, Escourrou MT, et al: Inhibition of angiotensin-converting enzyme for diagnosis of renal-artery stenosis. *N Engl J Med* 298:582, 1978.

Report of the Joint National Committee on Detection, Evaluation, and Treatment of High Blood Pressure: A cooperative study. JAMA 237:255, 1977.

Slater EE, Haber E: Hypertension, in Johnson RA, Haber E, Austen WG (eds): *The Practice of Cardiology*. Boston, Little, Brown, 1980, p 939.

Veterans Administration Cooperative Study Group on Antihypertensive Agents: Effects of treatment on morbidity in hypertension. Results in patients with diastolic blood pressures averaging 115 through 129 mm Hg. JAMA 202:1028, 1967.

Veterans Administration Cooperative Study Group on Antihypertensive Agents: Effects of treatment on morbidity in hypertension, II. Results in patients with diastolic blood pressure averaging 90 through 115 mm Hg. JAMA 213:1143, 1970.

Wenting GJ, DeBruyn JHB, Man In't Veld AJ, et al: Hemodynamic effects of captopril in essential hypertension, renovascular hypertension, and cardiac failure: Correlations with short and long-term effects on plasma renin. *Am J Cardiol* 49:1453, 1982.

Weinberger MH, Grim CE, Hollifield JW, et al: Primary aldosteronism. *Ann Intern Med* 90:386, 1979.

Woods JW: Oral contraceptives and hypertension. *Lancet* 2:653, 1967.

CHAPTER 24 | PULMONARY HYPERTENSION

Robert A. Kloner

Pulmonary hypertension is defined as the presence of pulmonary artery (PA) systolic pressure exceeding 30 mm Hg and PA mean pressure greater than 20 mm Hg. Normally, PA pressures are 18–25 mm Hg systolic, 6–10 mm Hg diastolic, and 12–16 mm Hg mean. Pulmonary hypertension is considered severe when PA pressures are greater than approximately 75% of systemic arterial pressures. There is recent evidence suggesting that prostaglandins may have a role in the development of pulmonary hypertension in some cardiac patients. Pulmonary hypertension may occur secondary to a variety of disorders, or it may be idiopathic.

The causes of secondary pulmonary hypertension are numerous and have recently been classified by Alpert et al. (1981). They describe 3 basic causes including (1) *precapillary pulmonary hypertension*, as occurs in primary pulmonary hypertension, disorders of ventilation, pulmonary embolism, Eisenmenger's physiology in congenital heart disease, schistosomiasis, collagen vascular disease, sickle cell disease, and the pulmonary hypertension associated with portal hypertension. Disorders of ventilation that may result in precapillary pulmonary hypertension include chronic obstructive lung disease, cystic fibrosis, restrictive lung disease (sarcoidosis, progressive systemic sclerosis, extensive lung resection), high altitude pulmonary hypertension, primary central hypoventilation, sleep apnea, myasthenia gravis, paralytic poliomyelitis, and kyphoscoliosis. (2) The second basic cause of pulmonary hypertension is *passive pulmonary hypertension*, as occurs with mitral valve disease, left ventricular failure, cor triatriatum, left atrial myxoma, and obstruction of pulmonary veins. (3) The third basic cause is *reactive pulmonary hypertension*, as occurs in some patients with mitral valve disease and venoocclusive disease.

Although the signs and symptoms associated with pulmonary hypertension vary to some extent depending on the associated illness, there are several common features. Patients typically complain of dyspnea, atypical chest pain, and weakness. With severe and long-standing pulmonary hypertension, symptoms of right ventricular failure emerge—with peripheral edema, gastrointestinal complaints, and ascites. Marked fatigue, dizziness, and sometimes syncope occur due to low forward cardiac output. If pulmonary hypertension is secondary to cardiac disease, such as left ventricular failure or mitral valve disease, the symptoms may predominantly reflect pulmonary congestion-orthopnea, dyspnea on exertion, and paroxysmal nocturnal dyspnea. If pulmonary hypertension is secondary to chronic obstructive lung disease, symptoms are predominantly related to pulmonary disease with dyspnea, cough, and frequent episodes of bronchitis.

Signs of pulmonary hypertension with right ventricular pressure overload include distended jugular venous neck veins, with a prominent a wave; a left parasternal lift due to right ventricular hypertrophy; a palpable P_2; and a palpable systolic pulsation in the second left intercostal space due to a dilated pulmonary artery. On auscul-

475

tation, the second heart sound (S_2) is closely split, the pulmonic component is louder than the aortic component, and a right ventricular S_4 is present. A systolic ejection click and flow murmur may be heard over the dilated pulmonary artery. As right ventricular failure occurs, peripheral edema, ascites, and hepatomegaly appear. In severe cases of pulmonary hypertension, signs of tricuspid regurgitation are present, including tall systolic regurgitant v waves in the jugular venous pulse, a holosystolic murmur along the left sternal border that increases with inspiration, and a right ventricular S_3. A high-pitched early diastolic murmur of pulmonary regurgitation may also be heard in severe cases. With reduced cardiac output, the carotid pulse is diminished in volume, and cyanosis may develop.

The chest x-ray film in pulmonary hypertension may help reveal the underlying disorder, such as calcification of the mitral valve and enlarged left atrium in mitral stenosis. The main pulmonary artery and the right ventricle typically are enlarged. The ECG shows evidence of right ventricular pressure overload with right axis deviation, tall p waves suggesting right atrial enlargement, and tall R waves in V_1 and V_2 suggesting right ventricular hypertrophy.

Echocardiography and cardiac catheterization help delineate the underlying cause for the pulmonary hypertension—for example, evidence of rheumatic mitral stenosis by echocardiogram and a gradient across the mitral valve at catheterization. Echocardiogram of the pulmonary valve may reveal a reduced a wave excursion and a midsystolic notch. In some cases, lung scans are performed to help diagnose pulmonary embolism. Serologic tests may aid in determining the presence of collagen vascular disease.

If the etiology of pulmonary hypertension is unclear, some authorities recommend lung biopsy in order to determine the severity and potential reversibility of the lesions as well as evidence of any active inflammatory process. Lung biopsy may also serve as a prognostic indicator.

Specific Clinical Disorders in Secondary Pulmonary Hypertension

CONGENITAL HEART DISEASE AND EISENMENGER'S SYNDROME

In the setting of congenital heart disease in which a left-to-right shunt is present, pulmonary hypertension simply may be due to increased pulmonary blood flow. This increased flow may act to secondarily cause pulmonary arteriolar vasoconstriction. If the shunt is large with markedly increased pulmonary flow and pulmonary hypertension is present over a long period of time, anatomic changes occur within the vascular bed. These anatomic changes initially are reversible (decreased pulmonary arteriolar cross-sectional area due to medial hypertrophy and vasoconstriction, and intimal cellular proliferation) or irreversible (necrotizing arteritis and plexiform lesions, which are capillary-like channels present in a dilated segment of the pulmonary artery). Grading systems have been developed in order to assess the severity of morphologic alterations. Surgical correction of the shunt during the reversible phase results in an immediate reduction in pulmonary artery pressure, followed by a more gradual reduction, as medial hypertrophy and intimal cellular proliferation regress.

However, as the vascular injury becomes irreversible with progressive anatomical obliteration of the pulmonary bed, there is reversal of the direction of the shunt. The term *Eisenmenger's syndrome* is used to describe patients with congenital communications between systemic and pulmonary circulations who have irreversible pulmonary hypertension due to anatomic changes in their pulmonary vascular bed, and in whom a previous left-to-right shunt has become a right-to-left shunt. These patients have a high pulmonary vascular resistance and pulmonary arterial pressures that often approach systemic arterial pressures. Examples of congenital heart disease that may lead to Eisenmenger's complex include ventricular septal defect, patent ductus arteriosus, atrial septal defect, and transposition of the great vessels. Patients with ventricular septal defect may develop Eisenmenger's complex in their teens or late adolescent years; patients with large patent ductus arteriosus may develop it from infancy; only occasional patients with atrial septal defect ever develop Eisenmenger's physiology. Further details of these congenital heart diseases are found in Chapter 18.

Patients with Eisenmenger's syndrome typically complain of dyspnea, fatigue, syncope, hemoptysis, and atypical chest pain. Physical examination reveals cyanosis, clubbing, and signs of severe pulmonary hypertension. Polycythemia is usually present. In patients with a patent ductus arteriosus and Eisenmenger's syndrome, the cyanosis and clubbing characteristically occur in the lower extremities but not in the upper extremities. In addition to the electrocardiographic features discussed above, patients with Eisenmenger's syndrome may develop supraventricular tachyarrhythmias, including atrial tachycardia, atrial fibrillation, and atrial flutter. Chest x-ray film reveals enlargment of the main pulmonary artery, proximal right and left pulmonary arteries with tapered peripheral pulmonary arteries, and an enlarged right ventricle and atrium. At cardiac catheterization, pulmonary vascular resistance is typically at least 75% of systemic vascular resistance, and arterial blood is desaturated. Cardiac catheterization rules out silent mitral stenosis and, in patients with Eisenmenger's syndrome, the pulmonary capillary wedge pressure (left atrial pressure) is usually normal. Patients with Eisenmenger's syndrome are at an increased risk of developing complications including cardiovascular collapse and sudden death with angiographic procedures. When pulmonary vascular resistance is equal to systemic resistance and irreversible anatomic changes in the vasculature are present, surgical closure of the intracardiac communication will fail to relieve the pulmonary hypertension and will result in severe right ventricular failure and very high mortality. Therefore, the treatment of these patients is medical and includes salt restriction, diuretics, and digitalis for treatment of right ventricular failure, phlebotomy, and chronic oxygen therapy. These patients should receive endocarditis prophylaxis; some physicians also treat these patients with chronic warfarin therapy to prevent pulmonary or paradoxical embolism. The use of vasodilators remains experimental. Pregnancy should be avoided in these patients, as it is associated with an increased risk of death. Overall prognosis is poor once Eisenmenger's syndrome develops, and most patients do not live past the fourth decade. Sudden death may occur or death may be secondary to severe heart failure, ventricular arrhythmias, pulmonary infection, thrombosis, brain abscess, endocarditis, or severe hemotysis.

PULMONARY HYPERTENSION DUE TO MITRAL STENOSIS

Initially, the pulmonary hypertension of mitral stenosis is passive and is due to impedance of pulmonary venous drainage secondary to high left atrial pressures. Over time, many patients develop a reactive component to their pulmonary hypertension with vasoconstriction and anatomic changes in the pulmonary vasculature. Hence, as stressed by studies of Dexter, a more proximal "second stenosis" at the level of pulmonary arterioles and small muscular arteries occurs, which results in high pulmonary artery pressures and signs of right ventricular failure. On the other hand, symptoms and signs of pulmonary congestion may actually be reduced somewhat during this stage of mitral stenosis, since the "second stenosis" is limiting blood flow to the left side of the heart. Anatomic changes that develop in the pulmonary vascular bed due to chronic venous hypertension of any cause include medial hypertrophy of small arteries and arterioles, distension of the pulmonary capillaries, swelling of capillary endothelial cells, intimal proliferation, thickening and rupture of the basement membrane of endothelial cells, transudation of red blood cells into the alveoli, distension of pulmonary lymphatics, and pulmonary hemosiderosis. In severe cases, pulmonary hemorrhage and fibrosis occurs. After mitral valve surgery, pulmonary artery pressure and resistance fall within the first postoperative week with reversal of many of the anatomic changes (medial hypertrophy, distension of capillaries and lymphatics, swelling of endothelial cells, intimal proliferation). Occasional patients will fail to eliminate their pulmonary hypertension following mitral valve surgery and develop a progressive course.

PULMONARY HYPERTENSION DUE TO PARENCHYMAL LUNG DISEASE

The most common situation in which parenchymal lung disease leads to pulmonary hypertension is chronic obstructive lung disease. It is well known that hypoxia causes pulmonary vasoconstriction and, thus, is probably an important factor in the development of pulmonary hypertension, although other factors, such as arterial PCO_2 and muscular hypertrophy of pulmonary arterioles, may play a role. Parenchymal lung disease also may result in an anatomic restriction or loss of the pulmonary vascular bed, which contributes to pulmonary hypertension. Eventually, cor pulmonale (dilatation and failure of the right ventricle due to pulmonary disease) may develop. Chronic administration of 28% O_2 for four to eight weeks will result in a substantial lowering of pulmonary artery pressures.

PULMONARY HYPERTENSION IN COLLAGEN VASCULAR DISEASES

Several collagen vascular diseases are associated with pulmonary hypertension. The pathology is usually a fibrous obliteration of the pulmonary vasculature. Pulmonary hypertension is especially severe in patients with the associated CREST variant of scleroderma (calcinosis, Raynaud's phenomenon, esophagitis, sclerodactyly, and telangiectasia); but it may also be severe in systemic lupus erythematosus, rheumatoid arthritis, dermatomyositis, mixed connective tissue disease, and in association with Raynaud's phenomenon.

PULMONARY EMBOLISM See Chapter 25.

Primary Pulmonary Hypertension

Primary pulmonary hypertension is the term used when there is no discernible cause for the hypertension. Several possible theories have been advanced to explain primary pulmonary hypertension, including recurrent occult pulmonary emboli, development of thrombi in small pulmonary arteries, congenital abnormalities of the media of the pulmonary arteries, and persistent fetal pulmonary architecture. Other theories include the possibility that primary pulmonary hypertension is an autoimmune phenomenon, a form of collagen vascular disease, a vasculitis, or due to some genetic predisposition toward increased vasospasm of the pulmonary bed. None of these theories has been shown to be the most likely cause. The pathologic features of primary pulmonary hypertension occur in small pulmonary arteries and arterioles and include intimal thickening and fibroelastosis, producing a characteristic "onion skin" appearance to the vessel, increased thickness of the media, plexiform lesions, necrotizing arteritis, and fibrinoid necrosis with eventual thrombosis and atherosclerosis.

The age of onset of the disease is variable (16–69 years, mean age 35) and the disease is four to five times more common in women than men. Symptoms include dyspnea, dizziness, syncope, fatigue, weakness due to low cardiac output, hypoxemia, and atypical chest pain that mimics angina. In early stages, these symptoms may be exercise-related; in the later stages of the disease, they occur at rest. When right ventricular failure occurs, peripheral edema, abdominal discomfort, nausea, vomiting, and ascites may be present. Other symptoms that occur during the late phase of the disease include cough, hemoptysis, and palpitations due to ventricular arrhythmias. The physical findings are those typical of severe pulmonary hypertension, as discussed above. Late cyanosis may be due to right-to-left shunting through a patent foramen ovale or to severely reduced cardiac output. Laboratory studies reveal arterial O_2 desaturation, polycythemia, and, with severe right ventricular failure, elevated liver enzymes. A hypercoagulable state may exist with abnormalities in fibrinolysis and platelet function. The chest x-ray film shows dilated proximal pulmonary arteries, with tapering of peripheral branches and relative oligemia of the lung fields. Right atrial and ventricular enlargement are present. ECG reveals tall peaked p waves and tall R waves in V_1 and V_2 (right ventricular hypertrophy). Echocardiography shows changes in the pulmonary valve motion, including reduction of the pulmonary valve a wave and midsystolic closure of the pulmonary valve, as well as an enlarged and hypertrophied right ventricle.

Cardiac catheterization delineates the severity of the pulmonary hypertension and rules out possible secondary causes of pulmonary hypertension. Some cardiologists consider cardiac catheterization mandatory, since primary pulmonary hypertension is a diagnosis of exclusion. Pulmonary artery pressure and right ventricular systolic pressure are elevated and may equal or sometimes exceed systemic arterial pressures, while left atrial and ventricular pressures are low or normal. Calculated pulmonary vascular resistance is markedly elevated. The right atrial pressure is also high with tall a waves; if tricuspid regurgitation is present, there may be tall regurgitant v waves. A small right-to-left shunt may be present if the foramen ovale has become patent, due to high right atrial pressures. Cardiac angiography is hazardous in advanced cases of primary pulmonary hypertension, and has resulted in cardiovascular collapse and sudden deaths. However, if the diagnosis is unclear and there is doubt whether the pulmonary hypertension is due to a secondary cause, such as pulmonary emboli, either a perfusion-ventilation lung scan or, in some cases, a cautious selective pulmonary angiography may be performed.

The prognosis of patients with primary pulmonary hypertension is notably poor; most patients die approximately 2–3 years after the onset of symptoms. Death may occur suddenly or be due to severe right ventricular failure and low cardiac output. Pulmonary vasodilators (sublingual isoproterenol, tolazoline, phentolamine, hydralazine) and O_2 administration may reduce pulmonary vascular resistance and provide some symptomatic improvement initially; but whether long-term mortality is improved remains to be determined. When vasodilators are first administered, patients should be closely monitored, as some will radically lower their cardiac output. In a recent study by Packer et al., four of 13 patients receiving hydralazine for pulmonary hypertension became symptomatically hypotensive within 24 hours of initiating treatment. Patients are commonly anticoagulated to prevent thromboembolism. Right ventricular failure is treated with digitalis and diuretics for control of edema and ascites.

Another valuable form of treatment is phlebotomy, in order to maintain the hemoglobin level under 20 and preferably at 16–18 grams per deciliter. There has been a recent promising report of heart-lung transplantation for pulmonary hypertension (Reitz et al.). Pulmonary hypertension is a relative contraindication to pregnancy, as there is a very high mortality rate in the puerperium (Sinnenberg).

Bibliography

Alpert JS, Braunwald E: Primary pulmonary hypertension. in Braunwald E (ed): *Heart Disease: A textbook of cardiovascular medicine.* Philadelphia, Saunders, 1980, p 1633.

Alpert JS, Irwin RS, Dalen SE: Pulmonary hypertension. *Curr Probl Cardiol* 5:1, 1981.

Bell WR, Simon TL, DeMets DL: The clinical features of submassive and massive pulmonary emboli. *Am J Med* 62:355, 1977.

Bower JS, Dantzker DR, Naylor B: Idiopathic pulmonary hypertension associated with nodular pulmonary infiltrates and portal venous thrombosis.

Braunwald E, Braunwald NS, Ross T Jr, et al: Effects of mitral valve replacement on pulmonary vascular dynamics of patients with pulmonary hypertension. *N Engl J Med* 273:509, 1965.

Buch J, Wennevold A: Hazards of diazoxide in pulmonary hypertension. *Br Heart J* 46:401, 1981.

Burrow B, Kettel LJ, Niden AH, et al: Patterns of cardiovascular dysfunction in chronic obstructive lung disease. *N Engl J Med* 286:912, 1972.

Connor PK, Bashour FA: Cardiopulmonary changes in scleroderma: A physiologic study. *Am Heart J* 61:494, 1961.

Daoud FS, Reeves JT, Kelley DB: Isoproterenol as a potential pulmonary vasodilator in primary pulmonary hypertension. *Am J Cardiol* 42:817, 1978.

Dexter L: Physiologic changes in mitral stenosis. *N Engl J Med* 254:829, 1956.

Ekici E, Olguntork R, Ilhan M, et al: Possible relationship between pulmonary hypertension and prostaglandins. *Prostaglandins Med* 7:71, 1981.

Fayemi A: Pulmonary vascular disease in systemic lupus erythematosus. *Am J Clin Pathol* 65:284, 1976.

Fishman AP: Hypoxia on the pulmonary circulation: How and where it acts. *Circ Res* 38:221, 1976.

Grossman W, Braunwald E: Pulmonary hypertension, in Braunwald E (ed): *Heart Disease: A textbook of cardiovascular medicine*. Philadelphia, Saunders, 1980, p 835.

Harris P, Health D: *The human pulmonary circulation*. ed 2. New York, Churchill Livingston, 1977, p 684.

Heath D, Edwards JE: The pathology of hypertensive pulmonary vascular disease: A description of six grades of structural changes in the pulmonary arteries with special reference to congenital cardiac septal defects. *Circulation* 18:533, 1958.

Heath D, Edwards JE: Histological changes in the lung in disease associated with pulmonary venous hypertension. *Br J Dis Chest* 53:8, 1959.

Hirschfeld S, Meyer L, Schwartz DC, et al: The echocardiographic assessment of pulmonary artery pressure and pulmonary vascular resistance. *Circulation* 52:642, 1975.

Inglesby TV, Singer JW, Gordon DS: Abnormal fibrinolysis in familial pulmonary hypertension. *Am J Med* 55:5, 1973.

James TN, Frame B, Coates ED: De subitaneis mortibus. III. Pickwickian syndrome. *Circulation* 48:1311, 1973.

Jones MB, Osterholm RK, Wilson RB, et al: Fatal pulmonary hypertension and resolving immune complex glomerulonephritis in mixed connective tissue disease. *Am J Med* 65:855, 1978.

Kleiger RE, Boxer M, Ingham RE, et al: Pulmonary hypertension in patients using oral contraceptives: A report of six cases. *Chest* 69:143, 1976.

Lebrec D, Capron JP, Dhumeaux D, et al: Pulmonary hypertension complicating portal hypertension. *Am Rev Respir Dis* 120:849, 1979.

Lew W, Karliner JJ: Assessment of pulmonary valve echogram in normal subjects and in patients with pulmonary arterial hypertension. *Br Heart J* 42:147, 1979.

Lupi-Herrera E, Bialostozky D, Sobrino A: The role of isoproterenol in pulmonary artery hypertension of unknown etiology (primary): Short- and long-term evaluation. *Chest* 79:292, 1981.

Lupi-Herrera E, Sandoval J, et al: The role of hydralazine therapy for pulmonary arterial hypertension of unknown cause. *Circulation* 65:645, 1982.

McDonnell PJ, Summer WR, Hutchins GM: Pulmonary veno-occlusive disease. Morphological changes suggesting a viral cause. *JAMA* 246:667, 1981.

Melman KL, Braunwald E: Familial pulmonary hypertension. *N Engl J Med* 269:770, 1963.

Morrison EB, Ganney FA, Eigenbrodt EH, et al: Severe pulmonary hypertension associated with macronodular (postnecrotic) cirrhosis and autoimmune phenomenon. *Am J Med* 69:513, 1980.

Packer M, Greenberg B, Massie B, et al: Deleterious effects of hydralazine in patients with pulmonary hypertension. *N Engl J Med* 306:1326, 1982.

Perloff JK: Auscultatory and phonocardiographic manifestations of pulmonary hypertension. *Prog Cardiovasc Dis* 9:303, 1967.

Reitz BA, Wallwork JL, Hunt SA, et al: Heart-lung transplantation: Successful therapy for patients with pulmonary vascular disease. *N Engl J Med* 306:557, 1982.

Rubin LJ, Handel F, Peter RH: The effects of oral hydralazine on right ventricular end-diastolic pressure in patients with right ventricular failure. *Circulation* 65:1369, 1982.

Rubin LJ, Peter RH: Oral hydralazine therapy for primary pulmonary hypertension. *N Engl J Med* 320:69, 1980.

Ruskin JN, Hutter AM Jr: Primary pulmonary hypertension treated with oral phentolamine. *Ann Intern Med* 90:772, 1979.

Salerni R, Rodman GP, Leon DG, et al: Pulmonary hypertension in the CREST syndrome variant of progressive systemic sclerosis (scleroderma). *Ann Intern Med* 86:394, 1977.

Santini D, Fox D, Kloner RA, et al: Pulmonary hypertension in systemic lupus erythematosus: Hemodynamics and effects of vasodilatory therapy. *Clin Cardiol* 3:406, 1980.

Shettigar UR, Hultgren HN, Specter M, et al: Primary pulmonary hypertension: Favorable effects of isoproterenol. *N Engl J Med* 295:1414, 1976.

Sinnenberg RJ Jr: Pulmonary hypertension in pregnancy. *South Med J* 73:1529, 1980.

Vogel JHK, Grover RF, Jamieson G, et al: Long-term physiologic observations in patients with ventricular septal defect and increased pulmonary vascular resistance. *Adv Cardiol* 11:108, 1974.

Wagenvoort CA: Hypertensive pulmonary vascular disease complicating congenital heart disease: A review. *Cardiovasc Clin* 5:43, 1973.

Wagenvoort CA: Lung biopsy specimens in the evaluation of pulmonary vascular disease. *Chest* 77:614, 1980.

Wagenvoort CA, Wagenvoort N: *Pathology of pulmonary hypertension*. New York, John Wiley & Sons, 1977, p 119.

Wagenvoort CA, Wagenvoort N: Primary pulmonary hypertension: A pathologic study of the lung vessels in 156 clinically diagnosed cases. *Circulation* 42:113, 1970.

Wagenvoort CA, Wagenvoort N: Pathology of Eisenmenger syndrome and primary pulmonary hypertension. *Adv Cardiol* 11:123, 1974.

Walcott G, Burchell HB, Brown AL: Primary pulmonary hypertension. *Am J Med* 49:70, 1970.

Walker WC, Wright V: Pulmonary lesions and rheumatoid arthritis. *Medicine* 47:501, 1968.

Wood P: The Eisenmenger syndrome, or pulmonary hypertension with reversed central shunt. *B Med J* 2:755, 1958.

Yamaki S, Wagenvoort CA: Plexogenic pulmonary arteriopathy: Significance of medial thickness with respect to advanced pulmonary vascular lesions. *Am J Pathol* 105:70, 1981.

PULMONARY EMBOLISM

Samuel Z. Goldhaber

Pulmonary embolism (PE) remains one of the most difficult conditions to diagnose accurately. PE can masquerade as or silently accompany congestive heart failure or pneumonia. In elderly patients, PE can be especially difficult to detect. When appropriate treatment for PE is instituted promptly, the prognosis is excellent. However, because of the risks inherent in the therapy of PE, overdiagnosis must be avoided.

Risk Factors, Symptoms, and Signs

The risk factors for PE are so numerous and diverse that they are not very useful clinically in the diagnosis of PE in the individual patient. Some of the more commonly cited risk factors are bed rest, cancer, cardiomyopathy, chronic obstructive pulmonary disease, congestive heart failure, deep venous thrombosis, hip fracture, myocardial infarction, obesity, oral contraceptives, pregnancy, sepsis, stroke, and surgery. When the clinical features of all 327 patients in the Urokinase or Urokinase-Streptokinase Pulmonary Embolism Trials were compiled, clues to PE from history and physical examination were sparse. The three most common symptoms were dyspnea (84%), pleuritic chest pain (47%), and apprehension (59%). The three most common signs were a respiratory rate of more than 16/minute (92%), rales (58%), and an increase in the intensity of the pulmonic component of the second heart sound (53%). Unfortunately, such nonspecific signs occur frequently in many acutely ill patients. Furthermore, three classic triads were virtually absent: (1) hemoptysis, cough, and sweating; (2) hemoptysis, chest pain, and dyspnea; (3) dyspnea, chest pain, and apprehension. Other "classic" signs were also infrequent: Allen's sign— fever, tachypnea, tachycardia (23%), hemoptysis (30%), and syncope (13%). When the subset of 215 patients without preexisting cardiopulmonary disease was analyzed separately, the clinical presentation of PE was equally nonspecific. In the Framingham Heart Study, obesity among women appears to be an important long-term risk factor (Goldhaber et al.).

Laboratory Tests

In the relatively small subset of patients with acute massive PE, the electrocardiogram (ECG) and chest roentgenogram may be useful. The finding of right heart strain by ECG, with a new right axis shift, S1Q3T3 pattern, or right bundle branch block, is highly suggestive of PE. These dramatic ECG changes tend to occur only in patients with more than 50% obstruction of pulmonary vasculature angiographically. In a series of 25 patients with massive PE, Kerr et al. found oligemia in at least one pulmonary segment of the chest x-ray film in every patient. Plump hilar shadows (56%), infiltrates (56%), hyperemic pulmonary segments (40%), and elevated hemidiaphragms (32%) were also observed. Unfortunately, unless the PE is massive, electrocardiographic and radiologic abnormalities are so nonspecific they are virtually useless as diagnostic aids.

Some physicians have routinely examined fluid from pleural effusions in patients suspected of PE. However, thoracentesis increases risk and discomfort to patients, precludes the use of fibrinolytic therapy, and yields pleural fluid with nonspecific findings. Of 26 patients in one series (Bynum et al.), 65% had bloody effusions and 35% had clear effusions. White blood cell counts and differentials had a wide range of values, as did fluid protein concentrations. Only 27% of effusions had the classic pattern of bloody appearance, polymorphonuclear predominance, and exudative characteristics. Therefore, routine thoracentesis cannot be recommended in patients suspected of PE.

The search for a sensitive blood screening test has been disappointing. In 1961, the triad of elevated lactic dehydrogenase and bilirubin with normal serum glutamic oxaloacetic transaminase was found in 71% of patients with autopsy or clinical evidence of PE (Wacker et al.). In 1971, after the introduction of pulmonary angiography, Szucs et al. found this triad of blood tests was observed in only 12% of patients with angiographically documented PE. Conversely, elevated fibrin split products and other disorders of fibrin metabolism are highly sensitive for PE but tend to be found in patients with many other acute illnesses.

Recently, plasma DNA detection has been proposed as a rapid, inexpensive, and accurate screening test for PE. However, in a recent study at the Brigham and Women's Hospital by Goldhaber et al., plasma DNA was detected in only 19% of patients with PE proven by high probability lung scan, pulmonary angiogram, or autopsy.

Arterial blood gases have a limited role in screening for PE and may have been overutilized for this purpose. Hypoxemia is a nonspecific finding that can be caused by pleural disease, splinting of chest wall muscles, acute bronchitis, and small airway disease, in addition to PE. Respiratory alkalosis, a frequent finding in PE, also occurs in a wide variety of acute illnesses. Thus, abnormal arterial blood gases are too nonspecific to be useful in diagnosing PE. Conversely, arterial blood gases that demonstrate mild hypoxemia do not exclude PE, especially in young adults. In a study reported by McNeil et al., of 97 patients 18–40 years of age who were suspected clinically of having PE, those with PE had a mean PO_2 of 81 mm Hg, compared to mean PO_2 of 77 mm Hg in those without PE. In the Urokinase-Streptokinase Pulmonary Embolism Trials, more than half the patients were older than 50 years, and 10% had a PO_2 greater than 80 mm Hg (Bell et al.)

Lung Scanning and Pulmonary Angiography

Any patient suspected clinically of PE should ordinarily undergo lung scanning (Fig. 1). A diagnostic strategy has been developed by McNeil to assess the probability of

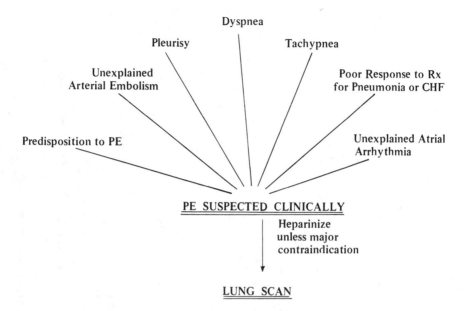

Figure 1 Initial diagnostic strategy for suspected PE.

PE using ventilation-perfusion lung scanning. Perfusion scans are usually performed with technetium-99m-iron hydroxide aggregates of human serum albumin. Xenon-133 is usually used for ventilation scans. When a perfusion scan is completely normal, clinically significant PE is excluded. When a perfusion scan shows multiple segmental or lobar defects, which ventilate normally, the probability of PE is high and pulmonary angiography can usually be obviated.

Nevertheless, a substantial group of patients (approximately 15% at the Brigham and Women's Hospital), will have multiple subsegmental defects with normal ventilation, abnormal chest roentgenograms with matching perfusion abnormalities, or single perfusion defects. Such patients have lung scans of moderate or indeterminate probability for PE. The optimal diagnostic and therapeutic strategy for these patients is controversial. Our approach, in most circumstances, is that patients with moderate or indeterminate probability scans undergo pulmonary angiography, the most accurate test for antemortem diagnosis of PE (Fig. 2). Another approach sidesteps the issue of whether PE is present and determines, instead, whether the patient has deep venous thrombosis (DVT), either by impedance plethysmography (IPG) or venography. If the physician is willing to anticoagulate such a patient, a positive IPG will be useful because of identical initial therapy (anticoagulation) for most patients with DVT or PE. The benefit of this approach is that the patient is spared the additional risk and discomfort of angiography. In a study at the West Roxbury Veterans' Administration Hospital by Sasahara et al., 90% of patients with positive IPGs had angiographically documented PEs. Conversely, in 90% of patients suspected of PE, angiography was normal when IPG was also normal. The disadvantages of this approach are: (1) the diagnosis of PE will remain uncertain, even if DVT is diagnosed; (2) even if DVT is excluded, the patient may still have PE. Furthermore, other

486

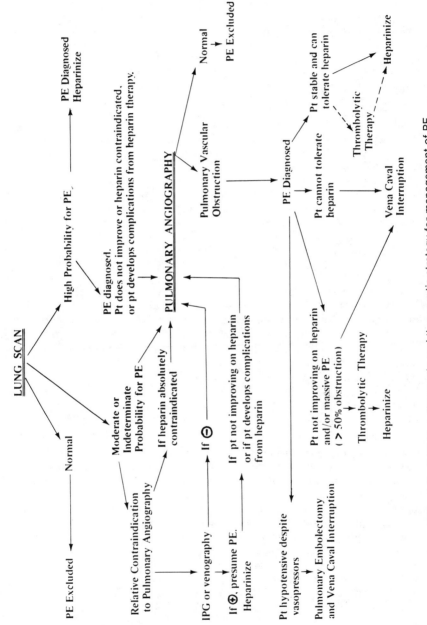

Figure 2 Definitive diagnostic and therapeutic strategy for management of PE.

investigators have found IPG to be much less sensitive and useful than did the Veterans' Administration group.

In a series of 248 pulmonary angiograms at the University of North Carolina, (Cheeley et al.), there was no mortality and a 2% serious morbidity. In 83 of the patients who were subsequently anticoagulated for angiographically documented PE and followed for an average of 11 months, 30% had significant bleeding complications, including two deaths. Approximately one-fifth of the bleeding episodes occurred during heparin therapy; the remainder occurred during chronic warfarin therapy. In 1979, Hull et al. published a study in which bleeding complications during warfarin therapy occurred in seven of 33 patients (21%); six of seven patients with bleeding had prothrombin times which were between one and a half and two times the control value, both three days or less before bleeding and at the time of bleeding. Thus, the dangers of anticoagulation outweigh the dangers of pulmonary angiography. It is especially unfortunate when bleeding complications occur in patients presumed to have PE who are subsequently found by angiography or autopsy to have no evidence whatsoever for PE.

Digital Subtraction Angiography

Digital subtraction angiography is a new approach to the diagnosis of PE. A relatively expensive computer system is integrated with existing fluoroscopic/cine radiographic apparatus to allow collection and storage of background and angiographic images. Imaging is initiated just prior to power injection of 40–70 ml of contrast material into an antecubital vein. Satisfactory images have been obtained of the cardiac chambers and pulmonary arteries. If initial studies can be confirmed, this process may eventually obviate pulmonary angiography in many clinical settings. However, it appears that digital subtraction angiography may have only limited value in identifying small peripheral pulmonary arterial emboli (Goldhaber and Markisz).

Therapy

The cardinal reason for an aggressive diagnostic approach to PE is that this illness can usually be treated successfully. Of 144 patients with angiographically documented PE at the Peter Bent Brigham Hospital, 86% survived and only 8% died with PE as a primary or secondary cause of death. The most important factor affecting mortality was shock from right ventricular failure secondary to massive PE (obstruction of more than 50% of pulmonary vasculature).

MEDICAL THERAPY

Standard therapy for patients suspected clinically of acute PE is intravenous heparin (Fig. 1). Prior to therapy, however, major contraindications to anticoagulation should be assessed and baseline stool guaiac, urine analysis, hematocrit, platelet count, prothrombin time (PT), and partial thromboplastin time (PTT) should be obtained. For average-sized adults, a heparin bolus of 5,000 units intravenously can be administered, followed by an intravenous infusion of approximately 1,000 units per hour. The infusion is usually regulated so that the patient's PTT is approximately twice the control value. A patient being treated presumptively for PE can undergo lung scanning within 24 hours to confirm or exclude the diagnosis. If PE is confirmed by lung scanning or pulmonary angiography, heparin is usually maintained for at least one week. Periodic platelet counts should be obtained because of possible immunologically-mediated heparin-induced thrombocytopenia. The hematocrit should be monitored frequently; urine and stool should also be checked routinely for occult blood. During this time, warfarin sodium can be administered orally, simultaneously with intravenous heparin. Warfarin should be given without a loading dose so that the patient's PT eventually stabilizes at approximately twice the control value. An excellent review of the science and art of using heparin has recently been published by Ryback and Handin.

For patients who can tolerate anticoagulation, the role of fibrinolytic drugs (urokinase and streptokinase) in the treatment of PE is controversial (Fig. 2). It is clear that the contraindications to thrombolytic agents are extensive (Table 1) and greatly restrict the number of patients to whom this therapy can be applied. For example, femoral arterial puncture (even with a small gauge needle) within 10 days of therapy or pulmonary angiography using the groin approach will preclude the use of these drugs. These agents may be best suited for patients with massive PE or for patients not improving rapidly on conventional heparin therapy. Detailed guidelines for the use of these drugs are provided elsewhere (Marder; Bell, Meek, Sharma et al.).

After acute anticoagulation, the duration of chronic treatment with warfarin is also controversial. Warfarin is frequently continued for six months. However, in the Urokinase-Streptokinase PE Trial, 26% of patients had a past history of PE. Of this group, 19% had a prior PE more than six months previously. These data raise ques-

Table 1. Contraindications to fibrinolytic therapy

Surgery within prior 10 days

Visceral carcinoma

Rheumatic valvular disease, severe hypertension, or subacute bacterial endocarditis

Recent trauma

Parturition within prior 10 days

Stroke within prior two months

Liver or kidney disease

GI bleeding within prior six months

Thrombocytopenia or evidence of defective hemostasis

Active tuberculosis

Ulcerative wound

Invasive procedures within prior 10 days, including liver or kidney biopsy, lumbar puncture, thoracentesis, paracentesis, intraarterial diagnostic procedure, or extensive or multiple venous cutdowns

SOURCE: From Dalen JE. The case against fibrinolytic therapy. *J Cardiovasc Med* 5: 799–814, 1980.

tions about the advisability of discontinuing oral anticoagulation routinely after six months of therapy. In patients without an obvious initiating cause for venous thrombosis or in patients whose predisposition to PE cannot be corrected (e.g., persistent massive obesity), serious consideration should be given to indefinite anticoagulation.

Chronic warfarin therapy does have substantial risk in patients with a previous episode of gastrointestinal or neurological hemorrhage. Elderly patients and alcoholics are frequently at increased risk for bleeding. For each person, the balance of benefits versus risks of anticoagulation should be weighed carefully. A special problem is warfarin's teratogenicity during the first trimester of pregnancy. Women who are pregnant or who may become pregnant should be treated chronically for PE with subcutaneous heparin. Occasionally, osteoporosis occurs following long-term heparin administration.

SURGICAL THERAPY

For patients judged to be poor candidates for anticoagulation, lung scanning should be obtained immediately. If PE is diagnosed definitively by lung scanning and pulmonary angiography, vena caval interruption is usually warranted (Fig. 2). Definitive treatment can be accomplished with an Adams-DeWeese clip placed below the renal veins. Such patients must be sufficiently stable to withstand a brief laparotomy. For poor risk patients, a Mobin-Uddin umbrella filter can be placed transvenously, with fluoroscopic guidance, through the right internal jugular vein to the inferior vena cava below the renal veins. The Kimray-Greenfield filter is becoming increasingly popular and may be technically easier to insert than the Mobin-Uddin umbrella filter. The Kimray-Greenfield filter has the advantages of potential placement from the right femoral vein as well as from the right internal jugular vein; in addition, the Kimray-Greenfield filter appears to have a higher patency rate than the Mobin-Uddin umbrella filter.

A few patients with PE will remain hypotensive despite vasopressors and anticoagulation. The prognosis of these patients, regardless of therapy, is extremely poor. In such patients, the combined operative procedures of pulmonary embolectomy and vena caval interruption may be appropriate.

Prophylaxis

PE prophylaxis has focused on preventing DVT, the most frequent source of PE. To diagnose DVT, the two most frequently used noninvasive tests are impedance plethysmography (IPG) and iodine-125-labeled fibrinogen scanning. IPG can identify accurately most venous thrombi proximal to the calf veins. The radionuclide fibrinogen scan is very accurate for assessment of calf vein thrombi, but is insensitive for diagnosing the clinically more important DVT of the iliac and femoral veins. Although replacement of venography with a combination of impedance plethysmography (for DVT above the knee) and iodine-125-fibrinogen scanning (for calf vein thrombi) has been advocated, venography remains the most accurate test for diagnosing DVT and is used routinely at the Brigham and Women's Hospital.

In 1975, investigators in the International Multicenter Trial, involving 4,121 patients, reported a significant reduction in PE as a primary cause of postoperative death, by using "minidose" heparin; 5,000 units subcutaneously two hours preoperatively and then every eight hours for at least seven days. Since then, a consensus has been reached that low-dose heparin is ineffective in DVT prophylaxis for surgical patients undergoing femoral fracture repair, hip and knee joint reconstruction, and open prostatectomy. However, for patients undergoing major elective abdominal or thoracic surgery, the Council on Thrombosis of the American Heart Association has recommended the prophylactic administration of heparin 5,000 units subcutaneously preoperatively and then every 12 hours until hospital discharge.

Much research needs to be devoted to the many questions surrounding DVT prophylaxis. For example, in patients undergoing total hip replacement, aspirin 0.6 grams twice daily decreased the occurrence of venographically documented postoperative DVT in men but unexpectedly showed no protective effect in women. In nonsurgical patients, the optimal regimen to prevent DVT remains uncertain. Finally, mechanical prophylaxis against DVT with electrical muscle stimulation intraoperatively, graded compression stockings, and external pneumocompression of the legs appears promising but will require further evaluation. Mechanical prophylaxis may be especially useful for patients undergoing intracranial or intraspinal surgery, where prophylactic anticoagulation carries an unacceptably high risk.

Conclusion

In diagnosing PE, careful history and physical examination should be followed by lung scanning, and at times, pulmonary angiography. Perhaps because of increased physician awareness and technological advances, hospital diagnosis of PE increased during the 1970s. The optimal treatment of PE necessitates frequent laboratory monitoring to minimize the risks of anticoagulation. A high clinical suspicion of PE in combination with appropriate reliance on medical technology should minimize the mortality rate from this elusive disease.

Bibliography

Alpert JS, Smith R, Carlson J, et al: Mortality in patients treated for pulmonary embolism. *JAMA* 236:1477, 1976.

Alpert JS, Smith RE, Ockene IS, et al: Treatment of massive pulmonary embolism: The role of pulmonary embolectomy. *Am Heart J* 89:413, 1975.

Bell WR, Meek AG: Guidelines for the use of thrombolytic agents. *N Engl J Med* 301:1266, 1979.

Bell WR, Simon TL, DeMets DL: The clinical features of submassive and massive pulmonary emboli. *Am J Med* 62:355, 1977.

Bynum LJ, Wilson JE III: Characteristics of pleural effusions associated with pulmonary embolism. *Arch Intern Med* 136:159, 1976.

Cheely R, McCartney WH, Perry JR, et al: The role of noninvasive tests versus pulmonary angiography in the diagnosis of pulmonary embolism. *Am J Med* 70:17, 1981.

Couch NP, Baldwin SS, Crane C: Mortality and morbidity rates after inferior vena caval clipping. *Surgery* 77:106, 1975.

Council on Thrombosis of the American Heart Association: Prevention of venous thromboembolism in surgical patients by low-dose heparin. *Circulation* 55:423A, 1977.

Crummy AB, Strother CM, Sackett JF, et al: Computerized fluoroscopy: Digital subtraction for intravenous angiocardiography and arteriography. *A J R* 135:1131, 1980.

Goldhaber SZ, Hennekens CH, Evans DA, et al: Factors associated with the correct antemortem diagnosis of major pulmonary embolism. *Am J Med* 104:325, 1982.

Goldhaber SZ, Hennekens CH, Markisz JA, et al: Low sensitivity of plasma DNA in screening for pulmonary embolism. *Am Rev Respir Dis* 126:360, 1982.

Goldhaber SZ, Hennekens CH: Time trends in hospital mortality and diagnosis of pulmonary embolism. *Am Heart J* 104:305, 1982.

Goldhaber SZ, Markisz J: Digital subtraction pulmonary angiography: An internist's and radiologist's view. *Cardiovasc Intervent Radiol* 1983 (in press).

Goldhaber SZ, Savage DD, Garrison RJ, et al: Risk factors for pulmonary embolism: The Framingham Study. *Am J Med* 74:1023, 1983.

Harris WH, Salzman EW, Athanasoulis CA, et al: Aspirin prophylaxis of venous thromboembolism after total hip replacement. *N Engl J Med* 297:1246, 1977.

Hull R, Hirsh J, Sackett DL, et al: Replacement of venography in suspected venous thrombosis by impedance plethysmography and I-125-fibrinogen leg scanning. *Ann Intern Med* 94:12, 1981.

Hull R, Delmore T, Genton E, et al: Warfarin sodium versus low-dose heparin in the long-term treatment of venous thrombosis. *N Engl J Med* 301:855, 1979.

Kerr IH, Simon G, Sutton GC: The value of the plain radiograph in acute massive pulmonary embolism. *Br J Radiol* 44:751, 1971.

International Multicentre Trial: Prevention of fatal postoperative pulmonary embolism by low doses of heparin. *Lancet* 2:45, 1975.

Marder VJ: The use of thrombolytic agents: Choice of patient, drug administration, laboratory monitoring. *Ann Intern Med* 90:802, 1979.

McNeil BJ: A diagnostic strategy using ventilation-perfusion studies in patients suspect for pulmonary embolism. *J Nucl Med* 17:613, 1976.

McNeil BJ: Ventilation-perfusion studies and the diagnosis of pulmonary embolism: Concise communication. *J Nucl Med* 21:319, 1980.

McNeil BJ, Hessel SJ, Branch WT, et al: Measures of clinical efficacy. III. The value of the lung scan in the evaluation of young patients with pleuritic chest pain. *J Nucl Med* 17:163, 1976.

Mobin-Uddin K, Callard GM, Bolooki H, et al: Transvenous caval interruption with umbrella filter. *N Engl J Med* 286:55, 1972.

Rickman FD, Handin R, Howe JP, et al: Fibrin split products in acute pulmonary embolism. *Ann Intern Med* 79:664, 1973.

Robin ED: Overdiagnosis and overtreatment of pulmonary embolism: The emperor may have no clothes. *Ann Intern Med* 87:775, 1977.

Romhilt DW, Holmes JC, Fowler NO: Mimicry in pulmonary embolism. *Geriatrics* 27:73, 1972.

Rybak ME, Handin RI: The science and art of using heparin. *J Cardiovasc Med* 6:265, 1981.

Sasahara AA, Dalen JE: Should fibrinolytic drugs be used to treat acute pulmonary embolism? *J Cardiovasc Med* 5:793, 1980.

Sasahara AA, Sharma GVRK, Parisi AF: New developments in the detection and prevention of venous thromboembolism. *Am J Cardiol* 43:1214, 1979.

Sharma GVRK, Cella, G, Parisi AF, et al: Thrombolytic therapy. *N Engl J Med* 306:1268, 1982.

Sipes JN, Suratt PM, Teates CD, et al: A prospective study of plasma DNA in the diagnosis of pulmonary embolism. *Am Rev Respir Dis* 118:475, 1978.

Szucs MM, Brooks HL, Grossman W, et al: Diagnostic sensitivity of laboratory findings in acute pulmonary embolism. *Ann Intern Med* 74:161, 1971.

Wacker WEC, Rosenthal M, Snodgrass PJ, et al: A triad for the diagnosis of pulmonary embolism and infarction. JAMA 178:108, 1961.

Young AE, Henderson BA, Phillips DA, et al: Impedance plethysmography: Its limitations as a substitute for phlebography. *Cardiovasc Radiol* 1:233, 1978.

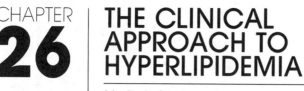

CHAPTER 26 | THE CLINICAL APPROACH TO HYPERLIPIDEMIA

Neil J. Stone

Knowledge of lipid (fat) and lipoprotein metabolism is important for understanding atherosclerosis and the clinical outcomes of angina pectoris, myocardial infarction, intermittent claudication, and thrombotic brain infarction. The hallmark of the atherosclerotic fibrous plaque is intra- and extracellular lipid deposited within and among smooth muscle cells and matrix elements of the vessel wall. Since lipids are insoluble in plasma water, they must be conveyed among intestine, liver, and peripheral tissues on macromolecules known as *lipoproteins*. Lipoproteins have in common an outer solubilizing coat of phospholipid, apoproteins (proteins that direct each lipoprotein to its metabolic site through interactions with either enzymes or cellular receptors), and free cholesterol and an inner oily core of lipids—cholesteryl ester and triglyceride in varying proportions. Either overproduction of lipoproteins or interference with their efficient removal systems can result in excess body cholesterol and accelerated atherosclerosis.

This chapter will present a rational approach to lipid and lipoprotein disorders. First, definitions and a brief overview of lipid metabolism will be presented. Next will follow a consideration of lipids and lipoproteins as risk factors for coronary heart disease (CHD). Then a practical approach to testing and classification will be given. After a description of familial syndromes of hyperlipoproteinemia, a rational approach to therapy will conclude this chapter.

Definitions and Lipid/Lipoprotein Metabolism

Cholesterol was discovered in bile by Chevreul in 1816, hence, *chole* meaning "bile" and *steros* meaning "solid." It has the multiring nuclear structure of the steroid family and is used for adrenal hormones and vitamin D. Unesterified or free cholesterol is used as a structural component of plasma membranes. Most tissues synthesize cholesterol, but in humans this occurs chiefly in the liver and intestine. Cholesterol concentrations in the plasma are tightly regulated by removal processes keyed to specific liver and extrahepatic cell receptors. These receptors bind and degrade the lipoproteins and internalize the cholesterol that can be used for cellular needs and also down-regulate cholesterol synthesis. Cholesterol is cleared from the body by excretion into bile or conversion to bile acids. Triglycerides consist of long chain fatty acids attached to a glycerol backbone. Since they provide 9 kcal/gram of energy, triglycerides are an economical means of energy storage.

Table 1. Composition and Metabolism of Lipoproteins in man

Weight (S_f values)	Size (relative size)	Name (origin)	Major Core/Surface Components	Interacts with	Fate
400	750–12,000 Å	Chylomicrons (gut)	Triglyceride/A, B (only 2% cholesterol)	Lipoprotein Lipase (C$_{II}$ as cofactor)	Triglyceride load to adipose stores. Chylo remnants carry Cholesterol/apo B to liver to modulate hepatic cholesterol synthesis.
100	300–700 Å	Very low density lipoproteins (VLDL) (liver, gut)	Triglyceride/B, E, C (only 15% cholesterol)	Lipoprotein Lipase (C$_{II}$ as co-factor)	Remodeled in plasma to intermediate density lipoprotein, then to form LDL.

S_f				
20	Low density lipoproteins (LDL) (from VLDL) 180–300 A	Cholesterol/B LDL carry about $\frac{2}{3}$ of total plasma cholesterol	High affinity cell receptors	LDL receptor degrades LDL, internalizes cholesterol, and regulates cell cholesterol synthesis.
0	High density lipoproteins (HDL) Nascent HDL secreted as discs (liver, gut) ↓ LCAT (apo A1) spherical HDL 50–120 A	Cholesterol/A, C, E	VLDL and chylomicrons during lipemic tides to provide apo C's needed for metabolism. Cholesterol from cell membranes, lipoproteins.	During triglyceride rich lipoprotein catabolism, HDL regenerated. Esterifies free cholesterol; Delivers it to liver, adrenals.

SOURCE: Stone NJ, Green D: Sustaining factors in atherosclerosis, in Moran, JM, Michealis LL (eds): *Surgery for the Complications of Myocardial Infarction*. New York, Grune & Stratton, 1980, pp. 47–66; and Fredrickson DS, Goldstein JL, Brown MS: The familial hyperlipoproteinemias, in Stanbury JB, Wyngaarden JB, Frederickson DS (eds): *The Metabolic Basis of Inherited Disease*, New York, McGraw-Hill, 1978, pp. 604–655.

S_f values from analytical ultracentrifuge.

LCAT is lecithin-cholesterol-acyltransferase.

apo is short from apolipoprotein; apo C stands for all apo C's (I, II, III).

The lipoproteins found normally in humans can be thought of as triglyceride-laden *chylomicrons* and very low density lipoproteins (VLDL) and cholesterol-laden chylomicron remnants, low density lipoproteins (LDL) and high density lipoproteins (HDL) (see Tables 1 and 2). Chylomicrons convey long chain dietary glyceride to adipose tissue and muscle capillaries via the thoracic duct. There they are metabolized by lipoprotein lipase generating fatty acids, which can be incorporated into adipose tissue sites for storage or used as fuel. Chylomicron remnants remain, which are rich in cholesterol and apoprotein B and apoprotein E. These proteins permit immediate recognition by hepatic receptors, which bind and degrade the particles and function to down-regulate hepatic cholesterol synthesis.

VLDL are produced in the intestine and liver. They carry endogenous glyceride and are processed by lipoprotein lipase as well. Chylomicrons have half-lives measured in minutes and VLDL have half-lives measured in hours; this explains the marked daily variation in triglyceride levels. Carbohydrate, fatty acids (catecholamine stimulation or diabetes), basal insulin levels (obesity, estrogen use) and augmented hepatic fatty acids (alcohol use) stimulate VLDL output. Impaired clearance as in uremia, myxedema, and poorly controlled diabetes causes raised VLDL as well.

LDL are formed through the intravascular modeling of VLDL. LDL are small cholesterol-laden particles that account for two-thirds of the plasma cholesterol. The concentration of LDL is regulated by high-affinity cellular receptors on peripheral cells, which recognize apoprotein B of LDL. These LDL receptors are specified by commonly inherited genes. Inheritance of a mutant copy (or copies) can result in deficient numbers or absent LDL receptors. This leads to increasing hypercholesterolemia, as LDL is less efficiently degraded and bound, with less LDL being internalized to down-regulate cellular cholesterol synthesis. When plasma LDL levels rise, scavenger cells are needed to degrade LDL; these macrophages soon become swollen with cholesterol ester and convert to foam cells, which give rise to plaques of atherosclerosis.

The HDLs are secreted from liver and intestine and are also formed from surface materials (apoproteins, phospholipids) generated by efficient chylomicron and VLDL metabolism. HDLs serve as reservoirs of activator apoproteins, such as apoprotein CII, which are required by chylomicrons for recognition by protein lipase. HDLs acquire free cholesterol from cell surfaces or lipoproteins and esterify it through the action of lecithin cholesterol acyl transferase (LCAT), which uses apoprotein AI found on HDL. This esterified cholesterol can be returned to the liver for disposal or use in further lipoprotein synthesis. HDL cholesterol levels vary inversely with body pools of cholesterol and so elevated levels may protect against total body cholesterol overload.

Risk Factors for CHD: Which Lipid/ Lipoproteins Do You Measure?

Risk factors are those personal traits or habits that convey an increased risk of developing CHD. The statement for physicians by the American Heart Association, "Risk factors and coronary heart disease," summarizes existing data well. Elevated blood lipids, elevated blood pressure, and diabetes mellitus are the personal traits;

while cigarette smoking, dietary intake of saturated fat, obesity, sedentary living, oral contraceptive use, and the type A behavior pattern are the habits most clearly associated with enhanced risk of CHD. On the other hand, moderate coffee or alcohol intake have not been shown to increase risk of CHD.

There is substantial experimental and epidemiologic data relating serum cholesterol levels to risk of CHD (as reviewed by Stamler). First, the risk of CHD rises exponentially with serum cholesterol level. There is no upper limit at which the risk of CHD begins. In the range between 220 mg/dl to 260 mg/dl, the risk of CHD for middle-aged men and women rises several-fold. Second, serum cholesterol appears to be a weak predictor of those persons above the age of 50 inclined to CHD. Third, the highest cholesterol levels in a large scale epidemiologic study occurred in those populations with the highest intakes of saturated fat (Keys). Moreover, the relationship between saturated fat intake and CHD was a strong one. The Finns were among the most active of those studied; nonetheless, they had the highest saturated fat intake and the greatest incidence of CHD. On the other hand, those populations who consumed diets with less than 10% of calories from saturated fat had the lowest rates of CHD.

The association between triglyceride levels and CHD has been recognized as a

Table 2. Mean and Percentile Values of LDL and HDL by Age[a] (expressed in mg/dl)

Age (years)	Men			Women (no hormones)		
	5	50	95	5	50	95
LDL Cholesterol Values						
20–24	66	101	147	—	98	—
25–29	70	116	165	70	103	151
30–34	78	124	185	68	109	148
35–39	81	131	189	76	117	173
40–44	87	135	186	89	122	174
45–49	98	141	202	81	127	188
50–54	89	143	197	90	140	214
55–59	88	145	202	101	148	212
HDL Cholesterol Values						
20–24	30	45	63	—	50	—
25–29	31	44	63	37	55	81
30–34	28	45	63	38	55	75
35–39	29	43	62	34	52	82
40–44	27	43	67	34	55	87
45–49	30	45	64	33	56	86
50–54	28	44	63	37	58	89
55–59	28	46	71	36	58	86

SOURCE: Heiss et al: Lipoprotein-cholesterol distributions in selected North American populations, *Circulation* 1980;61: 302–315.

[a] From Visit 2. Random Sample. Lipid Research Clinics Survey

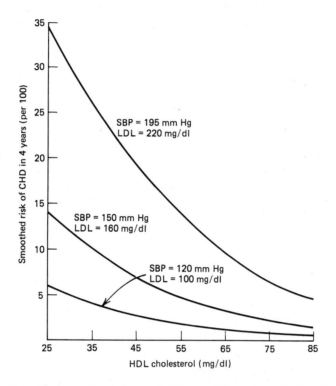

Figure 1 Risk of coronary heart disease in 55-year-old men from the Framingham Study as a function of HDL cholesterol level. (Kannel WB et al: *Ann Int Med* 1979:90; 85–91. Used with permission of American Heart Association.)

weak one for some time. A recent review (Hulley et al.) has convincingly summarized arguments holding that triglyceride levels are not independent predictors of CHD. Furthermore, it concluded that widespread screening and treatment of healthy persons for hypertriglyceridemia per se should be abandoned. This apparent departure from previous recommendations must be set in perspective; in those with a family history of either premature CHD or hyperlipidemia or both, the possibility of familial hyperlipidemia compels the determination of triglyceride levels. Some persons with elevated triglyceride may have increased apoprotein B as the major risk factor for enhanced atherosclerosis. In addition, severe hypertriglyceridemia—whether primary or secondary—predisposes to acute pancreatitis. It must be measured in those patients at risk for this problem. In patients undergoing aortocoronary bypass, hypertriglyceridemia has been found commonly in those with late developing graft atherosclerosis. Hypertriglyceridemia is also seen in diabetics and chronic dialysis patients who have excessive rates of CHD. It is still not clear whether these associations are causal or not.

High density lipoprotein cholesterol levels are powerful and independent predictors of CHD risk, especially in persons over age 50. In addition to large-scale population studies, smaller studies utilizing findings at coronary angiography as an end-point have verified the inverse association between HDL cholesterol and coronary artery disease (Havel). Even among kindred with familial hypercholesterolemia where risk of CHD occurs in proportion to LDL levels, HDL cholesterol is an independent risk indicator. Moreover, in kindred with inherited high levels of HDL, cases of CHD are infrequent.

Figure 1 shows that systolic blood pressure and LDL cholesterol level modify in an important way the prediction of CHD risk by HDL cholesterol. The clinician must realize that the entire risk profile—age, sex, blood pressure, cigarette smoking, family history of CHD, for example—must be utilized in assessing risk of CHD and not just a single risk factor. Thus, some patients with very low levels of HDL cholesterol do not invariably have premature CHD; these patients usually have low levels of LDL cholesterol as well.

Approach to Lipid/Lipoprotein Testing and Classification

Standardized sampling conditions are recommended to minimize confounding factors. Nonfasting cholesterol levels are adequate for screening purposes. A complete lipoprotein evaluation, however, should be performed after a 12–14 hour fast. Patients are counseled to minimize changes in diet and weight in the weeks before sampling. Moreover, remember that sampling in the upright position—as would be the case for outpatients—gives values 10% higher than those seen in patients sampled in the supine position—as would be the case for patients in the hospital.

What is a high cholesterol value? Figures 2 and 3 give ninety-fifth percentile limits

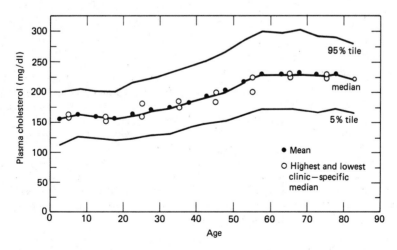

Figure 2 Plasma cholesterol for white males; mean and percentile values for 5-year age groups. LRC Program Prevalence Study Visit 1. (Used with permission of American Heart Association.)

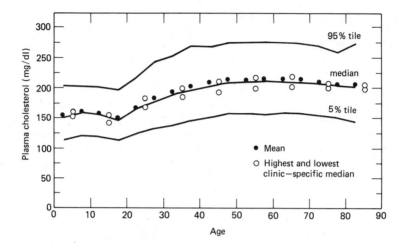

Figure 3 Plasma cholesterol for white females not taking sex hormones; mean and percentile values for 5-year age groups. LRC Program Prevalence Study Visit 1. (Used with permission of American Heart Association.)

based on age and sex. These data show the gradual increase in cholesterol levels after age 20. Please note that for those under age 20, the mean value for cholesterol is about 150 mg/dl and the ninety-fifth percentile cut-off is about 200 mg/dl. Since coronary atherosclerosis is infrequent in those populations where cholesterol values for adults are less than 200 mg/dl, values under 200 mg/dl give the lowest risk for CHD.

If a single value is elevated, it is prudent to obtain multiple samples before intervention is considered. Blackburn has shown that three or four samples substantially reduce the error in estimating the true mean. Even a single repeat value improves precision; when 326 children with elevated cholesterol values were resampled, only 58% were found to still have values exceeding the ninety-fifth percentile cut-off limits.

What is a high triglyceride value? Age and sex ninety-fifth percentile limits can be used. Some investigators require values greater than 300 mg/dl before they consider the triglyceride level to be elevated. Usually, above 300 mg/dl, the plasma is turbid (you cannot read newsprint through it). If triglyceride values exceed 1,000 mg/dl, there is often creamy plasma visible as a supernantant after overnight refrigeration at 4°C. These persons are at risk for acute pancreatitis.

How should lipoproteins be assessed? *Lipoprotein electrophoresis* has been used for almost two decades. Fredrickson, Levy, and Lees showed that lipoprotein patterns were useful in categorizing patients with clear cut disorders of lipoprotein metabolism. The phenotypes designated by electrophoretic patterns indicated lipoprotein excess, singly or in combination.

Type I   Chylomicron excess
Type IIa   LDL excess

Type IIb   LDL + VLDL excess
Type III   Intermediate density lipoprotein present
Type IV   VLDL excess
Type V   Chylomicron + VLDL excess

These rubrics are still useful shorthand notations of a person's lipoprotein status at any one time. They are not indications of genetic disease. Familial combined hyperlipidemia is a monogenic disorder, where multiple lipoprotein patterns are seen in family members as a rule. In addition, it is difficult to quantitate accurately the lipoprotein bands.

Table 3. Secondary Causes of Hyperlipidemia/Hyperlipoproteinemia

Secondary Cause	Major Lipid Change	Major Lipoprotein Change
Metabolic		
Weight gain after age 25	TG ↑↑	HDL ↓↓, VLDL ↑↑
Pregnancy	CHOL ↑↑, TG ↑↑	LDL ↑↑, HDL ↑↑, VLDL ↑↑
Exercise (distance)	CHOL ↓, TG ↓↓	LDL ↓, HDL ↑↑↑, VLDL ↓↓
After myocardial infarction	CHOL ↓, TG ↑↑	LDL ↓, HDL ↓, VLDL ↑↑
Diabetes mellitus	TG ↑↑	HDL ↓↓, VLDL ↑↑
Dietary		
Saturated fat and dietary cholesterol feeding	CHOL ↑↑	LDL ↑↑
Polyunsaturated fat feeding	CHOL ↓↓	LDL ↓↓, HDL ↓↓
High carbohydrate feeding	TG ↑↑	LDL ↓, HDL↓, VLDL ↑↑
Alcohol	TG ↑↑	HDL ↑↑, VLDL ↑↑
Medications		
Estrogens	TG ↑↑	HDL ↑↑, VLDL ↑↑
Steroids (high dose)	TG ↑↑↑	Chylomicrons, VLDL ↑↑
Thiazides/propranolol	TG ↑↑	HDL ↓↓, VLDL ↑↑
Chlorthalidone	CHOL ↑↑	LDL↑↑
Oral hypoglycemic agents		HDL ↓↓
Insulin	TG ↓↓	HDL ↑↑, VLDL ↓↓
Androgens	CHOL ↑↑	LDL ↑↑, HDL ↓↓,
Cigarette smoking	CHOL ↓	HDL ↓↓
Diseases		
Hypothyroidism	CHOL ↑↑, TG ↑	LDL ↑↑, HDL ↓, VLDL ↑
Nephrosis (mild)	CHOL ↑↑	LDL ↑↑, HDL ↓
Nephrosis (severe) (albumin less than 1 gm/dl)	CHOL ↑↑, TG ↑↑↑	LDL ↑↑, HDL ↓↓, VLDL ↑↑↑
Chronic renal failure (with or without dialysis)	TG ↑↑	HDL ↓↓, VLDL ↑↑
Obstructive liver disease	CHOL ↑↑	LDL ↑↑
Porphyria	CHOL ↑	LDL ↑↑
Pancreatitis	TG ↑↑↑↑	Chylomicrons

↑↑, increased; ↓↓, decreased
CHOL, cholesterol; TG, triglycerides

Measurement of HDL cholesterol is now the preferred addition to the measurement of total cholesterol and triglyceride levels. HDL cholesterol values are widely available, due to a precipitation method that measures cholesterol in the supranatant, after LDL and VLDL are precipitated by polyanions, such as heparin-manganese. The HDL cholesterol values so obtained can be inserted into the following formula:

$$\text{LDL cholesterol} = \text{total cholesterol} - (\text{HDL cholesterol} + \text{triglyceride}/5)$$

This formula is valid if the triglyceride level is less than 400 mg/dl and the rare intermediate density lipoprotein—as seen in familial type III—is not present.

Lipid and lipoprotein assessment is not complete until family screening has been accomplished, and secondary causes have been ruled out. Table 3 lists the common metabolic conditions, dietary factors, medications, and diseases responsible for hyperlipidemia. To avoid pitfalls in lipid assessment, it is important to determine foods consumed away from home, uncover estrogen use, which is often not regarded as medication, and adequately appraise thyroid status. Hypothyroidism can be subtle in the older person; tests of thyroid function should be performed always in the evaluation of hyperlipidemia.

A useful clinical classification is given in Table 4. It segregates lipid and lipoprotein patterns into three easily recognizable groups. In group A are those with *hypercho-*

Table 4. Classification of Hyperlipoproteinemia

Group A	Hypercholesterolemia only
Phenotypes:	2a
Primary:	Familial hypercholesterolemia, polygenic hypercholesterolemia
Secondary:	Dietary saturated fat and cholesterol excess, hypothyroidism, obstructive liver disease, mild nephrosis, porphyria
Caveat:	HDL cholesterol needed to determine if hypercholesterolemia owing to LDL excess
Group B	Mild-moderate hypertriglyceridemia or low HDL cholesterol (or both)
Phenotypes:	2b, 3, 4 or values for HDL cholesterol below 5 percentile cutoffs
Primary:	Familial combined hyperlipidemia, familial hypertriglyceridemia, familial dysbetalipoproteinemia
Secondary:	Adult onset weight gain, pregnancy, diabetes, chronic renal failure, severe nephrosis, estrogen therapy, diuretic therapy, steroid therapy, excessive use of alcohol, myxedema
Caveat:	Alcohol ingestion causes increased triglyceride and a rise in HDL cholesterol. Most secondary causes are associated with hypertriglyceridemia and a decline in HDL cholesterol
Group C	Severe hypertriglyceridemia (triglycerides exceed 1,000 mg/dl)
Phenotypes:	1, 5
Primary:	Familial chylomicronemia, familial mixed hyperlipoproteinemia
Secondary:	Diabetic lipemia, chronic high dose steroid therapy, pancreatitis, myxedema, excessive use of alcohol, estrogen therapy (especially in an obese women with mild type 4), SLE
Caveat:	Use chylomicron test for diagnosis. Observe cold plasma kept upright at 4°C; creamy supranatant indicates the presence of chylomicrons

lesterolemia alone. These patients require HDL cholesterol measurements to see if excess LDL cholesterol is present. In group B are those with *mild-moderate hypertriglyceridemia or low HDL cholesterol or both*. This pattern is quite common. In group C are those patients with severe *hypertriglyceridemia*. The plasma is creamy and the triglyceride level exceeds 1,000 mg/dl. This is not commonly seen. The diagnosis can be made by observing a substantial cream layer in upright cold plasma.

Syndromes of Familial Hyperlipoproteinemia

Studies of single cases of hyperlipidemia can not always identify those with familial syndromes. Only one in five with lipid levels elevated above ninety-fifth percentile cut-offs is found to have monogenic hyperlipidemia. An enriched sample of cases of familial hyperlipidemia is found in survivors of myocardial infarction (MI) under age 60 (as reported by Goldstein et al.). In this group, one out of five survivors is found to have a simply inherited form of hyperlipidemia. These are given in Table 5. A useful routine for pediatricians is to perform lipid tests on children whose family histories disclose myocardial infarction (MI) before age 60.

Familial hypercholesterolemia (FH) is inherited as an autosomal dominant trait with a high degree of penetrance. Heterozygotes have a single dose of a mutant allele specifying a receptor protein with either absent or defective binding or faulty internalization. In the United States, the minimum gene frequency is estimated at 1 in 225. Among survivors of MI under age 60, the frequency of FH (heterozygous form) is 4.1%. Homozygous cases have a double dose of one of the mutant alleles or rarely, have two differing mutant alleles with the same result; LDL binding and internalization is markedly impaired, preventing normal feedback of cholesterol synthesis by peripheral cells. These cases are rare; the gene frequency for homozygous FH is one in one million.

Heterozygous FH is diagnosed when LDL levels exceed 5% cut-off levels and similar degrees of LDL excess are seen in first degree relatives. Tendon xanthomas are seen in about 80% of cases. They characteristically involve the Achilles tendons and the tendons overlying the metacarpals (see Figs. 4 and 5). Many patients recall episodes of acute tendinitis in their teens.

The typical case of heterozygous FH has a cholesterol level of 350–450 mg/dl. In adults with FH, the most rigid restriction of dietary cholesterol and saturated fat fails to lower total cholesterol values below 300 mg/dl. Recognition of the heterozygous form of FH is important because of the predilection for premature CHD. In Framingham, only six subjects of the original cohort of 5,127 had cholesterol values exceeding 400 mg/dl and detectable xanthomas. All of these subjects had strong family histories of CHD and subsequently died of CHD before age 50.

Observations of 116 kindred with FH followed at the National Institute of Health further documented the striking risk of CHD (Stone et al., 1974). For those with the FH trait, 29.5% were found to have CHD, as compared to only 10.5% of adult relatives without the FH trait. The expectation of CHD by age 40 for affected male relatives was one in six; by age 60 it was more than one in two. When compared with nonaffected men in the same kindred, it was as if risk of CHD had developed

Table 5. Familial Forms of Hyperlipidemia Associated with an Increased Risk of CHD

Disorder	Age at Onset	Xanthomas	Characteristic (mg/dl)			Other
			Chol	Trig	CHD Risk	
Familial hypercholesterolemia		Tendon, tuberous				
Heterozygotes	Childhood	Occur in 80% or more	350	100	+ + + +	Common; 1 in 225
Homozygotes	Childhood	Onset before age 10	700	100	+ + + + +	Rare; 1 in one million
Familial combined hyperlipidemia	Adulthood	Not seen	300	275	+ + +	Commonest monogenic lipid disorder in MI survivors (11.3%)
			multiple lipid abnormalities or lipoprotein types seen			
Familial hypertriglyceridemia	Adulthood	Eruptive xanthomas (only in most severe cases)	250	350	+	Seen in 5% of MI survivors
Familial dysbetalipoproteinemia	Adulthood	Palmar and digital crease Tuboeruptive	450	500	+ + +	Rare; early peripheral vascular disease common
Polygenic hypercholesterolemia	Adulthood	No xanthomas	300	100	+ +	Family studies are needed for diagnosis

Chol, cholesterol; Trig, triglyceride; MI, myocardial infarction

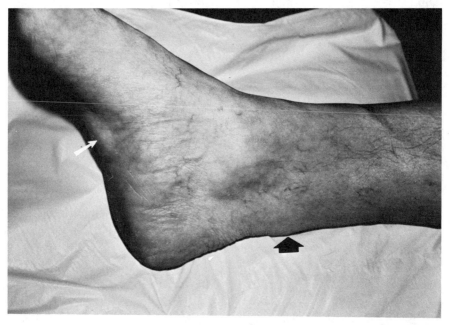

Figure 4 Achilles and flexor hallicus longus tendon xanthomas (arrows) in a patient with heterozygous FH.

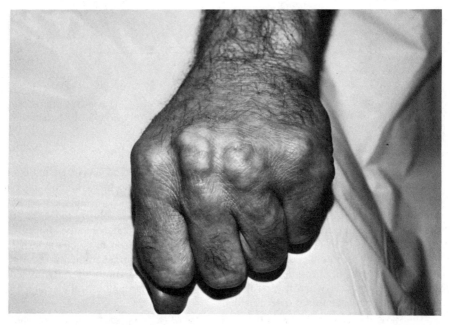

Figure 5 Extensor tendon xanthomas occurring in tendons overlying the metacarpals in a patient with heterozygous FH.

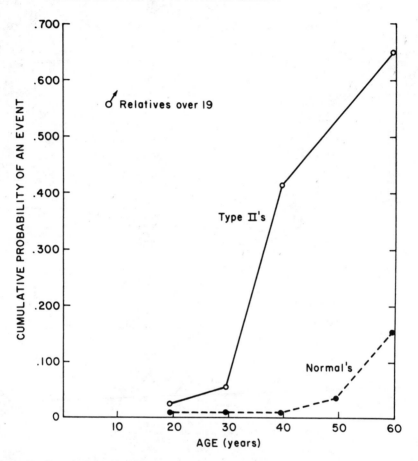

Figure 6 Cumulative probability by decade of fatal or nonfatal CAD events in first-degree male relatives with heterozygous FH. (Stone NJ et al: *Circulation* 49:476, 1974. Used with permission of American Heart Association.)

20 years prior to that expected (Fig. 6). Although CHD occurred less often and later in women as compared to men, affected female relatives also had a greater expectation of CHD after age 45 (Fig. 7).

Homozygous FH is diagnosed when cholesterol and LDL levels are twice that of the parents who are obligate heterozygotes. The serum cholesterol values for cases typically ranges from 600–1,000 mg/dl. Homozygous children have characteristic interdigital web xanthomas and tuberous and tendon xanthomas. When untreated, these lesions are quite prominent by age 10. Arcus corneae is not uniformly present in such children. Yet when it is visible in young caucasian children under age 15, cholesterol levels should be determined.

Homozygous children have distinctive cardiovascular findings. Basal systolic murmurs are invariably heard; with time, they progress to represent hemodynamically significant aortic stenosis. The aortic valve stenosis is unique and is due to intracellular lipid infiltration of the aortic cusps. In one case with a peak systolic gradient of 108 mm Hg, atherosclerotic plaquing was found to extend from the higher part of the sinuses of Valsalva to the aortic ring. In these cases there is almost always greater plaquing in the ascending aorta as compared to the abdominal aorta—the reverse of the usual situation. Coronary disease is often rapidly progressive in the untreated. Sequential studies in an 11-year-old homozygous boy documented complete occlusion of a previously patent right and left anterior descending artery in a two-year period of time. Of interest is the observation that atherosclerotic plaques have been noted in the pulmonary arteries; usually atherosclerosis is not seen in this low pressure circuit.

Familial combined hyperlipidemia is the newest monogenic lipid disorder to be described. It is the commonest genetic lipid disorder found among survivors of MI under age 60. In the Seattle study, 11.3% of young survivors were so affected. It is inherited as an autosomal dominant trait. The exact mechanism is not known. The disorder is usually expressed in adulthood, unlike FH, which can be detected from birth. Affected persons commonly have elevations of both cholesterol and triglyceride levels. The hypercholesterolemia is usually mild, however; and xanthomas are not seen. The diagnosis is made by observing many types of lipid excess in members of successive generations. Hypertriglyceridemia is commonly seen in affected members. In one small study, five relatives with this disorder had MI between the ages of 40 and 50 and five before age 40. Elevated apoB may be a useful marker.

Familial Type III or familial dysbetalipoproteinemia is a rare disorder. It was noted only once among 500 survivors of MI from Seattle. It is due to deficiency of a specific apoprotein E subclass (E3), with elevated total apoprotein E levels and the presence

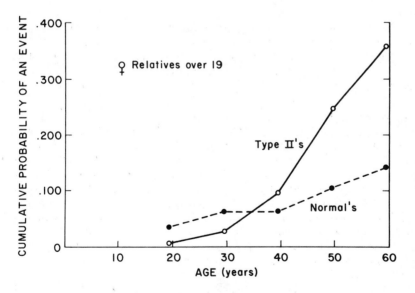

Figure 7   Cumulative probability by decade of fatal or nonfatal CAD events in first-degree female relatives with heterozygous FH. (Stone NJ et al: *Circulation* 49:476, 1974. Used with permission of American Heart Association.)

of an abnormal lipoprotein—the intermediate density lipoprotein (IDL). IDL results from the impaired conversion of VLDL to LDL in plasma. Estrogen therapy, which is one of the commonest causes of raised VLDL in young women, paradoxically improves the hypertriglyceridemia in this condition by enhancing VLDL removal.

Diagnosis requires sophisticated laboratory testing. The distribution of isoforms of apoprotein E should be determined; E2:E2 indicates dysbetalipoproteinemia. Additional suggestive laboratory findings are: (1) a VLDL cholesterol/VLDL triglyceride ratio exceeding 0.42; (2) a VLDL cholesterol/total triglyceride exceeding 0.3; and (3) elevated apoprotein E levels. For the clinician, a high index of suspicion is required for diagnosis. Important clues are the presence of premature CHD and peripheral vascular disease in a young man; tuboeruptive xanthomas, which look like sealing wax over extensor surfaces; digital crease and palmar xanthomas; and markedly elevated, but almost equal, levels of cholesterol and triglyceride. The peripheral vascular disease appears to respond to specific hypolipidemic therapy, so correct diagnosis is rewarding.

Familial Type IV or Familial Hypertriglyceridemia (FHTG) was identified in 5.2% of survivors of MI under age 60 in Seattle. It has an autosomal dominant mode of inheritance and is expressed in adulthood. Genetic and clinical studies of FHTG are impaired, however, by absence of distinguishing clinical features. When secondary causes of hypertriglyceridemia occur in several family members, FHTG can be simulated. In one study, relatives with FHTG did not show an increased frequency of MI as compared to control groups.

Should Lipid Levels Be Lowered?

To date, there is no rigorous proof that lowering lipid levels causes decreased progression or regression of atherosclerosis. Studies in rhesus monkeys have shown that regression with hypolipidemic therapy occurs; yet small scale clinical trials completed over the past two decades have given conflicting results. Two reviews of these trials emphasize flaws in trial design and/or preselection bias as possible sources for error (Ahrens; Cornfield and Mitchell).

The recently completed World Health Organization clofibrate trial did show that treated hypercholesterolemic men had an overall decreased incidence of nonfatal CHD as contrasted with men on placebo. Total mortality was not lowered, however, due to an increased mortality from noncardiovascular causes in those on the drug clofibrate. A diet trial from Oslo involved men aged 40–49 with cholesterol values of 290–380 mg% who were randomized into an intervention group (low saturated fat diet plus decreased cigarette smoking) and a control group. The treated group showed a significant lowering of MI and sudden death (Hjerman et al.). In addition, diet alone lowered cholesterol 13%. Analysis showed that cholesterol lowering was more potent than decreased smoking in determining the improved cardiovascular endpoints. This suggests the value of hypolipidemic therapy in middle-aged hypercholesterolemic men.

Finally, Blankenhorn et al., utilizing angiographic methods graded by computer technique, have shown regression of early lesions of the femoral arteries of human subjects who have effective lipid and blood pressure lowering. Moreover, lower lipid levels were associated with more rapid regression. Other large scale lipid intervention trials are near completion and should offer additional information on the value of lipid lowering in selected groups of patients.

A Rational Approach to Dietary and Drug Therapy See Table 6.

One dietary approach is to recommend a single diet with restriction of total fat, saturated fat, dietary cholesterol, total calories, simple sugars, and salt. Another approach is to tailor the diet to the patient. For those with hypercholesterolemia due to elevated LDL, the key step is to curtail intake of saturated fat and, perhaps less importantly, dietary cholesterol. Polyunsaturated fats do lower serum cholesterol levels, but they are only half as potent at changing serum cholesterol values as reducing saturated fats. Excessive use of polyunsaturated fats can lead to weight gain, gallstones, and possibly lowered HDL cholesterol. Practical pointers are to advise patients to read labels and avoid products with cocoa butter, palm oil, and coconut oil. These are potent saturated fats, which elevate serum cholesterol. Foods very high in dietary cholesterol, such as liver, shellfish, and egg yolks, should be restricted. Skim milk can be used instead of whole milk. Beef, pork, and lamb should be used sparingly, and the diet should have more chicken and fish. Egg white is an excellent source of albumin and its use should be encouraged. Vegetarians have markedly lower values for total and LDL cholesterol as compared with matched controls; this kind of a diet will give optimal dietary results.

Those patients with mild to moderate hypertriglyceridemia, often associated with a low HDL cholesterol, should begin with caloric restriction to attain ideal body weight. In some patients, especially those with type III, HDL cholesterol will rise concomitantly. The diet for those at ideal body weight should stress complex carbohydrate and restriction of alcohol and simple sugars. Diets high in carbohydrate do not elevate triglyceride when the source of the carbohydrate is not simple sugar. Alcohol does appear to elevate HDL cholesterol levels, but it cannot be recommended for this purpose.

For those with severe hypertriglyceridemia, the key dietary maneuver is to restrict total fat, often to less than 5–10 grams per day. Those patients with chylomicron excess alone are managed with a very low fat diet. For those with additional VLDL excess, the initial dietary maneuver is weight reduction to ideal weight and then a maintenance diet with avoidance of alcohol, simple sugars, and high fat foods.

Exercise is a useful adjunct to therapy in all groups with hyperlipidemia. It lowers triglyceride and raises HDL cholesterol. This is seen in middle-aged runners and even those patients recovered from MI participating in cardiac rehabilitation programs.

Hypolipidemic drug therapy is required for persons at substantial risk for premature CHD or acute pancreatitis. In the former category are those with diet-resistant familial hypercholesterolemia and familial combined hyperlipidemia and, possibly, patients with documented coronary atherosclerosis and/or peripheral artery atherosclerosis and diet-resistant lipid elevations. In the later category are those patients with triglyceride values above 800 mg/dl in whom a genetic abnormality

Table 6.   Treatment Plans Based on Type of Lipoprotein Overload

Group A	Hypercholesterolemia only: (Type 2a)		
	Dietary:	Restrict:	Cholesterol to less than 300 mg/day
			Saturated fat to less than 10% of calories
		Add:	Polyunsaturated fat for table and cooking fat; do not overdo—keep P/S at 1/1
	Medication:	Drug of choice:	Bile acid sequestering resins such as colestipol and cholestyramine
		Others:	Nicotinic acid
			D-thyroxine
			Probucol
			Neomycin
			Paraminosalicylic acid-C
Group B	Mild-moderate hypertriglyceridemia or low HDL cholesterol (or both) (Types 2b, 3, 4)		
	Dietary:	Restrict:	Calories to achieve ideal body weight
			Alcohol to one drink daily (1 oz hard liquor
			1 glass wine
			1 can of beer)
			Cholesterol to less than 300 mg/day
			Saturated fat to less than 10% of calories
		Add:	Polyunsaturated fat for table and cooking fat; do not overdo—keep P/S at 1/1
	Exercise:	Important adjunct to diet; distance run is best	
	Medication:	Drug of choice:	Nicotinic acid
		Others:	Clofibrate, Gemfibrozil
Group C	Severe hypertriglyceridemia (Triglycerides exceed 1,000 mg/dl) (Types 1, 5)		
	Dietary:	Restrict:	Total fat calories to 25 grams or less/day
			Calories to achieve ideal body weight
			Alcohol—best avoided
	Medication:	Drug of choice:	Nicotinic acid
		Others:	Clofibrate, Gemfibrozil
			Norethindrone acetate

predisposing to hypertriglyceridemia often coincides with diabetes, obesity, estrogen or steroid therapy, or excessive use of alcohol.

There are several guidelines that must be followed for effective and safe therapy. First, use medications that have a wide therapeutic/toxic ratio; therapy is supportive, not curative, and must be given chronically. Second, continue effective medications and promptly stop those that are not. Two or three baseline samples provide pre-treatment mean values that can be compared to a treatment value obtained four to six weeks after therapy is started. As a rule of thumb, require a 15% reduction of lipid values if therapy at the current dosage level is to continue. If this is not achieved, the dosage should be increased or an alternate therapy is required. Third, check periodically for side effects. Fourth, watch for a waning of drug efficacy with time; consider dietary as well as medication lapse.

For those with LDL excess, the bile-sequestering resins, either cholestyramine or colestipol, are the drugs of choice. These resins bind bile salts in the intestine, preventing their reabsorption and enterohepatic recirculation while promoting their fecal excretion. Cholesterol and LDL levels fall, while triglyceride values rise slightly. The cholesterol content in relation to apoprotein B is diminished, suggesting that resin therapy may lessen the delivery of cholesterol to peripheral cells. Also, resins appear to promote LDL catabolism via its specific receptor clearance pathway.

The usual dose for cholestyramine is 16–24 grams per day and for colestipol is 20–30 grams per day. These can be given twice daily. Resins have a gritty taste and cause hard, bulky, infrequent stools. A bowel regimen, often using stool softeners, is recommended. Resins can bind drugs (such as thyroid, phenylbutazone, digoxin, or dicumarol) in the intestine or reduce their absorption and augment their biliary excretion (digitoxin). Thus, other drugs should be given at times when resins are not.

For those with LDL excess only partially responsive to a resin (heterozygous FH) or for those with severe VLDL excess, the drug of choice is niacin or nicotinic acid. Niacin inhibits the release of fatty acids from adipose tissue, with a fall in VLDL and LDL production rates. Lowered values for cholesterol and triglyceride result. HDL values rise.

The initial dose of niacin is 100 mg three times daily. This is gradually increased to a total dose of 3–4 grams daily. Usually 1–3 grams is needed for most cases. All patients have an initial flush and pruritus; this can be lessened with a ½ tablet of aspirin, as the flush is prostaglandin mediated. Tachyphylaxis to the flush eventually occurs in about 80% of patients. Tests for liver function, blood sugar, and uric acid are required, as they can become abnormal. Avoid niacin in patients with active acid-peptic disease or those on ganglioplegic agents for hypertension.

Additional drugs for those with hypercholesterolemia are probucol and choloxin. Probucol is well-tolerated and, in usual dosages, may cause mild diarrhea. It may be useful in combination with a resin for those with FH. Probucol alone causes a decline in HDL as well as LDL, and this effect must be noted. Choloxin is D-thyroxin, the dextro rotary isomer of L-thyroxine. It is very useful in children and young adults with FH. It is contraindicated in those with a history of MI, ventricular ectopy, or active ischemic heart disease.

For those with hypertriglyceridemia, additional drugs are clofibrate and gemfibrozil. Clofibrate stimulates lipoprotein lipase. Clofibrate was widely used in the past decade. Since the WHO report documenting increased toxicity from noncardiac causes, its use has declined. It is still the drug of choice, however, for those with type III hyperlipoproteinemia. Gemfibrozil is a similar compound that appears to lower triglyceride and raise HDL. It is recommended for those with triglyceride values above 800 mg% so that acute pancreatitis can be avoided. All patients receiving these drugs should probably have a gallbladder ultrasound study to document whether silent gallstones are present at the start of therapy, as both drugs cause increased biliary cholesterol and incline the patient to cholelithiasis.

An excellent review of lipid disorders has recently been published and is worthy of review: Lipid Disorders: *The Medical Clinics of North America,* ed; RJ Havel, March 1982.

Bibliography

Ahrens EH: The management of hyperlipidemia: Whether, rather than how. *Ann Intern Med* 85:87, 1976.

Armstrong ML, Megan MB: Lipid depletion in atheromatous coronary arteries in rhesus monkeys after regression diet. *Circ Res* 30:675, 1972.

Bilheimer D, Stone NJ, Grundy SM: Metabolic studies in familial hypercholesterolemia: Evidence for a gene dosage effect in vivo. *J Clin Invest* 64:524, 1979.

Blackburn HL: Coronary risk factors: How to evaluate and manage them. *Eur J Cardiol* 2:249, 1975

Blankenhorn DH, Brooks SH, Selzer RH, et al: The rate of atherosclerotic change during treatment of hyperlipoproteinemia. *Circulation* 57:355, 1978.

Brown MS, Kovanen PT, Goldstein JL: Regulation of plasma cholesterol by lipoprotein receptors. *Science* 212:628, 1981.

Brunzell JD, Chait A, Bierman EL: Pathophysiology of lipoprotein transport. *Metabolism* 27:1109, 1978.

Cornfield J, Mitchell S: Selected risk factors in coronary disease: Possible intervention effects. *Arch Environ Health* 19:382, 1969.

dePalma RG: Atherosclerosis in vascular grafts, in Gotto AM, Paoletti R (eds): *Atherosclerosis Reviews*. New York, Raven Press, vol 6, 1979, p 147.

Falko JM, Schonfeld G, Witzum JL, et al: Effects of estrogen therapy on apolipoprotein E in type III hyperlipoproteinemia. *Metabolism* 28:1171, 1979.

Fredrickson DS, Goldstein JL, Brown MS: The familial hyperlipoproteinemias, in Stanbury JB, Wyngaarden JB, Fredrickson DS (eds): *The Metabolic Basis of Inherited Disease*. New York, McGraw-Hill, 1978, p 604.

Fredrickson DS, Levy RI, Lees RS: Fat transport in lipoproteins: An integrated approach to mechanisms and disorders. *N Engl J Med* 32:44,94, 148, 215,273, 1967.

Glomset J: HDL in human health and disease, in Stollerman G (ed): *Advances in Internal Medicine*. Chicago, Yearbook Medical Publishing Company, 1980, p 91.

Glueck CJ, Fallat RW, Millett F, et al: Familial hyperalphalipoproteinemia. *Arch Intern Med* 135:1025, 1975.

Goldstein JL, Brown MS: The low density lipoprotein pathway and its relation to atherosclerosis. *Ann Rev Biochem* 46:897, 1977.

Goldstein JL, Schrott HG, Hazzard WR, et al: Hyperlipidemia in coronary heart disease. II. Genetic analysis of lipid levels in 176 families and delineation of a new inherited disorder, combined hyperlipidemia. *J Clin Invest* 52:1544, 1973.

Goldstein JL, Hazzard WR, Schrott HG, et al: Hyperlipidemia in coronary heart disease. I. Lipid levels in 500 survivors of myocardial infarction. *J Clin Invest* 52:1533, 1973.

Gordon T, Castelli WP, Hjortland MC, et al: High density lipoprotein as a protective factor against coronary heart disease. *Am J Med* 111:707, 1977.

Havel RJ: High density lipoproteins, cholesterol transport, and coronary heart disease. *Circulation* 60:1, 1979.

Hjerman I, Velve BV, Holme I, et al: Effect of diet and smoking intervention on the incidence of coronary heart disease: Report from the Oslo study group of a randomized trial in healthy men. *Lancet* 2:1303, 1981.

Hulley SB, Rosenman RH, Bawol RD, et al: Epidemiology as a guide to clinical decisions. *N Engl J Med* 302:1383, 1980.

Kane JP, Malloy MJ, Tun P, et al: Normalization of low density lipoprotein levels in heterozygous familial hypercholesterolemia with a combined drug regimen. *N Engl J Med* 304:251, 1981.

Keys A: Coronary heart disease in seven countries (AHA monograph 29). *Circulation* (suppl I) 41:I-1, 1970.

Levy RI, Rifkind BM: The structure, function and metabolism of high density lipoproteins: A status report. *Circulation* (suppl IV) 62:IV-4, 1980.

Levy RI, Fredrickson DS, Shulman R, et al: Dietary and drug treatment of primary hyperlipoproteinemia. *Ann Intern Med* 77:267, 1972.

Lipid Disorders, in Havel RJ (ed): *The Medical Clinics of North America*. Philadelphia, Saunders, March 1982, p 550.

Miller GH, Miller NE: Plasma high density lipoprotein concentrations and development of ischemic heart disease. *Lancet* 1:16, 1975.

Morrison JA, Laskarzewski P, deGroot I, et al: Diagnostic ramifications of repeated plasma cholesterol and triglyceride measurements in children. *Pediatrics* 64:197, 1979.

Risk factors and coronary disease: A statement for physicians. *Circulation* 62:449A, 1980.

Roberts WC, Ferrans VJ, Levy RI, et al: Cardiovascular pathology in hyperlipoproteinemia. *Am J Cardiol* 31:557, 1973.

Ross R, Harker L: Hyperlipidemia and atherosclerosis. *Science* 193:1094, 1976.

Stamler J: Lifestyles, major risk factors, proof and public policy. *Circulation* 58:3, 1978.

Stone NJ: Type II hyperlipoproteinemia, in Rifkind B, Levy RI (eds): Hyperlipidemia: *Diagnosis and Therapy*. New York, Grune & Stratton, 1977, p 113.

Stone NJ: When to worry about plasma lipids. *Cardiovasc Med* 1:143, 1976.

Stone NJ, Levy RI, Fredrickson DS, Verter J: Coronary artery disease in 116 kindred with familial type II hyperlipoproteinemia. *Circulation* 49:476, 1974.

Tall AR, Small DM: Plasma high density lipoproteins. *N Engl J Med* 299:1232, 1978.

The Lipid Research Clinics Program Epidemiology Committee: Plasma lipid distributions in selected North American populations: The lipid research clinics program prevalence study. *Circulation* 60:427, 1979.

Wood PD, Haskell W, Klein H, et al: The distribution of plasma lipoproteins in middle-aged male runners. *Metabolism* 25:1249, 1976.

World Health Organization (WHO): Comparative trial on primary prevention of ischemic heart disease using clofibrate to lower serum cholesterol. *Lancet* 2:379, 1980.

Yeshurun D, Gotto AM: Drug treatment of hyperlipidemia. *Am J Med* 60:379, 1976.

CHAPTER 27 | CARDIAC DISEASE AND PREGNANCY

Carl E. Orringer

Approximately 1% of the pregnancies in this country occur in women with underlying cardiac disease. Although rheumatic heart disease used to account for about 90% of patients with cardiac diseases during pregnancy, the incidence of rheumatic disease has fallen in recent years. The survival to childbearing age of patients operated on for congenital heart disease and the increasing recognition of other types of heart disease have presented the practitioner with a changing spectrum of patients with heart disease during pregnancy.

This chapter will first address the alterations in cardiovascular function and the cardiovascular signs and symptoms that accompany normal pregnancy. The majority of the discussion will then be devoted to the discussion of specific cardiac disorders.

Alterations in Cardiovascular Function During Pregnancy

Pregnancy is characterized by dramatic alterations in the physiology of the cardiovascular system. A substantial elevation in the cardiac output has been documented as early as eight to twelve weeks of gestation, and the cardiac output peaks between 20 and 24 weeks, at a level about 30 to 40% above prepregnancy levels. During early pregnancy, the elevated cardiac output is achieved primarily by increased stroke volume. In the later stages, increased heart rate is the primary contributing factor. Other factors that contribute to the increased cardiac output include (1) a diminution in the afterload, largely due to the low resistance uterine and placental circulations, and (2) elevated estrogen levels, which increase cardiac output by expanding the blood volume and by enhancing cardiac contractility.

Maternal body position has been shown to exert a significant effect upon the cardiac output. The old clinical observation that some pregnant women develop hypotension and faintness upon assuming the supine position has been verified and is due to acute inferior vena cava obstruction by the gravid uterus. It has been estimated that complete obstruction of the inferior vena cava occurs in 90% of pregnant women at term when these women assume the supine position. Investigators who have measured the cardiac output in various positions have noted a 31% increase when pregnant women turn from the supine to the left lateral decubitus position.

Other characteristic physiologic changes include (1) an expansion in maternal blood volume, averaging 40%; (2) an increase in the resting heart rate by approximately 15 beats per minute near term; (3) a mild diminution in the systolic and a more marked lowering of the diastolic pressure, resulting in a widening of the pulse pressure; and (4) no significant change in intracardiac pressures.

515

Peripheral edema is observed in up to 80% of healthy pregnant women, and occurs as a result of the 8.5 liter increase in total body water and of the approximately 600 mEq increase in exchangeable sodium that characterizes a normal pregnancy. Uterine compression of the inferior vena cava also contributes to the edema.

Labor, delivery, and the postpartum period have substantial effects upon maternal hemodynamics. Each major uterine contraction is associated with a 10% rise in arterial pressure and an increase in the uterine blood volume of up to 500 ml. The increased venous return leads to an elevation in the cardiac output of about 20% and a secondary sinus bradycardia. Each contraction also compresses the distal aorta and the common iliac arteries, resulting in an increase in blood pressure in the upper extremities and diminution of that in the lower extremities.

Anesthesia and analgesia cause alterations in the above mentioned parameters. With the use of local anesthesia, the observed changes are virtually identical to those seen in the absence of medications. Caudal analgesia is associated with a less striking rise in the cardiac output, perhaps due to the more complete relief of pain. Cesarean section eliminates most of the hemodynamic changes of labor. In addition, the postpartum increase in the cardiac output may also be attenuated, at least in part, by the substantial blood loss that occurs during this operation. Studies of normal women undergoing cesarean section delivery under varying types of anesthesia have indicated that epidural anesthesia without epinephrine is the approach that best maintains maternal hemodynamic stability and is associated with the most minimal rise in the cardiac output at the time of delivery.

Cardiorespiratory Symptoms and Physical Signs During Normal Pregnancy

Normal pregnant patients frequently exhibit complaints which would, in nongravid patients, suggest cardiac or pulmonary disease. Dyspnea, diminished exercise tolerance, and fatigability are common. Palpitations are often reported; they may be related to increased cardiac awareness due to the elevated stroke volume, or they may result from atrial or ventricular dysrhythmias. These dysrhythmias are quite common during pregnancy and the puerperium and are, in the vast majority of cases, of no clinical importance.

On physical examination, the pulses are usually full, and occasionally bounding. The jugular venous pulsations are often prominent, particularly during the second and third trimesters. Venous hums are frequently present. These continuous systolic and diastolic sounds, which are best heard in the supraclavicular fossa, are produced by the rapid downward flow of blood in the jugular veins and are of no pathologic significance. However, their tendency to be loudest during early diastole and their occasional transmission to the upper chest may lead to the mistaken diagnosis of a patent ductus arteriosus or an arteriovenous fistula.

On auscultation of the heart, the first heart sound is often widely split and accentuated. The second sound retains its normal phasic respiratory changes. A third heart sound, best heard at the apex, has been reported in 84% of normal pregnant women. Rarely, an early apical diastolic murmur may be heard. This sound originates from one of the atrioventricular (AV) valves, and is probably a manifestation of increased transvalvar flow. Systolic ejection murmurs occur in almost all pregnant women, and are produced by a combination of the increased heart rate, blood volume and myocardial inotropy. One additional innocent murmur, the mammary souffle, may be heard over the breasts, particularly during the postpartum period. It is best heard with the patient supine and tends to diminish or disappear either with digital pressure at the site of auscultation or when the patient assumes the upright position.

Rheumatic Heart Disease During Pregnancy

Among pregnant patients with chronic rheumatic heart disease, 90% have pure or predominant mitral stenosis, 6 to 7% have predominant mitral regurgitation, and the remainder have aortic regurgitation with variable degrees of stenosis. With judicious medical management, most of these patients proceed safely through pregnancy and delivery.

Mitral stenosis is characterized by obstruction to left atrial emptying during diastole. In order to maintain cardiac output, left atrial pressure increases. Although this hemodynamic response generally serves to maintain the cardiac output at or near its normal resting level, it is also associated with a concomitant rise in the pulmonary capillary pressure. The increased heart rate and cardiac output of normal pregnancy result in an increased gradient across the stenotic mitral valve and may, therefore, result in elevated left atrial, pulmonary venous, and pulmonary capillary pressures, leading to pulmonary congestion. The elevated left atrial pressure may also result in atrial tachyarrhythmias, particularly atrial fibrillation. Atrial fibrillation predisposes to pulmonary congestion because the loss of atrial contraction, coupled with the accompanying rapid ventricular response with its shortened diastolic filling period, increases left atrial pressure. Patients with mitral stenosis may also develop pulmonary arterial hypertension, right ventricular failure, and systemic and pulmonary embolism.

A sound therapeutic program for these patients acts to maintain a safe margin of cardiac reserve and attempts to prevent infectious complications. Cardiac reserve may be maximized primarily by adherence to a low salt diet and by the avoidance of strenuous exercise. The patient should be instructed to inform her physician promptly if she develops palpitations, fever, or symptoms of pulmonary congestion. The physician should attempt to delineate the nature of the patient's palpitations either by electrocardiography, or by ambulatory electrocardiographic monitoring. Frequent paroxysmal atrial dysrhythmias should be managed with prophylactic digitalization so that the ventricular rate will be controlled if the dysrhythmia becomes sustained. The onset of a sustained supraventricular dysrhythmia without pulmonary congestion is an indication for therapy once the ventricular rate has been adequately controlled (generally to a rate of 110 per minute or less). For those sustained supraventricular dysrhythmias that are resistant to drug therapy, or that are associated with pulmonary congestion, cardioversion may be necessary. Several reports have indicated that this procedure may be performed safely for both the mother and the fetus (Vogel et al.; Sussman et al.; Schroeder and Harrison.).

Symptoms of pulmonary congestion, due to dysrhythmias and refractory to salt restriction, are often readily managed with small doses of oral diuretics. However, these drugs are best avoided due to the potentially adverse effects on the fetus of salt and water depletion, hypokalemia, neonatal jaundice, and thrombocytopenia.

In the pregnant patient with mitral stenosis, the effects of any infection may be devastating, predominantly due to the tachycardia and inceased cardiac output that accompanies fever. Killed influenza vaccine should be administered when the pregnancy occurs during the winter months, and repeated clean catch urinalyses should be obtained throughout pregnancy. Women who have small children may have increased risk of streptococcal infections, and should therefore receive rheumatic fever prophylaxis, preferably with penicillin. In view of the 20% incidence of positive blood cultures that have been reported following cesarean section delivery, it is advisable for patients with rheumatic valvular disease to receive bacterial endocarditis prophylaxis with penicillin or ampicillin and gentamicin or streptomycin. In those patients allergic to penicillin, vancomycin plus an aminoglycoside is substituted. Since endocarditis following spontaneous vaginal delivery is exceedingly rare, the American Heart Association does not recommend antibiotic prophylaxis in such patients.

There are occasional pregnant patients with mitral stenosis who exhibit marked hemodynamic deterioration, in spite of optimal medical therapy. Successful closed mitral commissurotomy during pregnancy was first reported in the United States in the 1950s, and several reviews in the 1960s reported maternal mortality rates less than 2% and a fetal mortality rate of less than 10% (Harkin and Taylor; Ueland). The era of open heart surgery led to the performance of mitral valve replacement in pregnant patients, using cardiopulmonary bypass. There are no large series, but fetal mortality has been substantial, and generally higher than that reported with closed commissurotomy (Snaith and Szekely). The use of mechanical prosthetic valves in these patients has been accompanied by their usual complications, particularly those related to anticoagulant therapy. Whether the mechanical mitral prosthesis is inserted prior to or during pregnancy, the risk of embolic events is higher in those patients who do not receive anticoagulants.

Although anticoagulant therapy benefits the mother, coumarin derivatives readily cross the placenta and their use has been felt by some physicians to be associated with a substantially increased risk of fetal mortality, primarily due to hemorrhage. Whereas some physicians have described an increased risk of teratogenicity with these drugs, others have maintained that such complications occur almost exclusively in patients whose clotting studies are outside of the therapeutic range. Heparin, which does not cross the placenta, is undesirable to use on a long-term basis, as it must be injected subcutaneously. When pregnancy is planned in the patient with a prosthetic valve and is diagnosed during the first trimester, it is advisable to use heparin for the remainder of the first trimester and then to switch to oral anticoagulants until term. The oral drug may be stopped just prior to delivery; 24 hours after delivery, simultaneous heparin and oral anticoagulants may be used until therapeutic clotting studies are obtained, at which time heparin may be discontinued. Another simpler option is to continue oral anticoagulants throughout pregnancy until labor begins, to stop the oral drug for 24 hours after delivery, and then to resume it once again. In either case, clotting studies should be maintained at a level just below two times the control level. Many of the problems related to anticoagulant therapy will be eliminated with increasing use of bioprosthetic valves for which anticoagulant therapy may, in many cases, not be required.

As the hemodynamics of rheumatic aortic and mitral insufficiency generally improve with pregnancy, primarily as a result of diminished afterload, these entities are usually not associated with symptomatic deterioration during pregnancy. Exceptions to this rule include those instances of spontaneous rupture of mitral chordae tendineae, or infective endocarditis involving either of these valves. Appropriate antibiotic prophylaxis for these lesions is indicated.

Congenital Heart Disease

Congenital heart disease is second in incidence to rheumatic heart disease during pregnancy. Those congenital cardiac defects in which adult female survival is likely are the following (in order of prevalence): ostium secundum atrial septal defect, patent ductus arteriosus, valvular pulmonic stenosis, ventricular septal defect with pulmonic stenosis, functionally normal bicuspid aortic valve, aortic stenosis, aortic regurgitation and coarctation of the aorta. Although a detailed discussion of each of these entities is beyond the scope of this chapter, several points should be emphasized. First of all, the great majority of pregnancies in patients with these conditions proceed satisfactorily and are unlikely to be associated with significant maternal or fetal complications. Second, hemodynamic and arrhythmic complications are more likely to occur in patients with preexisting pulmonary arterial hypertension. Third, all of these conditions, with the exception of atrial septal defect, may readily be complicated by bacterial endocarditis; and therefore, antibotic prophylaxis for bacterial endocarditis is indicated. In those patients with mitral valve prolapse associated with a murmur of mitral regurgitation, bacterial endocarditis prophylaxis is also indicated.

Cardiomyopathies

Although primary myocardial disease does not commonly affect the pregnant patient, the two types most likely to be seen are peripartal cardiomyopathy and hypertrophic obstructive cardiomyopathy.

Peripartal cardiomyopathy is an idiopathic congestive cardiomyopathy affecting previously healthy women during the last month of gestation, or in any of the five months following delivery. No definite etiology has been established, although an increased prevalence among women with poor nutrition, toxemia of pregnancy, and twin pregnancies has been reported. Findings at postmortem examination include four-chamber cardiac enlargement and mural thrombi. Clinically, the patients manifest biventricular failure, and their ultimate course takes either of two directions: in one group, the heart size returns to normal within six months of the onset of symptoms and the prognosis is generally good; in another group, cardiomegaly persists and the long-term prognosis is poor. Subsequent pregnancy is relatively contraindicated in those whose heart size has returned to normal, and is absolutely contraindicated in those women with persistent cardiomegaly. Appropriate management of peripartal cardiomyopathy includes activity restriction, dietary sodium restriction, digitalis, diuretics, and vasodilator therapy.

Hypertrophic obstructive cardiomyopathy may sometimes become clinically evident for the first time during pregnancy. These patients exhibit left ventricular hypertrophy with asymmetric hypertrophy of the ventricular septum. The mitral valve is demonstrated to exhibit abnormal anterior motion toward the ventricular septum during systole. Varying degrees of left ventricular outflow tract obstruction occur, and the degree of obstruction is determined by three major factors: (1) left ventricular end-diastolic volume; (2) systemic vascular resistance; and (3) the inotropic state of the left ventricle. Factors that increase the gradient include repeated Valsalva maneuvers, hypovolemia, and increased inotropy due to endogenous catecholamines produced during delivery. The usual clinical course of these patients is that they show mild functional deterioration, which resolves following delivery. Labor and delivery generally proceed well when the physician adheres to the following principles: (1) avoid digitalis glycosides, if possible; (2) avoid volume depletion and use diuretics sparingly; (3) advise the patient to maintain the left lateral decibitus position during labor to maximize venous return; (4) manage hypotension during delivery with blood replacement or pure vasoconstrictors; and (5) use intravenous propranolol, when necessary, to improve the patient's hemodynamics.

Preeclampsia and Chronic Arterial Hypertension

Pregnancy is generally associated with a diminution in arterial blood pressure. Hypertension during pregnancy has been defined as a rise in blood pressure of 30/15 mm Hg or more, or blood pressure levels of 140/90 or more on at least two separate readings taken at least six hours apart. Although most hypertensive pregnant women have essential hypertension, the development of new onset hypertension and proteinuria or edema after the twentieth week of pregnancy is consistent with the diagnosis of preeclampsia. Eclampsia is the clinical state in which preeclampsia is associated with seizures in the absence of other apparent etiologies for convulsions.

Several clinical features serve to distinguish preeclampsia from chronic hypertension. Generally, patients with preeclampsia are young primagravidas who suddenly develop hypertension and edema and gain weight after 20 weeks of gestation. On examination they have ocular funduscopic evidence of arteriolar spasm and, occasionally, papilledema. Laboratory findings include hyperuricemia and significant proteinuria. Their arterial blood pressures generally return to normal after delivery. Patients with chronic hypertension are generally older multiparous women who are noted to be hypertensive, even during early pregnancy. Their tendency to develop edema and to gain weight is more gradual. Their funduscopic examinations exhibit arteriovenous nicking and exudates. They usually have neither hyperuricemia nor significant proteinuria, and their blood pressure remains elevated upon the completion of pregnancy.

As hypertension during pregnancy is associated with an increased risk of fetal mortality, treatment should be initiated when the diagnosis is established. The initial mode of treatment is activity restriction and bed rest. Although most women respond favorably to such treatment, some do not and therefore require other agents, such as methyldopa or hydralazine. Salt restriction or diuretics are probably best avoided. Patients who exhibit eclampsia are treated with magnesium sulfate, which usually terminates seizure activity. Delivery should then be postponed until the blood pressure is controlled by the use of intravenous antihypertensive therapy. This mode of therapy is generally associated with minimal maternal risk and excellent fetal survival. Neither preeclampsia nor eclampsia appear to predispose to chronic hypertension.

Bibliography

Brock RC: Valvulotomy in pregnancy. *Proc R Soc Med* 45:538, 1952.

Chesley LC, Annitto JE, Cosgrove RA: The remote prognosis of eclamptic women. *Am J Obstet Gynecol* 124:446, 1976.

Cooley DA, Chapman DW: Mitral commisurotomy during pregnancy. *JAMA* 150:1113, 1952.

Csapo A: Actomyosin formation by estrogen action. *Am J Physiol* 162:406, 1950.

Cutworth R, MacDonald CB: Heart sounds and murmurs in pregnancy. *Am Heart J* 71:741, 1966.

Demakis JG, Rahimtoola SH, Sutton GC, et al: Natural course of peripartum cardiomyopathy. *Circulation* 44:1053, 1971.

Ehrenfeld EN, Brezizinski A, Braon K, et al: Heart disease in pregnancy. *Obstet Gyncol* 23:363, 1964.

Goodwin JF: Peripartal heart disease. *Clin Obstet Gynecol* 18:125, 1975.

Harken DE, Taylor WJ: Cardiac surgery during pregnancy. *Clin Obstet Gynecol* 4:697, 1961.

Hirsch J, Cade JF, Gallus AS: Anticoagulants in pregnancy: A review of indications and complications. *Am Heart J* 83:301, 1972.

Hytten FE, Leitch I: *The Physiology of Human Pregnancy*, ed 2. Oxford, Blackwell, 1971.

Hytten FE, Robertson EG: Maternal water metabolism in pregnancy. *Proc R Soc Med* 64:1072, 1971.

Hytten FE, Thompson AM: Water and electrolytes in pregnancy. *Br Med Bull* 24:15, 1968.

Kaplan NM: Systemic hypertension: Mechanisms and diagnosis, in Braunwald E (ed): *Heart Disease. A Textbook of Cardiovascular Medicine.* Philadelphia, Saunders, 1980, p 905.

Kaplan EL, Anthony BR, Bisno A, et al: Prevention of bacterial endocarditis. *Circulation* 56:139A, 1977.

Kolibash AJ, Ruiz DE, Lewis RP: Idiopathic hypertrophic subaortic stenosis in pregnancy. *Ann Intern Med* 82:791, 1975.

Lees MM, Taylor SH, Scott DB, et al: A study of cardiac output at rest throughout pregnancy. *J Obstet Gynecol Brit Comm* 74:319, 1967.

Logan A, Turner RWD: Mitral valvulotomy in pregnancy. *Lancet* 1:1286, 1952.

Metcalfe J, Ueland K: The heart and pregnancy, in Hurst JW, Logue RB, Schlant RC, et al (eds): *The Heart.* New York, McGraw-Hill, 1978, p 1721.

Perloff JE: Pregnancy and cardiovascular disease, in Braunwald E (ed): *Heart Disease. A Textbook of Cardiovascular Medicine*. Philadelphia, Saunders, 1980, p 1873.

Pritchard JA, Pritchard SA: Standardized treatment of 154 consecutive cases of eclampsia. *Am J Obstet Gynecol* 123:543, 1975.

Rose DJ, Bader ME, Bader RA, et al: Catheterization studies of cardiac hemodynamics in normal pregnant women with reference to left ventricular work. *Am J Obstet Gynecol* 72:233, 1956.

Schroeder JS, Harrison DC: Repeated cardioversion during pregnancy: Treatment of refractory paroxysmal atrial tachycardia during three successive pregnancies. *Am J Cardiol* 27:445, 1971.

Snaith L, Szekely P: Cardiovascular surgery in relation to pregnancy, in Marcus SL, Marcus CC (eds): *Advances in Obstetrics and Gynecology*. Baltimore, Williams and Wilkins, 1967, vol. I, p 220.

Sussman HF, Duque D, Lesser ME: Atrial flutter with 1:1 conduction. *Dis Chest* 49:88, 1966.

Swan DA, Bell B, Oakley CM, et al: Analysis of symptomatic course and prognosis of hypertrophic obstructive cardiomyopathy. *Br Heart J* 33:671, 1971.

Szekely P, Snaith L: *Heart Disease and Pregnancy*. Edinburgh & London, Churchill-Livingstone, 1974.

Turner GM, Oakley CM, Dixon HG: Management of pregnancy complicated by hypertrophic obstructive cardiomyopathy. *Br Med* 4:281, 1968.

Ueland K, Akamatsu TJ, Eng M, et al: Maternal cardiovascular hemodynamics. VI. Cesarean section under epidural anesthesia without epinephrine. *Am J Obstet Gynecol* 114:775, 1972.

Ueland K, Hansen JM: Maternal cardiovascular hemodynamics III. Labor and delivery under local and caudal analgesia. *Am J Obstet Gynecol* 103:8, 1968.

Ueland K, Hansen JM: Maternal cardiovascular hemodynamics II. Posture and uterine contractions. *Am J Obstet Gynecol* 103:1, 1969.

Ueland K: Cardiac surgery and pregnancy. *Am J Obstet Gynecol* 92:148, 1965.

Vogel JHK, Pryor R, Blound SG Jr: Direct current defibrillation during pregnancy. *JAMA* 193:970, 1965.

Vorys N, Ullery JC, Hanusek GE: The cardiac output in various positions in pregnancy. *Am J Obstet Gynecol* 82:1312, 1961.

CHAPTER 28

AORTIC AND PERIPHERAL ARTERIAL DISEASE

Marc A. Pfeffer

Aortic Disease

As with any other viable tissue, the aorta is subjected to systemic diseases, trauma, and degenerative changes, as well as congenital anomalies. Since even the grossly diseased aorta may perform the function of transmitting blood from the left ventricle to branch arteries, it is not uncommon for aortic diseases to be detected in asymptomatic people. On the other end of the spectrum, the first clinical manifestation of aortic disease may be the catastrophic interruption in the integrity of this major arterial conduit. This chapter will be concerned with diseases of the aorta that produce aneurysms and thereby threaten either rupture or the other serious manifestation of aortic disease—vascular occlusion.

The media of the large arteries have a high content of elastic fibers and smooth muscle cells. During the aging process, these cells and fibers degenerate and are replaced by fibrous tissue. This histologic change produces the well-known reduced aortic distensibility of aging and results in systolic hypertension and a greater work load on the left ventricle in elderly people. Medionecrosis, defined as a focal loss of nuclei in the media, also has been described as an aging process of the aorta. These changes of the aorta are believed to represent injury and repair processes resulting from the continuous hemodynamic impact to which the aorta is subjected.

Another important histological alteration of the media of the aorta is seen in idiopathic cystic medial necrosis. The histologic appearance of cystic medial necrosis is a focal loss of the normal elastic and fibromuscular elements of the media with replacement by amorphous ground substance. Although the etiology of cystic medial necrosis is truly idiopathic, the association with Marfan's syndrome has led to speculation that it is produced by a hereditary defect in elastic tissue formation. These histologic changes, whether degenerative or hereditary, are important in that they result in a weakening of the arterial wall. Such changes may result in localized dilatation of the vessel, or aneurysms. Once initiated, an aneurysm promotes its own expansion by the LaPlace relationship, in which wall tension is directly proportional to the product of the vessel radius and distending pressure. Thus, dilatation at a site of medial weakness increases wall tension, thereby promoting further expansion and thinning, which may lead to fatal rupture of a major vessel.

Aneurysms may occur at any location along the aorta, from the sinuses of Valsalva to the terminal bifurcation into the iliac arteries. The three important causes of aortic aneurysms are atherosclerosis, cystic medial necrosis, and syphilis. With the dramatic decrease in the incidence of tertiary syphilis, atherosclerotic aneurysms now are by far the most prevalent. Although atherosclerosis is an intimal process, secondary medial weakening is produced by destruction of elastic and fibromuscular support.

ABDOMINAL AORTIC ANEURSYMS

Most atherosclerotic aneurysms occur in the abdominal aorta, where over 90% of the aneurysms are caused by atherosclerosis. Typically, these aneurysms are fusiform, are located beneath the renal arteries, and may extend beyond the aortic bifurcation into the iliac arteries. Aside from the ever-present risk of rupture, these aneurysms usually contain mural thrombi and are potential sites for formation of emboli to the lower extremities.

Although the majority of patients with unruptured abdominal aortic aneurysms may be asymptomatic, the presence of dull abdominal or back pain, or awareness of an abdominal pulsation in an elderly person with other evidence of cardiovascular disease should alert the examiner to the possibility of aortic aneurysms. The physical examination may disclose a pulsatile abdominal mass, bruit, or evidence of peripheral arterial occlusive disease. In many instances, aortic aneurysms are first detected by abdominal roentgenograms performed for unrelated reasons. Not infrequently, the aneurysm is outlined by calcification of the atherosclerotic plaques. Abdominal ultrasound has become a reliable method of detecting and, indeed, sequentially following abdominal aortic aneurysms.

The major clinical problem concerning the asymptomatic abdominal aortic aneurysm or, for that matter, any asymptomatic aneurysm is to assess the comparative risks of an operation or a life-limiting rupture. Although there is controversy over the actual frequency of deaths due to rupture in patients with abdominal aortic aneurysms, compilations of both autopsy and clinical studies indicated that the death of about one-third of these patients was attributed to a ruptured aneurysm. One consistent conclusion is that the likelihood of rupture increased with the size of the aneurysm. The incidence of rupture of aneurysms larger than 6 cm in diameter approached 50%, whereas rupture of aneurysms less than 5 cm was considered uncommon. A recent autopsy series by Darling and coworkers confirmed this high rate of rupture of large aneurysms; however, the study also demonstrated a 23% rupture of aneurysms of only 4 to 5 cm in diameter.

Although a prospective randomized study was not conducted, most available information indicates that survival following resection and graft replacement is prolonged compared to that of unoperated controls. In one particularly careful study of 480 operated and 233 untreated patients, the five-year survival of the operated group was 47% compared to only 6% in the unoperated group. The leading cause of death in the unoperated patients was rupture of the aneurysm (45% of 174 deaths) followed by coronary atherosclerosis-related deaths (22%). Most patients surviving surgical resection eventually succumb to the associated cardiorespiratory problems so prevalent in this patient population.

With the progressive reduction in operative mortality, the surgical treatment of the asymptomatic patient with an abdominal aortic aneurysm has become even more attractive in recent years. The operative mortality in experienced centers is currently 2 to 5% for elective resection of an abdominal aneurysm. This figure is impressive when one considers that the operation is usually performed on elderly patients with diffuse atherosclerosis.

The clinical decision regarding resection of an aneurysm must be tailored to each patient. However, a reasonable framework would be to recommend surgery for patients with aneurysms 6 cm in diameter or larger, or for symptomatic patients with even smaller aneurysms. Aneurysms between 4 to 6 cm in diameter should not be considered entirely benign, since there is still a definite risk of rupture. One may recommend elective resection or a more conservative course of frequent evaluation of the size of the aneurysm by ultrasound.

In any event, the abdominal aortic aneurysm should be considered as a manifestation of diffuse atherosclerosis. Patients with abdominal aortic aneurysms are at high risk of serious cardiovascular events. All efforts should, therefore, be directed toward reducing those risk factors that can be treated.

THORACIC AORTIC ANEURSYMS

In the past half century, the etiology of the majority of the aneurysms of the thoracic aorta has undergone a dramatic shift from syphilitic to atherosclerotic. In a large autopsy series compiled from the mid-1920s to the mid-1950s, over 80% of the aortic aneurysms were attributed to syphilis. Over 90% of these syphilitic aneurysms were located in the thoracic aorta and most commonly involved the ascending aorta. However, in a more recent review of 100 consecutive cases of ascending aortic aneurysms operated on by Dr. DeBakey's group, only 9% were attributed to syphilis. Secondary degenerative changes in the media produced by atherosclerosis accounted for 69% of the ascending aortic aneurysms. In 22 of the 100 patients, the ascending aortic aneurysms were believed to be due to cystic medial necrosis, and six patients demonstrated skeletal stigmata of Marfan's syndrome.

Marfan's syndrome represents an autosomal dominant transmitted disorder of connective tissue, with a constellation of musculoskeletal, ocular, and cardiovascular abnormalities. These patients are usually tall, with long extremities (span exceeds height) and with elongated fingers and toes (arachnodactyly). High arched palate, pectus excavatum, and kyphoscoliosis are other musculoskeletal abnormalities associated with the syndrome. Lax ligaments including the suspensory ligament of the lens may result in subluxation of the lens (ectopia lentis). The cardiovascular abnormalities, which may include "floppy" redundant mitral valves and degenerative changes in the media of the major vessels, account for most of the premature mortality in these people. The medial degeneration characteristically involves the aortic ring and sinuses. Aortic regurgitation or rupture, and/or medial dissection of the aorta are grave consequences of the focal loss of elastic and fibromuscular elements in the aortic wall. The terms anuloaortic ectasia and idiopathic cystic medial necrosis are often used to describe people with similar aortic pathology who do not have other musculoskeletal stigmata of Marfan's syndrome.

The clinical approach to aneurysms of the thoracic aorta, whether atherosclerotic, luetic, or cystic medial necrosis, should be directed to the basic clinical question whether the aneurysm poses such a threat to longevity that surgical resection should be undertaken.

As found in abdominal aortic aneurysms, several associated factors appear to greatly reduce the five-year survival rate of individuals with thoracic aortic aneurysms. A vessel diameter of 6 cm or larger, associated atherosclerotic disease manifested in other regions, hypertension, and the presence of symptoms all appear to adversely alter the natural history of thoracic aortic aneurysms.

Because of their location, thoracic aneurysms have a greater tendency to produce symptoms than do abdominal aneurysms. Pain described as a deep throbbing or aching sensation was the presenting symptom of 18 of the 107 patients with aneurysms of the thoracic aorta reported by Joyce et al. Other presenting symptoms include cough and dyspnea from compression of the tracheobronchial tree, dysphagia from extrinsic compression of the esophagus, and hoarseness from involvement of the recurrent laryngeal nerve. Symptoms in patients with ascending aortic aneurysms may also reflect the commonly associated aortic regurgitation due to dilatation of the aortic ring.

In some diseases such as ankylosing spondylitis, very limited aortic involvement may lead to severe aortic insufficiency. In this relatively benign rheumatologic condition, a very limited area of aorta behind the sinuses and into the leaflets may be involved by an adventitial infiltrate clustering around the vasa vasora, similar to syphilitic aortitis. Because of the critical location of this limited aortic involvement, severe aortic regurgitation may be produced, which, if present, is the leading cause of cardiovascular morbidity in this otherwise benign disease.

Advances in prosthetic valves and synthetic grafts and in cardiopulmonary bypass procedures have reduced the mortality and morbidity of even complex aortic reconstruction by experienced thoracic surgeons. Surgical intervention is urgent in patients with large symptomatic aneurysms. In patients who have smaller asymptomatic aneurysms, but who do not have aortic insufficiency, the risk of surgery must be carefully compared to the risk of the continued presence of the aneurysm.

AORTIC DISSECTION

Perhaps the most catastrophic of all diseases of the aorta is acute dissection. A compilation of almost 1,000 untreated patients demonstrated a 50% mortality within 48 hours after the onset of pain. Moreover, before effective treatment was available, 90% of the patients died within three months of acute aortic dissection. During the past quarter of a century, complimentary strides in radiologic, medical, and surgical practices have so altered this grim prognosis that one can now expect to save 70 to 80% of patients presenting with acute aortic dissections.

The fundamental pathologic lesion in aortic dissection is a cleavage of the aortic media by a dissecting hematoma. Degenerative changes in the media of the aorta, whether from congenital defects or changes produced by aging and hypertension, are the predisposing factors for aortic dissection. With each cardiac contraction, the ascending aorta and the aorta just distal to the left subclavian are flexed by the sudden installation of the volume of blood into the arterial tree. In some people, these forces produce an intimal tear, permitting blood to enter the weakened media. Once initiated, the dissecting hematoma may propagate rapidly, involving a variable length of the aorta. The aortic media is cleaved into a thin outer wall surrounding a false channel. This thin outer wall is all that protects the aorta against fatal rupture and extravasation of blood. The propagation of the dissecting hematoma has been shown in experimental animals to depend on the rate of rise of arterial pressure (dP/dt) and the level of blood pressure. As the 90% three-month mortality indicates, a dissecting hematoma almost invariably progresses to rupture and death. Hemopericardium with cardiac tamponade and hemothorax are the most frequent fatal complications. Aside from outright rupture, the medial hemorrhage may distort the aortic anulus and produce aortic regurgitation. Occlusion of a major branch artery is yet another major complication of aortic dissection. The false channel may so compress the lumen of the true channel as to produce arterial insufficiency of the region supplied by the branch vessel. In aortic dissection, renal, splanchnic, cerebral, and even coronary ischemia may be encountered as a consequence of compression of the vital arteries.

As with other catastrophic disease processes, a rapid and accurate diagnosis is essential so that proper life-sustaining therapy can be immediately instituted. Severe pain is the outstanding clinical feature that should alert the physician to the possibility of aortic dissection. The quality of the pain is usually characterized as sharp and tearing; however, it may mimic the pain of a myocardial infarction. It may be localized in the anterior chest, interscapular region, and, particularly in distal dissections, it may occur simultaneously in several regions both above and below the diaphragm. In some instances, because of an altered state of consciousness, pain is not perceived, and therefore is not provided as a presenting symptom. Neurological symptoms indicative of cerebral ischemia represent an ominous presentation of aortic dissection.

Patients with acute aortic dissection characteristically appear in overt distress. Arterial pressure is usually elevated at the time of presentation. Hypotension is suggestive of proximal dissection or aortic rupture. Occlusion of an arterial branch of the aorta by compression of the true lumen produces the reduced or absent arterial pulse found in about one-third of the patients with aortic dissections. Therefore, careful examination of carotid, brachial, radial, and femoral arteries is quite important.

A murmur of aortic regurgitation is detected in about one-third of the patients with aortic dissection. When present, this murmur usually indicates proximal dissection, with loss of anular support.

The electrocardiogram is usually abnormal, but nonspecific. Left ventricular hypertrophy, with or without evidence of strain or ischemia, is common. Severe chest discomfort without electrocardiographic evidence of myocardial necrosis should raise the suspicion of an aortic dissection.

Plain films of the chest often provide radiographic findings suggestive of aortic dissection. The most common abnormalities are found in the region of the aortic knob. In one study of patients with aortic dissection, findings of an increased aortic diameter, double density as a result of posterior aortic enlargement, or deviation of the trachea to the right were reported in over one-half the cases of aortic dissection. Mediastinal widening or displacement of calcified intima by more than 1 cm was noted in only 11 and 7%, respectively, of the plain films of patients with confirmed dissections. It is important to note that in this same study, the plain chest films were not suggestive of aortic diseases in 20% of the patients with confirmed aortic dissection.

Aortography is required to confirm the diagnosis of aortic dissection. The objectives of the procedure are to determine the origin of the dissection and to define the extent of the dissecting hematoma. The most common angiographic finding is opacification of the false channel, creating a double lumen.

The treatment of aortic dissection has progressed admirably in the past 25 years.

In 1955, DeBakey and his coworkers reported a surgical approach to dissecting aneurysms. By the mid 1960s, this group was reporting a 74% survival rate in an extensive series of patients with dissections. Based on this experience, DeBakey defined specific surgical approaches to aortic dissection according to the origin and extent of the dissection. Type I dissections begin at the ascending aorta and extend to the abdominal aorta; type II dissections are localized to the ascending aorta and aortic arch; and type III dissections begin just distal to the left subclavian artery and extend to below the diaphragm. However, the results of other surgical series were not as impressive as the experience of the Houston group.

At the same time, Wheat and coworkers reported encouraging results with intensive medical therapy in patients with acute aortic dissection. They reasoned that the complications of aortic dissection were produced by the progression of the medial hematoma and not the initial intimal tear itself. Hydrodynamic forces in the arterial system, particularly the rate of rise of arterial pressure, as well as the level of blood pressure, are the major factors determining the propagation of the hematoma to rupture and death. Pharmacological attempts to halt the progression of the medial hematoma, therefore, are directed at reducing the steepness of the pulse wave (dP/dT) and reducing the arterial pressure. By the late 1960s, Wheat's experience had increased to over 50 medically treated patients with survival rates as impressive as the concurrent surgical series.

By the early 1970s, as more experience was gained with both surgical and medical therapies, it became apparent that neither blanket surgical nor medical strategies provided the optimal management of all patients with aortic dissection. The Stanford group introduced a new classification that is of therapeutic and prognostic importance: type A dissections originate in the ascending aorta (DeBakey I and II) and type B dissections begin after the left subclavian artery (DeBakey III). Roughly two-thirds of aortic dissections are type A and one-third are type B.

Recent results compiled from six separate centers indicate that surgery is the treatment of choice for proximal (type A) aortic dissections. Of the 46 patients with acute dissection originating in the ascending aorta who were treated medically, only 12 patients, or 26%, survived. In contrast, of the 71 patients with type A dissections who were treated surgically, 50 patients, or 70% survived. With ascending aortic involvement, the potential for retrograde dissection and fatal pericardial tamponade is great and prompt surgical intervention is indicated.

In contrast, patients with type B, or dissecting hematoma distal to the left subclavian artery not involving the ascending aorta, have a slight advantage with medical therapy. In this same report from six centers, 62 patients with type B dissections were treated medically and 50 patients, or 81%, survived. In patients with distal dissection, the surgical survival was not as good as in the medically treated group. Of the 40 patients with distal dissections undergoing surgical intervention, only 20 patients, or 50%, survived. Therefore, in the uncomplicated distal dissection, medical therapy provides an advantage over surgical intervention.

Using the carefully documented experiences of the recent past, it is possible to describe a unified plan that will provide for the optimal management of patients with acute aortic dissection. Patients suspected of having an aortic dissection should be treated immediately in an attempt to halt the progression of the dissecting hematoma. This therapy should reduce arterial pressure to the lowest level commensurate with organ perfusion and reduce the rate of rise of arterial pressure. The ganglionic blocker, trimethaphan, has been used effectively for this purpose. Alternatively, the use of the vascular smooth muscle dilator, nitroprusside, in combination with a beta-adrenergic blocking agent, such as propranolol, provides an alternate form of therapy designed to arrest the progression of the dissecting hematoma.

Once the patient's pain and blood pressure are under control, at best within the first four hours from presentation, an aortogram should be performed. The aortogram should confirm the diagnosis and determine whether or not the dissecting hematoma involves the ascending aorta. Attempts should also be made to define the distal circulation and determine if the dissection is producing an occlusion of a major branch of the aorta. The identification of a proximal dissection provides an urgent indication for surgical therapy.

On the other hand, distal dissections not involving the ascending aorta do somewhat better with medical therapy. If no complications are encountered in those patients with type B dissections, the intravenous antihypertensive agents can be replaced by an oral regimen, which should include a beta-adrenergic blocking agent. If a complication is encountered in a patient with a distal dissection on intensive medical therapy, surgical intervention would be required. Indications for surgical intervention in patients with distal dissection are evidence of continued propagation of the hematoma; continued pain, new aortic insufficiency murmur, and signs of occlusion of a major branch of the aorta, such as new neurologic findings, loss of an arterial pulse, or inability to control pressure. Indications of impending rupture of the dissecting hematoma, such as increasing size of the aneurysm and blood in the pleural space or pericardium, are other reasons to opt for surgical intervention, even in patients with type B acute dissections.

Once a medically or surgically treated patient has survived the acute phase of dissection, careful follow-up evaluations should be performed. Impressive five-year survival rates have been reported on both medically and surgically treated patients who have been successfully managed through the acute phase of the aortic dissection.

In summary, in the past 25 years, much progress has been made in the management of acute aortic dissection. One can now expect a 70 to 80% survival rate in what was an almost uniformly fatal disease.

Occlusive Diseases of Aorta and Peripheral Vessels

Of the causes of chronic occlusive disease of arteries, atherosclerosis is the disease process responsible for 95% of the cases. The infrarenal abdominal aorta and its iliac branches are the common sites of extensive atherosclerosis, which produces chronic ischemia of the lower limbs. A dynamic state exits between the progressive occlusive disease and the development of collateral channels. As with coronary artery disease, ischemia is a result of an imbalance between oxygen delivery and utilization.

Intermittent claudication, the discomfort in the limbs that occurs with exercise and is relieved by rest, is usually the first symptom of chronic occlusive arterial disease. This ischemic pain is usually indicative of severe multisegmental occlusive disease. With severe occlusive disease, nonobstructing factors that reduce oxygen delivery, such as reduced cardiac output, relative hypotension, and anemia, may enhance peripheral ischemia. In the patient awakened by an aching numbness from a distal limb, the slight increase in arterial inflow produced by the gravitational effect of hanging the extremity over the edge of the bed may be sufficient to relieve the ischemic pain. In its most severe form, chronic occlusive arterial disease may present as ischemic ulcers with gangrene as an end-stage. The hallmark of the physical examination of patients with chronic occlusive arterial disease is the diminished peripheral pulses. Bruits may or may not be heard. Postural color changes as pallor on elevation and rubor on dependency of the extremity are indicative of moderate to severe arterial insufficiency. Nutritional atrophy of skin and nails should be noted.

Noninvasive assessment of the arterial inflow to the extremity has provided a more standardized diagnostic assessment. A pressure index of Doppler-determined systolic pressures in tibial and brachial arteries has provided a quantitative assessment of the degree of chronic occlusive arterial disease.

In consideration of therapeutic courses, both the patient and physician must be aware that intermittent claudication does not alter life expectancy. The limitation of activity imposed by the exercise-induced pain may be acceptable to the patient. However, the intermittent claudication may so disable the patient that elective revascularization to improve the quality of life may be desired. On the other hand, revascularization may be urgently recommended to avoid the possible loss of a limb.

A detailed medical evaluation is of the utmost importance in all patients considered for arterial reconstructive surgery. This patient population with symptoms of atherosclerosis in the extremities usually has coexisting cardiac and respiratory disease. In obtaining a cardiac history from these patients, the physician must be aware that the functional limitations produced by the peripheral vascular disease may mask significant coronary artery disease. Indeed, it is our practice to perform exercise tests for ischemic cardiac changes prior to vascular reconstructive surgery, even though the test is usually limited by claudication. If there is clinical evidence of impressive myocardial ischemia at low exercise levels, coronary angiography is recommended.

Patients with chronic occlusive arterial disease should be instructed to provide meticulous care and avoid trauma to ischemic extremities. It is not uncommon for urgent bypass surgery or even amputation to be required in a person considered a relatively poor operative risk because of avoidable injury to the ischemic extremity. Cigarette smoking is strongly contraindicated, as evidenced by the ten-fold increase in amputation rate of patients with chronic occlusive arterial disease who continue to smoke over those who stop smoking. Vasodilator therapy is generally ineffective.

Arterial reconstructive surgery then should be considered in suitable candidates for surgery to improve a disabling lifestyle, relieve pain at rest, or—the most urgent indication—to prevent tissue necrosis and amputation.

Takayasu's arteritis, or pulseless disease, is a rare nonspecific inflammatory process of unknown etiology affecting segmental areas of the aorta and its main branches. The disease process results in a marked thickening of the arterial wall, which eventually produces occlusions of major branches of the aorta. Attempts have been made to link Takayasu's arteritis to rheumatic fever, syphilis, and tuberculosis; however, the evidence for each of these associations is sketchy. There is a very high predilection among women; the female to male ratio is 9:1. Unlike giant cell (temporal) arteritis, which usually afflicts elderly men, Takayasu's arteritis is a disease of young people. Although typically described as a disease of young Oriental women, Takayasu's arteritis has a worldwide distribution.

Several classifications of regional involvement of the aorta and major branches have been described. The most common areas of the arterial tree to be involved with the proliferative process are the aortic arch, including the origins of the brachiocephalic arteries, and the thoracoabdominal aorta, including the renal arteries.

The symptoms and signs of arterial occlusive disease are usually preceded by an initial systemic illness presenting with fever, weight loss, arthralgias, and fatigue. In the chronic phase, these young patients present with cardiovascular and neurologic symptoms related to arterial obstruction. Absent pulses and vascular bruits are almost uniformly found in these people. Hypertension was reported in 72% of a recent series of 107 patients with Takayasu's arteritis. Renal artery involvement caused hypertension in the majority of cases. The clinical course of this devastating arteritis is unpredictable. At present, therapy is only directed at the manifestations of the disease process: steroids for constitutional symptoms; antihypertensive therapy; possible anticoagulation therapy; and surgical vascular bypass procedures to reconstruct flow to vital organs.

Bibliography

Darling RC, Messina CR, Brewster DC: Autopsy study of unoperated abdominal aortic aneurysms. The case for early resection. *Circulation* 56, Supp 2:II-161, 1977.

Joyce JW, Fairbairn JF II, Kincaid OW, et al: Aneurysms of the thoracic aorta. *Circulation* 29:176, 1964.

Lindsay J Jr, Hurst JW: *The Aorta*. New York, Grune & Stratton, 1979.

Mannick JA: Surgical treatment of aneurysms of the abdominal and thoracic aorta. *Prog Cardiovasc Dis* 16:69, 1973.

Perdue GD, Smith RB III: Chronic aortoiliac occlusion, in Lindsay, Hurst (eds): *The Aorta*. New York, Grune & Stratton, 1979, p 189.

Pyeritz RD, McKusick VA: The Marfan syndrome: Diagnosis and management. *N Engl J Med* 300:772, 1979.

Roberts WC: Aortic dissection: Anatomy, consequences, and causes. *Am Heart J* 101:195, 1981.

Wheat MW Jr: Acute dissecting aneurysms of the aorta: Diagnosis and treatment-1979. *Am Heart J* 99:373, 1980.

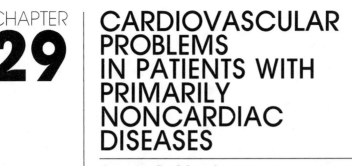

CARDIOVASCULAR PROBLEMS IN PATIENTS WITH PRIMARILY NONCARDIAC DISEASES

James D. Marsh

The internist or cardiologist is frequently asked to see patients in consultation who have primarily noncardiac disorders, but are suspected of having some cardiovascular complication arising from their primary disease or the therapy thereof. There are many disorders whose secondary manifestations may involve either the pericardium, myocardium, epicardium and valves, the great vessels, coronaries, or the neurohumoral regulation of the heart and circulation. It is the purpose of this chapter to outline the recognition and management of cardiovascular manifestations of primarily noncardiac diseases.

Paget's Disease

Paget's disease (osteitis deformans) is a skeletal abnormality that afflicts between 1 and 3% of the United States population over 40 years of age. In severe cases, important effects on the cardiovascular system may be present. Although the exact cause of the disorder is not entirely understood, the pathologic abnormalities are well described. To a greater or lesser degree, the bone marrow is replaced by vascular fibrous connective tissue and dense trabecular bone. The rate of bone turnover is accelerated, and although it was thought for many years that actual arteriovenous (AV) fistulae were present in the bone marrow of patients with this disorder, radio-labelled macroaggregated albumin studies have demonstrated that there are no true AV fistulae present. Instead, frequently there is cutaneous and soft tissue vasodilatation that accounts for increased flow to an extremity and the warmth of an extremity that is involved. Frequently, Paget's disease is asymptomatic; if one-third of the skeleton is involved, it is likely that cardiac output at rest or with exercise will be increased. In some patients, the blood flow through the involved extremity is nine times the normal level.

One direct cardiac consequence of Paget's disease is high output congestive heart failure. Pathophysiologically, this is a reflection of increased flow through soft tissues due to high metabolic rate and not due to true AV shunt flow. This is a disorder that most frequently presents in elderly patients; and it is important to note that, in patients with Paget's disease, by far the most frequent causes of congestive heart failure are the usual causes of congestive heart failure in an elderly population, such as ischemic heart disease or hypertensive heart disease, and not high output heart failure due to Paget's disease. One cardiac consequence of the high rate of calcium turnover in Paget's disease is metastatic calcification of the cardiac skeleton. There may be calcification of the valve rings, with extension into the interventricular septum, producing various degrees of conduction abnormalities.

Diagnosis of Paget's disease is made by typical radiographic findings; a markedly elevated alkaline phosphatase is often present as well. A high normal or high cardiac output will be present at cardiac catheterization.

Treatment of Paget's disease is not entirely satisfactory. Calcitonin, etidronate disodium, actinomycin-D, and mithramycin have been used with mixed results. High output symptoms respond quite well to a pulse of steroids in the range of prednisone 60 mg per day, with hemodynamic improvement within three or four days.

Rheumatoid Diseases See Table 1.

RHEUMATOID ARTHRITIS

Involvement of cardiac structures in rheumatoid arthritis is very common, but most frequently subclinical. Rheumatoid arthritis does frequently produce a pancarditis that is evident at necropsy. Nodular granulomas are the characteristic pathologic lesions involving the myocardium, endocardium, and valves. The pericardium is frequently involved as well, most commonly when there is diffuse systemic arteritis. Coronary arteritis is often present at necropsy, but rarely causes clinical myocardial ischemia.

Pericarditis is clinically evident in about 5% of patients with rheumatoid arthritis and usually follows a benign course, responding to moderate doses of steroids. However, pericarditis can be severe, producing either constriction or tamponade. Needle pericardiocentesis frequently is difficult technically to perform because of the markedly thickened pericardium and the tendency for loculation of pericardial effusions. When pericardial fluid is obtained, complement levels and glucose are frequently depressed, as they are in fluid from other serous spaces in rheumatoid arthritis. Myocarditis is present in 19% of patients at autopsy, but rarely is it of clinical importance. Granulomas, on occasion, involve the conducting system, and produce varying degrees of heart block. The most frequent electrocardiographic abnormality in patients with rheumatoid arthritis is first degree AV (atrioventricular) block; repolarization abnormalities are not particularly common. Rheumatoid granulomas may involve the cardiac valves, but very rarely cause enough distortion of the valve structure to cause regurgitation or stenosis of any hemodynamic significance. Delayed closing of the mitral valve on echocardiography has been attributed to either valvular or myocardial involvement with granulomata.

SYSTEMIC LUPUS ERYTHEMATOSUS

Cardiac manifestations of systemic lupus erythematosus (SLE) are numerous. The underlying pathologic abnormality is diffuse microvasculitis. Cardiac involvement

Table 1. Cardiovascular Manifestations of Rheumatoid Diseases

	Pericarditis	Myocarditis/ Fibrosis	Endocarditis	↑ BP	Valves Involved	Conduction Abnormalities	Arrhythmias	Treatment
Rheumatoid arthritis	+ +	+	+		AoV MV			Antiinflammatories
SLE	+ + + +	+ +	+ +	+ +	AoV MV	+	+ +	Steroids
Polyarteritis	+	+ +		+ + + +			+	Steroids
Scleroderma	+ +	+ + + +		+ + +		+ + +	+	Steroids ? Penicillamine
Ankylosing spondilitis				+	AoV	+ + +		
Dermatomyositis		+				+ + +		

Key: AoV, aortic valve; MV, mitral valve

is exceedingly common at necropsy, though clinical cardiac involvement is present in only about half of cases. SLE produces pancarditis with involvement of the pericardium most evident clinically. Approximately 30% of all patients with lupus will have clinical symptoms of pericarditis and another substantial proportion may have findings of pericarditis on auscultation or electrocardiography. Inflammation of the pericardium may be quite pronounced and involve the epicardium as well. The sinoatrial (SA) and AV node are occasionally involved with destruction of conducting fibers and resulting arrhythmias and conduction blocks. Pericardial constriction or tamponade occur in a small but important number of patients. Corticosteroids are quite effective, in most cases controlling the symptoms of pericarditis; but there is no evidence that administration of steroids prevents progression to constriction. For patients with refractory pericardial symptoms, pericardiectomy, rarely, may be necessary. The myocarditis of SLE is due to segmental arteritis of the small arteries in the myocardium. Subclinical myocarditis is quite common, producing fibrinoid necrosis of the interstitial tissue in blood vessels, though actual necrosis of myocardial cells is rare. In SLE, arteritis of the major coronary arteries leading to a clinical myocardial infarction (MI) is a very rare event. However, it is thought that the incidence of atherosclerotic coronary artery disease is somewhat higher in patients with SLE. In these patients, clinical myocardial ischemia or necrosis is far more likely to be due to typical large-vessel coronary artery disease than to arteritis. Thus, patients showing signs of myocardial ischemia would best be treated with conventional measures rather than with a pulse of steroids as a first approach.

Libman-Sacks endocarditis is observed at necropsy in 50% of cases. These verrucous excrescences on valve leaflets are comprised of degenerating valve tissue. These warty lesions are rarely large enough to have any hemodynamic effect. During a flare of SLE, various systolic and diastolic murmurs frequently seem to wax and wane; it is very unusual for these murmurs to be due to marantic endocarditis. Most often they represent the high flow state due to anemia and high metabolic rate; in some cases, they may actually originate from the pericardium.

Cardiomegaly on chest x-ray film is a frequent finding in SLE patients. This may be a reflection of pericardial effusion or frank chamber enlargement due to fibrosis or reflecting long-standing hypertension. In view of frequent minor valve abnormalities in SLE patients, as well as their frequent immunosuppression with steroids, antibiotic prophylaxis for endocarditis is recommended.

PERIARTERITIS NODOSA

Necrotizing vasculitis of muscular arteries is the pathologic hallmark of periarteritis nodosa. Gross nodularity of the involved vessels is apparent at necropsy. The vasculitis may produce infarction of an involved organ; and when coronary arteries are involved, as they frequently are, myocardial necrosis may occur. Clinically recognized acute MI caused by periarteritis nodosa is uncommon, though clinically unrecognized events are frequent, as patchy fibrosis of the myocardium is common and contributes to the dilation of the left ventricle that frequently occurs. Small aneurysms of coronary arteries are present, particularly at bifurcations, and, on occasion, may rupture and produce hemopericardium. Pericarditis is uncommon in the disorder, as is endocarditis.

The clinical picture of cardiac involvement with periarteritis nodosa is most frequently dominated by the effects of hypertension, resulting from renal involvement. Indeed, congestive heart failure secondary to hypertension and renal involvement is a very frequent cause of death. Atrial arrhythmias occur on occasion; conduction defects are not frequently recorded.

One variation of arteritis that is most prominent in children and adolescents is Kawasaki's disease. In this syndrome, aneurysms of the coronary arteries are prominent, and may rupture or produce clinical MIs.

Treatment of periarteritis nodosa includes immunosuppression with large doses of steroids and vigorous treatment of hypertension and congestive heart failure.

SCLERODERMA (PROGRESSIVE SYSTEMIC SCLEROSIS)

In this systemic fibrosing disease, visceral rather than skin involvement is the main determinant of the clinical course. There is gradual obliteration of small vessels with extensive fibrosis and scarring. Progressive systemic sclerosis (PSS) commonly involves the heart pathologically, though clinical involvement is less often appreciated. A pancarditis is produced, with pericarditis common but often asymptomatic, myocarditis quite frequent, and endocardial thickening unusual. There is intimal sclerosis of small intramural coronary arteries that produces ischemia and focal areas of myocardial necrosis and fibrosis. Focal fibrosis frequently causes conduction abnormalities; and, if fibrosis is extensive, cardiomyopathy may result. Direct cardiac involvement is often overshadowed by cardiac effects of both pulmonary and systemic hypertension. Both right and left ventricular failure are common. If congestive heart failure develops, due either to hypertension or to direct myocardial involvement, the prognosis is poor. It is worth noting that conduction abnormalities usually do indicate primary myocardial involvement.

Specific treatment is not entirely satisfactory. Corticosteroids do have a beneficial effect on pericarditis in scleroderma, and there have been reports of penicillamine being of value for myocardial involvement. Conduction disturbances occasionally require management with a permanent pacemaker.

ANKYLOSING SPONDYLITIS

Dilatation of the aortic root and incompetence of the aortic valve occurs in approximately 3% of ankylosing spondylitis patients. Aortic regurgitation may become severe and valve replacement may be necessary. Cardiac conduction abnormalities may be severe and require management with a permanent pacemaker.

DERMATOMYOSITIS

Dermatomyositis involves the skin and the skeletal muscles, primarily; and clinical cardiovascular manifestations are unusual, though pathologic abnormalities are frequently present. Edema of myocardial fibers is frequently present in patients, as well as lymphocytic infiltrations, necrosis, and fibrosis of myocardial tissue. The fibrosis seldom is extensive enough to cause distinct cardiovascular symptoms. Repolarization abnormalities on electrocardiogram are frequently present, however.

Connective Tissue Disorders See Table 2.

MARFAN'S SYNDROME

Cardiovascular manifestations of Marfan's syndrome (see also Chapter 28) are prominent and frequently determine the fate of patients with the syndrome. There is cystic medial necrosis in the aorta, with degeneration of the elastic elements. The ascending aorta frequently is dilated, with dilatation of the aortic anulus as well. Sinuses of Valsalva may become grossly enlarged; frequently, there is accompanying dilatation of the proximal pulmonary artery. Chronic aortic dissection and tears without dissection are frequently found. Dilatation of the aortic valve anulus leads to chronic aortic regurgitation, with left ventricular dilatation and hypertrophy as a consequence. The mitral valve has frequent intrinsic abnormalities as well. Redundancy of the mitral valve leaflets can very frequently be demonstrated by echocardiography. The chordae tendineae are often elongated; occasionally, there is frank fenestration of the mitral valve leaflets.

In patients with Marfan's syndrome, a cardiac cause of death is very frequent, with aortic dilatation, dissection, or rupture in most patients. Mitral regurgitation may be the dominant clinical feature, though somewhat less frequently than aortic regurgitation. In these patients, with markedly altered hemodynamics and turbulent blood flow, endocarditis may be a complication. Ventricular conduction abnormalities have also frequently been reported.

The cardiovascular management of a patient with Marfan's syndrome is directed toward minimizing the hemodynamic stress experienced by the arterial tree. To this end, beta-adrenergic blockers are frequently used. Cardiac surgical intervention in patients with Marfan's syndrome is frequently exceedingly difficult because of the friability of the arterial tissue, so prophylactic operations are seldom undertaken. Antibiotic prophylaxis for endocarditis is indicated for these patients.

OSTEOGENESIS IMPERFECTA

Skeletal manifestations of osteogenesis imperfecta include very brittle bones and severe osteoporosis. The syndrome has cardiac manifestations similar to that of Marfan's syndrome except that dissection of the aorta does not occur. However, there is some degree of cystic medial necrosis in the aorta, which produces abnor-

Table 2. Cardiac Manifestations in Connective Tissue Disorders

Syndrome	AoV	MV	Ascending Aorta	Peripheral Arteries	CHF
Marfan's	+ + + +	+ + +	+ + + +		+ +
Osteogenesis imperfecta	+ + +	+ +	+ + +		
Ehlers-Danlos		+	+ +	+ + +	
Pseudoxanthoma elasticum	+ +	+ + +		+ + + +	
Hurler's	+ +	+ +			+ + +

Key: AoV, aortic valve involvement; MV, mitral valve involvement

malities in the ascending aorta, aortic anulus, and aortic valve. Aortic regurgitation and mitral regurgitation frequently are present and respond to standard medical management.

EHLERS-DANLOS SYNDROME

In this heterogeneous group of connective tissue disorders, there are defects in collagen synthesis. There are seven subtypes of the syndrome recognized at present. The collagen defects can produce major weakness in arterial walls, leading to aortic dissection, spontaneous rupture of the aorta and other vessels. There is significant morbidity associated with arterial catheterization of these patients, and it is necessary to avoid the procedure if possible. As well as dilatation of the aortic root and the sinuses of Valsalva, there is widespread involvement of cardiac connective tissue, producing cardiomegaly and conduction abnormalities. Endocarditis prophylaxis is warranted in these patients.

PSEUDOXANTHOMA ELASTICUM

There is dysplasia of the elastic tissue in pseudoxanthoma elasticum. Four subtypes are recognized; and in one subtype, mitral valve prolapse is prominent. In addition, the endocardium of the atria and ventricles is thickened and pearly white. The valve cusps may be thickened and rolled, and the coronary arteries may be narrowed due to abnormal elastic elements. Peripheral arterial manifestations are often prominent, with intermittent claudication in the legs and fatigability of the arms and legs. The media of the involved arteries have a high affinity for calcium, and calcification of limb arteries appears on radiograph. Decreased pulses are particularly prominent in the upper extremities, and there may be frank occlusion of the radial or ulnar arteries. Angina pectoris and hypertension are common, and aortic and mitral regurgitation may occur. Antibiotic prophylaxis for endocarditis is indicated.

HURLER'S SYNDROME

This disorder of mucopolysaccharide metabolism produces thickening of cardiac valves with fibrous nodules at the lines of closure. Cardiac chambers are often dilated, and mild to severe narrowing of the coronary arteries is sometimes present. Systemic and pulmonary hypertension are common; and murmurs of mitral regurgitation, aortic regurgitation, and aortic stenosis may be noted. Congestive heart failure and symptoms of ischemic heart disease are frequently prominent and determine the survival.

Sickle-Cell Disease

Cardiac manifestations of sickle-cell disease are principally the sequelae of chronic anemia and chronic hypoxemia. Pulmonary arterial thrombosis in situ is frequent in patients with sickle-cell anemia, with resulting AV shunting and systemic desaturation. Cardiovascular physical findings are principally those of a hyperdynamic circulation, although—because of the additional burden of arterial desaturation for any given hemoglobin concentration—auscultatory findings are more prominent and cardiac output is increased more than in other forms of anemia.

Though pulmonary infarction is common and frequently causes a painful crisis, pulmonary hypertension due to pulmonary infarction is infrequent, and the incidence of cor pulmonale is not increased in patients with sickle-cell disease. MI due to sickling and thrombosis in situ is exceedingly rare, although it has been reported to occur in papillary muscles. Chest pain in painful crises may mimic the pain of myocardial ischemia, and repolarization abnormalities are very common on electrocardiogram; nevertheless, this frequent clinical picture is very unlikely to represent MI.

At necropsy, most hearts are found to have cardiac hypertrophy and ventricular dilatation. There appears to be increased fibrous tissue present that is attributed to the chronic anemia and hypoxemia. The right and left ventricle generally are able to remain compensated in a high cardiac output state until the appearance of an intercurrent problem, such as chronic renal failure, pulmonary thrombosis, severe hypertension, or infection. Clinical congestive heart failure is likely to become manifest at these times.

Long-term therapy for sickle-cell disease is generally not satisfactory. Hypertransfusion appears to be useful when clinical congestive heart failure is present, though the efficacy has not been fully established.

Cerebrovascular Disease

As well as participating in the cause of cerebrovascular disease, the heart frequently reflects active intracerebral processes. The manifestations are principally disturbances of cardiac conduction and of rhythm. In 90% of patients with cerebrovascular accidents who have been carefully monitored for the first three days, electrocardiographic abnormalities will be present. One common cardiac sign of increased intracerebral pressure is the Cushing reflex: elevation in blood pressure and bradycardia, at times marked. Acute subdural hematomas frequently have cardiac manifestations. Sinus bradycardia may be present and at times may be symptomatic and require pharmacologic or pacemaker intervention. In addition, sinus tachycardia, atrial fibrillation, atrial flutter, supraventricular tachycardia, and ventricular tachycardia occur. Conduction abnormalities have frequently been reported also. The conduction and rhythm disturbances often do require therapy. Perhaps the most characteristic electrocardiographic changes of cerebrovascular disease are caused by subarachnoid hemorrhage or spontaneous intracranial hemorrhage. Electrocardiographic changes may simulate acute myocardial ischemia quite closely. There can be ST elevation with symmetric T wave inversion, suggestive of transmural myocardial ischemia. The classic "cerebral T" waves occur in these disorders and are manifested by deep and markedly symmetric T wave inversion. Frequently, prominent U waves are present and there is QT prolongation. The exact etiology of these repolarization abnormalities is not clear, but it is not simply related to increased CSF pressure.

Intrinsic cardiac disease frequently causes, as well as reflects, cerebral events. Cerebral emboli frequently occur in patients with rheumatic heart disease, atrial fibrillation, left atrial myxomas, left ventricular aneurysms, and recent MIs. In rare cases, left heart catheterization produces cerebral emboli either from thrombi on the catheter of from atherosclerotic plaques. On occasion, a central nervous system event may result from a reaction to radiographic contrast media as well. Other causes of cerebral emboli include prosthetic heart valves, bacterial endocarditis, and paradoxical emboli from the venous system and right heart. It is often not appreciated that marantic endocarditis associated with chronic debilitating disease may also cause emboli in a small but important number of patients. In evaluating a patient with a recent cerebrovascular accident, one must be aware that 12 to 30% of these patients will have had a recent MI. The diagnosis of recent MI in this setting is sometimes subtle, as an accurate history frequently is not available and one may be inclined to attribute electrocardiographic abnormalities to the cerebral event. However, the MB fraction of the serum creatine kinase can be of substantial assistance in making the diagnosis. In the group of patients with a recent cerebrovascular accident as well as a recent MI, prognosis is poor, with a mortality that may exceed 50%.

Psychotropic Drugs

TRICYCLIC ANTIDEPRESSANTS

Tricyclic antidepressants may be very effective in the management of certain types of depression. They are frequently used in elderly patients, a population that has a substantial incidence of cardiovascular abnormalities as well. Tricyclic antidepressants (TCA) appear to block re-uptake of catecholamines from the synaptic clefts of central neurons, compensating for a relative deficiency of the neurotransmitters. This relative augmentation of neurotransmitters available at postsynaptic receptors is not limited to the central nervous system, however, and contributes to the peripheral vascular and cardiac effects of the TCA. There appears to be an increased incidence of sudden death in patients with cardiac disease receiving TCAs, particularly amitriptyline (Elavil). This has been attributed to the arrhythmogenic effects of the TCAs. In addition to the sympathomimetic action of TCAs, their pharmacologic effects include anticholinergic action, quinidine-like effects, and alpha-adrenergic blockade. This may be manifest on electrocardiograms by PR prolongation, QT prolongation, QRS widening, ST-T abnormalities, and AV and intraventricular conduction abnormalities. T wave abnormalities are exceedingly common and tachycardia is very frequent. Indeed, there is probably some increase in resting heart rate in all patients receiving TCAs. Postural hypotension, to some degree, is almost universal and 24% of cardiac patients receiving TCAs are symptomatic with postural hypotension. This is often attenuated after the first several days of therapy. It appears that TCAs may have positive inotropic effects at low and, perhaps, therapeutic doses and negative inotropic effects at high doses. Desipramine appears to have the least anti-cholinergic effect.

The TCAs, in varying degrees, have properties of a type I antiarrhythmic. This may be manifest by suppression of ventricular premature beats and, in higher doses, conduction abnormalities and myocardial depression. Imipramine appears to have the most prominent type I antiarrhythmic effects; doxepin depresses conduction the least.

It is common practice to decrease the dose of TCAs when QRS prolongation is noted on electrocardiography. Management of TCA toxicity includes physostigmine for atrial tachyarrhythmias; conduction abnormalities may require temporary transvenous pacing. If profound hypotension is present in a patient with an intentional overdose, an alpha-adrenergic agonist, such as methoxamine or dopamine, is the drug of choice. Acidosis potentiates the toxicity of TCAs and administration of sodium bicarbonate to correct the acidosis is occasionally quite beneficial.

MONOAMINE OXIDASE (MAO) INHIBITORS

This class of antidepressants commonly produces some degree of postural hypotension. Conversely, a hypertensive crisis is a major hazard with MAO inhibitors. This can be induced by ingesting food containing tyramine or from administration of sympathomimetic amines. The management of a hypertensive crisis for patients taking MAO inhibitors is the administration of an alpha-adrenergic blocker such as phentolamine. Alpha-methyldopa, reserpine, and guanethidine should be avoided in patients receiving MAO inhibitors.

ANTIPSYCHOTICS

In patients with heart disease receiving antipsychotic medication, there may be an increased incidence of sudden death that has been attributed to arrhythmias. The cardiovascular effects of antipsychotic medications are quite similar to that of TCAs. Prominent among the effects are alpha-adrenergic blockade producing orthostatic hypotension, tachycardia, and anticholinergic effects. This class of drugs also has a quinidine-like effect on the heart. Alpha-adrenergic blockade may be particularly prominent with phenothiazines, whereas this bothersome side effect is virtually absent with haloperidol. In addition, a specific toxic cardiomyopathy has been reported for phenothiazines. Of the phenothiazines, fluphenazine has minimal cardiovascular effects, whereas thioridazine (Mellaril) should be avoided in patients with cardiovascular disease. Electrocardiographic abnormalities that are particularly prominent in patients receiving phenothiazines include PR prolongation, QT prolongation, QRS widening, ST-T wave abnormalities, varying degrees of heart block, and ventricular arrhythmias. T wave abnormalities are almost universal, benign, and reversible. Management of toxic effects of phenothiazines is similar to that for TCAs. Of note, in TCA and phenothiazine toxicity, type I antiarrhythmics should be avoided, as they may worsen conduction abnormalities.

LITHIUM

Lithium carbonate is frequently a very effective agent for the management of manic depressive illnesses. It has minimal important cardiotoxicity and minimal blood pressure effects. Rare cases of sinoatrial node dysfunction have been reported, however.

Lithium does induce electrocardiographic abnormalities that appear similar to those of hypokalemia, as it partially displaces intracellular potassium. In patients with congestive heart failure, lithium toxicity is a particular risk, as glomerular filtration rate is frequently diminished and lithium clearance is dependent upon renal function, and thus may be cleared slowly. Thiazide diuretics significantly increase lithium concentration, and thus serum levels need careful monitoring in patients receiving thiazide diuretics.

SEDATIVE-HYPNOTICS

In therapeutic doses, this class of drugs has minimal cardiovascular effects. Intentional overdosing with them, however, is frequent and can result in hypotension and pulmonary edema due to increased capillary permeability. Pulmonary edema in this setting does not respond well to diuretics and in fact the left ventricular filling pressure is often normal or low. Diuretic therapy might further lower cardiac output and blood pressure. Management of pulmonary edema with assisted ventilation and positive end expiratory pressure is efficacious. Chloral hydrate in toxic doses may induce ventricular arrhythmias that respond to lidocaine and Type 1 antiarrhythmics.

NARCOTICS

Narcotic overdose produces centrally and peripherally mediated increases in vagal tone and decreases in sympathetic tone, producing bradycardia and hypotension as well as pulmonary edema. The specific narcotic antagonist naloxone is an important first line of therapy. As with the sedative-hypnotic class of drugs, pulmonary edema occurs in the face of normal or low pulmonary capillary wedge pressure and is due to increased capillary permeability. Therefore management may require assisted ventilation with positive end expiratory pressure. In this setting, diuretics are usually of little use and may worsen the hypotension.

STIMULANTS

Amphetamines, cocaine, phencyclidine (angel dust), and marijuana are psychotropic drugs that have similar cardiovascular effects, though their basic pharmacologic properties differ substantially. Excessive use of these agents produces hypertension and tachyarrhythmias. In the case of marijuana, this has been demonstrated to be due to increased levels of circulating catecholamines. When specific therapy is indicated, propranolol is frequently effective for the tachyarrhythmias and hypertension. If hypertension is severe, sodium nitroprusside may be required.

ETHANOL

Heavy ethanol consumption produces both acute and chronic effects on the heart. The acute "holiday heart" syndrome is acute episodes of tachyarrhythmias, principally atrial, occurring after a heavy bout of drinking. The arrhythmia most frequently seen is atrial fibrillation, followed by atrial flutter and supraventricular tachycardia. Frequent PVCs may also be present. These episodes are often self-limited, and occur in patients with no discernible cardiovascular abnormality. Transient hypokalemia is frequently present and may be a contributing cause.

Long-standing alcohol abuse produces a congestive cardiomyopathy that is distinct from disorders caused by malnutrition or drugs. It appears that the presence of ethanol or acedaldehyde interferes with a number of functions that involve transport and binding of calcium. The net result is biventricular failure, with abnormalities both in diastole and systole. Therapy includes strict abstinence from alcohol, as well as conventional therapy for congestive heart failure.

Renal and Electrolyte Abnormalities

Renal disease and cardiac function are inextricably linked, as the kidneys ultimately determine extracellular fluid volume and intravascular volume. It is the business of the heart to circulate the volume of the fluid that the kidneys have regulated.

ACUTE RENAL FAILURE

There are three principal aspects of acute renal failure that have cardiovascular sequelae: altered fluid volume, hypertension, and metabolic abnormalities. In oliguric acute renal failure, intravascular volume and extracellular fluid volume increase. Right and left heart filling pressures are frequently increased, which will eventually lead to pulmonary edema, elevation of pulmonary artery pressure; and manifestations of right heart failure, such as hepatic congestion. To some degree, it is frequently possible to manage fluid overload in acute renal failure by zealous attention to fluid intake and use of potent loop diuretics. If congestive heart failure is present and due to volume overload and refractory to these measures, phlebotomy or plasmaphoresis are safe and effective short-term methods of decreasing intravascular volume.

A very frequent concomitant finding in acute renal failure is hypertension. Hypertension may have been previously present in these patients and, in fact, may be a contributing cause to the renal failure; for those in whom it is a new finding, it is often a "volume dependent" form of hypertension. For these patients, blood pressure frequently is exquisitely sensitive to their intravascular volume status. If intravascular volume can be reduced by diuresis, limitation of salt and water intake, phlebotomy, or in severe cases, dialysis, hypertension is frequently readily controlled. In addition, the hypotensive medications methyldopa, propranolol, and hydralazine are very useful in acute, as well as chronic, renal failure; and because they do not depend importantly on renal function for their clearance, they can be used in usual doses.

The recognition and management of electrolyte abnormalities in acute renal failure is of critical importance, as electrolyte abnormalities in this setting may produce life-threatening arrhythmias and conduction abnormalities (see discussion of electrolytes on page 546).

CHRONIC RENAL FAILURE

End-stage renal disease presents a panoply of cardiovascular complications, and, indeed, the success or failure in management of the cardiovascular complications of renal disease often determine these patients' survival.

Hypertension is a significant problem in the majority of patients with end-stage renal failure. As in acute renal failure, the hypertension is frequently "volume dependent." Management of fluid status by dietary means, as well as by ultrafiltration by dialysis, can be a major factor in these patients' blood pressure control. There is a subset of patients with end-stage renal failure who have exceedingly high plasma renin activity and in whom alterations of intravascular volume make little difference for blood pressure control. Successful control of hypertension in these patients may require nephrectomy. An angiotensin converting enzyme inhibitor, such as captopril, may play an important role in management of hypertension in these patients in the future. It has been established that, in some patients with chronic renal failure, there is important alterations in baroreceptor function. There currently is no specific therapy for this other than control of plasma volume by ultrafiltration and use of antihypertensive medications.

Accelerated atherogenesis appears to be frequent in patients with end-stage renal disease. This is likely to be multifactorial, with probable contributions by the elevated triglyceride levels and decreased high density lipoprotein levels found in these patients, by hypertension, and by diabetes mellitus, which is present in about 25% of patients who come to dialysis. Atherosclerosis is a major contributor to morbity and mortality for these patients; but, unfortunately, their hypertension is often the only contributing factor that can be addressed with much success.

Dialysis patients frequently have several specific cardiovascular problems. At initiation of dialysis, there is often a rapid decrease in extracellular potassium concentration, with a rapid increase in extracellular ionized calcium concentration. These patients are frequently receiving a digitalis glycoside, and this combination of electrolyte shifts sets the stage very effectively for signs and symptoms of digitalis toxicity despite "normal" serum digoxin levels. This can best be managed by very cautious use of digoxin in these patients and maintenance of a relatively high potassium level in the dialysis bath at the initiation of dialysis. Most patients on chronic hemodialysis have one or more AV fistulas or shunts for circulatory access. In patients with little intrinsic ventricular dysfunction, this AV shunt flow, in the range of 250 to 750 ml per minute, combined with the chronic anemia, may contribute to high output cardiac failure. In patients with markedly depressed ventricular function, it has been proposed that the presence of these AV shunts are of physiologic benefit in that they may serve to "unload" the left ventricle. For a given patient, detailed hemodynamic investigation would be required to determine the effect of the shunt flow on their ventricular function. The presence of vascular access for dialysis also increases the incidence of infectious endocarditis, due to shunt or fistula infections. The organism is most frequently *Staphylococcus aureus*. The early diagnosis of infectious endocarditis may be quite subtle in these patients, as cardiac murmurs are almost invariably present, due to their relative high output state. Bacteremia is very frequent in shunt infections but does not uniformly indicate endocarditis, as the fistula or shunt may be the only source of the continuous bacteremia.

It has been well-documented that, during the first 30 minutes of dialysis, transient hypoxemia develops with a decrease in PO_2 of 10-15 mm Hg. In the presence of concominant rapid electrolyte shifts, important arrhythmias frequently appear. Supplemental oxygen during the first part of a dialysis will partially obviate this problem.

Pericarditis is a very frequent complication of both acute and chronic renal failure. Echocardiography frequently demonstrates a small asymptomatic effusion in many patients with chronic renal failure. A minor viral respiratory infection may trigger symptomatic pericarditis in these patients. This may be diagnosed by characteristic clinical symptoms of positional pleuritic precordial pain, by characteristic ECG abnormalities, with ST elevation but without reciprocal ST depression, and by the presence of a precordial friction rub. In patients on dialysis, one suggestive sign of some degree of constriction or tamponade is marked hypotension as their intravascular volume is reduced. The effusion tends to be fibrinous and hemorrhagic, and systemic heparinization for dialysis may augment hemorrhage into the pericardium and lead to tamponade. Therefore, in patients with active pericarditis, regional heparinization may help prevent this problem. When an effusion does produce tamponade, pericardiocentesis can rapidly relieve the symptoms; frequently catheter drainage of the pericardium may be needed. With vigorous ultrafiltration, the size of the infusion can usually be reduced, and it is unusual to need pericardiectomy.

A perplexing problem arises when a patient with hypertrophic cardiomyopathy requires dialysis. The rapid reduction in intravascular volume that occurs at the onset of dialysis will decrease left ventricular chamber size and may produce left ventricular outflow obstruction that is symptomatic. To manage these patients, administration of propranolol has been found useful, in addition to transfusing to keep the hematocrit over 30 and minimizing the extracorporeal fluid volume during dialysis.

Partly because of the hemodynamic ravages of chronic renal failure, as well as the rapid progression of atherosclerosis, chronic renal failure patients may, on occasion, benefit from cardiac valve replacement or coronary artery bypass grafting. When scrupulous attention is paid to electrolyte balance, fluid replacement, and arrhythmias, these procedures can be undertaken with only modest increase in morbidity and mortality over that expected for the general population. Surgical correction of these important cardiac lesions may make their subsequent clinical management substantially smoother.

ELECTROLYTE ABNORMALITIES

Abnormalities of calcium and potassium balance have critical cardiac manifestations; whereas alterations in sodium, hydrogen, and magnesium balance have little, if any, important direct cardiac effects. The presence of congestive heart failure itself alters potassium balance, as there is enhanced exchange of sodium for hydrogen and potassium ions in the renal distal tubule under the influence of excess aldosterone, which might be present in heart failure. In addition, all diuretics, with the exception of spironolactone and triamterene, increase sodium delivery to the distal tubal and enhance potassium wasting. It is important to note that potassium replacement in congestive heart failure should be in the form of potassium chloride, as potassium excretion is augmented and accompanied by alkalosis.

Hyperkalemia may have catastrophic cardiac effects. As well as being present in chronic renal failure, it may be produced by tissue necrosis and may at times be

Table 3. ECG Manifestations of Electrolyte Abnormalities

	Interval			T wave	U wave	Atrial Activity	VPB Frequency
	PR	QRS	QT				
↑ K	↑	↑		↑		↓ or ↑	↓
↓ K		↑	↑ [a]	↓	↑		↑
↑ Ca^{++}	↑	↑	↓				
↓ Ca^{++}	↓	↓	↑				

[a] QU prolongation

iatrogenic. The electrocardiographic effects of hyperkalemia (Table 3) include peaked symmetric T waves, followed by broadening QRS and prolongation of the PR interval. Atrial excitability is supressed when the potassium level exceeds eight to nine milliequivalents per liter; and with a potassium level of 10 to 14, there may be complete AV dissociation, ventricular fibrillation, or asystole. These electrocardiographic and electrophysiologic changes are potentiated by hyponatremia or hypocalcemia. Mild elevations in potassium decrease the rate of spontaneous diastolic depolarization of all pacemaker fibers; ectopic pacemakers are more sensitive than the SA node, with the resulting antiarrhythmic effect of mild hyperkalemia. When hyperkalemia has abolished atrial activity, broadened the QRS, and altered repolarization so that the electrocardiogram (ECG) has developed a sine wave pattern, treatment is a true medical emergency. Ten to 20 milliliters of 10% $CaCl_2$ should be administered intravenously while continuously monitoring the ECG. This helps correct some of the electrophysiologic abnormalities produced by hyperkalemia, but does not lower the serum potassium. Administration of $NaHCO_3$ (1–2 ampules, 44–88 mEq), followed by 50 ml of D_{50} W and 10 units of regular insulin, will lower extracellular potassium concentrations. The onset of this effect is within 15 minutes and lasts for a few hours. However, total body potassium has not been altered by this regimen. Sodium polystyrene sulfonate (Kayexalate), a cation exchange resin, should be administered orally or by rectum in the dose of 50 g two to three times a day. When it is administered orally, it should be combined with sorbital to avoid gastrointestinal inspissation. This resin will bind potassium and effectively lower total body stores.

Hypokalemia has important cardiac effects as well, though by itself is less life threatening than hyperkalemia. Low potassium has a mild negative inotropic effect. On ECG, T waves are flattened or inverted and U waves may become more prominent. TU fusion produces pseudo QT prolongation. The correlation between the serum potassium level and electrocardiographic findings both for hypo- and hyperkalemia are quite rough and are not an adequate substitute for determination of serum levels. It is important to note that hypokalemia increases the risk of digitalis toxic arrhythmias and should be particularly avoided in patients receiving cardiac glycosides.

Hypercalcemia may occur in primary hyperparathyroidism, secondary hyperparathyroidism of renal failure, multiple myeloma, sarcoidosis, Paget's disease, and may be associated with several tumors. Chronic elevations in serum calcium may produce ectopic calcification of the cardiac skeleton and produce varying degrees of heart block. The electrophysiologic effects of hypercalcemia include augmented contractility, shortened systole, and decreased automaticity. This is manifest electrocardiographically as slight increase in the PR and the QRS intervals and shortening of the QT interval. Indeed, the electrocardiographic findings mimic those of digitalis effect. Hypercalcemia can be managed in the short term by sodium chloride infusion and furosemide administration. Hypocalcemia may be due to hypoparathyroidism, chronic renal failure, or pancreatitis. This does not usually produce cardiac arrhythmias, though it may have a negative inotropic effect. Electrocardiographically, the QT interval may be prolonged with shortening of the PR interval and QRS duration.

Elevated serum magnesium levels experimentally decrease cardiac conduction and ventricular irritability. There are no diagnostic electrocardiographic findings of hypermagnesemia.

Alterations in serum pH have no direct electrocardiographic effects but are associated with alterations in potassium and calcium concentrations. Marked acidosis has an important negative inotropic effect and decreases ventricular response to epinephrine and lowers the ventricular fibrillation threshold. Correction of acidosis is frequently critical in successful cardiac defibrillation.

Hypophosphatemia depresses cardiac contractility and repleting phosphate stores has a rapid positive inotropic effect. The exact mechanism of this is uncertain, though it is suspected that hypophosphatemia is related to depressed intracellular high energy phosphate concentrations.

Thyroid Disease

HYPERTHYROIDISM

Cardiovascular signs and symptoms are quite frequent in hyperthyroidism and they can be found even in "apathetic hyperthyroidism." Palpatations, dyspnea, tachycardia, and hypertension occur in about 30% of these patients.

One physical finding helpful in making the diagnosis of hyperthyroidism is the minimal diminution in heart rate while the patient is asleep. Supraventricular arrhythmias are common, particularly atrial fibrillation. Atrial flutter, supraventricular tachycardia, and conducted atrial premature beats are also frequently seen. In 15% of patients without other evidence of heart disease, right bundle branch block is present. Echocardiographic or radionuclide assessment of ventricular function reveals hyperdynamic ventricles.

Pharmacologic management of cardiovascular signs and symptoms can be rather difficult until the underlying hyperthyroid state is treated. Patients are relatively refractory to the effects of digoxin. It is not uncommon for a patient to show signs and symptoms of cardiac glycoside excess as the digoxin dose is escalated, while there is minimal effect on the rate of atrial fibrillation. Conversely, rendering a patient euthyroid will cause 30% of patients in atrial fibrillation to convert to sinus rhythm. Indeed, treatment of the hyperthyroidism may be dramatically effective for many cardiovascular symptoms. In the short term, beta-adrenergic blockade with propranolol may ameliorate many of the signs of hyperdynamic circulation. Added to moderate doses of digoxin, propranolol in small doses may be quite effective in regulating the ventricular response in atrial fibrillation, while avoiding toxic effects of either medication. For patients with congestive heart failure while thyrotoxic, propranolol must be administered with great caution. However, if tachycardia is a major contributing factor to their congestive heart failure, judicious administration of propranolol may improve their heart failure.

HYPOTHYROIDISM

In severe, long-standing hypothyroidism, the heart may become pale and flabby and grossly dilated. Microscopically, there is myofibrillar swelling and interstitial fibrosis. It is uncommon for hypothyroidism to be prolonged and severe enough to produce this picture, however. Rather, it is more frequent to have mild cardiac dilatation with further enlargement of the cardiac silhouette on chest x-ray film, due to a large pericardial effusion. In addition, bradycardia, a weak arterial pulse, hypotension, distant heart tones, and low electrocardiographic voltage may be present, as well as pericardial and pleural effusions. The presence of effusions is more likely to represent altered capillary permeability rather than true myocardial failure. In hypothyroidism, cardiac output is depressed, bradycardia is present, and peripheral metabolism is depressed as well. Cardiac catheterization reveals normal pressures with normal response to exercise unless there is coexistent intrinsic cardiac disease. In addition, response to catecholamines is normal.

Serum cholesterol and triglyceride levels are very often elevated in hypothyroidism. There is considerable debate whether this contributes to an increased incidence of atherosclerosis in these patients. Hyperlipidemia may, in fact, not have the same implications in hypothyroidism as in euthyroid patients. Evaluation of chest pain in a hypothyroid patient can be perplexing, as hypothyroidism itself can cause modest elevations in serum creatine kinase, lactate dehydrogenase, and SGOT. Electrocardiographic abnormalities are also frequent and include sinus bradycardia, low voltage, and T-wave flattening or inversion. These electrocardiographic findings may be in part due to presence of pericardial effusions.

Hypothyroidism occurs frequently in elderly patients who may have underlying ischemic heart disease or other important cardiac disorders. Therefore, thyroid replacement therapy must proceed cautiously so as to not induce severe angina or myocardial necrosis. Though therapy with triiodothyronine (T3) may have more rapid onset of action than therapy with thyroxine (T4), this may not be desirable in patients with cardiac disease. Therefore, it is usually best to start replacement therapy with T4, 12.5 μg per day, doubling this dose every 14 days, with careful monitoring of the cardiovascular status. A stable thyroid replacement dose of 100 to 125 μg per day of T4 may be quite adequate in an elderly patient with cardiovascular disease. Should patients, during thyroid replacement, develop severe angina that is not manageable with beta blockers and nitrates, coronary artery bypass surgery can be successfully and safely performed by an experienced cardiac surgical team. Most cardiac signs and symptoms of hypothyroidism resolve entirely after thyroid replacement.

Bibliography

Aber CP, Thompson GS: The heart in hypothyroidism. *Am Heart J* 68:428, 1964.

Barron KD, Siqueira E, Hirano A: Cerebral embolism caused by nonbacterial thombotic endocarditis. *Neurology* 10:391, 1960.

Benowita NL, Rosenberg J, Becher CE: Cardiopulmonary catastrophies in drug over-dosed patients. *Med Clin N Amer* 63:267, 1979.

Bonfiglio T, Atwater EC: Heart disease in patients with seropositive rheumatoid arthritis. *Arch Intern Med* 124:714, 1969.

Bonfiglio TA, Botti RE, Hagstrom JWC: Coronary arteritis, occlusion, and myocardial infarction due to lupus erythematosus. *Am Heart J* 83:153, 1972.

Braunwald E (ed): *Heart Disease; A Textbook of Cardiovascular Medicine.* Philadelphia, Saunders, 1980. (For in-depth review of topics, see corresponding chapter.)

Cathcart ES, Spodick DH: Rheumatoid heart disease: A study of the incidence and nature of cardiac lesions in rheumatoid arthritis. *N Engl J Med* 266:959, 1962.

Criscitiello MG, Ronan JA, Besterman EMM, et al: Cardiovascular abnormalities in osteogenesis imperfecta. *Circulation* 31:255, 1965.

deDeuxchaisnes CN, Krane SM: Paget's disease of bone: Clinical and metabolic observations. *Medicine* 43:233, 1964.

Dimant J, Grob D: Electrocardiographic changes and myocardial damage in patients with acute cerebrovascular accidents. *Stroke* 8:448, 1977.

Doherty JE, Perkins WH: Digoxin metabolism in hypo and hyperthyroidism. *Ann Intern Med* 64:489, 1966.

Ettinger PO, Wu CF, DeLacruz C, et al: Arrhythmias and the "holiday heart": Alcohol associated cardiac rhythm disturbances. *Am Heart J* 95:555, 1978.

Furfar JC, Muir AL, Sawers SA, et al: Abnormal left ventricular function in hyperthyroidism: Evidence for a possible reversible cardiomyopathy. *N Engl J Med* 307:1165, 1982.

Fisch C: Relation of electrolyte disturbances to cardiac arrhythmias. *Circulation* 47:408, 1973.

Fletcher GF, Hurst JW, Schlant RC: Electrocardiographic changes in severe hypokalemia. *Am J Cardiol* 20:628, 1967.

Gerry JL, Bulkley BH, Hutchins GM: Clinicopathologic analysis of cardiac dysfunction in 52 patients with sickle cell anemia. *Am J Cardiol* 42:211, 1978.

Giardina EV, Bigger JT, Glassman AH, et al: The electrocardiographic and antiarrhythmic effects of imipramine hydrochloride at therapeutic plasma concentrations. *Circulation* 60:1045, 1979.

Goldman MR, Rogers EL, Rogers MC: Subarachnoid hemorrhage. *JAMA* 234:957, 1975.

Harvey AM, Shulman LE, Tumulty PA, et al: Systemic lupus erythematosus: Review of the literature and clinical analysis of 138 cases. *Medicine* 33:291, 1954.

Heistad DD, Abboud FM, Schmid PG, et al: Regulation of blood flow in Paget's disease of bone. *J Clin Invest* 55:69, 1975.

Hejtmancik MR, Wright JC, Quint R, et al: The cardiovascular manifestations of systemic lupus erythematosus. *Am Heart J* 68:119, 1964.

Holsinger DR, Osmundson PJ, Edwards JE: The heart in periarteritis nodosa. *Circulation* 25:610, 1962.

James TN, Rupe CE, Monto RW: Pathology of the cardiac conduction system in systemic lupus erythematosus. *Ann Intern Med* 63:402, 1965.

Lamberti JJ, Cohn LH, Collins JJ: Cardiac surgery in patients undergoing renal dialysis or transplantation. *Ann Thorac Surg* 12:135, 1975.

Landing BH, Larson EJ: Are infantile periarteritis nodosa with coronary artery involvement and fatal mucocutaneous lymph node syndrome the same? Comparison of 20 patients from North America with patients from Hawaii and Japan. *Pediatrics* 59:651, 1977.

Lessin LS, Jensen WN: Sickle cell anemia 1910–1973. *Arch Intern Med* 133:529, 1974.

Muers M, Stokes W: Treatment of scleroderma heart by D-penicillamine. *Br Heart J* 38:864, 1976.

Rhodes BA, Greyson ND, Hamilton CR, et al: Absence of anatomic arteriovenous shunts in Paget's disease of the bone. *N Engl J Med* 287:686, 1972.

Rubin E: Alcoholic myopathy in heart and skeletal muscle. *N Engl J Med* 301:28, 1979.

Rubler S, Fleischer RA: Sickle cell states and cardiomyopathy: Sudden death due to pulmonary thrombosis and infarction. *Am J Cardiol* 19:867, 1967.

Tilkian AG, Schroeder JS, Kao JJ, et al: The cardiovascular effects of lithium in man. *Am J Med* 61:665, 1976.

Surawicz B: Relationship between electrocardiogram and electrolytes. *Am Heart J* 73:814, 1967.

VanderArk GD: Cardiovascular changes with acute subdural hematoma. *Surg Neurol* 3:305, 1975.

Varat MA, Adolph RJ, Fowler NO: Cardiovascular effects of anemia. *Am Heart J* 83:415, 1972.

NONCARDIAC SURGERY IN THE CARDIAC PATIENT

Lee Goldman

Although cardiology consultants are often asked to "clear" a patient for general surgery, the proper role of the cardiology consultant is really far more complex. The consultant should be prepared to assess the patient's risk of cardiac complications with surgery, to address any ways in which such risk might be reduced preoperatively, to comment on the proper approach to any perioperative questions or complications that might be expected to develop, and to be prepared to assist in the postoperative medical management.

Assessment of Risk

The preoperative cardiac evaluation of an adult patient for noncardiac surgery should include an appropriate history and physical examination, as well as a laboratory data base that includes a chest x-ray, electrocardiogram, and either a blood urea nitrogen or a creatinine value. This general data base, which will help the consultant participate in the perioperative care of the patient, should specifically emphasize those factors that are known to be associated with an increased risk of anesthesia and surgery.

Although the risk of perioperative myocardial infarction (MI) in the general population is only about 0.15%, the risk of perioperative complications in patients with prior MIs or angina pectoris is about 6%. Perhaps the most dramatic risk factor is that of a recent preoperative MI. Pooled results from three recent studies (1–3) reveal that a recurrent MI or cardiac death may be expected in about 31% of patients operated on within three months after a prior MI, in about 15% of patients operated on between three and six months after a prior MI, but in only about 5% of patients operated on more than six months after the infarction. Once this six month interval is reached, there is no apparent benefit from further delay of surgery (Fig 1). Although early studies described a much lower risk after nontransmural as compared to transmural infarction, recent data suggest that risks are similar after both types of infarctions.

Patients with preoperative congestive heart failure are clearly at increased risk for a postoperative recurrence. The new onset of pulmonary edema will occur in no more than 2% of patients without a prior history of congestive heart failure, in about 6% of patients with congestive heart failure by history but not by preoperative examination, and in about 16% of patients whose signs or symptoms of congestive

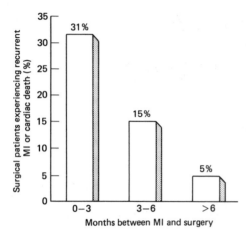

Figure 1 Pooled results of three recent studies show that the risk of cardiac death or recurrent myocardial infarction decreases significantly as the time increases between a preoperative MI and surgery. From Goldman L: Guidelines for evaluating and preparing the cardiac patient for general surgery. *Cardiovasc Med* 5:637, 1980.

heart failure persist up to the time of operation. At particularly high risk are patients who have histories of pulmonary edema or who have jugular venous distention or third heart sounds on preoperative examination. Patients with any such factor have a 25 to 35% chance of developing pulmonary edema in the preoperative period. When patients without a preoperative history of congestive heart failure develop new postoperative pulmonary edema, it is related to a postoperative MI in about 30% of cases;

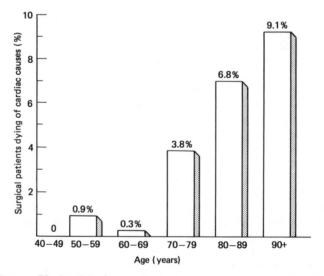

Figure 2 After age 70, the risk of cardiac death associated with surgery increases in a statistically significant linear fashion. From Goldman L: Guidelines for evaluating and preparing the cardiac patient for general surgery. *Cardiovasc Med* 5:637, 1980.

other patients usually will be over age 60, have major abdominal or thoracic surgery, and have baseline preoperative electrocardiographic abnormalities.

Patients with preoperative valvular heart disease have about a 20% risk of developing new or worsened congestive heart failure in the perioperative period. As with patients who have congestive heart failure on other bases, the severity of preoperative disease is probably the best predictor of the risk of developing postoperative heart failure. Patients with mitral stenosis are especially prone to develop supraventricular tachyarrhythmias that may precipitate congestive heart failure. Digitalis, which may not prevent new supraventricular tachyarrhythmias but which will make the rate of such new arrhythmias lower than if digitalis were not used, is usually recommended for such patients. Valvular aortic stenosis is also associated with difficulties in perioperative fluid management and with an increased risk of major cardiac complications.

Patients with preexisting rhythm disorders are also at increased risk for cardiac complications. Although such patients may develop specific arrhythmic complications, they are more prone to develop the same kinds of ischemic and congestive failure problems experienced by other patients with preoperative organic heart disease. This finding is consistent with other data suggesting that arrhythmias, especially ventricular arrhythmias, are often a marker of more severe coronary artery disease or of left ventricular dysfunction.

As the American population ages, older patients are subject to an increasing number of major surgical procedures. It is therefore noteworthy that the risk of cardiac complications increases in an almost linear fashion with age, and that the risk of perioperative cardiac death is about 10 times higher for patients over age 70 than for patients below age 70 (see Fig. 2).

The type of operative procedure is another major correlate of perioperative cardiovascular risk. Major intraabdominal, intrathoracic, or aortic procedures are associated with considerably higher risk than are other types of operations. The increased risk of such procedures is probably related to many factors: the seriousness of the surgery, the degree of respiratory compromise and postoperative pain, and the fluid and electrolyte shifts associated with major procedures.

Emergency operations are associated with about a four-fold increase in cardiac complications compared to the risks associated with elective operations. Part of this increased risk is probably related to general medical problems that cannot be corrected before emergency operations. Such abnormalities, including hypoxia, carbon dioxide retention, acidosis, hypokalemia, abnormal liver enzymes, or abnormal renal failure, are clearly associated with increased cardiac risk.

Although many factors may be associated with an increased risk of cardiac complications in noncardiac surgery, the consultant would like to be able to summarize these factors into an overall estimation of risk. Such a multivariable risk index, based on data from one hospital and subsequently shown to be valid at several other hospitals, is available to provide a rough estimate. As shown in Table 1, nine independently important factors were identified. After the appropriate number of ''points'' was assigned to each factor, patients could be placed into approximate risk classes (see Table 2). Note that over one-half of all patients were placed into risk class I, and that the risk of life-threatening or fatal cardiac complications in such patients was less than 1%. In risk classes II and III, the probability of a life-threatening cardiac complication increased, but the risk of perioperative cardiac death remained at 2%. Among the 18 patients in class IV, however, over 50% died of cardiac causes. These 10 cardiac deaths among the 18 class IV patients also represent over one-half of the cardiac deaths.

It is important to note that this multivariable approach to the assessment of cardiac risk was more accurate than reliance on any one risk factor. For example, the risk index could differentiate those patients who were less than six months after a preoperative MI into high-risk versus low-risk subgroups based on the presence or absence of other factors. It was also notable that factors such as stable hypertension, stable angina pectoris, or epidemiologic risk factors for the development of coronary artery disease were not independent predictors of the probability of life-threatening or fatal cardiac complications.

At the present time, there are insufficient data regarding the perioperative risks of patients who have unstable or class IV angina or who have had prior cardiac surgery to evaluate the importance of these factors precisely. As a rough guide to risk assessment, one might assume that a patient with unstable or class IV angina has at least as high a risk as a patient with a recent infarction, and that a patient

Table 1. Computation of Cardiac Risk Index from Factors Correlating with Perioperative Complications

Factors	Multivariate Discriminant-Function Coefficient	Points
History		
Age > 70 yr	0.191	5
MI in previous 6 mo	0.384	10
Physical examination		
S_3 gallop or JVD	0.451	11
Important VAS	0.119	3
Electrocardiogram		
Rhythm other than sinus or PACs on last preoperative ECG	0.283	7
>5 PVCs/min documented at any time before operation	0.278	7
General status		
PO_2 < 60 or PCO_2 > 50 mm Hg, K < 3 or HCO_3 < 20 mEq/l, BUN > 50 or Cr > 3 mg%, abnormal SGOT, signs of chronic liver disease, or patient bedridden due to noncardiac conditions	0.132	3
Operation		
Intraperitioneal, intrathoracic, or aortic operation	0.123	3
Emergency operation	0.167	4
Total possible		53

SOURCE: Reprinted by permission of the *New England Journal of Medicine* 297:845, 1977.

Key: JVD, jugular-vein distention; PACs, premature atrial contractions; PVCs, premature ventricular contractions; VAS, valvular aortic stenosis

Table 2. Correlation of Cardiac Risk Index with Complications in 1001 General Surgery Patients

Class	Point Total	No or Only Minor Cardiac Complication (N = 943)	Life-threatening Cardiac Complication[a] (N = 39)	Cardiac Death (N = 19)
I (N = 537)	0–5	532 (99)†	4 (0.7)	1 (0.2)
II (N = 316)	6–12	295 (93)	16 (5)	5 (2)
III (N = 130)	13–25	112 (86)	15 (11)	3 (2)
IV (N = 18)	≥26	4 (22)	4 (22)	10 (56)

SOURCE: Reprinted by permission of the *New England Journal of Medicine* 297:845, 1977.

Among the 532 patients with no more than 5 points, there was only one perioperative cardiac death as compared with 10 such deaths among 18 patients with 26 or more points.

[a] documented intraoperative or postoperative myocardial infarction, pulmonary edema, or ventricular tachycardia without progression to cardiac death; † figures in parentheses denote %

with prior cardiac surgery probably has a risk roughly equivalent to a patient without such surgery but with the same preoperative risk factors.

Preoperative Reduction of Risk

Of the factors associated with increased cardiac risks in non-cardiac surgery, at least several are potentially "controllable." For example, delaying an operation until at least three or perhaps six months after a preoperative MI will be associated with a reduction in risk. Unfortunately, most emergency surgeries and some semielective procedures, for example the surgical removal of a potentially curable cancer, cannot be delayed as long as one might like. Therefore, it is often important to compare operative to nonoperative risks, with the understanding that a patient with a high perioperative cardiac risk might have an even higher overall nonoperative risk.

There is a suggestion that preoperative control of congestive heart failure will greatly reduce the risk of postoperative pulmonary edema or worsened congestive heart failure, although there are no controlled data to prove such a contention. Because both general and spinal anesthetics often induce intraoperative hypotension, preoperative diuresis must not result in dehydration. Specifically, the aggressive diuresis that is usually suggested for a patient with chronic recurrent congestive heart failure would be too aggressive for a preoperative patient. Such overdiuresis can be avoided by monitoring the patient's blood urea nitrogen and creatinine and by carefully assessing postural blood pressure and pulse changes.

Because of the independent importance of valvular aortic stenosis, suspicious murmurs must be evaluated preoperatively. Such evaluation usually consists of a history, appropriate physical examination, and noninvasive tests, such as an echocardiogram and carotid pulse tracings. Sometimes such data will be inconclusive, and a cardiac catheterization will be recommended prior to nonemergency surgery. Some patients who deny cardiac symptoms may be so limited by noncardiac conditions, such as osteoarthritis or peripheral vascular disease, that symptoms normally induced by exercise are masked until these conditions are surgically corrected.

The value of cardiac catheterization and/or coronary artery bypass surgery in patients with stable but marked angina pectoris is uncertain. However, all agree that patients with unstable or crescendo angina should not be operated on until the angina is controlled, unless the surgery is absolutely imperative.

Effective treatment of a patient's general medical problems is also likely to decrease operative risk by reducing cardiac stress. The consulting cardiologist may appropriately recommend delay in surgery until such problems can be corrected.

Although recent studies suggest that hypertension per se is not an independent risk factor for perioperative cardiac complications, it has long been recognized that hypertensive patients have more labile blood pressures during anesthesia and surgery. At one time it was felt that this risk of lability could be reduced by discontinuing antihypertensive medications several days prior to surgery; conversely, others have suggested that such lability may be decreased by aggressively controlling blood pressure prior to surgery. Most recent data, however, suggest that neither of these extremes is correct. Although hypertensive patients do have more lability than do always normotensive patients, such lability seems to be independent of the degree of preoperative control of blood pressure as long as diastolic blood pressure is no higher than about 110 mm Hg. Thus, antihypertensive medications can be continued until surgery, and patients with persistent hypertension do not need to be brought under acute control preoperatively. Of course, the cardiology consultant should be sure that such hypertensive patients receive appropriate follow-up after hospital discharge.

Medical consultants often suggest that local or spinal anesthesia may be preferable to general anesthesia for cardiac patients. However, available data suggest that the advantages of local or spinal anesthesia may be limited to patients with substantial congestive heart failure, probably because such agents do not share the myocardial depressant action of general anesthetic agents. Spinal anesthesia causes just as much peripheral vasodilatation and subsequent hypotension as does general anesthesia. Furthermore, any anesthetic technique that does not effectively eliminate pain will be associated with markedly increased cardiac demands. Therefore, spinal anesthesia seems preferable from a cardiac standpoint only in patients in whom preexisting congestive heart failure is the overwhelming preoperative risk factor. Of course, spinal anesthesia may have substantial advantages for patients with important pulmonary disease in whom postoperative hypoxia or other pulmonary problems might markedly increase cardiac demands.

The choice among various general anesthetic agents is not nearly as critical as was originally believed. Halothane, which causes both myocardial depression and peripheral vasodilatation, is the agent most associated with hypotension; it should be used cautiously with patients who have other potential risk factors for intraoperative hypotension. In patients with idiopathic hypertrophic subaortic stenosis or with right-to-left shunts, peripheral vasodilatation during anesthesia may be especially hazardous. Ketamine, which has a sympathomimetic effect, is often recommended for such patients; alternatively, an alpha-adrenergic agent may be employed to increase systemic vascular resistance. Because anesthesiologists in most hospitals are fully aware of the risks and benefits of various agents and techniques, the cardiology consultant usually will not play a major role in such decisions.

Approach to Common Perioperative Questions and Complications

One of the major roles of the cardiology consultant is to anticipate common questions or problems that may develop in the perioperative period. In terms of the utility of the cardiology consultation for the surgeon and the anesthesiologist, the clear delineation of the approach to such issues is often more helpful than a calculation of the overall perioperative cardiac risk.

PREMATURE VENTRICULAR CONTRACTIONS

Patients with ventricular arrhythmias have an increased risk of cardiac complications with surgery, but most of these complications will be related to ischemia and congestive heart failure rather than to uncontrolled ventricular arrhythmias per se. Prophylactic lidocaine is usually recommended for patients with a history of symptomatic ventricular arrhythmias, a history of cardiac arrest, or very high-grade degrees of asymptomatic ventricular arrhythmias. For patients with lesser degrees of preoperative ventricular arrhythmias, lidocaine may still be given intraoperatively, for therapeutic rather than prophylactic purposes, if the ventricular arrhythmias compromise cardiac function. Because many ventricular arrhythmias during surgery are related to inadequate anesthesia, hypoxia, myocardial ischemia, or fluid and electrolyte imbalance, the identification and correction of such problems is more appropriate than is reliance on the antiarrhythmic properties of drugs such as lidocaine. It should be remembered that anesthesia may obscure the usual neurologic warnings of lidocaine overdose.

PROPRANOLOL WITHDRAWAL

It was originally feared that continuation of propranolol during the perioperative period would blunt the usual appropriate sympathetic response to the stress of surgery. However, more recent data suggest that patients on propranolol will usually respond appropriately to surgical stresses, and that supplemental isoproterenol can overcome the beta-blocking effects of the drug. Thus patients who require propranolol for the control of either angina or severe hypertension should remain on the drug until the morning of surgery; in other patients, the drug may be tapered over 48 hours prior to surgery. Hypotension or bradycardia in the patient on propranolol should not be treated intraoperatively or postoperatively with alpha-adrenergic agents; even epinephrine may cause hypertension, because its alpha-adrenergic effects will be unopposed while its beta-adrenergic effects will be blocked by propranolol.

Although the risk of a symptomatic rebound in sympathetic activity with the abrupt withdrawal of propranolol is small, recent studies suggest that patients are supersensitive to sympathetic stimuli after the drug is discontinued. Because the serum half-life of propranolol is only about six hours while its tissue half-life is substantially longer, withdrawal rebound, if it is to occur, will usually begin about 48 hours after discontinuation of the drug and persist for five to seven days. During the perioperative period, propranolol must be restarted immediately if the patient develops hypertension and tachycardia that are not related to postoperative problems such as pain, hypoxia, or fluid overload. The signs of propranolol withdrawal usually occur long enough after surgery so that the drug can be given orally. In some patients, propranolol can be given via a nasogastric tube that is then clamped for about one hour; sufficient absorption often will occur even though the gastrointestinal tract is not fully functional. Only an unusual patient will require intravenous propranolol, given as a 1 mg test dose, followed by 1 mg every five to ten minutes to control withdrawal, and then by either 1 mg every 20 to 60 minutes or a constant infusion of about 0.01 to 0.05 mg per minute.

PROPHYLACTIC DIGITALIS

In experimental animals, the myocardial depression caused by most general anesthetic agents can be prevented by digitalis. However, prophylactic digitalis for patients "at risk" for the development of heart failure has never been shown to be of benefit. Conversely, there are data showing that patients who develop new perioperative supraventricular tachyarrhythmias while on digitalis do so at a rate that is less than the rate noted in patients who have not taken digitalis. Those at risk for such arrhythmias include elderly patients undergoing pulmonary surgery, patients with valvular heart disease, and patients who have congestive failure but who are not yet on digitalis; in these patients, preoperative prophylactic digitalis may be of benefit.

CONTINUATION OF ANTICOAGULANTS

Patients who are on prophylactic anticoagulants for the prevention of systemic emboli in the setting of atrial fibrillation or rheumatic heart disease can usually have warfarin discontinued several days preoperatively, have the prothrombin time gradually return toward normal, and have anticoagulation restarted several days postoperatively. Most patients who are anticoagulated because of prosthetic heart valves can follow a similar regimen except that heparin should be started 48 hours postoperatively and continued until warfarin has resulted in an appropriate prothrombin time. Patients who have caged-disk valves, however, have an extremely high risk of thromboembolism with even the brief discontinuation of anticoagulants. In such patients, warfarin is usually reversed pharmacologically about 24 hours preoperatively, and low-dose heparin is begun at the same time; then, full-dose heparin is started about 12 to 24 hours postoperatively and continued until the patient can resume oral warfarin. If necessary, it is always easier to reverse heparin rapidly (with protamine) than it is to reverse rapidly the effects of oral vitamin K antagonists.

PACEMAKERS

Patients with asymptomatic bifascicular or trifascicular block are at risk for the eventual development of complete heart block, but such an event virtually never occurs during the perioperative period unless precipitated by new MI. Thus, there is no need for prophylactic pacemakers in such patients. Patients with symptomatic bradyarrhythmias that would normally require a pacemaker can have the pacemaker inserted preoperatively. If the operative procedure is likely to result in a substantial bacteremia, most physicians would recommend a temporary pacemaker during the perioperative period and then a permanent pacemaker after the infection has been cleared. Because some electrocautery equipment interferes with normal pacemaker function, such techniques should be used with caution. In the rare cases, in which a bradyarrhythmia requiring a pacemaker develops in the operating room, it is preferable for the patient to be maintained on atropine or isoproterenol until an experienced person can place the pacemaker under proper conditions.

PROPHYLACTIC ANTIBIOTICS

Patients with valvular heart disease or with prosthetic valves should receive appropriate high-dose antibiotic prophylaxis for the type of bacteremia that might be expected based on the site of surgery. In general, antibiotic prophylaxis should begin about six to 24 hours preoperatively and be continued for no more than about 48 hours postoperatively (also see Chapter 21).

SPEED AND EXTENT OF SURGERY

A debate often arises as to whether the planned operation in a cardiac patient should be briefer or more limited than the procedure that would be recommended for the patient with no cardiac problems. However, after controlling for the type of operation, there is no correlation between the length of surgery and the development of cardiac complications. In fact, postoperative MIs occur infrequently in the operating room or recovery room, but peak in incidence about four to six days postoperatively. Thus, cardiac complications are most common when patients are experiencing postoperative pain, fluid shifts, hypoxia, and other stresses. The operative technique, including the speed and extent of surgery, should be designed to minimize these postoperative risks.

INTRAOPERATIVE MONITORING

Many studies have substantiated the findings that marked reductions in blood pressure, especially reductions of 50% or more in systolic blood pressure or reductions of 33% or more that last for at least 10 minutes, are independent risk factors for the development of cardiac complications. Careful intraoperative monitoring can reduce the risk of such blood pressure changes. In patients without cardiac disease, blood pressure recordings, perhaps supplemented by central venous pressure lines, should be adequate. In patients with substantial left ventricular dysfunction, a recent preoperative MI, or class IV cardiac risk index scores, a Swan-Ganz catheter may be of additional benefit. Intraoperative hypotension is most commonly related to peripheral vasodilatation or bleeding, and can therefore usually be reversed by the rapid administration of fluids. Occasionally, brief doses of adrenergic agents may also be indicated, but one should be careful not to induce ischemia with such drugs.

INTRAOPERATIVE BRADYCARDIAS

Intraoperative bradycardias are most commonly the result of vagal stimulation. If such sinus bradycardias or nodal rhythms do not cause hypotension, ischemia, or inadequate perfusion, no therapy is necessary. Otherwise, these arrhythmias can be eradicated by changes in anesthetic technique, by small doses of intravenous atropine, or occasionally by small doses of beta-adrenergic agents. It should be emphasized, however, that most such arrhythmias are benign and short-lived, and that they do not correlate with more serious perioperative cardiac complications.

PERIOPERATIVE HYPERTENSION

Perioperative hypertension, as defined by an increase in systolic blood pressure of 50 mm Hg or more or as a systolic blood pressure above 200 mm Hg, will occur in about 5% of patients without a preoperative history of hypertension and in about 25% of patients with a preoperative history of hypertension. Adequate preoperative antihypertensive control does not clearly reduce this risk of perioperative hypertension. These hypertensive episodes commonly occur during intubation, during periods of inadequate anesthesia, or in the recovery room as the patient begins to wake up. The hypertension can often be reversed by changes in anesthetic technique in the operating room, or by correcting the hypoxia, fluid overload, or inadequate postoperative analgesia that has precipitated the hypertension. If these measures fail, specific antihypertensive medications can be given. Intravenous nitroprusside is the best way to control hypertension gradually and effectively, and it can be administered in the recovery room or intensive care unit setting. Intravenous Aldomet, usually given as 500 mg every six hours, will not have its pharmacologic affect for about six hours; but it is often enough to control patients whose perioperative hypertension is not in the potentially malignant hypertension range (diastolic blood pressure 120 mm Hg or higher). Hydralazine, which can be given intravenously, is an effective antihypertensive agent, but it often precipitates supraventricular tachycardia; its use should be discouraged unless other measures have failed, and it should usually be combined with small doses of intravenous propranolol (1 mg every 5 to 10 minutes) to control tachycardia. Again, it should be emphasized that perioperative hypertension usually can be kept in the nonmalignant range by appropriate analgesia, oxygenation, and fluid control.

VALVULAR HEART DISEASE

Careful perioperative fluid control is especially important in patients with valvular heart disease because of their increased risk of congestive heart failure. The issues pertinent to such patients have been discussed in other areas of this chapter.

IDIOPATHIC HYPERTROPHIC SUBAORTIC STENOSIS (IHSS)

Patients with IHSS will develop hypotension if they become volume depleted, receive beta-adrenergic agents, or develop tachyarrhythmias; these complications should be carefully avoided if at all possible. Intravenous propranolol is the preferred therapy for reducing left ventricular outflow obstruction in these patients, and it should be given to control congestive heart failure secondary to outflow obstruction. It must be emphasized that, in patients with IHSS, diuretics may worsen outflow obstruction and hence worsen congestive heart failure.

MITRAL VALVE PROLAPSE

There is no evidence that patients with mitral valve prolapse are at increased risk for cardiac complications with surgery; any slight increase in the likelihood of perioperative tachyarrhythmias does not justify antiarrhythmic prophylaxis. It is recommended, however, that prophylactic antibiotic coverage be given to patients whose prolapse is accompanied by an audible murmur.

Postoperative Medical Management

Because postoperative cardiac complications do not necessarily occur in the day or two after surgery, the cardiology consultant must continue to follow the patient for a minimum of five days after major surgery. During this postoperative period, the cardiology consultant can assist with the management of any acute postoperative complications and also help in the planning of the chronic therapy for conditions such as hypertension, congestive heart failure, or arrhythmias.

POSTOPERATIVE MYOCARDIAL ISCHEMIA AND INFARCTION

Only about one-half of postoperative infarctions will be accompanied by a complaint of chest pain, probably because many of the patients will be sedated or will have other severe types of postoperative pain. Nevertheless, most postoperative MIs will be associated with some symptoms: decreased blood pressure, congestive heart failure, arrhythmias, or a change in mental status. Routine daily postoperative ECGs may demonstrate presymptomatic ischemia in the patient at high risk for cardiac complications; but routine daily cardiac enzymes, in the absence of electrocardiographic changes have little to offer. Abdominal surgery, especially surgery on the biliary tract, or any surgery that involves prolonged manipulation of muscles will be associated with elevations of the usual "cardiac" enzymes; creatine kinase isoenzymes may be necessary to differentiate myocardial necrosis from these routine postoperative changes. In most series, postoperative MIs are associated with approximately a 50% mortality rate. Thus, patients who have evidence of infarction or of marked myocardial ischemia should receive the same kind of intensive care usually afforded to patients with unstable angina or MI.

POSTOPERATIVE HEART FAILURE

Congestive heart failure is often precipitated by postoperative surgical problems that increase myocardial demands, but some uncomplicated patients develop mild heart failure about 12 to 36 hours postoperatively, when the mobilization of intraoperative fluid occurs. One or two doses of diuretics are usually sufficient to manage fluid mobilization, but all patients with postoperative heart failure should be evaluated carefully regarding problems that may have precipitated the heart failure.

POSTOPERATIVE ARRHYTHMIAS

The new onset of supraventricular tachyarrhythmias, or the onset or worsening of ventricular arrhythmias, in the postoperative period is commonly related to coexistent medical problems. New supraventricular tachyarrhythmias will be associated with some cardiac condition in about 50% of cases, but only about one-third of these arrhythmias will be primarily related to a cardiac problem. Other major problems that must be investigated include infection (pneumonia, peritonitis, positive blood cultures), anemia, metabolic abnormalities, hypoxia, and new intravenous medications. In general, new postoperative supraventricular tachyarrhythmias do not require cardioversion, because most of them will resolve either with continuation of the patient's chronic cardiac medications or with the institution of digitalis. Electrical cardioversion should be used in emergencies only if the cardiac output is compromised; otherwise, cardioversion can be reserved until these predisposing medical problems have resolved, with the understanding that in most cases cardioversion will not be necessary.

Bibliography

Goldman L: Supraventricular tachyarrhythmias in hospitalized adults after surgery. *Chest* 73:450, 1978.

Goldman L: Noncardiac surgery in patients on propranolol: Case reports and a recommended approach. *Arch Intern Med* 141:193, 1981.

Goldman L: Cardiac risks and complications of noncardiac surgery. *Ann Intern Med* 98:504, 1983.

Goldman L, Caldera DL: Risks of general anesthesia and elective operation in the hypertensive patient. *Anesthesiology* 50:285, 1979.

Goldman L, Caldera DL, Southwick FS, et al: Cardiac risk factors and complications in noncardiac surgery. *Medicine* 57:357, 1978.

Goldman L, Caldera DL, Nussbaum SR, et al: Multifactorial index of cardiac risk in noncardiac surgical procedures. *N Engl J Med* 297:845, 1977.

Mahar LJ, et al: Perioperative myocardial infarction in patients with coronary artery disease with and without aortocoronary bypass grafts. *J Thorac Cardiovasc Surg* 76:533, 1978.

Prys-Roberts C: Hypertension and anesthesia: Fifty years on. *Anesthesiology* 50:281, 1979.

Selzer A, Walter RM: Adequacy of preoperative digitalis therapy in controlling ventricular rate in postoperative atrial fibrillation. *Circulation* 34:119, 1966.

Steen PA, Tinker JH, Tarhan S: Myocardial reinfarction after anesthesia and surgery. *JAMA* 239:2566, 1978.

Tarhan S, et al: Myocardial infarction after general anesthesia. *JAMA* 220:1451, 1972.

Tinker JH, Tarhan S: Discontinuing anticoagulant therapy in surgical patients with cardiac valve prostheses. *JAMA* 239:738, 1978.

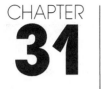

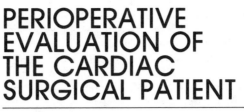

CHAPTER 31 | PERIOPERATIVE EVALUATION OF THE CARDIAC SURGICAL PATIENT

Gilbert Mudge

Cardiology is the most surgically oriented of all medical subspecialties. The properly trained cardiologist will always be assessing the timing of surgical intervention in patients with valvular heart disease or reappraising medical therapy and symptomatic status in patients with angina pectoris due to coronary artery disease. A firm working relationship between cardiologists and cardiothoracic surgeons is mandatory, for not only will patients receive expeditious surgical intervention when so indicated, but common cardiology problems can be easily addressed in the postsurgical patients when they arise. The purpose of this chapter is to review certain aspects of the perioperative care of patients undergoing both valvular replacement and coronary artery bypass grafting. Subtleties of perioperative care will be emphasized, to enhance the cardiologist's contribution to postoperative management.

Preoperative Evaluation

It will be assumed that the cardiologist is satisfied with the preoperative cardiac evaluation that has led to the decision for surgical intervention. The cardiac examination of patients with surgical valvular heart disease or coronary artery disease, with or without left ventricular dysfunction, will not be emphasized here. There are, however, several aspects of the general physical examination that must not be overlooked during final preoperative evaluation. In a patient being considered for valve replacement, there must be a careful oral examination, and carious teeth must be removed. Since one of the most serious complications of prosthetic valve replacement is superimposed bacterial endocarditis, all necessary dentistry should be completed before surgical intervention; a full mouth extraction and complete healing of the gum may be required in severe cases prior to elective valve replacement.

Patients undergoing coronary artery bypass surgery or mitral valve replacement should be carefully examined for the murmur of aortic insufficiency. One of the most severe complications that can occur during institution of cardiopulmonary bypass is significant distention of the left ventricle during the period of ventricular fibrillation. If such left ventricular distention is unattended, extensive subendocardial damage may well ensue. Patients with hemodynamically insignificant aortic insufficiency may have such ventricular distention when they are placed on bypass, for the aortic perfusion will distend the left ventricle. Accordingly, the surgeons should be advised when there is reasonable suspicion of such insufficiency.

The peripheral circulation should be carefully scrutinized in preoperative evaluation. Blood pressure should be assessed in both arms and peripheral pulses assessed in all extremities. Patients with asymptomatic carotid bruits should receive noninvasive evaluation of their carotids, with digital subtraction angiography or carotid angiography if so indicated. Since patients will often be perfused at a nonpulsatile pressure of 50 mm Hg while on cardiopulmonary bypass, questionable carotid circulation must be fully defined. Carotid endarterectomy, followed by cardiopulmonary bypass, can be effectively and safely done in patients with high grade carotid disease who require cardiac surgical intervention (Graver et al.). If this is not performed, major neurologic insult may occur, following the hypotension necessary for cardiopulmonary bypass technique. The abdominal aorta should be examined for bruits, and the competency of the iliofemoral system checked. This is particularly important in patients who may require transient use of the intraaortic balloon counterpulsation device following surgery. In addition, significant peripheral vascular disease may preclude femoral artery cannulation for initiation of cardiopulmonary bypass.

A careful gastrointestinal, renal, and neurologic history and examination is likewise required; the latter is of particular importance should any question regarding alteration in neurological status arise following surgery. The venous status should be carefully examined in patients who are to undergo aortocoronary artery bypass surgery. A history of venous ligation or past history of thrombophlebitis should be probably underscored in the admitting note. If arm veins are to be considered as potential conduits, intravenous therapy should not be administered through them during preoperative care.

Conventional laboratory studies are obviously mandatory in any preoperative evaluation. Patients with chronic obstructive lung disease or who have a history of many years of smoking should have pulmonary function tests. This will help in planning postoperative extubation and pulmonary care. Patients with advanced right heart failure should have the conventional indices of hepatic function carefully scrutinized. Thyroid studies should be checked in patients with underlying atrial fibrillation. Stool guaiacs for occult blood are mandatory, for they may help to dictate the choice of prosthetic valve. Chronic renal failure with hemodialysis is no contraindication to cardiopulmonary bypass, but compromised renal function that has not yet required such hemodialysis may be reason for surgical reconsideration. The hypotension and nonpulsatile blood flow that occurs during cardiopulmonary bypass may be sufficient to exacerbate renal dysfunction so much that hemodialysis will be required after surgery. There is preliminary evidence that a cardiopulmonary bypass machine capable of pulsatile blood flow will help in preserving borderline renal function.

The results of cardiac catheterization will obviously be carefully reviewed when the final decision regarding surgery is made. Patients with severely compromised left ventricular function with high left ventricular end-diastolic pressure and pulmonary capillary wedge pressure can certainly be expected to have persistent elevation of such pressure during the early postoperative stages. There are two other aspects to the results of the cardiac catheterization that might be emphasized when the cardiologist tries to anticipate postoperative complications. The right atrial pressure should be noted as a rough approximation of right ventricular function prior to coronary artery bypass surgery. Many patients with significant right coronary artery disease have sustained subclinical right ventricular infarctions. These patients may have exacerbation of right ventricular dysfunction in the early postoperative stages. This may be indicated by elevated right atrial pressures at cardiac catheterization. A right atrial pressure above 10 mm Hg should alert the cardiologist that right ventricular dysfunction is present, and that enhanced volume requirements may be necessary during the first 48 hours after surgery. In addition, the pulmonary artery pressure should be carefully measured. Many patients with mitral valve disease and pulmonary hypertension will have persistent elevation of such pulmonary artery pressures during the first days of their postoperative care. Such fixed pulmonary vascular resistance is identified when pulmonary artery diastolic pressure exceeds the mean pulmonary capillary wedge pressure. When this is the case, severe pulmonary hypertension may continue through the early postoperative days. This not only will necessitate extremely high right atrial filling pressures, but may also be easily exacerbated with hypoxia. It is mandatory that these patients be well oxygenated, and that a pulmonary vasodilator, such as isoproterenol, be considered in their early pharmacologic regimen. Patients with severe pulmonary hypertension, whose pulmonary artery diastolic pressure equals pulmonary capillary wedge pressure, can usually be expected to have rapid resolution of such pulmonary hypertension when the pulmonary capillary wedge pressure is reduced after mitral valve replacement.

Most medication can be safely continued right up until the time of surgery. Some centers institute digoxin during the last preoperative day, not only for its inotropic support, but also to control atrial fibrillation should it occur postoperatively (Burman, Selzer and Walter). Diuretic therapy can likewise be continued, bearing in mind that many patients with long-term diuretic use have relative total-body potassium depletion although the serum potassium levels are normal. Since hypokalemia may account for many early postoperative ventricular arrhythmias, additional potassium supplement should be considered in the final preoperative days for patients on high diuretic dosage.

A beta-adrenergic blocking agent is often administered to patients about to undergo coronary artery revascularization. In most patients with reasonable left ventricular function (an ejection fraction greater than 0.40), the beta-adrenergic blocking agent can be maintained until the time of surgery (Caralps et al.). By so doing, any potential "rebound" is avoided. In those patients with severely compromised left ventricular function, beta-adrenergic blocking agents are probably best discontinued for at least 24 hours prior to surgery, as long as the patient's activity is curtailed, and adequate nitrate administration is maintained.

Although clinical experience with the calcium channel blocking agents is in its early stages, there seems to be no current contraindication to continued use of nifedipine or verapamil right up to the time of surgery. This would be mandatory if part of a patient's clinical presentation was that of coronary artery vasospasm, superimposed upon a high-grade fixed obstructive lesion. Sudden withdrawal of a calcium channel blocking agent might exacerbate coronary artery vasospasm, provoking a preoperative myocardial infarction (Muller et al.). Each of the new calcium channel blocking agents must be reevaluated as it becomes clinically available. Since one of their potential pharmacologic effects is to uncouple myocardial excitation from its subsequent contraction, some of these calcium channel blocking agents may have profound negative inotropic effects during the early hours following cardiopulmonary bypass.

Conventional anticoagulation with Coumadin obviously must be discontinued so that the prothrombin time and partial thromboplastin time return to normal prior to surgery. Aspirin has been associated by some observers with significant postoperative bleeding, and probably should not be administered for at least 72 hours prior to surgery. The safety of other antiplatelet agents in the final preoperative hours is unclear. A recent investigation administered dipyridamole preoperatively to patients about to undergo myocardial revascularization, without excessive postoperative bleeding (Cheesebro et al.).

Conventional oral antiarrhythmics can be continued up to the time of surgery, and replaced with intravenous preparations if need be, as determined by the anesthesiologist.

Intraoperative Considerations

While inhalation anesthetics may be used in patients with low risk procedures, morphine has emerged as a safe and effective anesthesia, when used in conjunction with nitrous oxide. The dose of morphine may vary from 1–3 mg/kg, its primary benefit being the absence of any significant myocardial depression (Lowenstein et al.). Major disadvantages to morphine anesthesia are its vasodilating capacity and the prolonged postoperative intubation required. Since morphine may reduce both preload and afterload, patients may often require enhanced volume administration during the early postoperative hours. Such anesthesia is potentially dangerous in certain people whose cardiac output is dependent upon their preload status; this is particularly important in patients with critical aortic stenosis whose left ventricular stroke volume depends upon left ventricular filling. Patients with significant right-to-left shunts can have exacerbation of such shunts if peripheral vascular resistance is precipitously reduced during the induction of anesthesia. These two types of patient populations should be vigorously treated with both volume expansion and administration of pressor agents. Morphine anesthesia also requires a long intubation period after surgery, usually 12–18 hours after the patient has left the operating room. Fortunately, modern meticulous technique in respiratory care usually avoids the complications of such intubation.

While the cardiologist's presence is usually not required during surgery, he or she must be thoroughly familiar with the techniques of thoracotomy, of placing the patient on the pump oxygenator, of the surgical procedure itself, and of weaning the patient from cardiopulmonary bypass. The aortic arch is usually cannulated to receive the arterial input from the pump oxygenator, but the femoral artery can be used. Femoral artery cannulation is often indicated in patients with severely compromised left ventricular function, so that partial cardiopulmonary bypass support may be given as the patient's sternum is being opened. In addition, femoral artery cannulation may be required if the surgery involves the aortic arch itself. Cannulation of the aortic arch saves significant time by avoiding groin dissection, but it must be done with extreme care, particularly in elderly patients with fragile calcified aortas. Dissection from a proximal aortic cannulation usually has dire consequences. The venous return to the oxygenator is usually obtained from the vena cava via the right atrium. Once venous and arterial cannulae are in place, the patient may be cooled to approximately 28°C, with supplemental topical cardiac hypothermia applied during the time that the aorta is cross-clamped. The cardiologist should remember that left ventricular distention must be prevented during the time of aortic cross-clamp; a left vetricular vent may be required to decompress the left ventricle during this time. The cardiologist should also be familiar with the technique that the surgeon uses to remove air from the left heart and aorta before resumption of left ventricular ejection is permitted. The pump oxygenator will usually maintain a blood flow of 2.0–2.5 L/min/m², which generates a mean nonphasic blood pressure of 50–60 mm Hg. Lower blood flows are permitted with more intense cooling, and total circulatory arrest may be feasible for brief periods of time at 20°C.

When the surgical procedure is complete, monitoring lines are inserted before the patient is completely weaned from cardiopulmonary bypass. The exact line used will often depend upon the preference of the anesthesiologist or surgeon. While percutaneous pulmonary artery catheters are always feasible, direct left atrial lines inserted to the posterior aspect of the left atrium via the pulmonary veins provide a precise definition of hemodynamics for the first 48 postoperative hours. These can easily be brought out through a small skin incision and pulled before the chest tubes have been discontinued. Right atrial lines may be similarly inserted by the surgeons with minimal complications to their removal. Once measurement of both right and left heart pressures is performed, the surgeon will wean the patient from cardiopulmonary bypass. Anterior and posterior mediastinal chest tubes will then be inserted; additional chest tubes may be required if either of the pleural cavities have been entered. The pericardium is usually left open. Atrial and ventricular pacing wires are attached and brought out through the skin. The former wires are particularly helpful in the postoperative management of patients with hypertrophy, non-compliant ventricles that require pacing, and in the diagnosis and treatment of postoperative supraventricular tachycardias. The sternum is then reapproximated, the skin closed, and the patient returned to the recovery room intubated with need for continued ventilatory support.

Postoperative Care

The presence of an arterial line, right and left atrial lines, and perhaps a pulmonary artery catheter simplifies the close hemodynamic monitoring required for patients after cardiopulmonary bypass. While the right atrial line may be a venous access, the left atrial line must never be so used.

Postoperative hypotension is the most common hemodynamic problem in the first hours after surgery. Pharmacologic inotropic support does not need to be added to the patient's intravenous regimen until adequate right and left atrial filling pressures have been achieved. During the first hours after coronary artery bypass surgery, patients may have enormous volume requirements. Such enhanced fluid requirements are most often due to the morphine anesthetic used; a more remote etiology is transient right ventricular dysfunction. In addition to these two etiologies, the patients also vasodilate as their body temperature warms from 28°C. During the final phases of cardiopulmonary bypass, with a body temperature of 28°, there is a significant vasoconstriction with increased systemic vascular resistance. As the patients return to a more normal temperature, vasodilatation will beget further volume requirements. It is not at all unusual for patients with totally normal left ventricular function and an uncomplicated postoperative course to require 6 to 7 liters of volume expansion in the first several hours after surgery, before their hemodynamic status stabilizes. The choice or type of volume will obviously be made in conjunction with the surgeons; the patient should receive any blood left from the pump oxygenator. Daily weights during the first postoperative week and comparison to preoperative weight constitute an important means of assessing fluid balance.

Hypotension associated with high left atrial filling pressures should obviously be treated with appropriate inotropic support. Many patients may have inappropriately high systemic vascular resistance, with severely depressed left ventricular function and borderline hypotension; and combined inotropic support with afterload reduction in such a patient population is justified. During the first 24 hours after surgery, intravenous nitroprusside and dopamine are often adequate. Patients should be closely monitored for arrhythmias, which may be precipitated by inotropic agents such as dopamine and epinephrine. There is some evidence that in this patient population dobutamine has equal positive inotropic effect with greater afterload reduction capability when compared to equal doses of dopamine (DiSesa et al.). The latter point may form the rationale for single drug therapy in patients with severely depressed left ventricular function.

Significant hypertension after coronary artery bypass surgery has been reported to occur in 30–50% of patients undergoing myocardial revascularization (Viljoen et al.; Salerno et al.). Hemodynamic studies have indicated that this is related to an increase in total peripheral vascular resistance without any significant change in cardiac output, an increase in resting alpha-adrenergic vasoconstrictor tone postulated as a mechanism. Plasma epinephrine and norepinephrine levels have been documented to increase significantly in the early postoperative course; the renin-angiotensin system has also been incriminated, and converting enzyme inhibitors have been used successfully in controlling blood pressure (Niarchos et al.). There is no significant correlation with past history of hypertension or previous propranolol dosage. Most patients usually become significantly hypertensive within 2 hours after surgery, the hypertension abating 48 to 72 hours later. Aggressive therapy of this acute hypertension is indicated for several reasons. Not only is there a significant increase in myocardial oxygen consumption as a result of the enhanced blood pressure, but the degree of postoperative bleeding, both from the aortic cannulation site and from saphenous vein graft anastomosis, can be related to the blood pressure. Chest tube drainage often resolves when postoperative hypertension is brought under control. Since the postoperative hypertension is a transient hemodynamic phenomenon during the first 48 postoperative hours, intravenous therapy with sodium nitroprusside seems indicated, controlling the systolic pressure at 120 mm Hg. This can be easily tapered as the hypertension resolves. Should there be persistent elevation of blood pressure 48 hours postoperatively, alpha-methyldopa, captopril, or a beta-adrenergic blocking agent can be returned to the patient's medical regimen. Virtually all patients found to be normotensive during preoperative evaluation can be tapered off all antihypertensive medication before hospital discharge.

Postoperative bleeding should be carefully monitored by the anterior and posterior mediastinal chest tubes. Adequate protamine sulfate should be administered to reverse the heparin given when the patient was on the pump oxygenator. Protamine sulfate may produce peripheral vasodilatation and hypotension, thus enhancing the initial postoperative volume requirements. The platelet count should also be carefully monitored. In most patients with normal preoperative platelet counts, that count will drop to 60,000–70,000 due to destruction from the pump oxygenator. Platelet transfusions may be needed. Some surgeons will control mediastinal bleeding with positive-end expiratory pressure from the respiratory ventilator. If bleeding continues at 200–300 ml per hour for four hours after initial chest closure, surgical reexploration is usually required.

Significant ventricular arrhythmias are common after valvular or revascularization surgery (Angelini et al.). The etiologies for such dysrhythmias are many, including direct trauma to the ventricle, hypoxia, depressed left ventricular function, anesthetic agents, endogenous or exogenous catecholamine stimulation, electrolyte or acid-base abnormality, and, more commonly, the underlying disease process itself. Since the maximum depression of left ventricular function will not occur for 18–24 hours after cardiopulmonary bypass, it is perhaps best to treat all significant ventricular premature contractions, occurring more frequently than 10 per minute, with intravenous therapy, after corrective etiologies such as hypoxia, hypokalemia, acidosis, or alkalosis have been addressed. Digitalis toxicity must not be overlooked in this patient population. Lidocaine is preferred as the initial intravenous antiarrhythmic agent, for depression of myocardial contractility and peripheral vasodilatation are far less severe than with equivalent doses of procainamide or quinidine. If patients are refractory to lidocaine administration, intravenous procainamide can be administered, and the patient then switched to oral preparation when appropriate. Diphenylhydantoin or bretylium tosylate may also be considered as intravenous agents should patients have refractory high-grade and life-threatening ventricular ectopic activity.

All patients who have required intravenous antiarrhythmic therapy for ventricular ectopic activity should receive 24 hours of continuous monitoring in the last postoperative stages before discharge. It is common practice for significant ventricular ectopic activity, including couplets, multiform ventricular premature beats, or brief ventricular tachycardia, to be suppressed by oral therapy for at least six weeks after surgery. This is particularly important in those patients suspected of having a perioperative myocardial infarction after coronary artery revascularization.

Supraventricular tachycardias are also quite common after valvular or coronary artery bypass surgery. Atrial premature beats are typical, and transient atrial flutter or fibrillation has been reported to occur in as many as 30% of patients who were in normal sinus rhythm preoperatively. Fortunately, most of these atrial dysrhythmias can be easily converted and controlled with conventional antiarrhythmic therapy. Cardioversion is rarely needed. The atrial electrode should be used if the diagnosis of any supraventricular tachycardia is in question. An atrial wire can be connected to the precordial lead of an electrocardiogram, and atrial activity recorded. Etiologies for recurrent supraventricular tachycardia in the early postoperative course must be carefully considered. Hypoxia, persistent pulmonary infiltrates, pericarditis, gastric dilatation, anemia, fever, or right or left atrial cannulae can often be found. Rapid supraventricular tachycardias that cause hemodynamic embarrassment should be immediately treated with cardioversion. Little additional anesthesia is often required; 5–10 mg of intravenous diazepam is usually adequate. Supraventricular tachycardias in those patients who have had valve replacement are perhaps best treated with either quinidine or procainamide therapy. Among patients who demonstrate such dysrhythmia after coronary artery bypass surgery, low dose beta-adrenergic blockade or verapamil have been reported to be extremely effective and nontoxic antiarrhythmic agents (Mohr et al.). Rapid atrial pacing is safe, atraumatic, and can also be considered if an atrial wire is in place (Waldo et al.). The atrial rate should be increased to 125% of the underlying atrial arrhythmia. When this is abruptly terminated, normal sinus rhythm or atrial fibrillation often follows. The latter is more easily controlled than atrial flutter with intravenous digoxin or verapamil. Patients who are in normal sinus rhythm preoperatively and maintain normal sinus rhythm for six weeks after surgery can have all antiarrhythmic therapy discontinued at that time.

Many patients with mitral valve disease and chronic atrial fibrillation preoperatively may emerge from the operating room in normal sinus rhythm. In these patients, the left atrium has been inspected for the presence of thrombi. While most of these patients may revert to their basic atrial dysrhythmia during the first postoperative week, attempts should be made with appropriate antiarrhythmic therapy to maintain a sinus mechanism. In patients with aortic valve replacement and porcine heterograft, the maintenance of normal sinus rhythm may obviate the need for long-term anti-coagulation.

The possibility of digitalis toxicity should always be considered as an etiologic agent, and digoxin levels should be checked when clinically indicated. This is particularly important after the institution of quinidine therapy.

Third degree heart block is a rare complication of open heart surgery, more common following repair of ventricular septal defect and endocardial cushion defect. In adults, débridement of a heavily calcified aortic valve may produce complete heart block. This is often recognized in the operating room, and treated appropriately with ventricular wires. In patients with evidence of bifascicular conduction abnormalities, the treatment is often to place a permanent epicardial wire at the time of surgery, the wires brought down to a subcutaneous subxiphoid pouch. These can easily be retrieved if normal conduction is not restored after surgery. Nodal rhythms are a frequent conduction abnormality, most common after mitral valve and aortic valve replacement. These are usually well tolerated, with adequate rate, but can always be treated with overdrive pacing or isoproterenol infusion. Such nodal rhythm disturbances usually last 48–72 hours and resolve spontaneously.

Intraoperative myocardial infarctions are another potential problem that must be addressed within the first 48 hours after surgery. During this time, the appearance of new Q waves should be interpreted as evidence of infarction, with little emphasis placed on the ST segment or T wave contour. There can be marked ST segment elevation and T wave inversion that do not represent myocardial ischemia. Such ST segment elevation may resolve when the anterior and posterior mediastinal chest tubes are removed. ST-T wave abnormalities may persist for six months after surgery. Conventional myocardial enzymes are often elevated; a CK of 600–800 IU/L is not unusual; CK elevation may be associated with trace elevation to the CK-MB fraction. Presence of the CK-MB is frequently found in patients who have required direct conversion of ventricular fibrillation to sinus rhythm in the operating room with paddles placed upon the heart. An SGOT greater than 100 IU/L coupled with a CK greater than 1,000 IU/L should be considered evidence of a subendocardial myocardial infarction.

The incidence of perioperative myocardial infarction following coronary artery bypass surgery should not exceed 10–12%. Fortunately, most of these infarctions represent subendocardial damage, without major hemodynamic compromise, and these patients can usually be ambulated and progressed through their late postoperative management without undue complication. A perioperative myocardial infarction with major hemodynamic compromise should be treated by conventional therapy with proper inotropic support, and intraaortic balloon counterpulsation if necessary. Such patients are usually not considered reasonable candidates for emergency repeat revascularization.

Patients are usually slowly ambulated 48–72 hours after surgery, and if the postoperative course is uncomplicated, discharge can be anticipated on the seventh to tenth postoperative day. In patients who have undergone coronary artery bypass surgery, the leg incisions are often the primary source of discomfort. The physical examination should be directed toward evidence of congestive heart failure, pulmonary consolidation, atelectasis, pericardial rub, pericardial tamponade (evidence of pulsus paradoxus should be sought), and thrombophlebitis. The incidence of postpericardiotomy syndrome is low, approaching 5% in most series. Unexplained fever, chest pain, and pericardial rub are indication for nonsteroidal antiinflammatory agents. Other postoperative complications that may occur include wound infection, pulmonary embolism, cerebrovascular accident, urinary tract outlet obstruction, complications from use of intraaortic balloon pump, and hepatitis resulting from transfusion.

Indefinite anticoagulation is required on all mechanical prosthetic valves. A porcine xenograft valve, placed in the aortic position, does not require anticoagulation, but a patient with a porcine xenograft in the mitral position and normal sinus rhythm usually receives anticoagulation for six weeks after surgery. If normal sinus rhythm is maintained, then the anticoagulation can be discontinued without undue thromboembolic complications (Cohn et al.). In those patients with chronic atrial fibrillation, anticoagulation should be maintained indefinitely, irrespective of type of valve used. Such anticoagulation can be started 48 hours after surgery, once the chest tubes and atrial cannulae have been removed.

Recent evidence suggests that aggressive antiplatelet therapy should be initiated in patients with coronary artery disease (Cheesebro et al.; Baur et al.). Studies with sulfinpyrazone, and combined aspirin/dipyridamole therapy have indicated that graft closure rate can be reduced to 3% after coronary artery revascularization; those patients who received placebo therapy had a graft closure rate of 9%. In the latter study, dipyridamole was initiated before surgery, and aspirin instituted as soon as mediastinal bleeding ceased. The presence of antiplatelet therapy during the first 48 hours of surgery may be critical for its success. Additional controlled studies are pending.

Before discharge, patient's physical examination should be carefully noted in the record; a postoperative echocardiogram evaluating prosthetic valve function has been advocated by some observers as a baseline control observation. The physician should check the stability of the sternum, placing fingers on either side of the incision and asking the patient to cough. Patients clearly need to be instructed on complications of anticoagulation and proper prophylaxis for subacute bacterial endocarditis as so indicated. In patients with significant left ventricular dysfunction, diuretic regimen and sodium intake will have to be carefully adjusted.

Patients are encouraged to slowly increase their daily activity as comfort and energy permit. Most patients continue to experience variable degrees of fatigue for 4–6 weeks after surgery, with residual leg and sternal discomfort; resumption of totally normal activity usually is not practicable until the eighth postoperative week. An active rehabilitation program does not seem practical until such discomfort is fully resolved, and evaluation of operative success by exercise tolerance study is of little benefit until the surgically induced ST segment and T wave abnormalities have resolved and the patient is completely comfortable. Stress thallium studies may be indicated if surgically-induced ST segment abnormalities prevent a precise electrocardiographic analysis.

Most patients should be seen at least once a year after open heart surgery. Those with valve replacement must be carefully followed for evidence of paravalvular leaks or primary valve dysfunction. Recognizing that coronary artery bypass surgery is a palliative procedure, such patients should be carefully followed for evidence of recurrent myocardial ischemia. Risk factors that have contributed to the development of coronary artery disease cannot be ignored. Cigarette smoking must cease, blood pressure must be controlled, and lipid derangements must be lowered when possible.

References

Angelini P, Feldman MI, Lufochanowski R, et al: Cardiac arrhythmias during and after heart surgery: Diagnosis and management. *Prog Cardiovasc Dis* 16:649, 1974.

Baur HR, Van Tassel RA, Purach CA, et al: Effects of sulfinpyrazone on early graft closure after myocardial revascularization. *Am J Cardiol* 49:420, 1982.

Burman SO: The prophylactic use of digitalis before thoracotomy. *Ann Thorac Surg* 14:359, 1972.

Caralps JM, Mulet J, Wienhe HR, et al: Results of coronary artery surgery in patients receiving propranolol. *J Thorac Cardiovasc Surg* 67:526, 1974.

Cheesebro JH, Clements IP, Funster LR, et al: A platelet inhibitor drug trial in coronary artery bypass operations: Benefit of perioperative dipyridamole and aspirin therapy on early postoperative vein graft patency. *N Engl J Med* 307:73, 1982.

Cohn LH, Mudge GH, Pratter F, et al: Five to eight year follow-up of patients undergoing porcine heart-valve replacement. *N Engl J Med* 304:258, 1981.

DiSesa V, Brown E, Mudge GH, et al: Hemodynamic comparison of dopamine and dobutamine in the postoperative volume-loaded, pressure-loaded, and normal ventricle. *J Thorac Cardiovasc Surg* 83:256, 1982.

Graver JM, Murphy DA, Jones EL, et al: Concomitant carotid and coronary artery revascularization. *Ann Surg* 195:712, 1982.

Harris D, Segel N, Bishop JM: The relationship between pressure and flow in the pulmonary circulation in normal subjects and in patients with chronic bronchitis and mitral stenosis. *Cardiovasc Res* 1:73, 1968.

Lowenstein E, Hallowell P, Levine FH, et al: Cardiovascular response to large doses of intravenous morphine in man. *N Engl J Med* 281:1389, 1969.

Mohr R, Smolensky A, Goor DA: Prevention of supraventricular tachyarrhythmia with low dose propranolol after coronary bypass. *J Thorac Cardiovasc Surg* 81:840, 1981.

Muller JE, Gunther S: Nifedipine therapy in Prinzmetal's angina. *Circulation* 57:137, 1978.

Niarchos AP, Roberts AJ, Case DB, et al: Hemodynamic characteristics of hypertension after coronary artery bypass surgery and effects of the converting enzyme inhibitor. *Am J Cardiol* 43:586, 1979.

Salerno TA, Henderson M, Keith FM, et al: Hypertension after coronary operation. *J Thorac Cardiovasc Surg* 81:396, 1981.

Selzer A, Walter RM: Adequacy of preoperative digitalis therapy in controlling ventricular rate in postoperative atrial fibrillation. *Circulation* 34:119, 1966.

Viljoen JF, Estafanous FG, Tarazi RC: Acute hypertension immediately after coronary artery surgery. *J Thorac Cardiovasc Surg* 71:548, 1976.

Waldo AL, MacLean WAN, Karp RB, et al: Continuous rapid atrial pacing to control recurrent or sustained supraventricular tachycardia following open heart surgery. *Circulation* 54:245, 1976.

EFFECT OF EXERCISE ON CARDIOVASCULAR PHYSIOLOGY AND CARDIAC REHABILITATION

Peter H. Stone

Of the approximately 215 million persons in the United States, it has been estimated that 2.5 million under the age of 65 years have clinical manifestations of coronary artery disease. For every 100,000 citizens in an average community, over 1,100 people under 65 have angina, are postmyocardial infarction or exhibit cardiovascular insufficiency due to coronary heart disease. Over $\frac{1}{3}$ of the persons placed on the disability rolls of the Social Security Administration in 1973 were there because of cardiovascular disease.

The number of patients who may benefit from programs designed to restore an optimal level of function, therefore, is very high. The concept of cardiac rehabilitation has been gathering momentum in recent years, as the medical community has become more aware of the size of this patient population. If rehabilitative efforts were successful, the time and money spent for hospitalization and subsequent rehospitalization for these patients might decrease and the rehabilitated persons might return more rapidly to a productive and satisfying existence. The potential benefits to both the individual and society are obvious.

Before discussing the design of cardiac rehabilitation programs and their record of success or failure, it will be valuable first to review briefly the physiologic effects of bed rest and of exercise.

Physiologic Effects of Immobilization

The time course of the pathologic processes of myocardial infarction (MI) was described by Mallory in 1939, and he noted that 6–8 weeks are required until the major portion of the necrotic myocardium is removed and organized. The prolonged bedrest concept of six weeks, the healing time, originated from this information, and this concept became widely accepted. However, in 1951, Levine and Lown advocated the "chair treatment" of early mobilization after infarction and gradually this idea became more accepted.

Much of the impetus for early mobilization of post-MI patients came from an understanding of the deleterious effects of prolonged bed rest. For example, the early classic study by Saltin and coworkers showed that physical work capacity strikingly decreased after immobilization. Healthy normal volunteers were kept at

Table 1. Physiologic Effects of Immobilization

Decreased physical work capacity
  Decreased maximum oxygen uptake (VO_2 max)
Decreased circulatory blood volume
  Plasma volume decrease > RBC mass decrease
Decrease in lung volume and vital capacity
Negative nitrogen and protein balance
Decrease in skeletal muscle mass, contractile strength, and efficiency

bed rest for three weeks, and a 20–25% decrease in maximum oxygen uptake was observed on the basis of exercise testing. At least three weeks of physical activity training were required to restore the pre-test physical work capacity.

More recent information concerning the effects of immobilization has come from investigations on astronauts in preparation for the United States aerospace efforts. These studies have confirmed that the most marked alteration after immobilization at bed rest is a decrease in physical work capacity and maximal oxygen uptake (Table 1). Immobilization also causes a decrease in circulating blood volume of 700–800 ml, which leads to a significant tachycardia and orthostatic hypotension. Furthermore, the plasma volume decreases to a greater extent than does the red blood cell mass; this increases blood viscosity and predisposes to thromboembolism. A modest decrease in lung volume and vital capacity occurs with bed rest, but this appears of major significance only in the patient with associated pulmonary disease. A negative nitrogen and protein balance has been demonstrated, and perhaps this may be of significance in the healing phase of MI.

Finally, recent studies have documented a decrease in skeletal muscle mass and in muscular contractile strength and efficiency after strict bed rest. An inefficiently contracting muscle requires more oxygen than an efficient one in order to perform the same amount of work, and this imposes an increased oxygen demand on an already impaired oxygen transport system and myocardium.

Based on this extensive amount of data concerning the effects of bed rest, gradually progressive, low-level intensity, early-ambulation programs were designed to avert or lessen the deleterious effects of prolonged immobilization. Before reviewing the format and success of cardiac rehabilitation programs, it will be valuable first to mention briefly the physiologic benefits of exercise for the cardiac patient.

Physiologic Response to Exercise

In contrast to strength exercise of the isometric type (e.g., weightlifting), which results in hypertrophy of the muscle cells, "endurance" exercise does not result in muscle hypertrophy or an increase in strength. Instead, it brings about an increase in the capacity for aerobic metabolism. The most accepted physiologic index of total body fitness is the oxygen uptake at maximum exercise, or VO_2 max, which is determined by collecting the expired air at the individual's maximum exercise effort, measuring its volume per minute and the percentage of oxygen extracted. This capacity to take up oxygen is related not only to the effectiveness of the lungs, but also to the ability of the heart and circulatory system to transport oxygen, and to the ability of the peripheral tissues to metabolize it. VO_2 max is a reproducible figure; it increases and decreases directly with the degree of physical conditioning. The uptake of oxygen increases almost linearly with increases in heart rate or cardiac output.

Generally, the increase in VO_2 max observed after endurance exercise comes equally from cardiac factors, such as an increase in cardiac output, and from peripheral factors, such as an increase in peripheral tissue extraction of oxygen (i.e., widened arteriovenous oxygen difference) (Table 2). The resting cardiac output of a normal adult is about 5.6 L/min; and at maximum exercise, a well trained athlete may increase his cardiac output to about 36 L/min. This dramatic augmentation results from a number of cardiovascular mechanisms, such as an increase in heart rate, stroke volume, and contractility, as well as a marked net decrease in peripheral vascular resistance.

The initial increase in heart rate with exercise is thought to be due to an abrupt inhibition of vagal tone. Evidence in the dog indicates that about 50% of the cardiac acceleration is then due to sympathetic drive, primarily beta-adrenergic stimulation. The maximum heart rate attainable is limited by age, although the reason for this limitation is unclear. The heart rate progressively increases with exercise to a predetermined amount, and it then cannot accelerate further. If the person continues to exercise, however, and his or her peripheral tissues require more oxygen than the heart is capable of providing, lactate and other metabolites rapidly accumulate and soon render the cardiovascular system incapable of functioning. There is a direct linear relationship between the percent VO_2 max and the percent maximum heart rate, and this relationship provides a convenient means of comparing submaximal levels of exercise in a wide range of individuals, regardless of their state of cardiovascular fitness.

The stroke volume progressively increases with exercise, but it levels off somewhat before the maximal pumping capacity is achieved. The increased stroke volume is due both to an increase in venous return and to an increase in myocardial contractility. Immediately after the onset of exercise there is a reflex-mediated increase in venous tone that enhances venous return to the heart. In addition, the exercising leg muscles serve as a pump, which further augments venous return. This increase in venous return causes an increase in myocardial fiber stretch and thereby an in-

Table 2. Cardiovascular Responses to Exercise

Cardiac Factors	Peripheral Factors
Increased cardiac output	Decreased peripheral vascular resistance
Increased stroke volume	Enhanced capacity for aerobic
Increased venous return	metabolism
Increased myocardial contractility	
Decreased heart rate at rest and any given work load	

crease in contractility and stroke volume through the Frank-Starling mechanism. In normal people, the heart size gets slightly smaller near peak exercise, but stroke volume is maintained because the systolic volume decreases even more than the diastolic volume. Prolonged endurance conditioning leads to a progressive increase in stroke volume so that the stroke volume of conditioned athletes may be 50–75% higher than that of sedentary people. This response enables those who are conditioned to satisfy the oxygen requirements of the body at a slower heart rate.

In addition to the cardiac responses that enable the heart to pump more blood, there are major peripheral factors that enhance myocardial pump function. First, the increase in cardiac output is facilitated by a marked net decrease in peripheral vascular resistance. This unloading allows for a greater increase in cardiac output than would have been possible from increased heart rate and stroke volume alone. Systemic vascular resistance decreases primarily because of vasodilatation in the exercising muscle areas, while a concomitant mild decrease in blood flow to the splanchnic bed (hepatic, visceral, and renal) and nonworking muscles provide a shunt to the areas of demand. As a result of the increased cardiac output and decreased systemic resistance, systolic blood pressure increases, while diastolic blood pressure changes little or decreases slightly, creating a physiologic situation characteristic of an increased volume load.

The other major peripheral effect of endurance exercise is that of increasing the capacity for aerobic metabolism due to alterations in the biochemical content of skeletal muscle. When skeletal muscle adapts to endurance exercise it becomes more like cardiac muscle in that its content of mitochondria and its capacity to generate ATP from oxidation of pyruvate and fatty acids increases. Increases in both the size and number of mitochondria are responsible for the increase in total mitochondrial protein. Myoglobin content of skeletal muscle also increases as physical conditioning progresses. Because very little adaptive enhancement of carbohydrate metabolism occurs with exercise training, it appears that physical conditioning shifts the metabolic emphasis toward enhanced utilization of fatty acids, thus bringing about a glycogen saving effect.

A few words about coronary blood flow are important to this discussion, since patients with ischemic heart disease are clearly most compromised by limitations of this factor. Unlike the peripheral tissues capable of increasing their oxygen extraction from the blood in response to exercise, the cardiac muscle extracts the maximum amount of oxygen from the blood at rest. The resting arteriovenous oxygen difference across the coronary circulation is, therefore, much wider than that across the peripheral vascular beds. Since the myocardium cannot increase oxygen extraction during exercise, the only mechanism capable of providing more oxygen to the myocardium is an actual increase in coronary blood flow. In the normal individual, coronary blood flow is autoregulated by myocardial oxygen demand; and coronary flow therefore increases in a direct linear fashion as myocardial oxygen demand or consumption increases.

Myocardial oxygen demand or consumption (MVO_2) is dependent on a variety of factors, many of which can be noninvasively measured clinically. Such measurements are helpful in quantitating the cardiac performance in patients with coronary disease. The principal determinants of MVO_2 are heart rate, contractility, and ventricular wall tension, the latter being in turn determined by the peak ventricular systolic pressure and ventricular volume. Measurement of myocardial oxygen consumption is helpful in evaluating patients with ischemic heart disease, since it reflects the limits of the diseased coronary arteries to provide increased flow during stress. Initial estimates of MVO_2 were made using a triple product of heart rate, peak systolic blood pressure, and the systolic ejection time as calculated from the carotid pulse and ECG. More recent data, however, suggests that the double product of heart rate and peak systolic blood pressure alone is more reliable an estimation of MVO_2.

Effect of Exercise on Patients with Ischemic Heart Disease

An understanding of these physiologic responses to exercise is particularly germane for management of the cardiac patient. These physiologic mechanisms indicate how the patient with ischemic heart disease and myocardial dysfunction may be limited in his ability to perform exercise; and, equally important, they provide an understanding of the potential role of physical rehabilitation for the cardiac patient.

Figure 1 illustrates the effect of intensive physical training on maximal oxygen uptake in patients with ischemic heart disease. After training, there is a dramatic

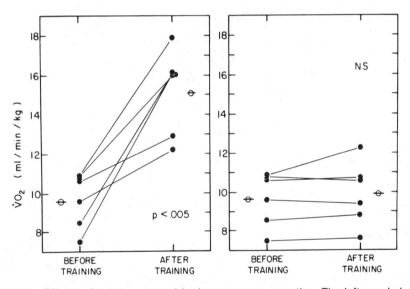

Figure 1 Effects of training on total body oxygen consumption. The left panel shows values obtained at the highest level of exercise that could be maintained before the onset of angina. In the right panel, points to the left represent the values obtained during the highest level of exercise that could be maintained without angina before training; points to the right represent values obtained after training when patients exercised at the identical pretraining exercise load. Mean values are represented by the barred circles. See text for further explanation. (DR Redwood et al: Circulatory and symptomatic effects of physical training in patients with coronary-artery disease and angina pectoris. *N Engl J Med* 286:959, 1972. Used with permission.)

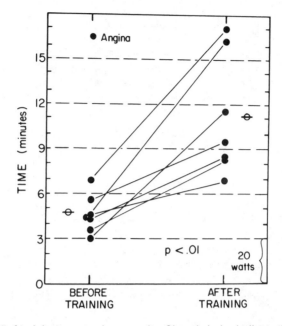

Figure 2 Effect of training on exercise capacity. Closed circles indicate the time at which angina occurred; barred circles indicate mean values. Dashed lines represent the intervals at which the work load was increased by 20 watts. (DR Redwood et al: Circulatory and symptomatic effects of physical training in patients with coronary-artery disease and angina pectoris. *N Eng J Med* 286:959, 1972. Used with permission.)

55% increase in maximal oxygen uptake in these patients, although at any given submaximal work load, the oxygen uptake is the same in trained and untrained patients. Also, since trained patients have increased their maximum capacity to consume oxygen, the cardiac patients are able to exercise for much longer periods of time after training (Fig. 2).

The effect of exercise training on the three major determinants of myocardial oxygen demand are noted in Figure 3. When compared to the level of exercise that provoked angina before training, the heart rate and systolic pressure after training decreased significantly, and the left ventricular ejection time increased. The net triple product for any given workload, however, was less after training (Fig. 4), indicating that the decreases in heart rate and blood pressure more than compensated for the tendency for the ejection time to increase. The myocardial oxygen demand, therefore, was less at any given workload after training. It should be emphasized that the physiologic benefit of physical conditioning, therefore, is similar to the physiologic benefit obtained from antianginal medications. Physical conditioning leads to a decrease in myocardial oxygen demand by decreasing heart rate and blood pressure; whereas antianginal medications decrease myocardial oxygen demand generally either by decreasing heart rate, blood pressure, or contractility.

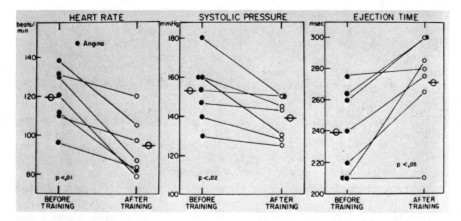

Figure 3 Effects of training on the response of heart rate, systolic aortic pressure, and ejection time to exercise. In each panel the points to the left represent pretraining values obtained during exercise at onset of angina, and points to the right represent posttraining values measured at the same intensity and duration of exercise as in the pretraining studies. Mean values are represented by the barred circles. (DR Redwood et al: Circulatory and symptomatic effects of physical training in patients with coronary-artery disease and angina pectoris. *N Eng J Med* 286:959, 1972. Used with permission.)

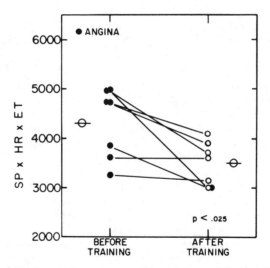

Figure 4 Effect of training on the response of the triple product of systolic arterial pressure (SP) × heart rate (HR) × Ejection time (ET) to exercise. Points to the left represent the values obtained during exercise at onset of angina before training. Points to the right represent posttraining values obtained at the same intensity and duration of exercise as in the pretraining studies. Means are indicated by the barred circles. (DR Redwood et al: Circulatory and symptomatic effects of physical training in patients with coronary-artery disease and angina pectoris. *N Eng J Med* 286:959, 1972. Used with permission.)

583

Organization of Cardiac Rehabilitation

With this background of basic exercise physiology, the organization and implementation of the cardiac rehabilitation process can be considered. From the outset, it should be emphasized that cardiac rehabilitation involves all efforts designed to restore and maintain the cardiac patient at an optimal level of function, and therefore attention is directed towards the physiologic, psychosocial, educational, and vocational areas of rehabilitation. Although this chapter concentrates primarily on the physiologic aspects of cardiac rehabilitation, it should be stressed that equally important to the cardiac patient are the nonphysiologic elements of rehabilitation; that is, those elements that help restore the sense of well-being and optimism. In a similar way, it should emphasize that the role of the physical therapists, social workers, occupational therapists, and dieticians are central to the functioning of a complete rehabilitation program.

The process of cardiac rehabilitation is generally divided into three phases. Phase I is the in-hospital phase, which begins during the patient's hospitalization for the acute event, be it an MI or cardiac surgery. The only patients that qualify for the rehabilitation program are those who have had an uncomplicated hospital course, that is, those without recurrent angina, arrhythmias, or congestive heart failure. Phase II begins when the patient leaves the hospital and continues approximately for the next three months. This is the hospital-based early outpatient rehabilitation phase, with close medical supervision. Phase III is the maintenance rehabilitation phase that continues indefinitely and generally requires only intermittent supervision and safety checks.

The exercise tolerance test (ETT) provides the objective basis for the serial determination of the patient's physical condition, as well as the safety monitor to insure that a particular degree of activity can be performed safely. If the acute MI has been uncomplicated, a low-level exercise test is generally performed before discharge. Usually an arbitrary end-point of a heart rate of 130 beats per minute is used to terminate the test. If the patient tolerates this degree of exercise well, then the patient is discharged and given an exercise prescription for phase II. It should be mentioned, however, that the use of a routine submaximal ETT in the early convalescent phase postinfarction is not considered accepted therapy by all cardiologists. There have been several law suits over untoward effects from low level exercise tests post-MI and patients who are exercised postinfarction need to be carefully selected. After two or three months of phase II training, a maximum symptom-limited exercise test is performed; and if that is safely tolerated, the patient progresses to phase III of rehabilitation, and exercise tests are then performed at six and 12-month intervals to assess safety and the degree of conditioning.

In order for physical conditioning, defined as an increase in the maximum oxygen uptake or aerobic capacity, to take place, exercise must be of a certain intensity, duration, and frequency. To make the greatest improvement in aerobic capacity with minimum of risk, 70 to 80% of maximum heart rate should be reached. The risk of complications from this degree of exercise is negligible. Exercise should last generally for at least 20–30 minutes at each work-out. Work-outs should be at least three times and preferably four or five times per week.

Sample recommendations for an exercise prescription for cardiac patients are shown in Table 3. During phase I, the patient should exercise two or three times a

Table 3. Recommendations for Exercise Prescription for Healthy Adults and Cardiac Patients

Prescription	Phase I (Inpatient Program)	Phase II (Discharge → 3 mo)	Phase III (3 mo →)	Healthy Adults
Frequency	2–3 times/day	1–2 times/day	3–5 times/wk	3–5 times/wk
Intensity	MI: RHR + 20 CABG: RHR + 30	MI: RHR + 20 CABG: RHR + 30	70%–85% max HR reserve	60%–90% max HR reserve
Duration	MI: 5–20 min CABG: 5–30 min	MI: 20–45 min CABG: 30–60 min	30–60 min	15–60 min
Mode-activity	ROM, TDM, bike, 1 flight of stairs	ROM, TDM, bike, arm erg	Walk, bike, jog, swim, cal, endurance sports	Walk, jog, run, bike, swim, endurance sports
GXT	MI: RHR + 20 CABG: RHR + 30	SL-GXT (8–10 wk)	SL-GXT (3–6 mo)	SL-GXT

SOURCE: ML Pollock, Ward A, Foster C: Exercise prescription for rehabilitation of the cardiac patient. *Heart Disease and Rehabilitation*, ML Pollock and DH Schmidt (eds), Boston, Houghton Mifflin 1979, p. 413, used with permission.

Key: GXT, graded exercise test; MI, myocardial infarction patient; CABG, coronary artery bypass graft surgery patient; HR, heart rate, beats/min; RHR, standing resting HR; ROM, range of motion exercise; TDM, treadmill; arm erg, arm ergometer; cal, calisthenics; SL-GXT, symptom-limited GXT.

day, with a target heart rate of about 20 beats per minute over the resting rate. Physical activity should be closely supervised, especially during the acute hospitalization, to insure that no untoward effects develop, such as angina, arrhythmias, or congestive failure. Duration of activity should be between about five and 20 minutes. During phase II, the frequency and intensity of the exercise do not change, but the duration of the activity doubles to 20 to 40 minutes. During phase III, in order to maximize conditioning, as noted earlier, exercise should be 3–5 times per week, with a heart rate of 70–85% of maximum predicted heart rate, for a duration of 30 to 60 minutes.

Value of Cardiac Rehabilitation

It is now important to analyze the results of rehabilitation programs. Is there a clear physiologic or psychologic benefit from these programs? Are the benefits worth the cost in both actual funds and in time committment of medical personnel?

The long-term benefits of cardiac rehabilitation remain quite controversial. Shown in Table 4 are some representative international studies concerning the effects of exercise training on recurrence of MI, total death rate, and cardiac death rate for patients following an acute MI. Participants in these exercise programs are those who experienced an acute MI and then became active in rehabilitation programs. Exercise training took place three to five times per week in a supervised setting, with peak heart rates about 75% of maximum predicted for age, with each exercise session lasting about $\frac{1}{2}$ hour. On the basis of these observations, many physicians consider that exercise improves the prognosis of the postcoronary patient. For example, the rate of recurrent MI is generally lower for the exercising group than it is for the nonexercising control patients. Similarly, the death rate and the cardiac death rate appear lower for the exercise group than for the nonexercising control group. However, the statistical interpretation of such reports is invalidated by the nonrandom selection of patients and uncertainties regarding the duration of exercise

Table 4. Estimate of the Value of Exercise To Reduce Morbidity and Mortality After Myocardial Infarction

Author	Exercise Group			Control Group		
	Recurrence Rate (%/year)	Death Rate (%/year)	Cardiac Death Rate (%/year)	Recurrence Rate (%/year)	Death Rate (%/year)	Cardiac Death rate (%/year)
Brunner	9.4	3.1	—	25.0	10.9	—
Heller	2.1	0.5	—	10.5	0.8	—
Kellerman	—	—	3.3	—	—	10.6
Kentala	9.7	7.1	5.8	8.6	6.8	6.2
Sanne	6.6	3.8	2.9	12.5	8.8	8.3
Wilhelmsen	8.4	4.4	3.6	10.0	5.6	5.3

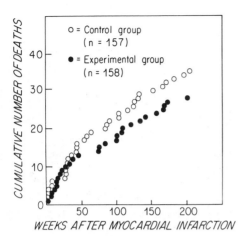

Figure 5 Total mortality after discharge from hospital and during four years of follow-up after myocardial infarction. (L Wilhelmsen et al: A controlled trial of physical training after myocardial infarction. *Preventive Medicine* 4:491, 1975. Used with permission.)

and the average follow-up period. The control groups, for example, have often consisted of arbitrarily selected populations, such as those patients not wishing to participate in an exercise class or those patients attending clinics that do not recommend exercise therapy.

Another major problem in assessing the benefit of organized cardiac rehabilitation is the lack of compliance to the exercise program. Experience from a number of large clinical investigations indicates that the drop-out rate varies between 30 and 85% over a period of about four years. In addition, from 10 to 35% of patients may develop medical contraindications to continued participation in an exercise program. It is obviously difficult to draw meaningful conclusions from a study when only 20–50% of the original cohort continue to participate.

There have been few closely controlled and randomized studies to evaluate the effects of exercise for the post-MI patients. Figure 5 illustrates the total mortality in 158 patients randomized to participate in an intensive physical rehabilitation program and 157 patients randomized to receive only the routine post-MI care (control patients). Over a four-year period, there were 35 deaths in the control group, and 28 deaths in the exercising group (difference not significant). In a similar manner, there was no difference in the number of nonfatal reinfarctions between the groups. Even when the data were analyzed by subgroups, looking only at those patients who actively trained after one year, and dividing the patients into categories based on the degree of risk and whether they continued to smoke or not, no significant differences in mortality were shown. One major source of difficulty for this study, similar to the ones mentioned earlier, however, is the poor compliance of the patients randomized to the exercise program. By the completion of the study only about 15% of the original cohort continued to train at the exercise center, and only another 15–20% claimed to be training by themselves at home. The majority of the patients randomized to the exercise program dropped out.

The National Exercise and Heart Disease Project recently reported quite favorable results of a three-year multicenter clinical trial of 651 men, postinfarction, who were randomized to a prescribed supervised exercise program or routine post-MI care. The results are encouraging, but unfortunately no convincing benefit was demonstrated. Overall mortality was reduced by 37%, cardiovascular deaths by 29%, non-sudden cardiovascular deaths by 56%, and all MIs, fatal and nonfatal, by 25%. Yet none of these differences achieved statistical significance. These investigators concluded that exercise rehabilitation following MI appeared to be valuable, but suggested a large scale trial to provide definitive confirmation. Given the extremely high cost of such a study, however, it is questionable whether such an undertaking will ever be funded.

The effect of exercise on risk factors is important to consider, since the benefits of exercise, if there are any, may be due more to a decrease in risk factors than to an actual enhancement of cardiorespiratory fitness. A composite of recent data indicates that the change in risk factors from exercise training programs may, unfortunately, be quite small. Over a three-year period of observation, changes in body weight and skin fold thickness are negligible. The resting systolic blood pressure shows a small decrease, possibly associated with increased habituation to the test laboratory, but the maximum systolic pressure tolerated during exercise actually increases as myocardial contractility improves.

Changes in serum lipids again are not striking. Cholesterol values remain essentially unchanged. It should be pointed out, though, that the recently reported multicenter Lipid Research Clinics North American Prevalence Study indicated that strenuous exercise may increase the protective plasma HDL levels. Although neither treadmill exercise test duration nor heart rate response to submaximal exercise was significantly related to HDL cholesterol levels, participants who reported strenuous physical activity at home had higher HDL cholesterol levels than those who reported none. Although there is a decrease of triglycerides, for some unexplained reason, the triglycerides often decrease almost equally in the control groups. The significance of the decreased triglycerides is unknown. The percentage of cigarette smokers is also a little lower in exercised than in nonexercised groups of postcoronary patients, although, in some studies, over a third of the exercising patients who continued to smoke claimed to have made substantial reductions in their cigarette consumption.

The psychologic effects of exercise training are important to explore, since exercise rehabilitation programs may be justifiable if the patients' sense of well-being and employment activities are improved, even if true physiologic benefits cannot be documented. The psychologic benefits from rehabilitation, however, do not appear to be major. For example, psychologic factors seem to play a relatively minor role in whether coronary patients return to work. Most studies that have investigated the typical course of return to vocational function in coronary patients suggests that 80% generally resume their preillness work status within the first year after the onset of symptoms. The principal factors affecting return to work are age, severity of illness, and the preillness level of activity. Psychologic factors contribute only to a small degree. For example, in a recent study, 46% of patients followed after discharge from a coronary care unit failed to return to work as soon as one might expect, but only 10% of these patients (5% of the total sample) listed anxiety as a primary reason for this. Other investigators estimate that psychological problems post-MI are the reason for only 3–12% of the patients not returning to work. Therefore, the possible benefits of exercise to make patients psychologically better able to return to work appear to be quite small.

A number of investigators have reported that a program of physical exercise leads to a significant reduction in self-reported anxiety and, to a somewhat lesser degree, in depression. It also appears to increase self-esteem and perception of one's health, thus providing reinforcement and increased motivation for further adherence to the rehabilitation regimen. In perhaps the best study of this type, Ibrahim and associates investigated the effect of group psychotherapy on post-MI patients during the 18 months after the illness. They noted that most patients were eager and faithful participants in this type of rehabilitation program. Results suggested that patients receiving such therapy experienced less social alienation after their MI than patients receiving no therapy. Therapy patients also showed a decrease in levels of competition and in the exaggerated sense of responsibility. Interestingly, however, such effects were short-lived, in that the majority of the post-MI patients returned to their preillness levels of stressful behavior within six months after the end of therapy.

Shephard and colleagues from Toronto have also become somewhat skeptical of the psychological benefits of cardiac rehabilitation. They note that almost all of the participants in their training programs say that they feel better as a result of exercising. Yet these changes are difficult to demonstrate objectively by formal psychologic testing. After 12–15 months of rehabilitation, as many as a third of the cohort showed the neurotic triad on the Minnesota Multiphasic Personality Inventory: high scores for hysteria, hypochondriasis, and psychasthenia, as well as very high depression scores. Over four years of rehabilitation, the investigators observed some favorable changes in those who complied with the prescribed exercise regimen. Gains were relatively small, however, even in those who trained themselves to the point of participating in marathon events. The Toronto group is currently exploring the use of other psychologic tests in an attempt to pinpoint the elusive exercise euphoria. However, the consensus of a number of investigators is that postcoronary patients remain severely depressed and that statements that they feel better are merely a denial of their problem.

Summary

In summary, it is quite clear that a long-term program of intensive physical training enables cardiac patients to perform more work with a decreased physiologic expenditure. Patients are, therefore, capable of performing their daily activities with fewer symptoms and less disability. Exercise may prolong life and decrease reinfarction in such patients, but the few controlled trials of long-term exercise training do not confirm that concept. The effects of exercise on coronary risk factors are slight. Psychological scars from an acute MI appear to exist and persist in most cardiac patients, although return-to-work status is generally not affected by these psychological factors. The improvement in psychologic well-being from exercise programs, if actually present, has been extremely hard to document.

Many investigators in the field of cardiac rehabilitation acknowledge that a more definitive study of the possible benefits of long term rehabilitation may be prohibitively expensive, and that a judgment on the overall value of cardiac rehabilitation may need to be made on the basis of currently available information. If the actual benefits and the limitations of cardiac rehabilitation are explained openly and clearly to cardiac patients, and the options offered to patients accordingly, we can provide these patients with a very helpful service. To those interested patients, cardiac rehabilitation programs will enable them to live a more active, comfortable, and perhaps fruitful life.

Bibliography

Dehn MM, Mullins CB: Physiologic effects and importance of exercise in patients with coronary artery disease. *Cardiovasc Med* 2:365, 1977.

Haskell WL: Mechanisms by which physical activity may enhance the clinical status of cardiac patients, in Pollock ML, Schmidt DH (eds): *Heart Disease and Rehabilitation.* Boston, Houghton Mifflin, 1979, p 276.

Haskell WL, Taylor HL, Wood PD, et al: Strenuous physical activity, treadmill exercise test performance and plasma high-density lipoprotein cholesterol. *Circulation* 62(Suppl IV):IV-53, 1980.

Hellerstein HK: Cardiac rehabilitation: A retrospective view, in Pollock ML: Schmidt DH (eds): *Heart Disease and Rehabilitation.* Boston, Houghton Mifflin, 1979, p 701.

Ibrahim MA, Feldman JG, Sultz HA, et al: Management after myocardial infarction: A controlled trial of the effect of group psychotherapy. *Int J Psychiatry Med* 5:253, 1974.

Kavanagh T: Intervention studies in Canada: Primary and secondary intervention, in Pollock ML, Schmidt DH (eds): *Heart Disease and Rehabilitation.* Boston, Houghton Mifflin, 1979, p 317.

Kavanagh T, Shephard RJ, Qureshi S, et al: Prognostic indexes for patients with ischemic heart disease enrolled in an exercise-centered rehabilitation program. *Am J Cardiol* 44:1230, 1979.

Levine SA, Lown B: The chair treatment of acute coronary thrombosis. *Trans Assoc Am Physicians* 64:316, 1951.

Mallory GK, White PD, Salcedo-Salgar J: The speed of healing of myocardial infarction: A study of the pathologic anatomy in 72 cases. *Am Heart J* 18:647, 1939.

Mitchell JH: Exercise training in the treatment of coronary heart disease. *Adv Intern Med* 20:249, 1975.

Pollock ML, Ward A, Foster C: Exercise prescription for rehabilitation of the cardiac patient, in Pollock ML, Schmidt DH (eds): *Heart Disease and Rehabilitation.* Boston, Houghton Mifflin, 1979, p 413.

Rechnitzer PA, Pickard HA, Paivio A, et al: Long-term follow-up study of survival and recurrent rates following myocardial infarction in exercising and control subjects. *Circulation* 45:853, 1972.

Redwood DR, Rosing DR, Epstein SE: Circulatory and symptomatic effects of physical training in patients with coronary artery disease and angina pectoris. *N Engl J Med* 286:959, 1972.

Saltin B, Blomqvist G, Mitchell JH, et al: Response to exercise after bed rest and after training. *Circulation* 38(Supp VII):1–78, 1968.

Sanne H: Risk factors modification studies in Europe, in Pollock ML, Schmidt DH (eds): *Heart Disease and Rehabilitation.* Boston, Houghton Mifflin, 1979, p 352.

Shephard RJ: Cardiac rehabilitation in prospect in Pollock ML, Schmidt DH (eds): *Heart Disease and Rehabilitation.* Boston, Houghton Mifflin, 1979, p. 539.

Wenger NK: Research related to rehabilitation. *Circulation* 60:1636, 1979.

Wilhelmsen L, Sanne H, Elmfeldt D, et al: A controlled trial of physical training after myocardial infarction. *Preventive Med* 4:491, 1975.

Wohl AJ, Lewis HR, Campbell W, et al: Cardiovascular function during early recovery from acute myocardial infarction. *Circulation* 56:931, 1977.

CHAPTER **33** | # CARDIOPULMONARY RESUSCITATION

Richard F. Wright
Wilson S. Colucci

Resuscitation has been attempted for thousands of years, but only in the last century has any measure of success been achieved. Despite early reports of success with external chest compression and artificial ventilation in the late nineteenth century, direct internal cardiac massage remained the standard of therapy until Kouwenhoven et al. rediscovered the utility of external chest compression in 1960. Standard cardiopulmonary resuscitation has changed little since that time.

More than 500,000 people experience sudden cardiac death in the United States each year. Prompt institution of appropriate resuscitative efforts could save many of these lives. Reported success rates for cardiopulmonary resuscitation vary widely, from 10% to 90%. In general, low success rates are achieved with critically ill patients and in those cases in which institution of resuscitation is delayed; high success rates occur in patients in whom primary ventricular fibrillation is rapidly identified and treated, as in anesthesia-induced cardiac arrest. Out-of-hospital victims with ventricular fibrillation typically have successful resuscitation about 40% of the time.

It is important to remember that external chest compression and mouth-to-mouth ventilation are temporizing measures, designed to prevent irreversible ischemic deterioration in the patient while awaiting the institution of definitive therapy. While there can be no absolute rules predicting the success of resuscitation, it is known that, if institution of resuscitation is delayed beyond approximately four to five minutes, the success rate is very low. If more advanced resuscitative efforts, beyond chest compression and ventilation, are delayed by seven to eight minutes, survival is still lower. Certain causes of cardiac arrest, notably hypothermia, may violate these guidelines; therefore, patients may occasionally be successfully revived despite much longer delays. In general, however, time is of the utmost importance.

Causes of Cardiac Arrest

The predominant causes of sudden death are ventricular tachycardia and ventricular fibrillation. Other tachyarrhythmias, such as atrial fibrillation in the patient with accelerated atrioventricular conduction or hypertrophic cardiomyopathy, may occasionally cause sudden death. The bradyarrhythmias are much less frequent precipitating events; sinus arrest, with inappropriate escape rhythm, and complete heart block are the usual causes.

Other causes of sudden death include primary respiratory arrest; electromechanical dissociation (the absence of effective mechanical systole despite persistent electrical complexes); and acute mechanical lesions, such as massive pulmonary embolism, acute disruption of the cardiac valves or great vessels, pericardial tamponade, and myocardial rupture. Regardless of the etiology of cardiac arrest, the initial approach to the victim is the same.

Mechanisms of Blood Flow During Resuscitation

Successful cardiopulmonary resuscitation is, in large part, dependent upon achieving adequate blood flow to the heart and brain. Kouwenhoven et al. described external chest compression as "closed-chest cardiac massage." As this implied, the mechanism of resuscitation-induced blood flow invoked was the obvious one: the heart was squeezed between the sternum and spine, mimicking the action of internal cardiac compression and propelling blood forward by increasing intramyocardial pressure above aortic pressure. However, recent work by many investigators casts doubt on the universal validity of this proposed mechanism.

It is now apparent that cardiac output during sternal compression is primarily due to an increase in intrathoracic pressure during each compression. According to this hypothesis, the heart acts as a conduit for blood flow rather than as a pump. When intrathoracic pressure is elevated by chest compression, blood is squeezed out of the pulmonary vascular bed. Retrograde flow is prevented by the pulmonic valve, possibly by the tricuspid valve and systemic venous valves, and probably by collapse of the systemic veins as they exit from the thorax. Thus, as intrathoracic pressure rises, blood is forced from the lungs, through the heart, and into the aorta. As pressure on the sternum is released, blood flows back into the pulmonary vascular bed from the systemic veins. Flow from the aorta back into the heart is prevented by the aortic valve.

Evidence for such a flow pattern was originally based on clinical observation. Patients with flail chests, in whom the unstable chest segment precluded the attainment of positive intrathoracic pressure with sternal compression, could be successfully revived only after stabilization of the chest wall. Emphysematous patients were not more difficult to resuscitate despite the increased distance between their sternum and spine. Coughing, which substantially raises intrathoracic pressure, was noted to generate remarkable cardiac output in the absence of cardiac systole; in fact, repetitive coughing has been found to maintain consciousness in humans with ventricular fibrillation. Recent attempts to duplicate the physiology of the cough, by increasing abdominal pressure (with binding, for example) and by inflating the lungs simultaneously with sternal compression, have resulted in marked increases in forward blood flow.

Hemodynamic data also support the chest pump hypothesis. It has been shown that measured pressures in the great vessels and the intracardiac chambers are equal during sternal compression; if forward blood flow were due to direct squeezing of the heart, intracardiac pressures should exceed pressures elsewhere in the thorax. However, the best data supporting the chest pump hypothesis are the recent angiographic and two-dimensional echocardiographic demonstrations that the majority of patients exhibit flow from the lungs to the aorta through *open* mitral and aortic valves during sternal compression. It is likely that, at least in a minority of patients, both proposed mechanisms of flow are operating.

Supplemental maneuvers, such as abdominal binding and simultaneous lung inflation, have been shown to further increase intrathoracic pressure and carotid blood flow during sternal compression in humans. However, they can not yet be recommended for general use until documentation of their safety and efficacy become available.

Technique of Cardiopulmonary Resuscitation

Figure 1 is a diagram of this process of resuscitation.

VENTILATION

Once a patient is discovered to have suffered a cardiac arrest, the first priority is to ensure the presence of a patent airway. This is accomplished most quickly by placing the patient supine and tilting the head back, while simultaneously pulling the jaw forward and opening the mouth slightly. These maneuvers preclude airway obstruction by the tongue and pharynx and allow inspection of the pharynx if ventilatory difficulties indicate the presence of upper airway obstruction.

Mouth-to-mouth resuscitation at a rate of about 12 breaths per minute is then instituted. Adequate ventilation is easily gauged by the presence of chest expansion and the sounds of the victim's exhalations. Mouth-to-mouth ventilation should be a temporizing measure, as the fractional inspired oxygen tension being administered is only 0.17. In a prolonged resuscitation, this will usually be insufficient to achieve adequate oxygenation. Therefore, the use of a respirator bag and a tight-fitting mask, esophageal airway, or endotracheal tube will be necessary to administer supplemental oxygen if initial attempts at restoring spontaneous ventilation are unsuccessful.

The adequacy of ventilation should be followed by arterial blood gas determinations. Hyperventilation frequently will be necessary to compensate for the metabolic acidosis commonly seen in the patient with cardiac arrest. The arterial pH should be maintained in the range of 7.30–7.45, if possible. Hypoxia is invariably present due to the presence of intrapulmonary shunting; therefore, 100% oxygen should always be administered. There is no danger in using high levels of oxygen for such brief periods.

Upper airway obstruction due to foreign body aspiration, as in the so-called café coronary syndrome caused by aspiration of food, may be treated successfully by use of the Heimlich maneuver. The rescuer stands behind the victim with the fists clenched beneath the victim's xiphoid, and delivers a swift thrust upwards and inwards. This usually will drive the diaphragm up and expel the offending agent from the airway.

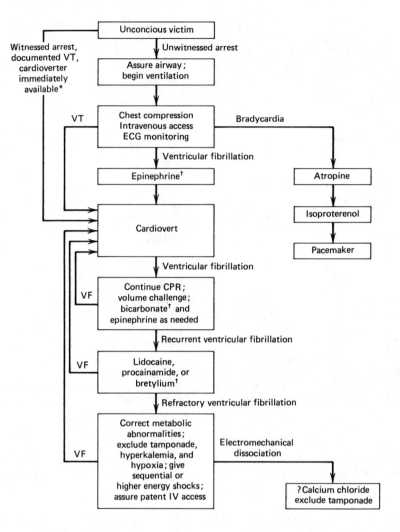

Figure 1 Schematic diagram showing the steps instituted during a typical cardiopulmonary resuscitation. *If the electrocardiogram reveals ventricular tachycardia, a chest thump may be attempted. See text for further discussion of the use of the chest thump. †See text for dosage and dosing intervals.

CIRCULATION

Simultaneous with restoration of effective ventilation, adequate circulation must be achieved. External chest compression usually results in 25% or less of the normal cardiac output. Fortunately, this reduced output is directed predominantly cephalad and is often sufficient to perfuse the brain adequately, at least temporarily. My-ocardial perfusion is less optimal. It is not unusual for coronary blood flow during resuscitation to be less than 10% of normal. Insufficient myocardial blood flow is a frequent cause of the inability to achieve a stable cardiac rhythm. This is due, in large part, to low diastolic blood pressure during resuscitation, and thus a low driving force for cardiac perfusion.

The proper technique of chest compression is very important for maximizing blood flow. The rescuer kneels or stands beside the victim and places his interlocked hands, one atop the other, on the lower half of the sternum. The exact position of the hands is not critical as long as they are above the xiphoid process (pressure on the xiphoid may result in ineffective thoracic compression and/or hepatic lacerations). If sternal placement is impossible, positioning of the hands anywhere on the thorax can be effective and should be utilized. For instance, one hand can be placed on each hem-ithorax. Each compression is accomplished by depressing the sternum 4–6 cm. This is most easily done by locking the elbows and leaning over the victim's chest, thereby transmitting the weight of the upper torso to the hands. A force of 40–120 pounds is usually needed. A firm surface beneath the patient makes the job easier and more effective, but successful compressions can be performed with a patient in bed, if necessary.

There has been much controversy concerning the optimal rate of compression. Some observers note no significant change in blood flow with rates between 40–120 compressions per minute, whereas others report a linear rise in output over this range. Sixty to 80 compressions per minute usually suffice and limit rescuer fatigue. The duration of compression is important. Fifty to 60% down-time results in im-proved flow compared to briefer periods of compression; therefore, sharp, short compressions should be avoided. In sum, 60–80 compressions per minute, with 50–60% of the time spent in the compression phase, is sufficient. Ventilations should be interposed between every fourth or fifth compression; if a rescuer is alone this pattern can be modified so that two ventilations are administered between every 12–15 compressions.

Internal cardiac massage results in demonstrably better cardiac output than sternal compression but is used infrequently due to the invasiveness of the technique. Never-theless, it is indicated in certain cases of penetrating cardiac trauma; in the post-operative cardiac surgical patient; in mechanical lesions, such as severe aortic sten-osis; in the patient with a grossly unstable chest; possibly in some patients with prosthetic valves (it has been observed that external pressure applied over prosthetic valve rings may cause severe cardiac trauma during chest compression); and oc-casionally, as a measure of last resort in patients who have failed to respond to more routine measures.

The precordial thump is no longer recommended in the unwitnessed arrest, due to its low rate of success. It still may be useful for the patient with witnessed ven-tricular tachycardia, in which a single thump may convert the patient to sinus rhythm, or with severe bradycardia, in which repetitive thumps may induce spontaneous cardiac contractions. From a height of 20–30 cm above the victim's chest, the fleshy portion of the fist is used to deliver a swift blow to the midsternum. Conscious patients will not like this maneuver, and other modes of therapy, such as intravenous lidocaine for the patient with ventricular tachycardia, should be considered.

Electrical Cardioversion

The most useful element in successful resuscitation has been electrical cardioversion. When instituted promptly, it has a very high rate of successful conversion of a diversity of dysrhythmias. Alternating current defibrillators are now obsolete, and direct current (DC) devices are used almost exclusively. These machines deliver a monophasic depolarization of several thousand volts over a period of about 10 milliseconds. The delivered energy is variable up to a maximum of 360 joules (watt seconds) on most defibrillators.

The optimal power setting for external cardiac defibrillation has been debated. Advocates of high-energy shocks maintain that body weight is an important variable in determining the power requirements for successful defibrillation, but this has not been borne out by clinical studies. High-energy shocks result in increased electrical injury to the myocardium and a higher incidence of postshock asystole and atrioventricular block. Current evidence indicates that 175–200 joules is optimal for initial attempts at defibrillation; much less energy is usually required for the conversion of ventricular tachycardia (e.g., 10–50 joules).

The technique of cardioversion is straightforward. The machine is set to the desired power level and the paddles charged. Exact paddle placement is less critical than ensuring that adequate electrode paste (or saline pads) and firm paddle pressure are used, as these simple maneuvers will maximize the amount of energy delivered to the victim. One paddle is placed just below the right clavicle; the other is placed just lateral to the cardiac apex (or below the left scapula, when a flat posterior paddle is used). When everyone stands clear of the patient and the bed, the shock is delivered.

In the monitored patient with witnessed ventricular tachycardia or ventricular fibrillation, cardioversion, if immediately available, should precede chest compression and ventilation. In the unwitnessed arrest, it is usually preferable to administer cardiopulmonary resuscitation and appropriate pharmacologic intervention for one to two minutes prior to attempting countershock. This will increase the likelihood of successful conversion, although, even in an unwitnessed arrest, a rapidly administered shock is potentially beneficial.

Some patients have recovered even after several hours of ventricular fibrillation and cardiopulmonary resuscitation; therefore, attempts at defibrillation should continue until irreversible cardiac asystole appears. If several attempts at defibrillation have failed, more intensive pharmacologic therapy, closer attention to metabolic abnormalities, and higher energy shocks may be useful. Rapid sequential shocks, spaced a few seconds apart, are occasionally of benefit as the first shock lowers skin impedance and allows a higher delivery of energy by the second shock.

Asystole is rarely, if ever, responsive to cardioversion. Although successful shocks have been reported in cases of asystole, it is likely that ventricular fibrillation was actually present in these patients. If asystole appears on the electrocardiographic monitor, the electrodes should be changed to obtain a lead 90° to the first lead. This will ensure that the isoelectric tracing is not actually ventricular fibrillation, which occasionally may be isoelectric in a particular ECG lead.

Pharmacology of Resuscitation

Restoration of effective circulation is often dependent upon pharmacologic manipulation and volume expansion (see Table 1). Rapid placement of an intravenous line is crucial. Any vein can be used, but, in theory, it is preferable to use a vein above the diaphragm. Blood flow during chest compression is preferentially directed cephalad; infusion into the saphenous or femoral veins may, therefore, result in delayed entry of instilled medications into the central circulation.

If an arm vein is palpable, it should be used. Frequently this is not possible, due to marked venospasm that may accompany cardiac arrest. In this situation, the external or internal jugular vein should be cannulated with a 16 gauge catheter. The subclavian vein also may be used, but it carries a higher incidence of potentially serious complications and is difficult to cannulate while the patient is undergoing chest compression.

If technical problems preclude the rapid establishment of intravenous access, many drugs can be instilled effectively into the tracheobronchial tree via an endotracheal tube. Epinephrine, atropine, and lidocaine can be safely used in this manner, in doses equal to initial intravenous doses. Sodium bicarbonate should not be instilled into the lungs.

Except during open chest massage, intracardiac injection of medications is indicated only if intravenous or intratracheal administration is unavailable. Potentially serious complications of this route include coronary artery laceration, intramyocardial injection, and pericardial tamponade. Epinephrine is inherently no more effective when administered by the intracardiac route. When intracardiac administration is indicated, the subxiphoid approach is preferable to the parasternal approach.

Volume expansion with one to two liters of normal saline or other volume expander is often helpful in elevating systolic and diastolic pressure during resuscitation. It is especially critical in the volume-depleted patient, but should also be utilized in the patient who appears to be normovolemic.

ADRENERGIC DRUGS

The most useful drug for resuscitation is epinephrine. Unfortunately, it frequently is underutilized. Since epinephrine has both alpha and beta-adrenergic agonist activity, in doses given during resuscitation it increases both peripheral vasoconstriction (alpha effect), and myocardial contractility (beta effect). In animals the success rate of resuscitation is unaffected by increasing myocardial contractility. For this reason, other beta agonists, such as isoproterenol, dopamine, and dobutamine, have essentially no role in the acute phase of cardiac resuscitation. Increasing peripheral vasoconstriction, on the other hand, results in higher rates of successful resuscitation, presumably due to augmented myocardial blood flow resulting from the increase in diastolic blood pressure. Other alpha agonists, such as methoxamine, phenylephrine, and norepinephrine, are also effective in this regard, but are less frequently used and less readily available than epinephrine. An alpha-adrenergic agonist should be administered as soon as possible during cardiac resuscitation. Epinephrine, 1 mg

Table 1. Drugs Commonly Used during Cardiopulmonary Resuscitation

Drug	Dose	Route	Mechanism of action	Comments and precautions
Epinephrine	0.5–1.0 mg every 5 min or 1–4 µg/min (1 amp = 1 mg)	IV ET IC	Increases blood pressure and contractility	Inactivated by sodium bicarbonate; drug of choice for resuscitation
Sodium bicarbonate	1 mEq/kg, then 0.5 mEq/kg as needed (1 amp = 44.6 or 50 mEq)	IV	Helps reverse acidosis	May result in alkalemia, hypernatremia, hyperosmolar state; inactivates epinephrine; precipitates with calcium
Calcium chloride	250–1,000 mg (1 amp = 1 gm)	IV IC	Increases contractility ?Helps electromechanical dissociation	Causes transient hypercalcemia; intracardiac injection may cause severe bradycardia; precipitates with bicarbonate; contraindicated in digitalis toxicity
Atropine	0.5–1.0 mg every 5 min, up to 3 mg (1 amp = 1 mg)	IV ET IC	May reverse bradycardia	Low doses may cause paradoxical bradycardia; rarely may elicit ventricular tachycardia or fibrillation
Lidocaine	100–300 mg in 50–100 mg boluses; then 1–4 mg/min	IV	May prevent ventricular fibrillation	High doses cause central nervous system toxicity
Procainamide	100–1,000 mg at 20–50 mg/min then 1–5 mg/min	IV	May prevent ventricular fibrillation	Can cause hypotension
Bretylium	5 mg/kg every 10 min, up to 30 mg/kg; then 1–2 mg/min	IV	May prevent or convert ventricular fibrillation; lowers threshold for successful cardioversion	Can cause hypotension

Key: IV, intravenous; ET, endotracheal; IC, intracardiac.

intravenously every 4–5 minutes throughout the duration of the resuscitation, or as a continuous infusion at 1–4 µg/min, is the usual choice. Frequent administration is necessary, due to the rapid metabolism of epinephrine.

SODIUM BICARBONATE

Sodium bicarbonate is frequently overused during resuscitation. Although valuable for the temporary correction of metabolic acidosis, excessive use of this drug may result in hypernatremia, the hyperosmolar state, and/or severe alkalemia. These conditions can be quite dangerous and may actually preclude successful resuscitation. Therefore, caution must be used whenever bicarbonate is administered. In the witnessed arrest, none need be given for the first 5–10 minutes of the resuscitation, as long as the patient is being adequately ventilated and metabolic acidosis did not precede the cardiac arrest. In the unwitnessed arrest, and in the patient with known metabolic acidosis, correction of systemic acidosis may, in large part, be accomplished by hyperventilation-induced hypocarbia. Sodium bicarbonate may still be necessary, usually at an initial dose of 1 mEq/kg (ampules of bicarbonate contain 44.6 or 50 mEq of the drug). Subsequent doses should be gauged by maintaining the arterial pH between 7.30 and 7.45. If arterial blood gas determinations are unavailable, half the initial dose can be administered empirically every 10–15 minutes until spontaneous circulation reappears. Sodium bicarbonate inactivates epinephrine and precipitates calcium chloride; therefore, these drugs should not be administered concurrently through the same intravenous line.

CALCIUM CHLORIDE

Although calcium is necessary for myocardial contraction, there are few data indicating that calcium salts are therapeutically useful in cardiac resuscitation. Indications for calcium administration include hypocalcemic states, such as after transfusion with large quantities of citrated blood, and hyperkalemia. Although frequently used in patients with asystole and electromechanical dissociation, it is of no proven benefit in these conditions and should be given with caution. Calcium salts are specifically contraindicated in the patient with digitalis toxicity, since ventricular dysrhythmias may be exacerbated or precipitated by calcium administration in such patients.

ATROPINE

This parasympatholytic drug occasionally is useful in transiently reversing sinus bradycardia and high degree atrioventricular block. It has no role in the initial stages of resuscitation unless bradycardia has been identified as the initial rhythm. The usual dose is 0.5–1.0 mg every five minutes as needed, to a total of 3 mg. Smaller doses, 0.2 mg or less, should be avoided as they may cause a paradoxical increase in vagal tone.

ISOPROTERENOL

Isoproterenol is sometimes effective in accelerating the heart rate of patients who remain bradycardic despite atropine and in patients with complete heart block. The usual dose is 1–10 µg/min, titrated down to the lowest dose capable of maintaining an adequate heart rate.

ANTIARRHYTHMIC DRUGS

Antiarrhythmic agents can be valuable adjuncts in maintaining sinus rhythm after successful defibrillation. With the exception of bretylium, they do not contribute to restoring sinus rhythm and, in fact, may raise the threshold for successful cardioversion. For this reason, antiarrhythmics need not be administered during the first stages of resuscitation. If ventricular tachycardia or ventricular fibrillation are persistant or recurrent, lidocaine (50–75 mg IV every five minutes for three doses, followed by a continuous infusion at 1–4 mg/min), procainamide (300–1,000 mg IV loading dose at an initial infusion rate of 20 mg/min, followed by continuous infusion at 1–5 mg/min), or bretylium (5 mg/kg loading dose IV repeated in 10–15 minutes, if necessary, to a total dose of 30 mg/kg, followed by a continuous infusion at 1–2 mg/min, if needed) may be useful. These drugs are often used in this sequence. Bretylium has the unique effect of lowering the defibrillation threshold and, occasionally, producing defibrillation directly without electrical countershock; for these reasons, it is sometimes used as a first-line drug. Phenytoin is rarely of use as an antiarrhythmic.

Other drugs, such as morphine, metaraminol, propranolol, diuretics, nitrates, and calcium channel antagonists have little role in cardiac resuscitation. High-dose corticosteroids and glucose-insulin-potassium infusions have been reported to be useful occasionally in the treatment of the patient with refractory ventricular fibrillation.

Mechanical and Electromechanical Support

Emergent placement of a pacing wire is frequently useful in the symptomatically bradycardic patient, but is unlikely to resuscitate the asystolic patient. Transvenous pacers are preferable to transthoracic wires, as the latter are less often effective and can be associated with serious complications.

The antishock garment (MAST suit) directs blood flow toward the central circulation and, thus, may have a role in cardiac resuscitation; its exact place remains to be defined. Mechanical devices to compress the sternum are effective, when properly used, but are probably no more effective than an experienced rescuer. The use of such devices may limit rescuer fatigue.

When Resuscitation is Failing

When resuscitative efforts are failing, there is often little that can be done to avert the victim's death. However, potentially treatable causes do exist and must be thoroughly excluded. Ineffective ventilation may be present, perhaps due to improper endotracheal tube placement or tension pneumothorax. Unreliable intravenous access is often a problem; during frenetic resuscitation efforts, the subcutaneous infiltration of an intravenous line may go unnoticed. Severe metabolic abnormalities, such as hyperkalemia, or volume depletion may be unsuspected and may need empiric treatment if suspicion warrants. Rarely, pericardial tamponade may be present; in such instances, the removal of 50 ml of blood from the pericardial space may result in dramatic hemodynamic improvement. Resuscitation should not be abandoned until all potentially reversible causes are investigated.

Cerebral Protection and Resuscitation

In spite of successful cardiac resuscitation, many patients suffer severe and irreversible ischemic encephalopathy following cardiac arrest. This is due to long periods of cerebral ischemia, as well as to delayed cranial reperfusion after successful restoration of spontaneous circulation. Despite early hopes for effective cerebral protection utilizing high-dose barbiturates, phenytoin, corticosteroids, anticoagulation, hypothermia, and a variety of other measures, there is little evidence that these interventions have benefited post-resuscitation patients. More recent data indicate that calcium channel antagonists may have an important role in preventing the no-reflow phenomenon, but further studies will be needed before this approach can be recommended for routine use.

Bibliography

Standards and guidelines for cardiopulmonary resuscitation and emergency cardiac care. *JAMA* 244:453, 1980.

Thirteenth Bethesda Conference: Emergency cardiac care. *Am J Cardiol* 50:365, 1982.

Babbs CF: New versus old theories of blood flow during cardiopulmonary resuscitation. *Crit Care Med* 8:191, 1980.

Bishop RL, Weisfeldt ML: Sodium bicarbonate administration during cardiac arrest: Effect on arterial pH, pCO_2, and osmolality. *JAMA* 235:506, 1976.

Chandra N, Rudikoff MT, Weisfeldt ML: Simultaneous chest compression and ventilation at high airway pressure during cardiopulmonary resuscitation. *Lancet* 1:175, 1980.

Chandra N, Snyder LD, Weisfeldt ML: Abdominal binding during cardiopulmonary resuscitation in man. *JAMA* 246:351, 1981.

Kouwenhoven WG, Jude JR, Knickerbocker GG: Closed chest cardiac massage. *JAMA* 173:94, 1960.

Niemann JT, Rosborough JP, Hausknecht M, et al: Pressure-synchronized cineangiography during experimental cardiopulmonary resuscitation. *Circulation* 64:985, 1981.

Rosborough JP, Hausknecht M, Niemann JT, et al: Cough supported circulation. *Crit Care Med* 9:371, 1981.

Rudikoff MT, Maughan WL, Effron M, et al: Mechanisms of blood flow during cardiopulmonary resuscitation. *Circulation* 61:345, 1980.

Safar P: *Cardiopulmonary Cerebral Resuscitation*. Philadelphia, Saunders, 1981.

Taylor GJ, Tucker WM, Greene HL, et al: Importance of prolonged compression during cardiopulmonary resuscitation in man. *N Engl J Med* 296:1515, 1977.

Werner JA, Greene HL, Janko CL, et al: Visualization of cardiac valve motion in man during external chest compression using two-dimensional echocardiography. *Circulation* 63:1417, 1981.

White BC, Gadzinski DS, Hoehner PJ, et al: Effect of flunarizine on canine cerebral cortical blood flow and vascular resistance post cardiac arrest. *Ann Emerg Med* 11:119, 1982.

INDEX